METABOLISM

Metabolism

Carole J. Coffee, Ph.D.

Professor of Biochemistry

Department of Molecular Genetics and Biochemistry

University of Pittsburgh School of Medicine

University of Pittsburgh

Pittsburgh, Pennsylvania

Fence Creek Publishing

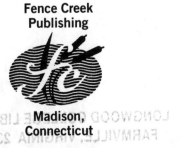

Madison, Connecticut

This book is dedicated to the hundreds of medical students from whom I have been privileged to learn over the last 25 years. They have patiently taught me how to think about basic science concepts from the perspective of a future physician, and collectively they have contributed significantly to the style and scope of this book.

Typesetter: Pagesetters, Brattleboro, VT
Printer: Port City Press, Baltimore, MD
Illustrations by Visible Productions, Fort Collins, CO
Distributors:

United States and Canada

Blackwell Science, Inc.
Commerce Place
350 Main Street
Malden, MA 02148
Telephone orders: 800-215-1000 or 781-388-8250
Fax orders: 781-388-8270

Australia

Blackwell Science, PTY LTD.
54 University Street
Carlton, Victoria 3053
Telephone orders: 61-39-347-0300
Fax orders: 61-39-347-5001

Outside North America and Australia

Blackwell Science, LTD.
c/o Marston Book Service, LTD.
P.O. Box 269
Abingdon Oxon, OX 14 4XN England
Telephone orders: 44-1-235-465500
Fax orders: 44-1-235-465555

2 3 4 5 6 7 8 9 10

TABLE OF CONTENTS

Chapter 24 335

Introduction to Amino Acid Metabolism: Digestion and Absorption
of Dietary Protein

Chapter 25 347

Amino Acid Catabolism: Disposal of Nitrogen and Carbon Skeletons

Chapter 26 363

One-Carbon Metabolism and the Synthesis of Nonessential Amino Acids

Chapter 27 375

Specialized Products Derived from Amino Acids

Chapter 28 393

Nucleotide Metabolism

Index 411

PREFACE

Human metabolism, a subject of prime importance to medical students and physicians, integrates biochemical pathways with themes traditionally covered in physiology, cell structure, histology, and nutrition courses. Due to the rapid expansion of knowledge in human biology that has occurred over the last several years, the medical student no longer has time to master the details of any basic science discipline. The two questions most frequently posed by students are: "What do I need to know?" and "What is the significance of this information?" It is my hope that this book will make answers to these questions obvious. This book is predicated on two assumptions: (1) that medical students learn any discipline more readily when it is presented in a context that can be applied to solving critical problems, and (2) that our role as educators is to provide a conceptual framework within which students can begin to solve problems rather than to provide all of the details that we believe they will need for problem-solving.

The preparation of this book was motivated by a change in our medical school curriculum from a traditional discipline-based curriculum to a fully integrated curriculum that relies heavily on problem-based learning. In integrating multidisciplinary concepts into a concise format, emphasis has been placed on basic principles, function, and regulation at the expense of many metabolic intermediates and tedious structural details. For example, consideration of a particular pathway includes a statement of the function the pathway plays in the cell or the organism as a whole, a description of the key reactions in the pathway, where the reactions occur in the cell, the organ specificity of the pathway, how it is regulated, and how it is coordinated with other pathways so that homeostasis is maintained. Clinical examples are used frequently to emphasize the connection between disease and abnormalities in metabolism.

Carole J. Coffee

ACKNOWLEDGMENTS

I want to thank Matt Harris for his encouragement and Jane Edwards for her tireless editorial assistance and good humor throughout the preparation of this manuscript.

INTRODUCTION

Metabolism is one of ten titles in the *Integrated Medical Sciences (IMS) Series* from Fence Creek Publishing. These books have been designed as course supplements and aids for board review for first- and second-year medical students. Rather than focusing on the individual basic science disciplines, the books in the *IMS Series* have been designed to highlight the points of integration between the sciences, including clinical correlations where appropriate. Each chapter begins with a clinical case, the resolution of which requires the application of basic science concepts to clinical problems. Extensive use of margin notes, figures, tables, and questions illuminates core biomedical concepts with which medical students often have difficulty.

Each book in the *IMS Series* shares common features and formats. Attempts have been made to present difficult concepts in a brief and focused format and to provide a pedagogical aid that facilitates both knowledge acquisition and review.

Given the long gestation period necessary to publish a book, it is often impossible for publishers to keep pace with the changes and advances that occur so rapidly. However, the authors and the publisher recognize the need to have access to the most current information and are committed to keeping *Metabolism* as up to date as possible between editions. As the field of metabolism evolves, updates to this text may be posted periodically on our web site at http://www.fencecreek.com.

We hope that the student finds the format and the text material relevant, interesting, and challenging. The author, as well as the Fence Creek staff, welcome your comments and suggestions for use in future editions.

1

THE CELL: THE FUNDAMENTAL UNIT OF METABOLISM

CHAPTER OUTLINE

INTRODUCTION OF CLINICAL CASE

Cheryl, the first child of healthy parents, was placed in the neonatal unit shortly after birth because of seizures. She remained there until she died at 22 weeks of age as a result of cardiac failure. At birth, she had dysmorphic facial features, an unusually high forehead, redundant folds of skin at her neck, and eye abnormalities. She had difficulty feeding because of poor ability to suck. Her liver was enlarged, and her heart showed severe malformation. Analysis of plasma taken from the patient showed that the concentration of very long-chain fatty acids (C_{24} and C_{26} in length) was tenfold higher than normal, while the concentration of fatty acids that were C_{22} and shorter was markedly decreased. Biochemical analysis of tissues taken at autopsy revealed the accumulation of cholestanoic acid (the precursor for bile acids) in the liver and low levels of plasmalogens in the brain, heart, and kidney. Morphologic analysis by electron microscopy of liver tissue showed the absence of peroxisomes but the presence of several unusual membranous structures that are not seen in normal tissue. Enzyme analysis of the tissue showed normal levels of catalase, but it was all located in the cytosol.

OVERVIEW OF CELL STRUCTURE AND FUNCTION

Metabolism
The sum of all of the enzyme-catalyzed reactions that occur in cells, metabolism includes synthetic pathways for assembling small molecules into more complex macromolecules, and degradative pathways for breaking down complex nutrients into simpler molecules. The synthetic pathways usually require energy that is supplied by ATP hydrolysis, and the degradative pathways release energy that is used to synthesize ATP.

The fundamental unit of *metabolism* is the cell. The periphery of the cell is defined by the plasma membrane that separates the contents of the cell from the external environment (Figure 1-1). Eukaryotic cells have an internal membrane system that organizes the cell into several subcellular compartments, each having discrete metabolic functions. Cells are composed of four types of macromolecules, proteins, nucleic acids, polysaccharides, and lipids, each of which is assembled from a small number of universal building blocks. All cells use nutrients from their environment for generating the building blocks and the energy necessary for cell maintenance, growth, and division. The most abundant component of living organisms is water. It provides both the extracellular medium for transporting nutrients to cells and the intracellular medium required for metabolism. The external surface of cells has specific structural features that allow cells to adhere to one another and form tissues.

FIGURE 1-1
Structural Features of a Typical Eukaryotic Cell. *Membranes surround the nucleus, mitochondria, lysosomes, and peroxisomes in eukaryotes. An internal membrane system forms a series of contiguous compartments, including the endoplasmic reticulum and Golgi complex. The volume of eukaryotic cells is several thousand times larger than that of prokaryotic cells. Because specific metabolic functions are restricted to specific cellular compartments enclosed by membranes, the need for enzymes and substrates to diffuse through long distances is minimized.*

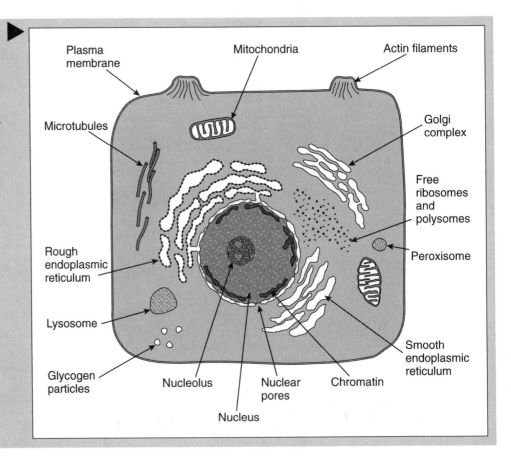

STRUCTURE AND FUNCTION OF MEMBRANES

Biologic membranes are *bilayers* that are assembled from a mixture of lipids and proteins. Lipids provide the structural framework, while the proteins perform the dynamic functions associated with the membrane. The relative proportion of lipid to protein varies with different membranes. In general, the more metabolic activity associated with the membrane, or the greater the need to respond to external stimuli, the greater the proportion of protein. The red blood cell (RBC) membrane and key features of the lipid bilayer are illustrated in Figure 1-2.

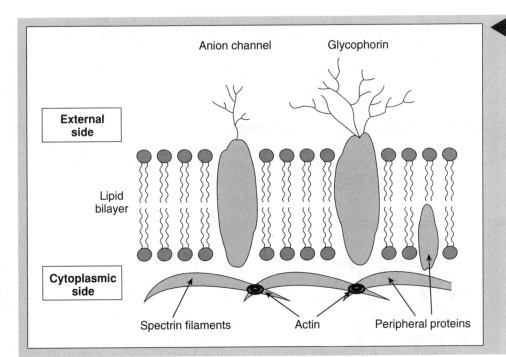

FIGURE 1-2
Lipid Bilayer Surrounding the RBC. *The model of the RBC membrane shows the arrangement of phospholipids and proteins. The two major integral membrane proteins are glycophorin and the anion channel protein. Both are glycoproteins, having branched carbohydrate chains extending from the outer leaflet into extracellular space. Glycophorin contains the blood group determinants of the ABO system. The anion channel allows HCO_3^- to leave the cell in exchange for chloride (Cl^-). Spectrin is the major peripheral membrane protein and is loosely associated with the lipid bilayer and with actin filaments in the cell.*

Membrane Lipids

Lipids that are found in membranes are *amphipathic* molecules, having one end that is hydrophilic and another that is hydrophobic. In biologic systems, the most stable arrangement for amphipathic lipids is in *bilayers* where the hydrophobic ends associate with one another and are protected from the aqueous environment. Membrane lipids consist of phospholipids, glycolipids, and cholesterol. The proportion of these lipids affects the properties of the membrane and may vary considerably from one membrane to another.

Phospholipids. The universal building blocks of all biologic membranes are phospholipids. They comprise between 50% and 60% of the total membrane lipid. The four major membrane phospholipids are phosphatidylcholine, phosphatidylethanolamine, phosphatidylserine, and phosphatidylinositol.

Cholesterol. A major component of the plasma membrane, cholesterol comprises between 15% and 25% of the total lipid, but membranes of the subcellular organelles contain very little, if any, cholesterol. Membrane cholesterol is always unesterified.

Glycolipids. This class of lipids is found primarily in plasma membranes and usually makes up less than 10% of the total membrane lipid. The carbohydrate portion of glycolipids is always on the noncytoplasmic side of the plasma membrane, extending into the extracellular space.

Membrane Proteins

Whereas lipids provide the structural framework of membranes, proteins are responsible for the dynamic functions of membranes. They serve as hormone receptors, ion channels, transport proteins, and enzymes. Membrane proteins are classified in two groups based on the ease with which they can be released from the lipid bilayer.

Integral Membrane Proteins. These proteins are embedded in the membrane, and their removal usually requires detergents. Integral membrane proteins usually span the lipid bilayer one or more times. The sequence of amino acids spanning the lipid bilayer is usually a segment of alpha-helix (α-helix) consisting of approximately 20 amino acids, most of which are hydrophobic. The association of integral proteins with the membrane is stabilized by *hydrophobic interactions* between amino acid side chains and the internal, hydrophobic portion of the lipid bilayer.

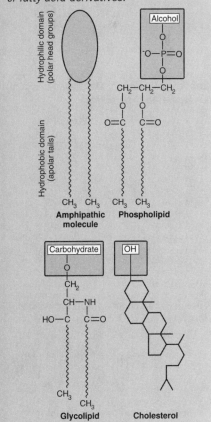

Amphipathic Properties of Phospholipids, Cholesterol, and Glycolipids
All of the membrane lipids have hydrophilic (polar) domains that interact favorably with water and hydrophobic (apolar) domains that are insoluble in water. Most of the hydrophobic domains are fatty acids or fatty acid derivatives.

Peripheral Membrane Proteins. The proteins that are found near the surface of the membrane can often be removed from the membrane by altering the pH or ionic strength of the solution. The association of peripheral proteins with the membrane is stabilized primarily by *ionic interactions* between the protein and the polar head groups of phospholipids or the polar groups on other proteins.

Transport of Molecules Across Membranes

Membranes form selective barriers that maintain distinct internal and external environments. Several mechanisms exist for moving substances from one side of the membrane to the other (Figure 1-3).

FIGURE 1-3

Mechanisms for Transporting Molecules Across Membranes. Simple diffusion is the only mechanism that does not require a protein. In both facilitated transport and active transport, the solute that is being transported binds to its transport protein on one side of the membrane and is released on the opposite side. In active transport, the solute moves from a region of low concentration to a region of high concentration, a process that requires energy.

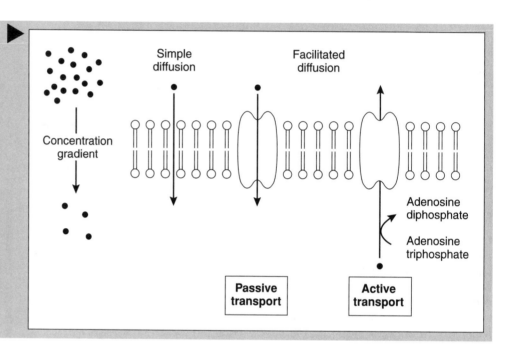

Passive Transport. By definition, passive transport describes the process by which molecules move across a membrane without energy supplied by the hydrolysis of adenosine triphosphate (ATP). The direction of passive transport is always from a region of higher concentration to one of lower concentration. There are two types of passive transport, simple diffusion and facilitated diffusion.

In *simple diffusion*, the rate of transport of a molecule across a membrane is directly proportional to its concentration, and the process is not saturable at high concentrations. The smaller the molecule and the fewer hydrogen bonds it forms with water, the more rapidly it diffuses across the membrane. Some small uncharged molecules like molecular oxygen and carbon dioxide readily dissolve in the membrane. Other small molecules such as water, ethanol, and urea diffuse across the membrane much more slowly. In contrast, charged molecules, regardless of how small they are, cannot enter the hydrophobic bilayer, and they do not cross membranes by simple diffusion.

In *facilitated diffusion*, proteins aid in the transport of molecules across membranes. A *transport protein* binds to a specific molecule on one side of the membrane and releases it on the other side. The rate of transport by facilitated diffusion is limited by the number of transport proteins in the membrane. Therefore, the rate plateaus at high concentrations of solute. Transport proteins are classified as *uniporters*, *symporters*, or *antiporters*.

Active Transport. The transport of a molecule against a concentration gradient (from a lower to a higher concentration) requires both a *carrier protein* and a source of *energy*. The energy is supplied either directly or indirectly by the hydrolysis of ATP. Active transport of a molecule is always unidirectional.

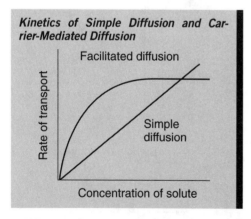

Kinetics of Simple Diffusion and Carrier-Mediated Diffusion

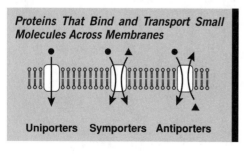

Proteins That Bind and Transport Small Molecules Across Membranes

Uniporters   Symporters   Antiporters

Endocytosis and Exocytosis. Endocytosis describes the transport of *macromolecules* from the outside to the inside of cells. Invagination of the plasma membrane around the macromolecule occurs, resulting in the release of a vesicle that contains the macromolecule inside the cell. The reverse process, exocytosis, is used to transport macromolecules to the exterior of the cell. The macromolecules are packaged into secretory vesicles that fuse with the plasma membrane, releasing their contents outside the cell.

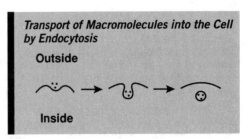

Transport of Macromolecules into the Cell by Endocytosis

Outside

Inside

SUBCELLULAR COMPARTMENTS AND THEIR METABOLIC FUNCTIONS

The division of labor in eukaryotic cells is very pronounced with specific subcellular organelles performing one or more discrete functions. This type of organization allows the cell to function much more efficiently by partitioning different metabolic pathways into different cellular compartments (Table 1-1). In many cases, opposing pathways are found in different subcellular compartments. A brief summary of the subcellular organelles and their functions is provided below.

◀ **TABLE 1-1**
Compartments of Eukaryotic Cells and Their Functions

Subcellular Compartment	Major Functions
Plasma membrane	Transport of molecules in and out of cell, hormone receptors, and receptors for macromolecules
Nucleus	DNA storage, replication, and repair; and RNA synthesis and processing
Nucleolus	Ribosomal RNA synthesis and ribosome assembly
Mitochondria	ATP synthesis; tricarboxylic acid (TCA) cycle; fatty acid oxidation; and some steps in urea, heme, and glucose synthesis
Lysosomes	Cellular digestion; and hydrolysis of nucleic acids, proteins, glycosaminoglycans, glycolipids, sphingolipids
Peroxisomes	Oxidation of very long-chain fatty acids and branched-chain fatty acids, bile acid synthesis, plasmalogen synthesis, ethanol oxidation, and hydrogen peroxide metabolism
Endoplasmic reticulum	Synthesis of proteins for organelles and secretion, membrane synthesis, phospholipid and triglyceride synthesis, steroid hydroxylation, and cytochrome P-450 detoxification reactions
Golgi	Post-translational modification and sorting of proteins; and export of proteins
Cytosol	Carbohydrate metabolism, purine and pyrimidine nucleotide synthesis, and fatty acid synthesis
Cytoskeleton	Cell morphology, cell motility, cell division, and intracellular movements
Polysomes	Synthesis of cytosolic proteins

Plasma Membrane

The plasma membrane serves as a *selective barrier* that limits the exchange of materials between the inside and the outside of cells. The plasma membrane contains a number of *transport proteins* that control entry of molecules. Ions are frequently found at different concentrations on the inside and outside of cells, creating *ion gradients* across the plasma membrane. The transport of any molecule from a lower to a higher concentration requires energy. For example, the intracellular and extracellular concentrations of sodium (Na$^+$) and potassium (K$^+$) are very different. The energy for maintaining the gradient across the membrane is provided by coupling ion transport with ATP hydrolysis. The plasma membrane also participates in signal transduction pathways. The plasma membrane contains both *receptors* that bind specific peptide hormones or neurotransmitters and *enzymes* that generate second messengers inside cells.

Nucleus

The nucleus is the largest of the organelles. It contains the components of the genetic apparatus, including DNA, RNA, and nuclear proteins. The metabolic functions of the nucleus include the *synthesis of DNA and RNA*. Also present are enzymes that correct mistakes introduced during DNA synthesis. The transport of molecules in and out of the nucleus is facilitated by pores in the nuclear membrane that are created by a complex of proteins. The *nucleolus* is a region within the nucleus where ribosomal RNA (rRNA) is synthesized and the *assembly of ribosomes* occurs.

Mitochondria

Mitochondria are oblong structures that have a smooth outer membrane and a highly folded inner membrane. The folds in the inner membrane, called *cristae*, increase the surface area of the inner membrane. Although the outer membrane is porous and allows many molecules to pass through it, the inner membrane is highly impermeable and contains many specific transport proteins that allow molecules to enter or exit the mitochondrial matrix. One of the major functions of mitochondria is to oxidize fuels, using the energy released to synthesize ATP. More than 95% of the oxygen consumed by humans is used for mitochondrial oxidation reactions. The inner surface of the cristae are tightly packed with particles that contain all of the proteins and enzymes needed for *oxidative phosphorylation*. In any particular cell, the number of mitochondria depends on the need of that cell for energy. As much as 25% of the volume of some cells is occupied by mitochondria. Mitochondria contain their own DNA as well as enzymes that synthesize DNA, RNA, and protein. Defects in mitochondrial function are associated with *ammonia toxicity*, *viral infections*, and *cirrhosis* of the liver.

Lysosomes

Lysosomes are membrane-bound vesicles, including more than 50 different *acid hydrolases* that degrade nucleic acids, complex carbohydrates, and proteins. The pH in the lysosome is low compared to that of the cytosol. The low pH is maintained by an ATP-dependent proton (H$^+$) pump that pumps H$^+$ from the cytosol into the interior of the lysosome. More than 35 inherited diseases have been associated with defects in degradative lysosomal enzymes, resulting in a family of *lysosomal storage diseases*.

Peroxisomes

Peroxisomes are small membrane-bound vesicles that specialize in *oxidation reactions* that produce *hydrogen peroxide* as a side product. These reactions are particularly important in the liver and kidney, where several hundred peroxisomes may be found per cell. A major function of peroxisomes is the oxidation of very long-chain fatty acids and branched-chain fatty acids. Some of the hydrogen peroxide produced in these reactions is used by the liver to oxidize *toxic molecules* that enter the bloodstream. For example, about 30% of ethanol oxidization occurs in peroxisomes. Peroxisomes also contain *catalase*, an enzyme that degrades excess hydrogen peroxide to water and oxygen. Defects in peroxisomal function are associated with *Zellweger syndrome* and *adrenoleukodystrophy (ALD)*.

Endoplasmic Reticulum (ER)

The extensive intracellular membrane network, known as the ER, is continuous with the nuclear membrane and the Golgi. It stores, segregates, and transports substances within the cell and is involved in the assembly of subcellular organelles. The ER exists in rough and smooth forms. The *rough ER (RER)* has ribosomes attached and is involved in the *synthesis of proteins* that are destined for secretion or incorporation into subcellular organelles. The *smooth ER (SER)* plays a central role in *lipid synthesis*. Most of the lipids found in the mitochondrial and peroxisomal membranes are synthesized in the ER. Additionally, the SER contains many cytochrome P-450 enzymes that catalyze a variety of *detoxification reactions*, rendering highly insoluble compounds sufficiently soluble to be excreted.

Golgi Complex

The Golgi complex consists of a stack of flat, closed-membrane sacs that are continuous with the ER. The Golgi is responsible for *sorting* newly synthesized proteins and *targeting* them to specific destinations. The synthesis of glycosaminoglycans (GAGs) also occurs in the Golgi.

Cytosol

The cytosol is defined as the aqueous medium that is located inside a cell but outside the nucleus and other organelles. It is a concentrated solution or suspension that contains many of the substrates and enzymes involved in *carbohydrate metabolism, fatty acid synthesis, nucleotide synthesis, and protein synthesis*.

Other Subcellular Structures

Other entities found inside cells, but not surrounded by membranes, include the cytoskeleton and polysomes. The *cytoskeleton* is an organized network of filamentous structures that give a cell its *shape* and *motility*. The major components of the cytoskeleton include actin filaments, microtubules, and intermediate filaments. Intermediate filaments form a diverse family of proteins that provide rope-like networks in cells. More stable than actin filaments and microtubules, they provide cells with mechanical strength. *Polysomes* are complexes of messenger RNA (mRNA) and ribosomes that are actively involved in the *synthesis of cytosolic proteins*.

MACROMOLECULES AND BUILDING BLOCKS

The major structural and functional components of cells are the macromolecules, a diverse set of polymers that are assembled from a relatively small number of simple building blocks (Figure 1-4). There are *four major classes of macromolecules*: nucleic acids, proteins, polysaccharides, and lipids. Macromolecules have molecular weights

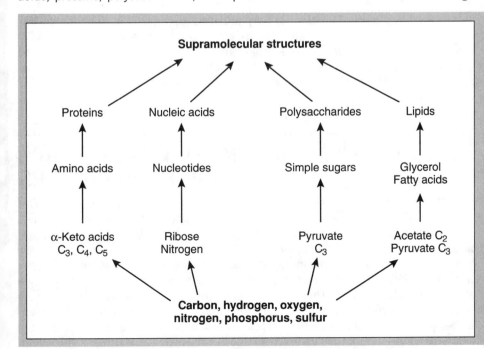

FIGURE 1-4
Molecular Hierarchy in Cell Structure. *The elements hydrogen, oxygen, nitrogen, carbon, phosphorus, and sulfur make up more than 99% of the mass of most cells. These elements are combined in various ways to form almost all of the compounds found in cells. Some of these compounds are used to synthesize a small number of building blocks that are, in turn, used for constructing a diverse family of macromolecules. The building blocks for proteins, nucleic acids, polysaccharides, and lipids are linked together by covalent bonds. Membranes, organelles, and other supramolecular structures are formed by association of macromolecules into larger complexes that are held together by many noncovalent interactions. The structures of the small building blocks have a profound effect on the structure and function of macromolecules and supramolecular complexes.*

ranging from approximately 10^3 to 10^9 and are assembled by the polymerization of *building blocks* that have molecular weights in the range of 200–500. The synthesis of macromolecules involves the formation of *covalent bonds* between building blocks, a process that requires *energy*. Two major functions of metabolism are to provide the energy needed for the synthesis of macromolecules and to provide simple, universal intermediates that can be converted into the building blocks for macromolecules. Macromolecules can be assembled into larger functional complexes such as membranes, organelles, chromatin, and ribosomes. These supramolecular complexes are held together by noncovalent interactions.

Nucleic Acids

Nucleic acids are polymers of *nucleotides* that store and transmit genetic information. The building blocks for both DNA and RNA synthesis consist of a set of four nucleotides. DNA requires deoxyadenosine triphosphate (dATP), deoxyguanosine triphosphate (dGTP), deoxycytidine triphosphate (dCTP), and deoxythymidine triphosphate (dTTP), while RNA requires ATP, guanosine triphosphate (GTP), cytidine triphosphate (CTP), and uridine triphosphate (UTP). The nucleotides, in turn, are synthesized from simpler compounds that are intermediates in metabolic pathways found in all cells.

Proteins

Proteins are polymers of *amino acids* that are responsible for carrying out most of the instructions dictated by the genetic code. There are 20 different amino acids that are the building blocks for proteins. About half of these amino acids can be synthesized from intermediates in metabolism, and the remainder are supplied by dietary protein.

Polysaccharides

Polysaccharides are polymers containing a large number of *simple sugars*. Some are homopolymers that contain only one kind of sugar, while others are complex heteropolymers that contain 8–10 types of sugars. Polysaccharides function both as structural components of cells and as storage forms of energy. Glycogen is a storage form of glucose in animal tissues, whereas the GAGs are structural components of the extracellular matrix. The 8–10 monosaccharides that are the building blocks for polysaccharides can be synthesized from glucose or from other simpler intermediates in metabolism.

Lipids

The major building blocks for lipids are *fatty acids* and *glycerol*. Lipids function both as structural components of membranes and as a storage form of energy. The two major classes of lipids are triglycerides, the storage form of fatty acids, and phospholipids, the major building blocks for all membranes. Both fatty acids and glycerol can be synthesized from small intermediates in metabolism that are present in all cells.

CELLULAR ENVIRONMENT: WATER, ACIDS, BASES, AND BUFFERS

Body Water
About 55% of the weight of a normal adult is water. Approximately two-thirds of the body water is found inside the cells (intracellular fluid), and the remaining one-third is found outside cells (extracellular fluid). The extracellular fluid includes both the blood plasma and the water in between cells (interstitial fluid).

Homeostasis can be defined as the maintenance of a constant cellular environment. This is a remarkable feat, considering that each cell obtains nutrients from the surrounding interstitial fluid and releases its waste products into the same fluid. The H^+ concentration in both the *extracellular and intracellular fluids* must be maintained within a narrow concentration range to be compatible with life. A constant H^+ concentration in body fluids and subcellular compartments, as reflected by a constant pH, is achieved by a number of buffering systems. These systems, consisting of a weak acid and its conjugate base, are able to donate and accept protons from the surrounding medium. The relationship between H^+ concentration, the dissociation constant of weak acids (pK_a), and the concentration of the conjugate acid–base pair of a buffering system is an important concept in understanding the regulation of normal pH and the abnormal states of *acidosis* and *alkalosis*.

Acids and Bases

Acids can be defined as proton donors and bases as proton acceptors. Many important compounds found in biologic fluids, including amino acids, lactic acid, propionic acid, and acetoacetic acid, are weak acids.

Properties of Weak Acids. In contrast to strong acids, such as hydrochloric acid (HCl) and sulfuric acid (H_2SO_4), weak acids are not completely dissociated under physiologic conditions. The dissociation of a weak acid can be described by the equation below.

$$HA \rightleftharpoons H^+ + A^-$$

Conjugate acid   **Conjugate base**

The undissociated form of the acid is known as the *conjugate acid* (*HA*), whereas the corresponding form that has lost its proton is known as the *conjugate base* (A^-). Since H^+ is released in this reaction, the relative proportion of conjugate acid and conjugate base is dependent on the pH of the solution, which is inversely related to the H^+ concentration.

The Henderson-Hasselbalch Equation. The relationship between the pH and the concentration of a weak acid and its conjugate base is described by the Henderson-Hasselbalch equation shown below. In this equation, pH is defined as the negative log of [H^+], and pK_a is defined as the negative log of the dissociation constant, K_a, for the acid.

$$pH = pK_a + \log \frac{[A^-]}{[HA]}$$

The pK_a is a constant that describes the inherent ability of an ionizing group to lose its proton. This equation can be used to calculate the amounts of the conjugate acid and its conjugate base at any given pH. Additionally, it provides two useful concepts relative to acid–base balance.

First, the Henderson-Hasselbalch equation predicts a simple and useful definition of pK_a. *The pK_a of any ionizing group is the pH where the concentration of the conjugate acid (HA) and its conjugate base (A^-) are equal.* When [HA] = [A^-], the last term of the equation becomes zero, and the equation simplifies to pH = pK_a.

Second, small changes in pH produce large effects. Because of the logarithmic nature of the Henderson-Hasselbalch equation, *a change of one pH unit results in approximately a tenfold change in the conjugate acid/conjugate base ratio*. This effect, where the weak acid is acetic acid whose carboxyl group has a pK_a of 4.7, is illustrated in Table 1-2. The ratio of the concentration of acetic acid to its conjugate base, acetate, are given for integral changes in pH. When the pH decreases, the H^+ concentration increases, and the concentration of conjugate acid increases; whereas when the pH increases, H^+ concentration decreases, and the concentration of conjugate base increases.

pH of Biologic Fluids
The pH of both extracellular and intracellular fluids is maintained within a narrow pH range in living systems. The range shown below for intracellular fluid is for different cell types. Within a particular type of cell, the range is much narrower.

Extracellular fluids	
Arterial blood	7.40
Venous blood	7.35
Interstitial fluid	7.35
Intracellular fluid	6.0–7.4
Lysosomal matrix	5.5–6.5

Acidosis: Blood pH less than 7.36
Alkalosis: Blood pH greater than 7.44

◄ **TABLE 1-2**
Effect of pH on Relative Amounts of Acetic Acid and Acetate

pH	Acetic Acid: Acetate
2.7	100
3.7	10
pK_a 4.7	1
5.7	0.1
6.7	0.01

Titration of Weak Acids

The addition of a base to a weak acid results in an increase in both the pH of the solution and the relative proportion of its conjugate base. The addition of sodium hydroxide (NaOH) to a weak acid (HA) is described by the following equation.

$$HA + NaOH \rightleftharpoons Na^+A^- + H_2O$$

The protons that are released from the acid combine with the hydroxide ions to form water. Therefore, as the addition of NaOH continues, the concentration of H^+ decreases, and the pH of the solution increases. A *titration curve* for any acid can be generated by plotting the pH of the solution versus the equivalents of NaOH that have been added. *The pK_a value of the acid can be deduced from the titration curve.* The titration curve for acetic acid is shown in Figure 1-5. At the midpoint of the titration, half of the acid has been converted to acetate, and $[HA] = [A^-]$. As predicted by the Henderson-Hasselbalch equation, the pH of the solution at the halfway point in the titration is equal to the pK_a of the acid.

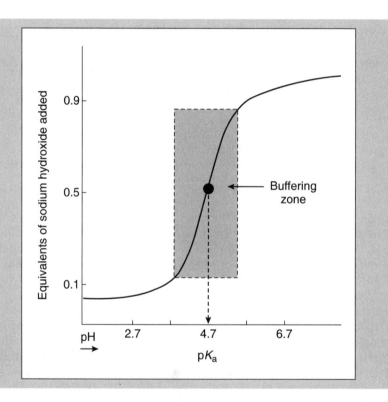

FIGURE 1-5 ▶

Titration Curve for Acetic Acid. The midpoint in the titration (●) of acetic acid occurs when half of the acid is present in the dissociated form, acetate. The pH at which this occurs is pH 4.7 and is equal to the pK_a for the carboxyl group of acetic acid. The shaded area corresponds to the pH range where this conjugate acid–base pair has a high buffering capacity.

Buffering Properties of Weak Acids

Buffers are mixtures of weak acids and their conjugate bases. The buffering capacity of any conjugate acid/conjugate base pair depends on both the pH and the concentration of the buffer. A buffer resists changes in pH most effectively when it is used at a pH near its pK_a. Buffers are usually chosen with pK_a values within one pH unit of the desired pH. In this region (see *shaded area* in Figure 1-5), the addition of acid or base results in minimal change in the pH.

Important Buffers in Biologic Systems

The three most important buffering systems in humans are the bicarbonate, phosphate, and protein systems. The conjugate acid–base pairs and the pK_a for these buffers are summarized in Table 1-3.

◀ **TABLE 1-3**
Properties of Major Buffering Systems in Humans

Buffer	pK_a	Major Compartment
Protein systems		
Histidine side chains	5.6–7.0	Intracellular fluid
Bicarbonate system		
$CO_2/H_2CO_3/HCO_3^-$	6.1	Extracellular fluid
Phosphate system		
$H_2PO_4^-/HPO_4^{-2}$	6.8	Intracellular fluid

Bicarbonate Buffer System. The most important *extracellular* buffer is the bicarbonate system described by the following equation.

$$CO_2 + H_2O \rightleftharpoons H_2CO_3 \rightleftharpoons H^+ + HCO_3^-$$

Carbon dioxide (CO_2), produced as a result of metabolism, combines with water to form carbonic acid (H_2CO_3), which has a pK_a of 6.1. The dissociation of H_2CO_3 produces a proton and bicarbonate ion (HCO_3^-). In response to an increase in H^+ concentration (a decrease in pH), the equilibrium of this system shifts to the left, producing more CO_2. Conversely, in response to a decrease in the H^+ concentration (an increase in pH), the equilibrium shifts to the right, producing more HCO_3^-. The concentrations of CO_2 and HCO_3^- are carefully regulated by the lung and kidney. The lung releases CO_2, and HCO_3^- is excreted by the kidney.

Phosphate Buffer System. The phosphate buffer system plays a major role in buffering *intracellular* fluids but is of little importance in buffering extracellular fluid. The pK_a of dihydrogen phosphate ($H_2PO_4^-$) is 6.8, and depending on the type of cells, the pH of the intracellular fluid may range from 6.0 to 7.4. Therefore, the phosphate system is ideally suited as a buffer in this pH range.

Protein Buffer System. Proteins are important *intracellular* buffers where they are present in high concentrations. Some of the amino acid side chains (particularly the imidazole side chains of histidine) have pK_a values that are close to intracellular pH. In the RBC, hemoglobin is the most important buffer because of its histidine content and its high concentration. The protein buffering system is also important in maintaining a constant pH in serum where its concentration is much higher than in interstitial fluid.

RESOLUTION OF CLINICAL CASE

The infant described at the beginning of the chapter was born with Zellweger syndrome, a rare autosomal recessive disorder characterized by abnormalities of brain, liver, heart, kidney, and skeletal muscle. Death usually occurs within a few months. The biochemical abnormalities observed with plasma and tissues taken at autopsy can be attributed to the absence of peroxisomes. These organelles are required for several metabolic pathways, including synthesis of bile acids and plasmalogens, and oxidation of very long-chain fatty acids. The oxidation of very long-chain fatty acids normally starts in peroxisomes where they are degraded to shorter fatty acids that are released and further oxidized by mitochondria. Mitochondria are unable to oxidize fatty acids that are greater than C_{22} in length. Therefore, patients with Zellweger syndrome accumulate fatty acids that are greater than C_{22} in length, while fatty acids that are less than C_{22} in length are oxidized by the mitochondria. An increase in the plasma ratio of $C_{26}:C_{22}$ is an important parameter in the diagnosis of this disorder. In the absence of peroxisomes, these patients cannot convert cholestanoic acid to bile acids, accounting for the accumulation of cholestanoic acid in the liver. Similarly, plasmalogen levels are undetectable because of the absence of the peroxisomal enzymes required for their synthesis. Oxidation reactions that occur in peroxisomes result in the formation of hydrogen peroxide, most of which is degraded by catalase. Normally, 50%–65% of the catalase found in cells is located in peroxisomes. However, in this patient, all of the catalase was in the cytosol. In some cases of Zellweger syndrome, membranous structures referred to as "peroxisome ghosts" have been identified in liver and kidney cells. These structures contain peroxisomal membranes but lack catalase and other enzymes normally found in the matrix. The peroxisomal matrix proteins have a specific sequence of three amino acids near the carboxyl end that acts as a signal that they are to be imported into peroxisomes. It has been postulated that a deficiency in the import process may be the underlying cause of Zellweger syndrome [1]. This disease can be diagnosed prenatally by assaying amniotic fluid cells for peroxisomal enzymes or by analyzing the fatty acid content in amniotic fluid.

REVIEW QUESTIONS

Directions: For each of the following questions, choose the **one best** answer.

1. Which of the following is both a weak acid and a weak base?
    (A) Carbonic acid (H_2CO_3)
    (B) Hydrochloric acid (HCl)
    (C) Bicarbonate ion (HCO_3^-)
    (D) Dihydrogen phosphate ($H_2PO_4^-$)
    (E) Sulfuric acid (H_2SO_4)

2. Blood was drawn from a patient who was admitted to the emergency room with a suspected drug overdose. Analysis of the blood sample showed that the [H^+] was 5×10^{-8}M. The pH of this blood sample is
    (A) 7.30
    (B) 7.35
    (C) 7.40
    (D) 7.45
    (E) 7.50

3. Both active transport and facilitated diffusion are characterized by
    (A) transport from a high concentration to a low concentration
    (B) hydrolysis of ATP
    (C) movement through channels formed by membrane proteins
    (D) saturation in the rate of transport at very high concentrations of solute
    (E) transport in only one direction

Directions: The group of questions below consists of lettered choices followed by several numbered items. For each numbered item, select the appropriate lettered option with which it is most closely associated. Each lettered option may be used once, more than once, or not at all.

Questions 4–9
For each of the following metabolic functions, select the subcellular compartment where it is most likely to occur.
    (A) Mitochondria
    (B) Peroxisomes
    (C) Lysosomes
    (D) Nucleus
    (E) Cytosol
    (F) Endoplasmic reticulum
    (G) Plasma membrane
    (H) Golgi

4. RNA processing

5. Fatty acid oxidation

6. Carbohydrate metabolism

7. Synthesis of plasma proteins

8. Detoxification of drugs

9. ATP synthesis

ANSWERS AND EXPLANATIONS

1. The answer is D. Weak acids and bases are only partially dissociated in solution. Weak acids can donate protons, and weak bases can accept protons from the solution. $H_2PO_4^-$ releases a proton forming monohydrogen phosphate (HPO_4^-), and can accept a proton forming $H_3PO_4^-$. H_2CO_3 can donate but cannot accept a proton, and HCO_3^- can accept but cannot donate a proton. Both HCl and H_2SO_4 are strong acids and are completely dissociated in solution.

2. The answer is A. Since pH = $-\log[H^+]$, then pH = $-\log 5 \times 10^{-8} = -(\log 5 + \log 10^{-8}) = (0.7 - 8) = 7.3$.

3. The answer is D. For both active transport and facilitated diffusion, the molecule binds to a transport protein, and the rate of transport plateaus when all the binding sites are occupied. Active transport occurs against a concentration gradient and requires ATP hydrolysis, which supplies the energy for transport from a low to a high concentration. While facilitated diffusion always moves down a concentration gradient, active transport is unidirectional and moves up a concentration gradient. Active transport always requires a transport protein, whereas facilitated diffusion can either involve a transport protein or movement of solute through a membrane channel.

4–9. The answers are: 4-D, 5-A, 6-E, 7-F, 8-F, 9-A. RNA processing occurs in the nucleus. Fatty acid synthesis and most pathways of carbohydrate metabolism are localized in the cytosol of the cell. Synthesis of plasma proteins occurs in the rough endoplasmic reticulum. The only proteins that are synthesized on polysomes are proteins that remain in the cytosol. Most drugs are detoxified by cytochrome P-450 enzymes that are found in the smooth endoplasmic reticulum. Most of the ATP synthesis in cells occurs in mitochondria.

REFERENCES

1. Lazarow PB, Moser HW: Disorders of peroxisome biogenesis. In *Metabolic and Molecular Bases of Inherited Disease*, 7th ed. Edited by Scriver CR, Beaudet AL, Sly WS, et al. New York, NY: McGraw-Hill, 1995, pp 2287–2314.

2

PROTEINS: THE WORKHORSES OF THE BODY

CHAPTER OUTLINE

INTRODUCTION OF CLINICAL CASE

Ellen, a 16-year-old, was admitted to the hospital with pneumonia. She was the third child born to healthy parents. One of her brothers died of emphysema at 10 years of age. The other brother appears to be healthy. At the time of her admission to the hospital, her liver was enlarged. Laboratory tests showed an abnormal serum electrophoresis pattern, with the α_1-globulin peak barely detectable. The protein concentration in this fraction was tenfold below the normal level. Further electrophoretic analysis of the α_1-globulin fraction showed that the mobility of this protein fraction was abnormally slow. Electron micrographs of liver tissue obtained by needle biopsy, showed large granular inclusion bodies within the endoplasmic reticulum. These granules stained positive for carbohydrate and were cross-reactive with antibodies to α_1-antitrypsin. When protein was solubilized from the liver granules, it was found to bind to and inhibit the activity of elastase. The patient was treated with antibiotics, and when the pneumonia had cleared, she was released from the hospital. She was urged to avoid smoking and was given vitamin E supplements.

OVERVIEW OF PROTEINS

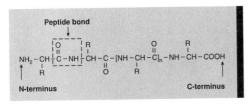

Peptide bond

$NH_2-CH-C-NH-CH-C-[NH-CH-C]_n-NH-CH-COOH$

N-terminus   C-terminus

Proteins comprise the most abundant and versatile class of macromolecules found in living systems. They are responsible for almost every function that occurs in the body. They are linear chains of amino acids that are linked together by *peptide* (amide) bonds. Protein polymers have a *polarity* that is indicated by a free amino group at one end and a free carboxyl group at the other end. The amino acids found in proteins are referred to as amino acid *residues*, and the ends are known as the *N-terminus* and the *C-terminus* of the *polypeptide chain*. Each protein has a specific and unique sequence of amino acids that defines both its three-dimensional structure and its biologic function. Approximately 1500 human diseases have been traced to the production of abnormal proteins, and in about one-third of these, the change of a single amino acid residue leads to the disease.

Number of Amino Acid Residues

Peptides	2–10 amino acid residues
Polypeptides	10–100 amino acid residues
Proteins	> 100 amino acid residues

Classification of Proteins

Proteins are classified in numerous ways based on their chemical and physical properties. Five of the classification methods that are useful from a clinical perspective are summarized below.

Shape. Proteins that are highly folded and *globular* in shape tend to be responsible for the dynamic functions of the cell, whereas the more extended *fibrous* proteins usually are associated with structural roles in cells and tissues. Because of the asymmetric structure of fibrous proteins, they behave more like larger molecules than do globular proteins of equal molecular weight.

Solubility. The *albumins* are soluble in water, whereas the *globulins* are insoluble in water but soluble in dilute salt solutions. *Scleroproteins* are insoluble in both water and salt solutions but are soluble in dilute acid.

Composition. *Simple proteins* are composed only of amino acids, whereas *complex proteins* contain additional components. For example, *glycoproteins* contain carbohydrate, *lipoproteins* contain lipid, and *metalloproteins* contain metal ions.

Density. The classification of *lipoproteins* into chylomicrons, very low-density lipoproteins (VLDLs), low-density lipoproteins (LDLs), and high-density lipoproteins (HDLs) is based on increasing density.

Charge. Proteins that have a net negative charge at physiologic pH are known as *acidic proteins*, while those with a net positive charge are known as *basic proteins*.

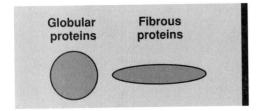

Globular proteins   Fibrous proteins

Protein Function

A typical cell contains thousands of different proteins. In general, each of these proteins is encoded by a specific gene and performs a unique function in the cell. *The function of a specific protein is determined by its structure.* The versatility and specificity of proteins can be illustrated by summarizing some of the major biologic functions of proteins.

Catalytic Proteins. The largest and most diverse class of proteins are the *enzymes* that serve as the biologic catalysts. These proteins accelerate the rate at which reactions occur in the cell. A single cell may contain thousands of different enzymes, each highly specific for the reaction it catalyzes.

Transport Proteins. Blood contains many proteins that bind specific molecules and transport them from one site in the body to another. For example: (1) *hemoglobin* binds oxygen as the blood circulates through the lungs and releases it to tissues engaged in oxidative metabolism; (2) *transferrin* transports iron (Fe^{3+}) to various tissues; and (3) *lipoproteins* act as vehicles for transporting cholesterol esters and triglycerides, molecules that are insoluble in aqueous solutions.

Storage Proteins. Some proteins are designed to store small molecules and release them as needed. Cardiac muscle is enriched in *myoglobin*, a protein that stores oxygen inside muscle cells and releases it when the oxygen tension begins to decrease. Liver, muscle, and intestinal cells are enriched in *ferritin*, an intracellular protein that stores iron.

Structure Determines Function

Oxytocin and vasopressin are two hormones whose structures differ by a single amino acid. Although the structural differences are small, the sites at which the hormones act and the effects they elicit are very different.

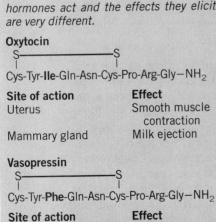

Oxytocin

Cys-Tyr-**Ile**-Gln-Asn-Cys-Pro-Arg-Gly—NH$_2$

Site of action	**Effect**
Uterus	Smooth muscle contraction
Mammary gland	Milk ejection

Vasopressin

Cys-Tyr-**Phe**-Gln-Asn-Cys-Pro-Arg-Gly—NH$_2$

Site of action	**Effect**
Coronary arteries	Constriction
Kidney	Reabsorption of H_2O

Defense Proteins. Many of the proteins found in blood and on the surface of cells play protective roles. For example, the *clotting proteins* prevent loss of blood, and the *immunoglobulins* protect against disease by binding foreign proteins associated with bacteria and viruses.

Regulatory Proteins. A few proteins are responsible for maintaining hemostasis. For example, metabolic pathways are usually regulated by the enzyme that catalyzes the slowest step in the pathway.

Contractile and Motile Proteins. The major proteins responsible for cellular movement are polymeric forms of *actin, myosin,* and *tubulin.*

Structural Proteins. Some proteins perform structural roles, acting as the mortar and bricks that provide cells and tissues with strength and extensibility. *Collagen,* the major component of tendons, has high tensile strength. *Elastin,* found in the connective tissue of the major arteries and lungs, provides elasticity.

AMINO ACIDS: BUILDING BLOCKS OF PROTEINS

A set of 20 amino acids is used to synthesize the thousands of proteins found in biologic systems. Of the 20 amino acids, 19 can be represented by the generic structure shown in Figure 2-1. Attached to the α-carbon is an amino group, a carboxyl group, and a hydrogen

$$R - C_\alpha - COOH$$
(with NH_2 above and H below the C_α)

FIGURE 2-1
General Structure for Amino Acids Found in Proteins. *The α-carbon of an amino acid is defined as the atom to which the carboxyl ($-COOH$) group, the amino ($-NH_2$) group, and the hydrogen atom ($-H$) are attached. The amino acids differ in the chemical nature of their side chain group ($-R$).*

atom. The amino acids differ from one another in the nature of the R group, commonly referred to as the *side chain.* Proline is the one exception to this general structure. The α-carbon of proline is part of a cyclic structure formed between the R group and the amino group. The structures of the 20 amino acids that are used for synthesizing proteins are shown in Figure 2-2. Both the three letter code and the one letter code for each amino acid are given in the figure.

The aromatic amino acids (tryptophan, tyrosine, phenylalanine) absorb ultraviolet light. The absorbance at 280 nm is frequently used to monitor the purification of proteins.

D- and L-Amino Acids

The D- and L- designation for amino acids refers to the absolute configuration around the α-carbon atom. The absolute configuration is relative to D- and L-glyceraldehyde, which are the universal standards for stereoisomers. The D- and L-amino acids are mirror images of one another. *Only L-amino acids are used for protein synthesis.* D-Amino acids are found in bacterial cell walls and in some antibiotics produced by microorganisms.

Classification of Amino Acids

There are many ways of classifying amino acids, depending on the nature of the side chains. When describing protein structure, it is most useful to classify them in two major groups, the hydrophilic (polar) and hydrophobic (apolar) amino acids.

Hydrophilic Amino Acids. The hydrophilic amino acids interact favorably with water. They are usually found on the surface of proteins where they are exposed to the aqueous medium. The side chains of the hydrophilic amino acids contain polar groups that may be either charged or uncharged.

D-Amino Acids and L-Amino Acids
The configurations around the α-carbon atoms are mirror images of one another.

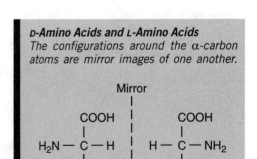

L-Amino acid   D-Amino acid

FIGURE 2-2

Structures of the 20 Common Amino Acids Found in Proteins. Beside the name of each amino acid, the one-letter code word is given in parentheses. Below the name, the more commonly used three-letter code word is shown. The amino acids are grouped on the basis of the hydrophilicity or hydrophobicity of their side chains. Five of the hydrophilic amino acids have charged side chains, and five have uncharged side chains. Those with uncharged side chains have atoms with unshared pairs of electrons (O, N, S) that can form hydrogen bonds with water. The hydrophobic amino acid side chains are either aliphatic or aromatic. The side chain groups are shaded to emphasize their differences.

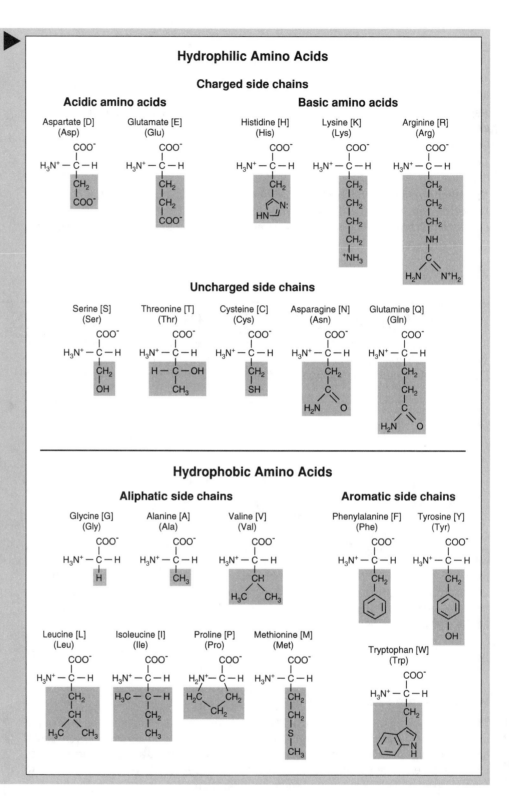

The *charged side chains* are of two types. The side chains of the acidic amino acids, *aspartic acid* and *glutamic acid*, have carboxyl groups that are *negatively charged* within the physiologic pH range. The side chains of the basic amino acids, *lysine, arginine, and histidine*, have a *positive charge* at physiologic pH. The positive charge is due to the presence in the side chains of nitrogen atoms that are protonated.

The *uncharged side chains* of other amino acids have *oxygen, sulfur,* and *nitrogen atoms*, enabling them to form hydrogen bonds with water. Although they are uncharged, these amino acids are hydrophilic. Included in this group are *serine* and *threonine* with side chain hydroxyl groups; *asparagine* and *glutamine* with side chain amide groups; and *cysteine* with a side chain sulfhydryl group. In general, most of these side chains are found on the surface of proteins where they interact with water.

Hydrophobic Amino Acids. The side chains of hydrophobic amino acids interact poorly with water. They are usually found buried in the interior of proteins where they are protected from the aqueous environment and stabilized by hydrophobic interactions with one another. The hydrophobic amino acids have either aliphatic or aromatic side chains.

   Aliphatic side chains of varying lengths are found in *alanine, valine, isoleucine,* and *proline.* These side chains are more stable in a nonaqueous environment. *Methionine* has an aliphatic side chain that contains a sulfur atom. It is found in the interior of proteins more frequently than on the surface. *Glycine*, having a hydrogen atom for a side chain, can fit into many spaces and is found both on the surface and in the interior of proteins.

   Aromatic side chains are found in *phenylalanine, tyrosine,* and *tryptophan*. All of these side chains are usually found in the interior of proteins where their ring systems are stabilized by stacking one on top of another.

Modified Amino Acids

In addition to the common amino acids, small amounts of several other amino acids are found in proteins. These amino acids are formed by the modification of one of the 20 common amino acids *after incorporation* into the protein. Hundreds of modification reactions have been described that produce the *modified amino acids* found in proteins. The following modified amino acids are of particular significance.

Cystine. Cystine is formed by the linkage of two cysteine side chains through a *disulfide bond.* This modified amino acid is found in many proteins, where it provides stability to the three-dimensional structure.

Hydroxyproline and Hydroxylysine. The hydroxylation of selected lysine and proline residues is found primarily in the connective tissue protein, collagen.

Desmosine and Isodesmosine. These two amino acids are formed by the oxidation and crosslinking of four lysine side chains. Desmosine and isodesmosine are found in the connective tissue protein, elastin.

γ-Carboxyglutamate. Carboxylation of glutamic acid side chains occurs in many of the clotting proteins found in the blood. The inability to form γ-carboxyglutamate results in bleeding disorders.

Phosphoserine, Phosphothreonine, and Phosphotyrosine. The hydroxyl groups found in the side chains of serine, threonine, and tyrosine residues can be phosphorylated. These modified amino acids are of particular importance in regulatory proteins.

Ionic (Acid–Base) Properties of Amino Acids

In neutral solutions, amino acids exist as dipolar ions, also known as *zwitterions*. In zwitterions, the α-amino group is protonated and has a positive charge, while the α-carboxyl group is ionized and has a negative charge. The effect of pH on the structure of an amino acid is shown in the following equation:

$$
\underset{\substack{\textbf{pH 1.0}\\\textbf{Net charge} = +1}}{R-\overset{\overset{\displaystyle N^+H_3}{|}}{C}H-COOH} \rightleftharpoons \underset{\substack{\textbf{pH 7.0}\\\textbf{Net charge} = 0}}{R-\overset{\overset{\displaystyle N^+H_3}{|}}{C}H-COO^-} \rightleftharpoons \underset{\substack{\textbf{pH 11.0}\\\textbf{Net charge} = -1}}{R-\overset{\overset{\displaystyle NH_2}{|}}{C}H-COO^-}
$$

If acid is added to a neutral solution of an amino acid, the α-carboxyl group becomes protonated, and the equilibrium between these various ionic forms is shifted to the left. If base is added, the proton on the α-amino group dissociates, and the equilibrium is shifted to the right.

pK_a for Ionizing Groups. All amino acids have at least two ionizing groups, and each ionizing group has a characteristic *dissociation constant* (K_a) that is usually expressed in terms of pK_a (the negative log of K_a). The pK_a of the α-carboxyl group of the amino acids is between 2.0 and 2.5, while the pK_a of the α-amino group is between 9.0 and 10.0. The predominant ionic form of an amino acid varies with the pH. The concentration that exists at a specific pH can be calculated from the Henderson-Hasselbalch equation (see Chapter 1).

The acidic and basic amino acids have an additional ionizing group in their side chains. These amino acids have a third characteristic pK_a. The pK_a of the side chain carboxyl group of aspartic and glutamic acid is approximately 4.0, whereas the pK_a for the basic side chains of lysine and arginine is between 10 and 12. At pH values below the pK_a for an ionizing group, the protonated form predominates; while at pH values above the pK_a, the ionized (deprotonated) form predominates. Therefore, in the physiologic pH range, aspartic acid and glutamic acid side chains are negatively charged, while lysine and arginine side chains are positively charged.

Isoelectric Point. The pI is defined as the pH at which a molecule is at its isoelectric point. At the pI, the molecule has no net charge and will not move in an electric field. For a simple amino acid that has no ionizing group in its side chain, the pI is the average of the pK_a for the α-carboxyl group and the α-amino group.

$$pI = \frac{pK_a^{\,a\,COOH} + pK_a^{\,a\,N^+H_3}}{2}$$

For amino acids that have an ionizing group in the side chain, however, the pI is the average of the two pK_a values that are on each side of the isoelectric species. This can be illustrated by the following equation that describes the equilibria between the ionic forms of aspartic acid. In this particular case, the pI for aspartic acid is the average of pK_a for the α-carboxyl group and the pK_a for the side chain carboxyl group.

Net charge = +1   Net charge = 0
                                Isoelectric species

Net charge = -1   Net charge = -2

Titration of Amino Acids. Titration curves for representative amino acids are shown in Figure 2-3. The upper curve is for glycine, a simple amino acid having no ionizing group in its side chain. The lower curve is for histidine, a basic amino acid with an additional ionizing group in its side chain. The ionic form of the amino acid that predominates at various pH values is shown below each titration curve.

Ionic Properties of Proteins

Almost all of the charge on proteins is due to the side chains of the acidic and basic amino acids. For every protein chain, there is only one free α-amino group and one free α-carboxyl group, since all others have been incorporated into peptide bonds that hold amino acids together. The pK_a of each ionizing side chain has a range of values, depending on its microenvironment in the protein, as shown in Figure 2-4.

The burial of an ionizing side chain in the interior of a protein can significantly alter its pK_a. The ionic properties of the side chains have important implications with respect to protein function.

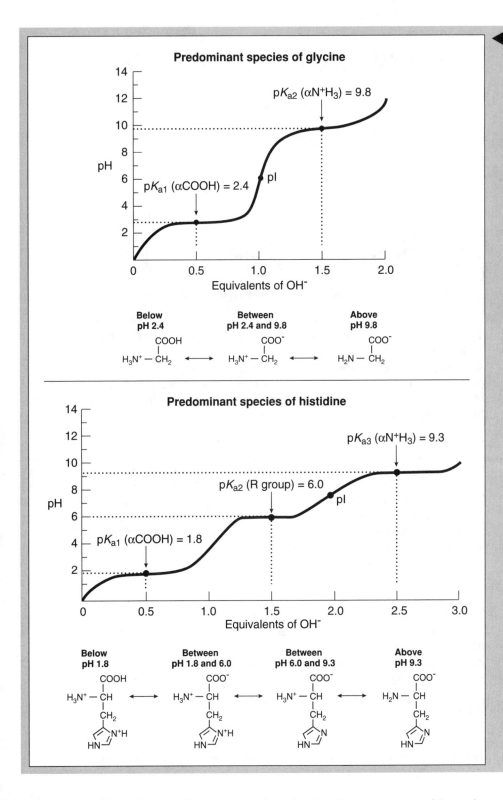

FIGURE 2-3
Titration Curves for Glycine and Histidine.
The upper curve demonstrates the change in both the pH, and the predominant ionic species of glycine as base (OH⁻) is added to a solution of the amino acid. The point indicated by pI is the pH where the molecule has zero net charge. The pK_a of the α-carboxyl group (αCOOH) and the α-amino group (αN⁺H₃) are shown in the graph. The titration curve for histidine is shown in the lower curve. The three phases in the titration curve of histidine reflect the presence of three ionizing groups. In addition to αCOOH and αN⁺H₃ groups, histidine also has a side chain structure (imidazole ring) that ionizes with a pK_a equal to 6.0.

Buffering Capacity of Proteins. Proteins as a class of molecules serve as one of the major intracellular buffers. The ability to donate and accept protons within the physiologic pH range is due almost entirely to the histidine content of proteins (see Chapter 1).

Specialized Functions of Acidic and Basic Proteins. Proteins that are enriched in acidic amino acids are negatively charged at physiologic pH, and they often serve as chelators of divalent cations. *Calsequesterin*, a protein found in the sarcoplasmic reticulum that stores calcium ions (Ca^{2+}), contains a large amount of aspartic and glutamic acid residues. Proteins that are enriched in the basic amino acids are positively charged at physiologic pH and are frequently found associated with negatively charged macro-

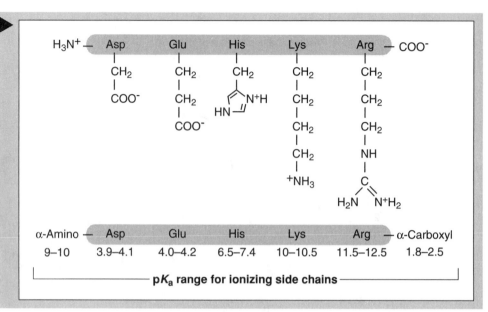

molecules. *Histones*, the major proteins associated with DNA in chromatin, have a high content of lysine and arginine residues.

Separation Methods for Proteins. Many of the methods used to separate complex mixtures of proteins are based on the fact that different proteins have different ionic properties. Clinical laboratories routinely use *electrophoresis* and *ion exchange chromatography* to separate various classes of serum proteins from one another.

PROTEIN STRUCTURE AND CONFORMATION

The *native conformation* of a protein is defined as the three-dimensional structure that is biologically active. Both covalent and noncovalent bonds stabilize the structure of proteins. The amino acids are linked together into linear polymers by *covalent* bonds, whereas the overall three-dimensional structure, which is unique to each protein, is stabilized by a large number of *noncovalent* interactions that occur between the amino acid side chains.

Covalent Bonds

Two major types of covalent bonds are found in proteins, peptide bonds, and disulfide bonds.

Peptide (Amide) Bonds. The backbone of the protein chain is formed by the reaction of the α-carboxyl group of one amino acid with the α-amino group of the next amino acid in the linear chain. As shown in the following equation, this reaction results in the elimination of water.

$$H_2N-\underset{\underset{R'}{|}}{CH}-\underset{\underset{O}{\parallel}}{C}-OH + H_2N-\underset{\underset{R''}{|}}{CH}-\underset{\underset{O}{\parallel}}{C}-OH \xrightarrow[H_2O]{} H_2N-\underset{\underset{R'}{|}}{CH}-\underset{\underset{O}{\parallel}}{C}-NH-\underset{\underset{R''}{|}}{CH}-\underset{\underset{O}{\parallel}}{C}-OH$$

Disulfide Bonds. The reaction between two cysteine residues, resulting in the formation of *cystine*, is shown below.

Not all proteins contain disulfide bonds. They are more prevalent in extracellular proteins than in intracellular proteins. Disulfide bonds may be either intrachain or interchain bonds. *Insulin* is a small polypeptide hormone having both intrachain and interchain disulfide bonds (Figure 2-5). Both polypeptide chains, A and B, are held together by interchain disulfide bonds, but the A chain also contains an intrachain disulfide bond.

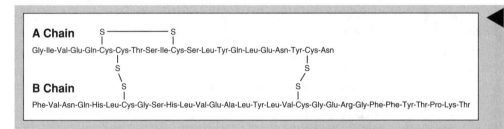

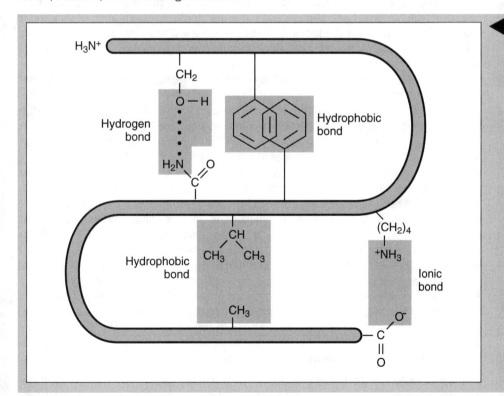

FIGURE 2-5
Structure of Human Insulin. The A and B polypeptide chains are linked by disulfide bonds, and the A chain has an intrachain disulfide bond. Insulin is synthesized as a single polypeptide and subsequently cleaved into two chains, releasing a peptide (the C peptide) that joins the end of the B chain with the beginning of the A chain.

Noncovalent Bonds and Interactions

The folding of proteins into a three-dimensional structure is stabilized by the formation of a *large number of weak noncovalent interactions* between the side chains of amino acids. These interactions include *hydrogen bonds, hydrophobic bonds,* and *ionic interactions* (Figure 2-6). The strength of the noncovalent bonds ranges from 0.6 kcal/mol to 7.0 kcal/mol. These interactions are all much weaker than the covalent bonds found in proteins, which are usually more than 50 kcal/mol. The overall significance of the noncovalent bonds, however, is in their large numbers.

FIGURE 2-6
Types of Noncovalent Bonds Found in Proteins. The tertiary and quaternary structures are stabilized by a large number of hydrogen, ionic, and hydrophobic bonds that are formed by interactions between different side chains.

Denaturation of Proteins

The denaturation of a protein is defined as the loss of its native conformation. The covalent bonds remain intact, but the noncovalent interactions that stabilize the three-dimensional structure are abolished. Conditions that disrupt noncovalent interactions include extremes of pH, exposure to heat, organic solvents, and detergents. Frequently denaturation results in decreased solubility, loss of catalytic activity, or a change in antigenic properties of the protein.

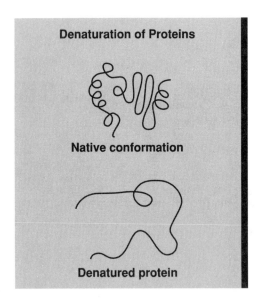

Denaturation of Proteins

Native conformation

Denatured protein

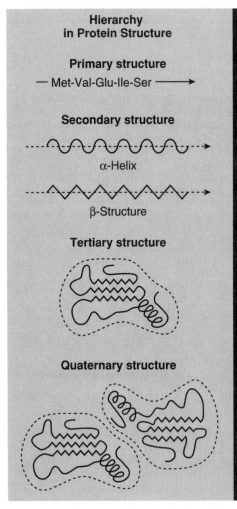

Hierarchy in Protein Structure

Primary structure

— Met-Val-Glu-Ile-Ser ——→

Secondary structure

α-Helix

β-Structure

Tertiary structure

Quaternary structure

Hydrogen Bonds That Stabilize Secondary Structure
The oxygen atom and the hydrogen atom come from different peptide bonds

$$\rangle C = O \cdots\cdots H - N \langle$$

Levels of Protein Structure

A hierarchy exists in protein structure that is described at four levels: primary, secondary, tertiary, and quaternary structures. These structural levels are distinguished from one another by the kinds of bonds and interactions that stabilize each level of structure. *Anfinsen's law* states that the secondary, tertiary, and quaternary structures of a protein are determined by the primary structure.

Primary Structure. The primary structure is defined as the *sequence* of amino acids that is linked together by *peptide bonds*. By convention, the amino acids are numbered from the N-terminal to the C-terminal residue. Two features of the primary structure have profound effects on higher orders of protein structure.

First, the linear *sequence of amino acids* dictates the types of interactions that can occur between side chains as the protein folds into higher orders of structure. Second, the peptide bonds that form the backbone of the protein profoundly influence the secondary structure. *The four atoms of the peptide bond (C, O, N, and H) are coplanar in nature*, and therefore, rotations are restricted to the bonds involving the α-carbon atoms (Figure 2-7). Additionally, the *carbonyl oxygen ($\rangle C = O$) and amide hydrogen ($\rangle N - H$) atoms of the peptide bond are at opposite corners of the plane*, a condition that maximizes the number of hydrogen bonds that can be formed between these atoms of the peptide bond. These properties of the peptide bond influence the types of secondary structures that can be formed in proteins.

Secondary Structure. The secondary structure of proteins is defined as repeating structures that can be formed by making permissible rotations in the polypeptide backbone. These repeating structures are stabilized by *hydrogen bonds* that are formed between the carbonyl oxygen atom of one peptide bond and the amide hydrogen atom of another. In many fibrous proteins, secondary structure is the highest order of structure observed. There are three major types of secondary structure found in proteins: α-helix, β-sheets, and β-bends.

α-Helical structures are stabilized by *intrachain hydrogen bonds* that are formed between the carbonyl oxygen of one peptide bond and the amide hydrogen of another peptide bond that is four amino acid residues downstream toward the carboxy end (Figure 2-8). Examples of proteins that are rich in α-helical structure are α-keratin, myosin, and fibrinogen. Almost all of the amino acids in α-keratin, the major protein in hair, skin, and nails, are found in an α-helix. The only amino acid that has not been found in the α-helix is proline. In globular proteins, *proline terminates the α-helical segments* of their structure.

Another secondary structural motif is the *β-sheet structure* that is stabilized by *interchain hydrogen bonds* formed between the carbonyl oxygen of a peptide bond in one chain and the amide hydrogen of a peptide bond in another chain. Parallel β-sheets are formed when the two chains are both aligned in the same direction from the amino to the carboxyl end. *Antiparallel β-sheets are formed* when the two chains have opposite polarities (Figure 2-9). The best known example of protein found in human tissues that contain the β-sheet structure is *amyloid*, a protein that accumulates in *amyloidosis* and *Alzheimer's disease*. Amyloid is highly enriched in antiparallel β-sheet structure.

In tightly folded globular proteins, the direction of the polypeptide chain is reversed by *β-bends*. A β-bend consists of four amino acid residues. The bend is stabilized by a *hydrogen bond* that is formed between the first carbonyl oxygen and the last amide hydrogen in the bend. Frequently, β-bends contain glycine, proline, or both.

Tertiary Structure. The tertiary structure of a protein refers to the overall three-dimensional arrangement of the polypeptide chain. It may contain segments of both α-helical and β-sheet structures that are folded into a more compact globular protein. The tertiary structure is stabilized by *hydrogen bonds, ionic bonds,* and *hydrophobic interactions* between amino acid side chains. The interacting side chains may come from amino acid residues that are far apart in the linear sequence but are close together in the three-dimensional structure because of compact folding patterns. The contribution of any one of these noncovalent interactions to the stability of the protein is small, but the total number of noncovalent interactions is large. In most globular proteins, the *hydrophobic interactions* make the most important contribution to the stability of the native conformation.

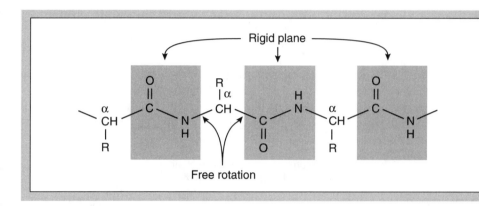

FIGURE 2-7
The Peptide Bond. *The four atoms of the peptide bond lie in a plane that is rigid, prohibiting rotations around the carbon–oxygen, carbon–nitrogen, and nitrogen–hydrogen bonds. The only rotations in the polypeptide backbone that are permissible are around the bonds that connect the α-carbon atoms to the carbon and nitrogen atoms of the peptide bonds.*

The *folding* of globular proteins into their native conformation begins while the polypeptide is still being synthesized. The protein is guided through the folding process by *chaperons*, a family of proteins that bind to hydrophobic patches and prevent premature aggregation into nonfunctional complexes. The protein is folded so that most of the hydrophilic (polar) side chains are located on the outside of the molecule, where they can interact with the aqueous medium, whereas the hydrophobic side chains are buried in the interior of the molecule, creating a structure similar to an "oil drop."

Globular proteins usually consist of several *domains*, each having its own characteristic three-dimensional structure and are usually associated with a *specific function*. Domains consist of α-helices, β-sheets, or a mixture of the two. The domains of a globular protein are separated from one another by stretches of polypeptide that lack regular secondary structure. Domains are encoded by an *exon* in the DNA, and a particular domain may be used in many different proteins that share a common functional property. The "zinc finger" is a domain that is found in many proteins that bind to DNA (Figure 2-10).

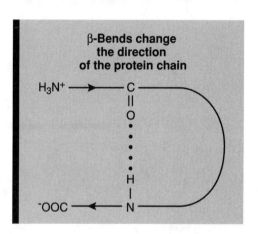

FIGURE 2-8
α-Helical Structure in Proteins. *The right-handed α-helix is the most common form of secondary structure found in proteins. There are 3.6 amino acid residues in each complete turn of the helix. Each carbonyl oxygen atom forms a hydrogen bond with the amide nitrogen atom four residues away in the linear sequence.*

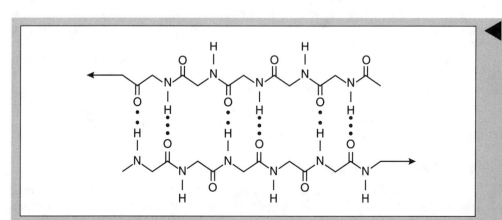

FIGURE 2-9
β-Sheet Structure in Proteins. *The arrows indicate the direction from the amino- to the carboxyl-terminus for two segments of protein that form antiparallel β-sheets. Hydrogen bonds are formed between the carbonyl oxygen atoms in one segment and the amide hydrogen atom in an adjacent segment.*

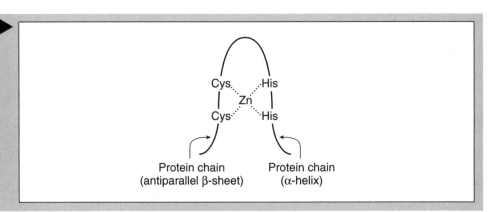

FIGURE 2-10 ▶

The Zinc Finger Domain of DNA-Binding Proteins. *Each zinc finger contains 30 amino acid residues, including 2 cysteine and 2 histidine residues that directly bind to the zinc atom (Zn). The finger contains two antiparallel β-strands and one α-helical strand of secondary structure. The cysteine residues are found in the antiparallel β-strands, and the two histidine residues are in the α-helical region.*

Quaternary Structure. Proteins that have more than one polypeptide chain (subunit) in their native conformation have a quaternary structure. Not all proteins have subunits. Quaternary structures are usually stabilized by hydrophobic, hydrogen, and ionic bonds.

ELECTROPHORESIS OF PROTEINS

One of the most powerful tools for separating mixtures of proteins is electrophoresis, a procedure that is used routinely in clinical laboratories. The basic principles and the clinical application of electrophoresis are briefly described in the following discussion.

Principles

Proteins are *polyelectrolytes*, having different amounts of charge at a particular pH, and when placed in an electric field, different proteins move at different rates. The rate of movement is determined by the *charge:size ratio* and is directly proportional to the charge and inversely proportional to the size of the protein. Since the charge is dependent on the pH, the electrophoretic mobility of a protein will also vary with the pH. At its pI, a protein has no net charge and will not move in an electric field; but at a *pH above the pI*, the protein will have a *net negative charge*, whereas at a *pH below the pI*, the protein will have a *net positive charge*.

Clinical Application

*The presence of α_1-fetoprotein in nonfetal serum is a marker for **liver carcinoma**.*

In a clinical laboratory, electrophoresis of serum proteins is usually carried out at pH 8.6. Most serum proteins with a pI between 4 and 8 have a net negative charge at pH 8.6. When placed in an electric field, they will migrate toward the positive electrode (anode). The electrophoretic mobility of serum proteins is shown in Figure 2-11.

Electrophoresis at pH 8.6 separates serum proteins into five major fractions. Except for albumin, which is pure, each of these fractions contains a complex mixture of proteins. Most of the serum proteins are synthesized in the liver with the notable exception of the γ-globulins, which are synthesized in the lymphocytes. Further separation of the proteins in each fraction can be achieved by techniques that are based on other physical or chemical properties.

Serum electrophoretic patterns provide *useful diagnostic information*. The patterns are not necessarily indicative of any one disease, but an increase or decrease in any one fraction may provide important clues about the disorder. The appearance of a high, narrow peak of protein in the γ-globulin region is consistent with *multiple myeloma*, whereas a low albumin level, combined with an elevation in the α_2-globulins and a decrease in the γ-globulins, is consistent with *kidney disease*.

Variations on the Theme of Electrophoresis

Many variations of protein electrophoresis can be made that alter either the type of *inert support* (polyacrylamide gels, agarose gels, or cellulose acetate strips), the *buffer condi-*

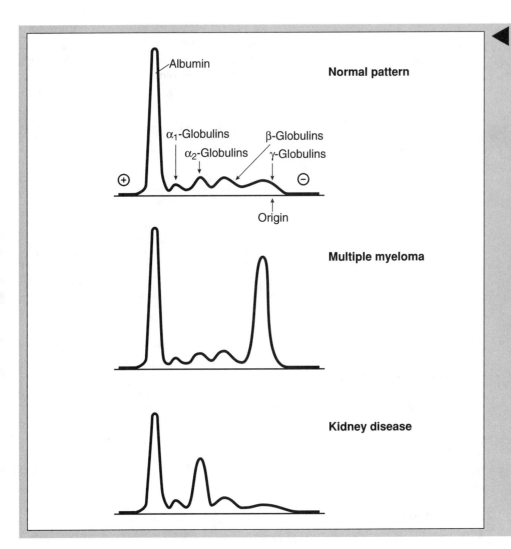

◄ FIGURE 2-11
Electrophoresis of Serum Proteins. A sample of normal serum was applied to a strip of cellulose acetate at the point indicated as the origin in the top figure. Following electrophoresis, the strip was stained for protein, and the amount of protein in each peak was quantitated by densitometry. The most rapidly moving peak is albumin, which is followed by the α_1-globulins, the α_2-globulins, the β-globulins, and the γ-globulins. The center figure shows an electrophoretic pattern for serum taken from a patient with multiple myeloma. The most significant change is the presence of a large peak of protein in the γ-globulin region. The serum in the lower figure was obtained from a patient with kidney disease. Albumin is decreased, the α_2-globulins are increased, and the γ-globulins are decreased.

tions (denaturing or nondenaturing conditions), or the *detection method* (protein stain, enzyme activity, or immunochemical detection). The choice of conditions depends on the purpose of the analysis. The two most useful variations are discussed briefly below.

Sodium Dodecyl Sulfate–Polyacrylamide Gel Electrophoresis (SDS-PAGE). This type of electrophoresis uses polyacrylamide gels as an inert support and is performed in the presence of SDS, a detergent that denatures proteins. SDS is a negatively charged detergent that coats the protein with a *uniform negative charge*. The intrinsic charge on the protein is swamped out by the large negative charge of the detergent. Consequently, the *electrophoretic mobility* of the protein-SDS complex *is dependent only on the mass of the protein*. This technique can be used to determine the minimum molecular weight of a protein.

Western Blots. Western blots can be used to *detect a very small amount of a specific protein in a complex mixture of proteins*. The proteins are separated from one another by SDS-PAGE, as described above. The ability to detect one specific protein in the complex mixture depends on the use of a *radiolabeled antibody* that only binds to the protein of interest.

FUNCTIONS OF SELECTED PLASMA PROTEINS

Centrifugation of blood removes the cellular components, leaving a supernatant that is known as *plasma*. If blood is allowed to clot prior to centrifugation, the clotting proteins are also removed, resulting in a supernatant known as *serum*. Electrophoretic patterns of plasma show a sharp peak of protein that is not seen in serum. Located between the β-globulins and the γ-globulins, this peak consists of fibrinogen and other clotting factors.

The protein concentration of normal plasma is 6–8 g/dL with albumin comprising more than 50% of the total protein. The percentage of protein found in each of the major electrophoretic classes, along with one or more specific proteins in each class, is summarized in Table 2-1.

TABLE 2-1 ▶
Major Classes of Plasma Proteins

Class	Total Protein (%)	Selected Proteins
Albumin	55	Albumin (essentially pure)
α_1-Globulins	5	α_1-Antitrypsin and α_1-fetoprotein
α_2-Globulins	9	Ceruloplasmin and haptoglobulin
β-Globulins	13	Transferrin and hemopexin
ϕ-Proteins	7	Fibrinogen and clotting factors
γ-Globulins	11	Immunoglobulins G, M, and A

Albumin

Albumin is the major serum protein, having a concentration of 3–5 g/dL. Two major functions are associated with albumin. It is important in *regulating the fluid balance between plasma and the interstitial fluid*. The distribution of fluid between these compartments depends on a balance between the hydrostatic pressure and the osmotic pressure of the blood. Albumin is responsible for about 75% of the osmotic pressure of the blood. Therefore, a decrease in serum albumin can result in the accumulation of water in the interstitial space, a condition known as *edema*. A second important function of albumin is to bind and *transport many small hydrophobic molecules*, including fatty acids, steroid and thyroid hormones, bilirubin, and tryptophan. Additionally, about 50% of the total Ca^{2+} in plasma is bound to albumin.

α_1-Antitrypsin

α_1-Antitrypsin is a glycoprotein that normally accounts for 70%–90% of the protein found in the α_1-globulin fraction. Its function is to *inhibit elastase*, an enzyme that is released from neutrophils in lung tissue. Elastase degrades *elastin*, the major connective tissue protein that gives the lung its elasticity. In the normal lung, the destructive power of elastase is kept in check by α_1-antitrypsin.

A genetic deficiency in α_1-antitrypsin can lead to *emphysema*, an obstructive lung disease. In many cases of α_1-antitrypsin deficiency, large inclusion bodies containing α_1-antitrypsin are found in the liver. The ability of this protein to inhibit elastase is normal, but it has a strong tendency to aggregate, thereby decreasing the rate of secretion into the plasma. Analysis of the amino acid sequence of the α_1-antitrypsin that accumulates in the liver of individuals with serum α_1-antitrypsin deficiency shows a single amino acid difference compared to normal α_1-antitrypsin. Normal α_1-antitrypsin has a glutamic acid residue at position 342 in its amino acid sequence, whereas the protein with impaired secretory properties has a lysine residue in this position.

Haptoglobulin and Hemopexin

Both of the serum proteins, haptoglobulin and hemopexin, play important roles in the *conservation of iron* by preventing its loss in the urine. Much of the extracellular iron in the body is found in hemoglobin where it is a part of the heme molecule. Intravascular hemolysis of red blood cells (RBCs) releases hemoglobin. *Haptoglobulin binds free hemoglobin*, whereas *hemopexin binds free heme*. Both the haptoglobulin–hemoglobin complex and the hemopexin–heme complex are too large to be filtered by the kidney. Therefore, they are taken up by phagocytic cells, and the iron can be recycled. In cases of hemolytic anemia, the level of haptoglobulin is decreased because the haptoglobulin–hemoglobin complex is degraded much more rapidly than free haptoglobulin. The serum level of hemopexin is elevated in cases of iron deficiency.

Cigarette Smoke and Lung Disease
Cigarette smoke: (1) oxidizes a specific methionine residue in α_1-antitrypsin, and the oxidized form of the protein can no longer inhibit elastase; and (2) increases the number of neutrophils in the lung and, therefore, increases the amount of elastase.

Wilson's Disease
This is a disease of copper storage, resulting from a genetic deficiency in ceruloplasmin, a copper transport protein that migrates with the α_2-globulins during serum electrophoresis. Copper accumulates in various tissues, including the iris of the eye where it is responsible for the characteristic Kayser-Fleischer rings.

RESOLUTION OF CLINICAL CASE

The problem that brought the 16-year-old patient described at the beginning of the chapter to the hospital was pneumonia, which was treated with an antibiotic. The family history of lung disease, however, suggested an additional problem, a possible deficiency in α_1-antitrypsin. A deficiency in this protein results in an imbalance in the ratio of elastase to α_1-antitrypsin, thereby allowing elastase to degrade elastin in the alveolar walls of the lung. Electrophoretic analysis of serum from this patient showed a marked decrease in the amount of protein found in the α_1-globulin fraction. This finding is consistent with a deficiency in α_1-antitrypsin, since as much as 90% of the α_1-globulin fraction is normally contributed by α_1-antitrypsin. Several lines of evidence suggested that this patients' enlarged liver could be attributed to the accumulation of α_1-antitrypsin. Electron micrographs of liver tissue taken by needle biopsy showed the accumulation of a glycoprotein that reacted with an antibody to α_1-antitrypsin. Extraction of this protein from the tissue sample confirmed that it was as effective as normal α_1-antitrypsin in inhibiting elastase. Therefore, the patient was able to synthesize active α_1-antitrypsin, but the secretion into the plasma was impaired. The decreased electrophoretic mobility of the α_1-globulin fraction in this patient suggests a decrease in the negative charge on the protein. Although structural analysis on the protein was not available for this patient, the amino acid sequence of α_1-antitrypsin found in the liver of several other patients who died from emphysema has been determined. In these patients, the amino acid at position 342 had been changed from glutamic acid to lysine, resulting in a decreased negative charge.

The most important therapy for individuals with α_1-antitrypsin deficiency is preventing lung destruction, primarily by avoiding smoking. Smoking enhances the oxidation and inactivation of α_1-antitrypsin in the lung. Smokers have a considerably higher rate of lung destruction and a poorer survival rate than nonsmokers with the deficiency. Vitamin E is commonly given to maintain maximal antioxidant activity in the lung tissue.

REVIEW QUESTIONS

Directions: The groups of questions below consist of lettered choices followed by several numbered items. For each numbered item, select the appropriate lettered option with which it is most closely associated. Each lettered option may be used once, more than once, or not at all.

Questions 1–5

For each of the following descriptions, select the amino acid with which it is most closely associated.

(A) Serine

(B) Isoleucine

(C) Phenylalanine

(D) Histidine

(E) Glutamine

(F) Cysteine

(G) Aspartic acid

1. The aliphatic amino acid most likely to be buried inside a globular protein

2. The amino acid that contributes most to the buffering properties of proteins

3. The amino acid that contributes most to the negative charge on a protein

4. The amino acid most likely to become phosphorylated in regulatory proteins

5. The amino acid that forms covalent crosslinks in proteins

Questions 6–9

For each of the following descriptions, select the type of bonds with which it is most closely associated.

(A) Hydrogen bonds

(B) Ionic bonds

(C) Peptide bonds

(D) Hydrophobic bonds

(E) Disulfide bonds

6. Stabilization of the polypeptide backbone

7. Stabilization of α-helix

8. Stabilization of tertiary structure

9. Stabilization of β-sheet

Questions 10–15

For each of the following clinical conditions, select the protein with which it is most closely associated.

   (A) Albumin

   (B) Hemopexin

   (C) α-Fetoprotein

   (D) Ceruloplasmin

   (E) Amyloid

   (F) α_1-Antitrypsin

   (G) γ-Globulin

   (H) Haptoglobulin

10. Liver carcinoma

11. Multiple myeloma

12. Wilson's disease

13. Edema

14. Hemolytic anemia

15. Alzheimer's disease

ANSWERS AND EXPLANATIONS

1–5. The answers are: 1-B, 2-D, 3-G, 4-A, 5-F. Hydrophobic amino acids tend to be buried inside globular proteins. Only two hydrophobic amino acids are listed, isoleucine and phenylalanine, but only isoleucine is an aliphatic amino acid. Histidine contributes most to the buffering properties of proteins because the pK_a of the side chain is closest to the physiologic pH. Negative charge on proteins comes from the side chain carboxyl groups of aspartic and glutamic acids. The hydroxyl group of serine is often phosphorylated in regulatory proteins. The other hydroxylated amino acids, threonine and tyrosine, can also be phosphorylated. Disulfide bonds, created by the reaction of two cysteine side chains, form covalent crosslinks in proteins.

6–9. The answers are: 6-C, 7-A, 8-D, 9-A. The polypeptide backbone is formed by a series of peptide bonds that join amino acids together in a linear chain. All types of secondary structure, including α-helix, β-sheet, and β-bends are stabilized by hydrogen bonds. Tertiary structure of proteins is stabilized by a combination of hydrogen bonds, ionic bonds, and hydrophobic bonds. The most important contribution, however, comes from hydrophobic bonds that create a structure for globular proteins resembling an oil drop. Many of the side chains that form hydrogen bonds and ionic bonds are found on the surface of the protein where they interact with the aqueous medium.

10–15. The answers are: 10-C, 11-G, 12-D, 13-A, 14-H, 15-E. The presence of α-feto-protein in nonfetal serum is closely associated with primary carcinoma of the liver. However, during pregnancy, this protein is synthesized by the fetal liver, and small amounts gain access to the maternal circulation. Multiple myeloma is characterized by the presence of high concentrations of γ-globulins in the serum. A deficiency in ceruloplasmin results in Wilson's disease, a disease of copper storage and accumulation in many tissues. Edema can result from a decrease in the concentration of serum albumin. The distribution of water between the plasma and interstitial space is regulated, in part, by the osmotic pressure of the plasma. The major contributor to the osmotic pressure of the plasma is albumin. A decrease in albumin concentration results in a decrease in the osmotic pressure of the blood, a condition that allows fluid to accumulate in the interstitial space. In hemolytic anemia, the concentration of haptoglobulin in serum is decreased. Hemoglobin that is released by lysis of RBCs binds to haptoglobulin; and the haptoglobulin–hemoglobin complex is degraded much more rapidly than free haptoglobulin, thereby decreasing the concentration in serum. Amyloid, a fibrous protein enriched in antiparallel β-sheet structure, accumulates in the brain of patients with Alzheimer's disease.

REFERENCES

1. Cox DW: α_1-Antitrypsin deficiency. In *Metabolic and Molecular Bases of Inherited Disease*, 7th ed. Edited by Scriver CR, Beaudet AL, Sly WS, et al. New York, NY: McGraw-Hill, 1995, pp 4125–4191.

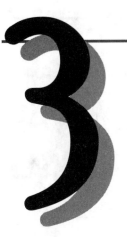

ENZYMES: THE CATALYTIC AGENTS OF METABOLISM

CHAPTER OUTLINE

INTRODUCTION OF CLINICAL CASE

A 40-year-old man was admitted to the hospital for evaluation of chest pain. He had a history of diabetes and 2 years earlier had been diagnosed with atherosclerotic heart disease with angina. A similar episode of chest pain 5 months earlier had been diagnosed as myocardial infarction. However, 3 months ago, myocardial infarction had been ruled out. At the time of the current admission, electrocardiograms (ECGs) were equivocal. Analysis of serum enzyme levels were determined at the time of admission and over the next 3 days. These analyses included total serum creatine kinase (CK) and lactate dehydrogenase (LDH) activity. Separation of CK and LDH isozymes was carried out by serum electrophoresis to determine the percentage of CK activity that was due to the MB isozyme, as well as the percentage of LDH activity that was due to the LDH_1 isozyme. A summary of the enzyme analyses are shown in Table 3-1. The time of admission is set at 0 hours. The patient was released from the hospital a week after admission with a list of foods and physical activities to avoid, and he was scheduled to return for a checkup 3 weeks later.

TABLE 3-1 ▶

Summary of Enzyme Analyses of Creatine Kinase (CK) and Lactate Dehydrogenase (LDH)

	Total CK (IU/L)	% MB	Total LDH (IU/L)	% LDH$_1$
0 hours	242	5.6	188	15
8 hours	361	5.1	200	17
12 hours	193	3.2	287	42
24 hours	151	2.0	365	59
48 hours	147	1.7	348	56
60 hours	143	1.7	216	37

INTRODUCTION

Enzymes are a special class of proteins that serve as catalysts in all living cells. They increase the rate of chemical reactions without changing the equilibrium of the reaction. Under the mild conditions of pH and temperature that exist in cells, most reactions would not proceed at rates sufficient for survival without the assistance of enzymes. Enzymes differ from other catalysts in three major ways. (1) They are specific for the reaction they catalyze. In general, each enzyme catalyzes a different reaction. (2) They have greater catalytic power than other catalysts and are typically able to transform 10^3 to 10^4 molecules of reactant to product per second. (3) Their catalytic action can be regulated to ensure that the rate at which a product is formed is not in excess of the amount needed. Many enzymes have a characteristic organ, tissue, cellular, and subcellular localization, a property that has been used as a diagnostic tool. The structure of enzymes varies in complexity, with some enzymes consisting of a protein subunit while others are multi-subunit complexes requiring additional cofactors. All enzymes can be classified into six groups based on the type of reaction that is catalyzed (Table 3-2). The reactant in an enzyme-catalyzed reaction is referred to as the substrate.

TABLE 3-2 ▶

The Six Classes of Enzymes

Class	Type of Reaction Catalyzed
Oxidoreductases	Oxidation and reduction reactions that transfer electrons from one compound to another
Transferases	Transfer of a functional group (i.e., amino, acyl, phosphate, methyl) from a donor molecule to an acceptor molecule
Hydrolases	Cleavage of bonds between carbon and some other atom by the addition of water across the bond
Lyases	Nonhydrolytic cleavage of C—C, C—S, and some C—N bonds by the addition of a group to a double bond
Isomerases	Interconversion of isomers by the transfer of a group from one position to another within the same molecule
Ligases	Formation of C—O, C—S, C—C, and C—N bonds by joining two molecules together in reactions requiring energy, which is usually supplied by adenosine triphosphate hydrolysis

THE ACTIVE SITE

An enzyme-catalyzed reaction is initiated when the substrate binds to a specialized region of the enzyme known as the active site. The active site is a three-dimensional cleft or crevice that is created by the side chains of several amino acids. These amino acids come from different regions in the linear sequence of the enzyme, but the enzyme is folded in such a way that their side chains are close at the active site. The amino acid residues that form the active site can be classified into two functional groups, binding residues and catalytic residues.

Binding Residues. The binding residues recognize and bind the correct substrate, a property known as *specificity*. In general, enzymes are specific for a single substrate, and they catalyze reactions that form a specific product.

Catalytic Residues. The catalytic residues create a chemical environment that enhances the reaction rate, a property known as *catalysis*. Enzymes can increase the rate of chemical reactions by a factor ranging from 10^3- to 10^8-fold over the rate of the uncatalyzed reaction.

> **Lead** is a potent enzyme inhibitor, particularly of enzymes involved in heme synthesis. Lead binds to thiol groups at the active site of these enzymes and can lead to anemia.

ENZYME SPECIFICITY

Substrates are bound to enzymes through multiple noncovalent interactions between the binding residues at the active site and chemical groups on the substrate. Two models for substrate binding have evolved to explain the high degree of specificity that an enzyme has for its substrate, the template model and the induced-fit model.

Template Model

In the template model, the active site has a rigid structure that is complementary to that of the substrate (Figure 3-1). This model is also known as the *lock-and-key model*, in which the substrate fits into the active site in much the same way that a key fits into a lock. This model has been useful in understanding how some enzymes will bind one substrate but will not bind another compound with an almost identical structure. For example, most enzymes in carbohydrate metabolism will bind the D-isomer of hexoses but will not bind the corresponding L-isomer, which differs only in the configuration around a single carbon atom.

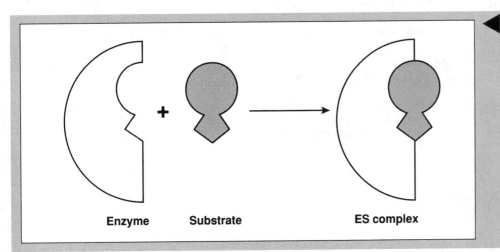

Enzyme   Substrate   ES complex

◀ *FIGURE 3-1*
Template Model of Enzyme Specificity.
The shape of the enzyme active site is rigid and complementary to the shape of the substrate. The substrate (S) is anchored to the enzyme (E) through multiple noncovalent interactions.

Induced-Fit Model

In the induced-fit model, the active site is more flexible than in the template model, and its structure changes when the substrate binds (Figure 3-2). This model is also known as the *hand-in-glove model*. When the substrate binds to the active site, a conformational change is induced that leads to an exact fit between the enzyme and the substrate. These structural changes are analogous to the way a glove takes on the shape of the hand. This model is believed to describe more accurately the specificity of substrate binding than does the template model. A key feature of the induced-fit model is the flexibility of the active site, that is, its ability to change shape in response to the binding of some molecule.

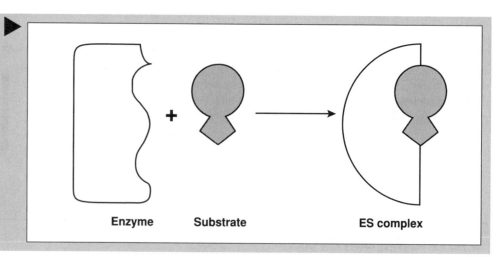

FIGURE 3-2 ▶

Induced-Fit Model of Enzyme Specificity. *The shape of the enzyme active site is flexible and conforms to the shape of the substrate after binding. The interaction of substrate (S) with enzyme (E) induces a conformational change in the enzyme.*

ENZYME CATALYSIS

Enzymes increase the rate of a reaction by decreasing the *activation energy* for the reaction (Figure 3-3). As a reactant is converted to a product, a series of intermediates are formed that have structures resembling both the reactant and product. The intermediate with the highest energy content is defined as the *transition state*. It is also the intermediate that most resembles both the reactant and the product. The difference in the energy content of the initial reactant and the transition state is defined as the activation energy (ΔG^*) of the reaction. The ΔG^* forms a barrier that all reactants must cross to be converted to products. The magnitude of ΔG^* determines how many molecules of reactant will cross the energy barrier and be converted to a product during a given period of time. The larger the ΔG^*, the fewer the number of molecules that will be able to achieve an energy state equal to that of the transition state. Therefore, the *rate of a reaction is inversely related to the ΔG^** of the reaction. Enzymes function as catalysts by decreasing the magnitude of ΔG^*. This property can also be described as a stabilization of the transition state. Enzymes affect the rate of the forward and reverse reactions equally; therefore, they have no effect on the equilibrium of the reaction.

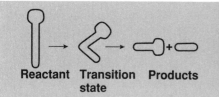

Reactant   Transition   Products
state

FIGURE 3-3 ▶

Energy Diagram of a Catalyzed and Uncatalyzed Reaction. *The rate of a chemical reaction is inversely related to the free energy of activation (ΔG^*). A catalyst decreases the ΔG^*. The difference in free energy between reactant and product (ΔG) is unchanged by a catalyst. The magnitude of ΔG is related to the equilibrium constant for the reaction.*

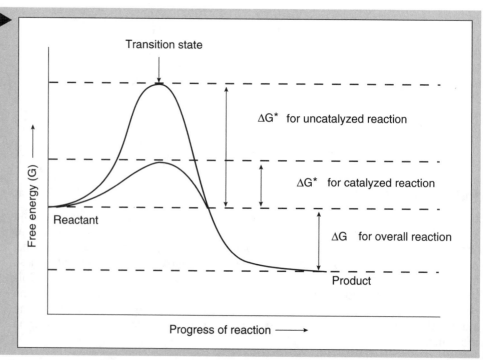

The ability of an enzyme to accelerate a reaction is due to catalytic residues in the active site. These amino acid residues have functional groups in their side chains that participate in the conversion of substrate to product. There are four major factors that contribute to the ability of an enzyme to increase the rate of a reaction: (1) proximity and orientation effects, (2) substrate strain, (3) acid and base catalysis, and (4) covalent catalysis.

Proximity and Orientation. The binding of substrate by the enzyme increases the "effective concentration" of the substrate by removing it from the solution and placing it near the catalytic groups in the active site. The proximity of the substrate and catalytic residues increases the probability of overcoming the energy barrier posed by the transition state. The binding of substrate induces a conformational change that orients the substrate with respect to the catalytic residues in the active site.

Substrate Strain. The conformational change that occurs when the substrate binds to the enzyme results in a distortion of bond lengths and angles. The bound substrate has a higher energy content than the unbound substrate, and its structure resembles that of the transition state. The overall effect of inducing strain in the substrate is one that achieves an energy level closer to that of the transition state.

General Acid–Base Catalysis. Some of the catalytic residues found in the active site can participate in general acid–base catalysis by donating and accepting protons during the catalytic cycle. Amino acid residues having side chains that can participate in catalysis are shown in Table 3-3. Each of these side chains can act as either a conjugate acid or a conjugate base.

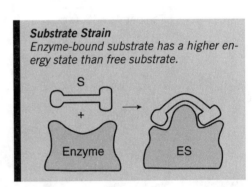

Substrate Strain
Enzyme-bound substrate has a higher energy state than free substrate.

◀ **TABLE 3-3**
Amino Acid Side Chains That Commonly Participate in Enzyme Catalysis

General Acid–Base Catalysis	Conjugate Acid	Conjugate Base
Histidine	$R\text{-Imidazole-N}^+H$	$R\text{-Imidazole-N}$
Aspartic acid	$R\text{-COOH}$	$R\text{-COO}^-$
Glutamic acid	$R\text{-COOH}$	$R\text{-COO}^-$
Lysine	$R\text{-N}^+H_3$	$R\text{-NH}_2$

Covalent Catalysis	Nucleophilic Group	
Histidine	Imidazole-N	
Serine	$R\text{-OH}$	
Cysteine	$R\text{-SH}$	

Covalent Catalysis. Some catalytic residues have nucleophilic groups that can assist in cleavage of covalent bonds. Typically, the nucleophilic group attacks an electron-deficient center in the substrate. In the first part of a catalytic cycle, a portion of the substrate becomes transiently and covalently bound to the enzyme, while the other portion of the substrate is released into solution. In the second part of the cycle, the group that is attached to the enzyme is released. Examples of *nucleophilic groups* found in enzymes are amino acid side chains having oxygen, sulfur, or nitrogen atoms with unshared pairs of electrons (see Table 3-3).

FACTORS THAT AFFECT THE RATE OF ENZYME-CATALYZED REACTIONS

Enzyme kinetics is the study of the rate (velocity) of enzyme-catalyzed reactions. Since enzymes act as catalysts, this property is also referred to as *enzyme activity*. There are a number of factors that influence enzyme activity including temperature, pH, and the concentration of enzyme.

Temperature. The velocity of all chemical reactions increases with temperature. The fold increase in velocity that occurs with an increase of 10°C is defined as the *temperature coefficient* (Q_{10}) of the reaction. For many biologic processes, including most enzyme-

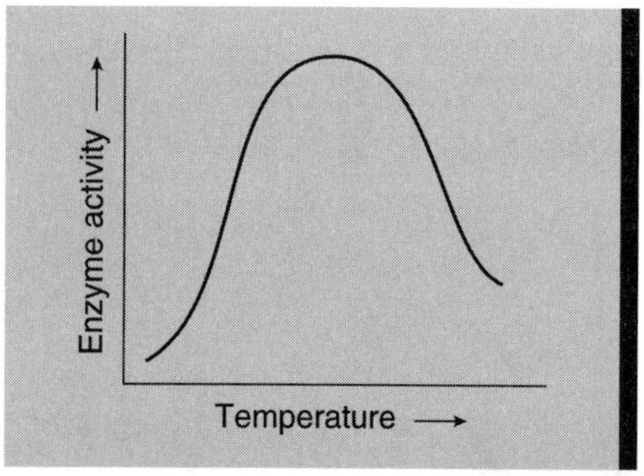

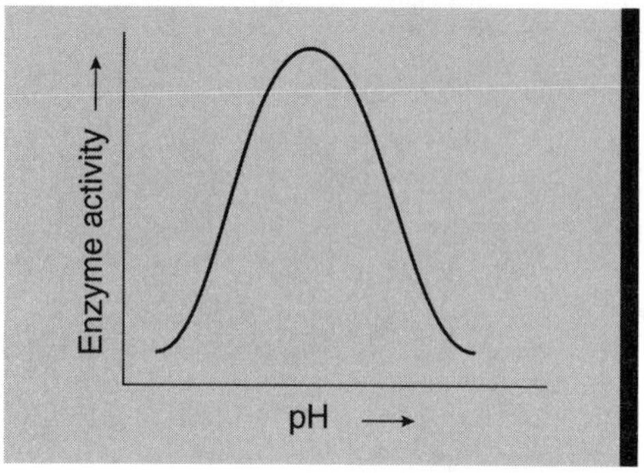

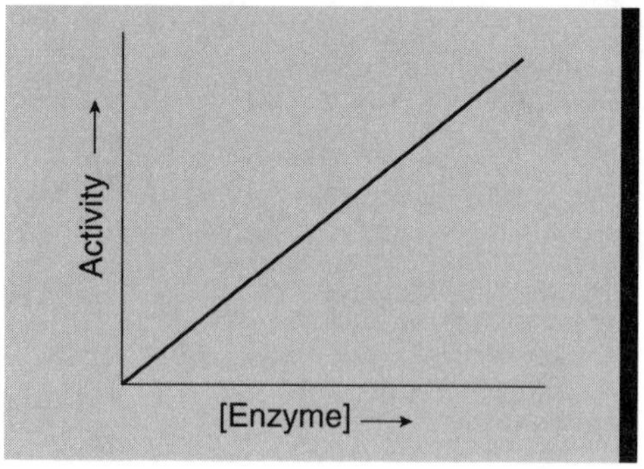

catalyzed reactions, the Q_{10} is approximately 2. Thus, the rate of enzyme-catalyzed reactions doubles for every 10°C increase in temperature until denaturation begins, and then the rate begins to decline. All enzyme-catalyzed reactions have an optimal temperature (frequently between 30°C and 40°C) at which the maximal rate of product formation occurs.

pH. The effect of pH on the activity of most enzyme-catalyzed reactions is described by a bell-shaped curve that shows an optimal velocity between 5 and 9. The shape of the curve is usually determined by changes in the ionization state of catalytic residues in the active site. This effect is illustrated by the following equation, where X—H and Y—H represent two functional groups in the active site that can exist in different ionic forms, depending on the pH.

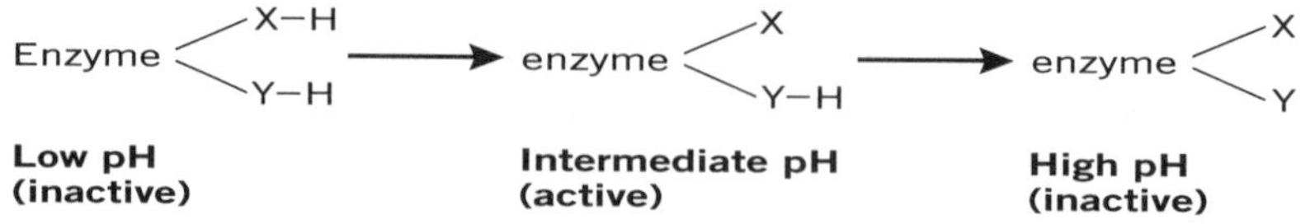

The three forms of enzyme in the equation above represent the ionic forms that predominate at low pH (*left*), intermediate pH (*middle*), and high pH (*right*). A pH-activity profile that first increases and then decreases indicates that the active form of the enzyme has one ionizing group that has lost a proton and another that retains its proton.

Enzyme Concentration. The velocity of a reaction is directly proportional to the amount of enzyme present, as long as the amount of substrate is not limiting. The substrate must be present at a concentration sufficient to ensure that all of the enzyme molecules have substrate bound to their active sites.

RELATIONSHIP BETWEEN VELOCITY AND SUBSTRATE CONCENTRATION

Enzyme-catalyzed reactions occur in two stages, as shown in the following equation. First, the substrate (S) binds to the enzyme (E), forming a complex (ES) that is stabilized by multiple noncovalent interactions. The enzyme-bound substrate is then transformed to a product (P) that dissociates from the enzyme. The rate constants k_1 and k_2 describe the formation and dissociation of the ES complex, while k_3 and k_4 describe the second phase of the reaction.

$$E + S \underset{k_2}{\overset{k_1}{\rightleftharpoons}} ES \underset{k_4}{\overset{k_3}{\rightleftharpoons}} E + P$$

The effect of substrate concentration on the reaction rate is shown in Figure 3-4. This curve has the shape of a rectangular hyperbola. At very low concentrations of substrate, the rate is directly proportional to the substrate concentration, a condition known as *first-order kinetics*. At high concentrations of substrate, the rate becomes essentially independent of substrate concentration, a condition known as *zero-order kinetics*.

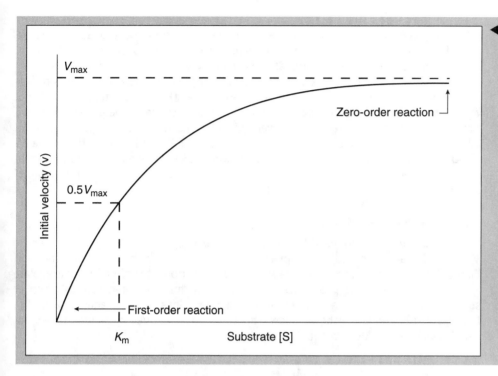

FIGURE 3-4
Effect of Substrate Concentration on the Initial Velocity of an Enzyme-Catalyzed Reaction. At any point on the curve, the rate is related to the amount of the enzyme-substrate (ES) complex. At low substrate concentration, the velocity is directly proportional to the concentration (obeys first-order kinetics). At high substrate concentration, the velocity is essentially independent of substrate concentration (zero-order kinetics). The K_m is defined as the concentration of substrate that results in half-maximum velocity and the concentration where half of the enzyme exists as the ES complex.

Michaelis-Menten Equation

The relationship between reaction rate and substrate concentration in Figure 3-4 is described mathematically by the Michaelis-Menten equation:

$$v = \frac{V_{max}[S]}{K_m + [S]}$$

In this equation, the maximum velocity (V_{max}) is observed when all active sites on the enzyme are filled with substrate. Under these conditions $[E_{total}] = [ES]$. The Michaelis constant (K_m) can be defined as the substrate concentration that results in half-maximum velocity.

Significance of V_{max} and K_m

The Michaelis-Menten equation defines two kinetic parameters that are related to intrinsic properties of the enzyme. Every enzyme has a characteristic V_{max} and K_m.

V_{max}. The V_{max} of a reaction is an index of the catalytic efficiency of an enzyme. The V_{max} is defined as the rate that occurs when all of the active sites are filled with substrate; therefore, at a saturating concentration of substrate, the value of V_{max} is directly proportional to the enzyme concentration. V_{max} is sensitive to changes in pH, temperature, and ionic strength. The units for V_{max} are always rate units.

K_m. The K_m of an enzyme is a measure of the affinity of the enzyme for its substrate. It can be defined as the concentration of substrate that is required to achieve half-maximum velocity. Therefore, a low K_m indicates a high affinity for the substrate, whereas a high K_m indicates a low affinity. The K_m is sensitive to changes in pH, temperature, and ionic strength. The units for K_m are always concentration units.

Assumptions Underlying the Michaelis-Menten Equation

The derivation of the Michaelis-Menten equation is based on four assumptions. Therefore, the validity of K_m and V_{max} measurements depends on whether the assumptions are valid under the conditions used for the kinetic measurements. The four assumptions are: (1) The substrate concentration is very large relative to the enzyme concentration. Under these conditions the formation of ES does not significantly alter the concentration of substrate. (2) At the beginning of the reaction, the concentration of product is insignificant. Therefore, if initial velocity measurements are made, the concentration of product is essentially zero, and the reaction rate described by k_4 can be ignored. (3) The rate at which ES is transformed into E + P is the rate-limiting (slowest) step in the reaction. This assumption can be expressed mathematically as $v = k_3$ [ES]. This rate equation is not very useful because it is difficult and, in some cases impossible, to measure the concentration of the ES complex. It does, however, define V_{max} as the rate that occurs when all of the enzyme has substrate bound to it or when $[E_{total}] = [ES]$. (4) The formation of the ES complex is rapid and reversible, and the rate at which ES is formed is equal to the rate at which ES disappears. This allows the concentration of ES to be expressed in terms of parameters that can be easily measured.

Lineweaver-Burk Plots

Lineweaver-Burk plots are used to obtain values for V_{max} and K_m. Rough estimates for V_{max} and K_m can be extrapolated from a substrate saturation curve such as that shown in Figure 3-4. However, these values are subject to large errors: it is difficult to extrapolate an accurate value for V_{max} because it occurs at an infinitely large concentration of substrate. A more accurate method of determining values for V_{max} and K_m uses the Lineweaver-Burk equation shown below. This equation is obtained by taking the reciprocal of the Michaelis-Menten equation.

$$\frac{1}{v} = \frac{K_m}{V_{max}} \cdot \frac{1}{[S]} + \frac{1}{V_{max}}$$

When $1/v$ is plotted against $1/[S]$, a straight line is obtained (Figure 3-5). Inspection of the equation shows that the slope of the line is equal to K_m/V_{max}. The point at which the line intersects the y-axis is numerically equal to $1/V_{max}$, and the point at which the line intersects the x-axis is numerically equal to $-1/K_m$. Therefore, the values of K_m and V_{max} can be readily calculated from the values of these two intercepts.

FIGURE 3-5 ▶
Lineweaver-Burk Double Reciprocal Plot. A plot of 1/v versus 1/[S] for an enzyme-catalyzed reaction gives a straight line with a slope equal to K_m/V_{max}. The values of K_m and V_{max} can be calculated from the points at which the line intersects the x-axis and y-axis, respectively. v = initial velocity; [S] = the substrate concentration.

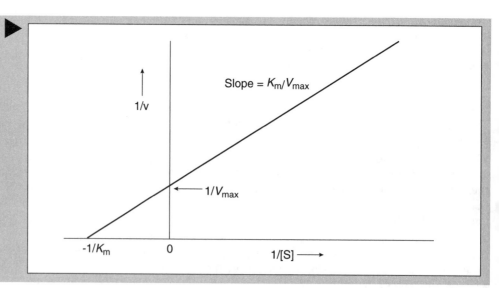

INHIBITION OF ENZYME-CATALYZED REACTIONS

Many compounds bind to enzymes and decrease their catalytic activity. The therapeutic action of many drugs is based on the principles of enzyme inhibition. Inhibitors can produce either reversible or irreversible effects on the catalytic activity of an enzyme.

Reversible Inhibitors

Compounds that reversibly inhibit enzymes can be classified in two major categories, competitive and noncompetitive inhibitors.

Competitive Inhibitors. Competitive inhibitors are structural analogues of the substrate and compete with the substrate for the same binding site on the enzyme. Therefore, the inhibitor and substrate cannot be bound to the enzyme at the same time. Since both compounds compete for the same site, the effects of a competitive inhibitor can be reversed by increasing the substrate to a concentration sufficiently high to occupy all of the binding sites. The effect of a competitive inhibitor on the kinetic parameters is illustrated in Figure 3-6. The V_{max} is unchanged by a competitive inhibitor. However, the apparent K_m (K_{app}) for the substrate is increased, since a higher concentration of substrate is required to achieve half-maximum velocity. The K_{app} is equal to K_m (1 + [I]/K_i), where I is the concentration of the inhibitor and K_i is the dissociation constant of the EI complex.

> *Ethanol is used to treat toxicity related to ingestion of wood alcohol (methanol). Methanol itself is not toxic, but it is metabolized to formaldehyde, which is very toxic and can lead to blindness and severe acidosis. Ethanol slows down the metabolism of methanol by acting as a competitive inhibitor.*

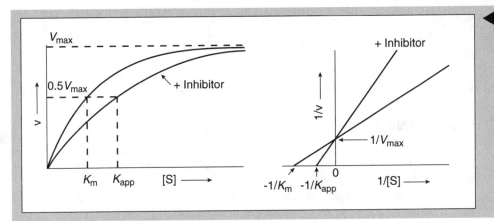

FIGURE 3-6
Effect of a Competitive Inhibitor on the Substrate Saturation Curve and the Lineweaver-Burk Plot. The substrate saturation curve is shown on the left and the Lineweaver-Burk plot on the right. The concentration required to give half-maximum velocity in the absence of the inhibitor is the K_m and in the presence of the inhibitor is K_{app}. K_{app} is equal to K_m (1 + I/K_i), where I is the concentration of the inhibitor and K_i is the dissociation constant for the enzyme inhibitor (EI) complex.

Noncompetitive Inhibitors. Structurally unrelated to the substrate, noncompetitive inhibitors bind to a site that is independent of the substrate binding site. Therefore, both the inhibitor and the substrate can bind to the enzyme at the same time. The effect of a noncompetitive inhibitor cannot be reversed by increasing the concentration of substrate. Since the binding sites for substrate and inhibitor are independent, a noncompetitive inhibitor has no effect on the K_m for the substrate. However, the binding of the inhibitor results in a decreased V_{max} (Figure 3-7). The binding of the inhibitor alters the conformation of the catalytic residues in the active site but has no significant effect on the binding residues.

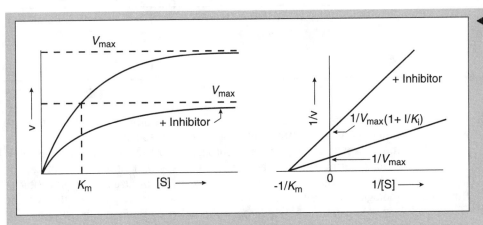

FIGURE 3-7
Effect of a Noncompetitive Inhibitor on the Substrate Saturation Curve and the Lineweaver-Burk Plot. The substrate saturation curve is shown on the left, and the Lineweaver-Burk plot on the right. A noncompetitive inhibitor decreases the V_{max} and has no effect on the K_m. The intercept on the 1/v axis of the Lineweaver-Burk plot for the inhibited reaction is numerically equal to $1/V_{max}$ (1 + I/K_i), where I is the concentration of the inhibitor and K_i is the dissociation constant for the enzyme inhibitor (EI) complex. Since the inhibitor does not bind to the active site and has no effect on substrate binding, the apparent K_m is unchanged.

Irreversible Inhibitors

Irreversible inhibitors react covalently with an amino acid side chain on the enzyme to form a stable complex that is permanently inactivated. Some irreversible inhibitors are also known as *mechanism-based inhibitors*. These inhibitors are structurally similar to the substrate and inactivate the enzyme by reacting with a catalytic residue in the active site. Mechanism-based inhibitors are also known as *suicide substrates*. They bind to the active site and start to undergo a cycle of catalysis, but they become covalently bound to the enzyme, and therefore, the catalytic cycle cannot be completed. The kinetic effect of an irreversible inhibitor is similar to that of a noncompetitive inhibitor, resulting in a decrease in V_{max} but having no effect on the K_m. An irreversible inhibitor has the same kinetic effect as decreasing the amount of enzyme. A summary of the effects of the major types of inhibitors on the kinetic parameters of enzymes is shown in Table 3-4.

Aspirin
Used prophylactically to inhibit aggregation of platelets and blood clotting, aspirin is an irreversible inhibitor of cyclooxygenase, an enzyme required for the synthesis of prostaglandins.

TABLE 3-4 ▶
The Effects of Inhibitors on the Kinetic Properties of Enzymes

Type of Inhibitor	K_m	V_{max}
Competitive	Increased	No effect
Noncompetitive	No effect	Decreased
Irreversible	No effect	Decreased

Use of Enzyme Inhibitors as Therapeutic Agents

Many drugs exert their effects by inhibiting specific enzymes. Most inhibitors that are used therapeutically are either competitive inhibitors or mechanism-based suicide substrates. Most of modern pharmacology is based on the principles of enzyme kinetics and the mechanisms of enzyme inhibition. Some commonly used drugs that exert their effects by inhibiting enzymes are described in Table 3-5.

TABLE 3-5 ▶
Commonly Used Drugs That Are Enzyme Inhibitors

Drug	Therapeutic Use	Target Enzyme	Type of Inhibitor
Mevinolin	Hypercholesterolemia	HMG–CoA reductase	Competitive
5-Fluorouracil	Cancer	Thymidylate synthase	Suicide
Methotrexate	Cancer	Dihydrofolate reductase	Competitive
Allopurinol	Gout	Xanthine oxidase	Suicide
Coumadin	Anticoagulant	γ-Glutamylcarboxylase	Competitive
Aspirin	Anti-inflammatory	Cyclooxygenase	Suicide
Captopril	High blood pressure	Angiotensin-converting enzyme	Competitive

Note. HMG = 3-hydroxyl-3-methylglutaryl; CoA = coenzyme A.

ISOZYMES

Isozymes are enzymes that catalyze the same reaction but differ in chemical structure and kinetic properties. Isozymes frequently have an organ-specific localization, a property that has been exploited for diagnostic purposes. Most of the enzymes present in serum are released during the normal turnover of cells and tissues. Therefore, the increase of a particular isozyme in serum can frequently be used as an indicator of trauma or pathologic damage to the organ or tissue that normally houses the isozyme (Table 3-6). Isozymes can be separated from one another by serum electrophoresis. Two of the isozymes most commonly used for diagnostic purposes are CK and LDH.

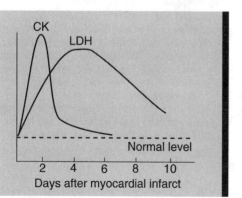

▼ TABLE 3-6
Serum Enzymes Used in Clinical Diagnosis

Enzyme	Major Diagnostic Use
Acid phosphatase	Prostate cancer
Alkaline phosphatase	Liver and bone disease
Amylase	Acute pancreatitis
Aspartate aminotransferase	Liver and heart disease
Alanine aminotransferase	Viral hepatitis
Creatine kinase	Muscle disorders and myocardial infarction
Lactate dehydrogenase	Myocardial infarction
Lipase	Acute pancreatitis

Creatine Phosphokinase (CK)

CK isozymes are dimers that are assembled from two types of subunits, the M (muscle-type) and B (brain-type) subunits. Three combinations of the M and B subunits are the basis for the MM, MB, and BB isozymes of CK. Skeletal muscle CK is almost entirely the MM isozyme; brain CK is entirely the BB form; and cardiac muscle contains approximately 15% MB and 85% MM. The only source of the MB isozyme in serum is cardiac muscle. Therefore, an elevation of the MB isozyme in serum is useful in the diagnosis of a myocardial infarct. An increase in the MB isozyme in serum is measurable within 6 to 8 hours following damage to the myocardium. The increase reaches a peak within 12 to 24 hours and returns to normal within another 48 to 72 hours. Both total serum CK activity and the contribution of the MB isozyme to the total activity should be evaluated. If the activity of the MB isozyme constitutes more than 4% of the total CK activity, a myocardial infarct should be suspected.

Lactate Dehydrogenase (LDH)

LDH is a tetramer that is assembled from two different types of subunits, the M (muscle-type) and H (heart-type) subunits. Five different LDH isozymes can be separated by electrophoresis. The relative amount of each LDH isozyme found in the serum of a normal person and in the serum of a patient with a myocardial infarct is shown in Figure 3-8. LDH_2 normally is higher than LDH_1, but following a myocardial infarct, the activity of LDH_1 will exceed that of LDH_2. The release of LDH_1 from the heart into the serum begins from 1 to 2 days after the appearance of elevated CK in the serum. If LDH_1 constitutes more than 40% of the total serum LDH, a myocardial infarct should be suspected.

LDH Isozymes

Designation	Subunit composition	Tissue distribution
LDH_1	H_4	Heart, kidney, RBC
LDH_2	H_3M	Heart, kidney, RBC
LDH_3	H_2M_2	Brain, pancreas
LDH_4	HM_3	Lung, spleen
LDH_5	M_4	Skeletal muscle, liver

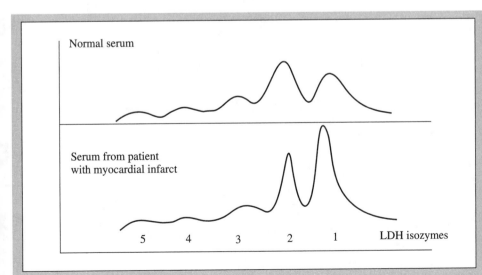

▼ FIGURE 3-8
Separation of Serum Lactate Dehydrogenase (LDH) Isozymes by Electrophoresis. *The isozymes of LDH are separated at pH 8.6 by electrophoresis. The upper graph shows the relative amount of the isozymes in normal serum, and the lower graph represents a patient with a myocardial infarct. The five isozymes are designated LDH_1, LDH_2, and so on, with LDH_1 being the form that migrates most rapidly toward the positive electrode under the conditions of the electrophoresis. The subunit composition of the five isozymes is as follows: $LDH_1 = H_4$, $LDH_2 = H_3M$, $LDH_3 = H_2M_2$, $LDH_4 = HM_3$, and $LDH_5 = M_4$.*

RESOLUTION OF CLINICAL CASE

The patient described at the beginning of the chapter was admitted to the hospital because of chest pain and was diagnosed with acute myocardial infarction (AMI). Chest pain is a nonspecific presentation; therefore, patients are further evaluated by ECG and by serial measurements of serum CK and LDH activity. Diagnosis is usually based on two of the following three criteria: chest pain, characteristic ECG changes, and abnormalities in serum levels of cardiac enzymes. In this patient, the ECG results were equivocal. However, the serum enzyme levels, together with the chest pain, provided sufficient evidence for making the diagnosis. Following a myocardial infarct, the maximum activity of the MB isozyme in serum precedes that of the total CK. If the total CK is greater than 200 IU/L, and the percentage of MB is greater than 4% of the total, AMI is suspected. In this patient, the maximum total CK (361 IU/L) occurred 8 hours after admission. The maximum contribution of MB (5.6%) to the total CK activity was found at the time of admission and decreased over the next 60 hours. Both the total LDH activity and the contribution of LDH_1 peaked at 24 hours after admission. In 95% of all normal subjects, the total LDH activity is less than 170 IU/L, and LDH_1 constitutes between 20% and 30% of the total [1]. Therefore, AMI is suspected if the total serum LDH is greater than 170 IU/L and LDH_1 contributes more than 40% of the total activity. In this patient the total LDH at 24 hours after admission was 365 IU/L, and 59% of the total was attributable to LDH_1.

REVIEW QUESTIONS

Directions: For each of the following questions, choose the **one best** answer.

1. Enzymes have which of the following characteristics?
   - **(A)** They increase the activation energy of a reaction
   - **(B)** They increase the equilibrium constant of a reaction
   - **(C)** They decrease the free energy of the transition state
   - **(D)** They increase the free energy of the product
   - **(E)** They decrease the free energy of the substrate

2. The Michaelis constant (K_m) is best described by which of the following statements?
   - **(A)** It is the concentration of substrate required for maximum velocity
   - **(B)** It is increased when the concentration of enzyme is increased
   - **(C)** It is a measure of the catalytic efficiency of the enzyme
   - **(D)** It is an index of the affinity of an enzyme for its substrate
   - **(E)** It is decreased by a competitive inhibitor

3. Which of the following amino acid side chains is most likely to act as both a weak acid and a nucleophile in enzyme-catalyzed reactions?
   - **(A)** Glutamine
   - **(B)** Histidine
   - **(C)** Serine
   - **(D)** Lysine
   - **(E)** Threonine

Questions 4–6

The Lineweaver-Burk plot below shows lines that describe two kinds of enzyme inhibitors.

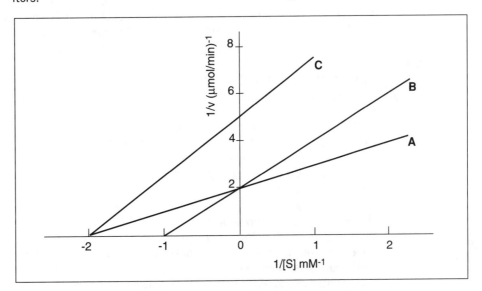

4. The Michaelis constant (K_m) for the enzyme described by line A is which of the following values?

  (A) 4.0 mM

  (B) 2.0 mM

  (C) 1.0 mM

  (D) 0.5 mM

  (E) 0.1 mM

5. The maximum velocity (V_{max}) for the reaction described by line C has which of the following values?

  (A) 5.0 µmol/min

  (B) 2.5 µmol/min

  (C) 2.0 µmol/min

  (D) 0.2 µmol/min

  (E) 0.1 µmol/min

6. The effect of an inhibitor on this enzyme is shown by line B. This inhibitor produces the effect by which of the following actions?

  (A) It binds to a site distinct from the active site

  (B) It decreases the K_m for the substrate twofold

  (C) It increases the V_{max} of the reaction

  (D) It inactivates the enzyme by irreversibly binding to the active site

  (E) It increases the concentration of substrate required for maximum velocity

ANSWERS AND EXPLANATIONS

1. The answer is C. Enzymes increase the rates of reactions by decreasing the free energy of the transition state. The transition state is the intermediate in a reaction having the highest amount of free energy. All substrate molecules must go through the transition state to be converted to product. Enzymes have no effect on the equilibrium constant for the reaction, but they increase the rate at which equilibrium is achieved. The equilibrium constant is related to the difference in the free energy of the substrate and the product, both of which are unchanged by the presence of an enzyme.

2. The answer is D. The K_m is an index of the affinity of an enzyme for a substrate. It can be defined as the concentration of substrate required for half-maximum velocity. When comparing the affinity of two substrates, the substrate with the lower K_m will have the higher affinity for the enzyme. The K_m is independent of the concentration of enzyme. The catalytic efficiency of an enzyme is related to the V_{max} but not to the K_m. A competitive inhibitor increases the K_m for a substrate by binding to the same site as the substrate, and therefore, a higher concentration is required to achieve half-maximum velocity.

3. The answer is B. Amino acid side chains that act as weak acids must have a proton that will ionize in the physiologic pH range, whereas side chains that act as nucleophiles must have a nitrogen, oxygen, or sulfur atom with an unshared pair of electrons. The only amino acid whose side chain meets both of these requirements is histidine. Although lysine has a protonated nitrogen that is capable of ionizing, its pK_a is at least 3 pH units higher than that of the histidine side chain and is much less likely to act as a weak acid. Glutamine, serine, and threonine all have atoms with unshared electron pairs in their side chains, but they do not have groups that ionize within the physiologic pH range.

4. The answer is D. The intercept of line A on the x-axis is numerically equal to $-1/K_m$, and the units are mM^{-1}. Therefore, $-1/K_m = -2\ mM^{-1}$, and $K_m = 0.5\ mM$.

5. The answer is D. The intercept of line C on the y-axis is numerically equal to $1/V_{max}$ and the units are $(\mu mol/min)^{-1}$. Therefore, $1/V_{max} = 5\ (\mu mol/min)^{-1}$, and $V_{max} = 0.2\ \mu mol/min$.

6. The answer is E. The inhibitor described by line B is a competitive inhibitor, which binds to the same site as the substrate. The V_{max} is unaltered by this inhibitor. However, since both substrate and inhibitor compete for the same binding site, a higher concentration of substrate is required to saturate the active site and achieve V_{max}. The fact that the same V_{max} is obtained in the presence as well as the absence of an inhibitor indicates that the binding of an inhibitor is reversible.

REFERENCES

1. Walmsley RN, White GH: *A Guide to Diagnostic Clinical Chemistry*, 3rd ed. Boston, MA: Blackwell Scientific, 1994, pp 300–310.

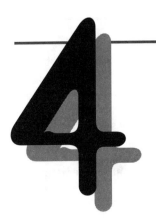

4

OXYGEN TRANSPORT AND STORAGE: HEMOGLOBIN AND MYOGLOBIN

INTRODUCTION OF CLINICAL CASE

A 43-year-old man was working alone in a warehouse when he began to experience a severe headache, lightheadedness, and nausea. The manager advised him by phone to go home, but 13 hours later, he was discovered unconscious with the door of the warehouse open. He had fixed, constricted pupils, cherry-red skin and nails, and muscle rigidity [1]. Soon after arriving in the emergency room, the patient experienced respiratory arrest and was started on mechanical ventilation. His hemoglobin–carbon monoxide (HbCO) level was 42%, and oxygen therapy was started. After 4 hours of receiving 100% oxygen, his pupils were reactive to light, and he was breathing spontaneously, but there was no improvement in his central nervous system (CNS) status. His HbCO level had dropped to 2.9%. After an additional 6 hours of treatment with 100% oxygen, he showed signs of movement but still could not follow verbal commands. The patient was kept in the critical care unit for the following 48 hours, during which time ventilatory assistance was gradually terminated. Seventy-two hours after admission, he was able to follow verbal commands, was oriented to time and place, but was totally amnesic about the warehouse incident. The patient was released from the hospital 7 days after the incident. A week later, his family felt that he had returned to normal.

INTRODUCTION

The mechanism by which humans extract energy from their environment involves the oxidation of foods by molecular oxygen, resulting in the production of carbon dioxide and water. Since most oxidation reactions occur in the mitochondria, which are remote from an atmosphere of oxygen, mechanisms have evolved for providing tissues with a constant supply of oxygen and for constant removal of carbon dioxide. Hemoglobin (Hb) transports oxygen from the lungs to the tissues and is responsible, either directly or indirectly, for transporting most of the carbon dioxide from the tissues to the lungs where it is exhaled. Hb also serves as a buffer for transporting protons (hydrogen ion [H^+]) from the tissues to the lungs. Myoglobin (Mb), an oxygen-storage protein, is found in the cytoplasm of cardiac and striated muscle cells, ensuring that an adequate supply of oxygen is present for oxidative metabolism in these cells. The major oxygen-binding protein in mitochondria is cytochrome oxidase, the terminal component of the electron transport chain, which reduces oxygen to water. Since oxygen moves readily across membranes, the uptake of oxygen by cells is influenced by the concentrations and the relative affinities of Hb, Mb, and cytochrome oxidase for oxygen. Cytochrome oxidase has the highest affinity and Hb the lowest. The hemoproteins consist of two components: heme and a protein component that binds heme.

HEME: THE PROSTHETIC GROUP OF MYOGLOBIN AND HEMOGLOBIN

Heme is a prosthetic group that reversibly binds and releases oxygen from Hb and Mb, a property essential for oxygen transport and storage. The structure of heme is shown in Figure 4-1.

Heme Structure

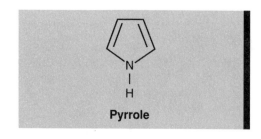

Pyrrole

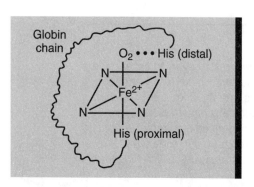

Heme is a hydrophobic molecule that contains a planar porphyrin ring and an iron atom. The porphyrin ring is assembled from four pyrrole rings, which are connected to one another by single carbon groups. The iron atom forms six coordinate bonds. Four bonds are formed between the iron and the nitrogen atoms that are at the center of the porphyrin ring system. A fifth bond is formed between a nitrogen atom that is contributed by a histidine residue in the globin, known as the *proximal histidine*, and the sixth bond is formed with oxygen. The oxygenated forms of Mb and Hb are stabilized by a hydrogen bond between the oxygen and the side chain of another histidine residue, the *distal histidine*.

Oxidation State of Iron

Functional Mb and Hb contain iron in the ferrous (Fe^{2+}) state. Oxidation to the ferric (Fe^{3+}) state results in the inability of Mb or Hb to bind oxygen. The oxidized form of heme is known as *hemin*, and the oxidized form of Hb is *methemoglobin*.

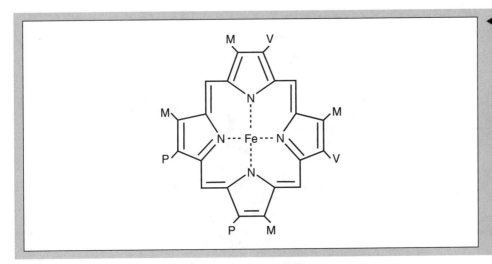

Structure of Heme. The pyrrole rings, the methylene carbons that connect them, and the iron atom are all planar. Each pyrrole ring has two substituents, which are either methyl (M), vinyl (V), or propionyl (P) groups.

GLOBIN: THE PROTEIN COMPONENT OF HEMOGLOBIN AND MYOGLOBIN

The globin chains are relatively small proteins, having molecular weights of about 16,000. They have no biologic activity in the absence of heme. The globin component alone is frequently referred to as the *apoprotein*, and when it combines with heme, it becomes a *holoprotein*. This nomenclature is widely used to describe proteins that depend on prosthetic groups, or cofactors, for their biologic activity.

Function

The primary function of the globin chain of Mb and Hb is to form a *protective hydrophobic pocket for binding heme* that shields the iron atom from the aqueous environment. Exposure of the heme iron to water results in oxidation and loss of oxygen-binding capacity.

Structure

The globin chain is tightly folded into a globular molecule with little space in the interior. About 75% of the polypeptide chain is folded into eight segments of an α-helical structure (Figure 4-2). The folding of the helical segments creates a V-shaped pocket that binds heme between the E and F helices. This crevice is lined with hydrophobic amino acid side chains, which exclude water and provide a protective pocket for heme. The only two hydrophilic amino acids in the heme crevice are the distal and proximal histidine residues that are in the E and F helices, respectively.

COMPARISON OF MYOGLOBIN AND HEMOGLOBIN

There are many similarities in the tertiary structures of globin chains found in Mb and Hb, a reflection of the fact that the globin chains are designed to bind heme and protect it from the aqueous medium. The major difference in Mb and Hb structure is in their quaternary structure.

Subunit Structure

Mb is a *monomer*, consisting of a single globin subunit, whereas Hb is a *tetramer*, containing two types of globin chains. All of the globin chains of Hb fold into a tertiary structure that is essentially identical to that of Mb, with each subunit binding a molecule of heme. The Hb subunits are held together by numerous electrostatic interactions between positively and negatively charged amino acid side chains.

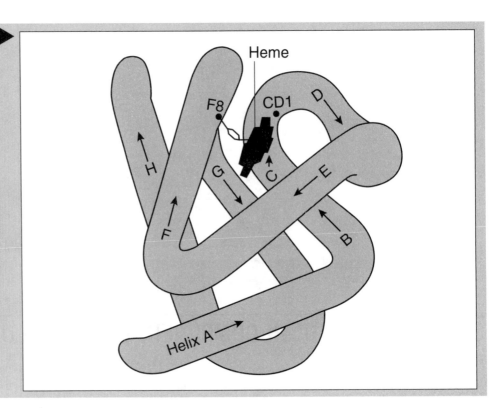

FIGURE 4-2 ▶

Tertiary Structure of the Globin Chain. *The globin chain is folded into eight helical segments (A–H). The arrows indicate the direction of the peptide chain from the amino terminus to the carboxyl terminus. Heme is bound in a hydrophobic crevice created by the E and F helices. The proximal histidine, which is bound to the iron of heme, is located in helix F. The distal histidine, which stabilizes oxyhemoglobin by hydrogen bonding with oxygen, is in helix E. (Source: Reprinted with permission from Thompson, MW, McInnes, RR, Willard, HF: Genetics in Medicine, 5th ed. Philadelphia, PA: W. B. Saunders, 1991, p 250.)*

Differential Expression of Globin Gene

The expression of different globin genes throughout the course of human development results in the presence of different types of Hb in embryonic, fetal, and adult blood. These different types of Hb differ in their subunit composition (Table 4-1). The major form of Hb in adults (HbA) contains two α- and two β-subunits, designated as $\alpha_2\beta_2$. The globin genes are organized into two clusters that are located on different chromosomes (Figure 4-3). The genes for the "alpha-like globins" are located on chromosome 16, and the genes for the "beta-like globins" (β, γ, Δ, and ε) are located on chromosome 11.

Oxygen Binding

Oxygen-binding curves are generated by plotting the percentage of oxygenated hemoglobin (percent saturation) against the partial pressure of oxygen (Po_2). The oxygen-

TABLE 4-1 ▶

Human Hemoglobins at Different Stages of Development

Stage of Development	Hemoglobins	Subunit Composition
Embryonic (0–8 weeks)	HbE	$\alpha_2\varepsilon_2$
Fetal (3–9 months)	HbF	$\alpha_2\gamma_2$
Adult (after birth)	HbA	$\alpha_2\beta_2$
	HbA$_2$	$\alpha_2\Delta_2$

FIGURE 4-3 ▶

Organization of the Globin Genes. *The genes for alpha and alpha-like globin chains are located on chromosome 16. There are two copies of the alpha gene, designated as α_1 and α_2, and one copy of the zeta gene. The genes for beta and beta-like globins are located on chromosome 11. There is one copy each of the beta, delta, and epsilon genes, and two copies of the gamma gene, designated G_γ and A_γ*

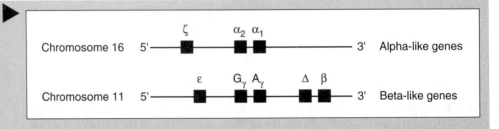

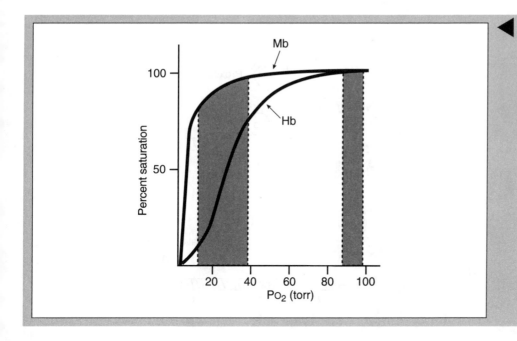

FIGURE 4-4
Oxygen-Binding Curves for Myoglobin (Mb) and Hemoglobin (Hb). The percentage of oxygenated Mb and Hb molecules is shown with increasing oxygen tension. The Po_2 in arterial blood is about 100 torr and in venous blood between 20 torr (active muscle) and 40 torr (resting muscle). Half-saturation occurs at 3 torr for Mb and 25 torr for Hb. The shaded areas *represent the range of* Po_2 *in the venous and arterial blood, respectively.*

binding curves for Mb and Hb differ in the shape of the saturation curves and in the partial pressure of oxygen required for 50% saturation (P_{50}) [Figure 4-4]. Both of these differences have significant physiologic implications.

Shape of Oxygen-Saturation Curves. The shape of the curve that describes the binding of oxygen to Mb is *hyperbolic*, while that for Hb is *sigmoidal*, a difference that reflects the characteristic subunit structure of each protein. Mb, having only one subunit, contains a single site for oxygen, whereas Hb has four oxygen-binding sites. The sigmoidal saturation for Hb indicates positive cooperativity between the oxygen-binding sites. As the blood passes through the lungs, the binding of oxygen to the first site facilitates the binding to other sites. Similarly, as the blood passes through the tissue bed, the release of oxygen from the first subunit facilitates the release from other subunits.

P_{50} for Oxygen Binding. Mb has a higher affinity for oxygen than Hb, as indicated by the lower value for P_{50}. Mb is half-saturated at a partial pressure of about 3 torr, while a partial pressure of about 25 torr is required for half-saturation of Hb.

Physiologic Significance. The significance of the differences in the oxygen-binding curves for Mb and Hb are apparent when considered in the context of the conditions that exist in the lungs and tissue bed. The Po_2 in the lungs is approximately 100 torr, a pressure at which Hb is almost totally saturated. In the tissue bed, the Po_2 is between 20 torr and 40 torr, depending on the metabolic activity of the tissue. Within this range, the binding and release of oxygen is very sensitive to small changes in oxygen pressure, a property that facilitates the release of oxygen from Hb. At a Po_2 of 20 torr, Mb is almost totally saturated with oxygen. Therefore, Hb is saturated at the oxygen tension that exists in the capillaries of the lungs, and Mb is saturated at the oxygen tension in the capillaries of the peripheral tissues.

Molecular Basis of Cooperativity. The trigger for cooperative binding of oxygen occurs when the first molecule of oxygen binds to deoxyhemoglobin. In the deoxygenated state, the bulky iron atom occupies a position slightly outside the plane of the heme ring (Figure 4-5). Upon oxygenation, there is a change in the spin state of the iron and a slight reduction in size, which allows it to move into the plane of the heme ring. The movement of iron is accompanied by the movement of the proximal histidine of the globin chain.

This localized conformational change initiates a ripple effect that spreads throughout the globin chains, resulting in an enhanced affinity of the unoccupied hemes for oxygen. Oxygen binds to the fourth subunit of Hb with an affinity that is about 300 times greater than that of the first subunit. The differences in the conformations of deoxyhemoglobin and oxyhemoglobin are shown schematically in Figure 4-6. Deoxyhemoglobin is described as having a *taut conformation* that impedes the binding of oxygen,

Units
The most commonly used unit for expressing the concentration or tension of oxygen is the torr (mm Hg).

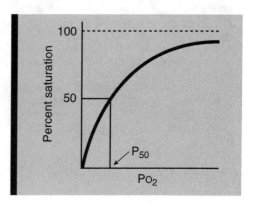

	Lungs	Peripheral Tissues
Po_2	100 torr	20–40 torr
pH	7.4	7.2

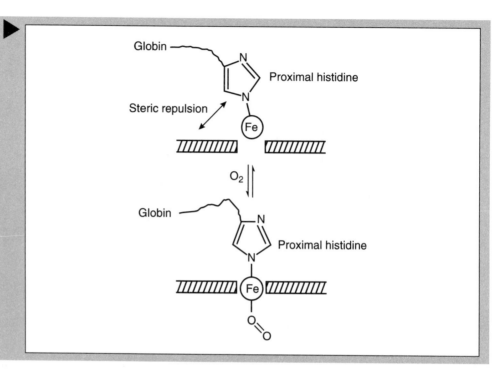

FIGURE 4-5
Trigger for Cooperativity of Oxygen Binding to Hemoglobin. In the deoxygenated state, the iron atom occupies a space slightly outside the plane of the heme ring. Upon oxygenation, it moves into the plane of the ring and pulls the proximal histidine along with it. The movement of the proximal histidine is transmitted throughout the globin chains, resulting in increased affinity of the other hemes for oxygen.

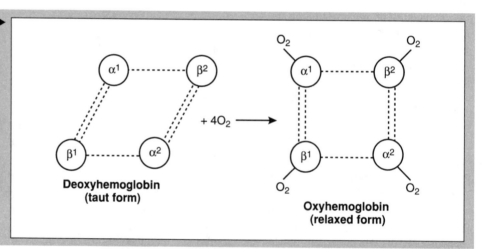

FIGURE 4-6
Structural Differences in Oxygenated and Deoxygenated Hemoglobin (Hb). The structure of deoxygenated (and partially oxygenated) Hb is described as taut and that of totally oxygenated Hb as relaxed. Upon oxygenation, the positions of the subunits shift relative to one another. The bonding between subunits is strong in the $\alpha^1\beta^1$ and $\alpha^2\beta^2$ pairs, and each of these pairs acts as a unit in the transition between the taut and relaxed forms. The affinity for oxygen is low in deoxyhemoglobin and increases progressively as each subunit becomes oxygenated.

whereas fully oxygenated Hb has a *relaxed conformation* with no impediments to oxygen binding.

Carbon Monoxide Binding and Toxicity

Carbon monoxide (CO) is an odorless gas that combines with Hb to form HbCO, a complex having a distinctive cherry-red color that can be seen in the skin and tissues of victims of carbon monoxide poisoning. Carbon monoxide binds to heme in a manner analogous to oxygen and exerts its toxic effects by interfering with the normal function of hemoproteins. The affinity of Hb for carbon monoxide is about 210 times greater than for oxygen, and once it is bound, it does not readily dissociate. The affinity of Mb for carbon monoxide is about 15 times greater than for oxygen.

In the presence of carbon monoxide, the *oxygen-saturation curve is shifted to the left*, indicating a higher affinity for oxygen in the presence of carbon monoxide. The binding of carbon monoxide to one or more of the hemes shifts the conformation of Hb from the taut to the relaxed state and enhances the binding of oxygen to the unoccupied sites. The more avid binding of oxygen by HbCO compromises the ability of Hb to deliver oxygen to the tissues.

Carbon monoxide poisoning may occur in the presence of automobile exhaust fumes, poorly oxygenated coal fires, or any other situation in which incomplete oxidation of carbon-containing compounds occurs. The catabolism of heme in humans produces one molecule of carbon monoxide for every molecule of heme degraded. This carbon

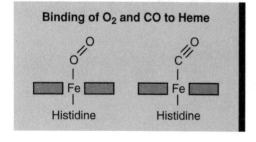

Binding of O_2 and CO to Heme

monoxide is ultimately released by the lungs, and there are no known cases where endogenous carbon monoxide was toxic.

REGULATION OF HEMOGLOBIN FUNCTION

There are two principal mechanisms for regulating the release of oxygen by Hb. The first mechanism involves changes in the partial pressure of carbon dioxide (P_{CO_2}), a property known as the Bohr effect, which is mediated by a small decrease in the pH of the blood in the capillaries of peripheral tissues. The second mechanism is mediated by 2,3-bisphosphoglycerate (2,3-BPG), a metabolite found in red blood cells (RBCs).

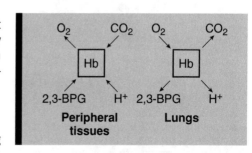

Bohr Effect

A decrease in pH (an increase in H^+) results in a lower affinity of Hb for oxygen, resulting in the release of oxygen from Hb (Figure 4-7). The same effect is produced by an increase in the P_{CO_2}.

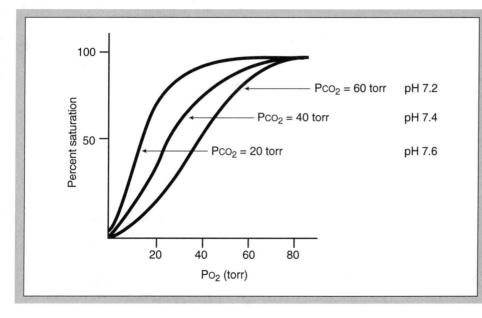

FIGURE 4-7
Effect of pH and Carbon Dioxide on the Oxygen-Saturation Curve for Hemoglobin (Hb). A decrease in pH (an increase in H^+ concentration) decreases the affinity of Hb for oxygen, shifting the oxygen-binding curve to the right. An increase in the P_{CO_2} creates the same qualitative effect as it undergoes hydration and dissociation to protons and bicarbonate ions. A decrease in the pH of blood from pH 7.4 to pH 7.2 is seen in working muscle, with some of the acidification resulting from carbon dioxide production by the tissue.

Molecular Basis. The molecular basis for the Bohr effect resides in the fact that oxygenated hemoglobin ($H\text{-}Hb\cdot O_2$) is a stronger acid than deoxyhemoglobin ($H\text{-}Hb$) and has a greater tendency to dissociate protons from the side chains of ionizable amino acids. This concept can be described by the following equation:

$$H\text{-}Hb + O_2 \rightleftharpoons [H\text{-}Hb\cdot O_2] \rightleftharpoons HbO_2 + H^+$$

Clearly, any condition that results in an increase in the H^+ concentration will shift the equilibrium of the above equation to the left, resulting in the release of oxygen from Hb. The H^+ concentration is greater in the capillaries of metabolically active tissues than in the capillaries of the lungs, thereby facilitating oxygen delivery to peripheral tissues.

Source of H^+. The increased H^+ concentration in the capillaries of peripheral tissues is related to the production of carbon dioxide and can be described by the following equation:

$$CO_2 + H_2O \rightleftharpoons H_2CO_3 \rightleftharpoons H^+ + HCO_3^-$$

The carbon dioxide diffuses out of the tissues and into the RBCs where carbonic anhydrase catalyzes its hydration, resulting in carbonic acid (H_2CO_3), which readily dissociates to protons (H^+) and bicarbonate (HCO_3^-) ions. Since the pK_a (i.e., the negative logarithm of the ionization constant of an acid) of H_2CO_3 is 6.1, most of the H_2CO_3 is dissociated at physiologic pH (see Chapter 1). From the combined effects of these two equations, it is clear that the Bohr effect can be described either as the effect

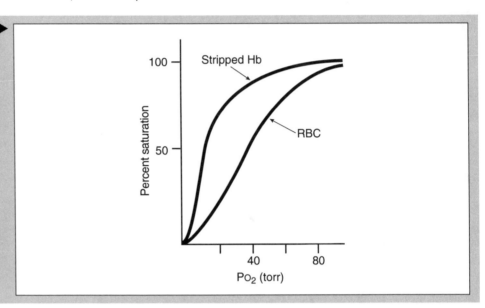

COO⁻
|
H — C — O — PO₃⁼
|
CH₂ — O — PO₃⁼

2,3-BPG

of carbon dioxide or the effect of H⁺ on the affinity of Hb for oxygen. An increase in the P_{CO_2} results in an increase in the H⁺ concentration, which, in turn, promotes the release of oxygen from Hb.

2,3-Bisphosphoglycerate (2,3-BPG) Effect

The presence of 2,3-BPG in the RBCs markedly decreases the affinity of Hb for oxygen (Figure 4-8). 2,3-BPG is formed as an intermediate in glycolysis, but it accumulates only in the RBC, where it is present at about the same concentration as Hb.

FIGURE 4-8
Effect of 2,3-Bisphosphoglycerate (2,3-BPG) on Oxygen-Saturation Curve for Hemoglobin (Hb). 2,3-BPG decreases the affinity of Hb for oxygen, as indicated by a shift in the oxygen-saturation curve to the right. In RBCs, the concentration of 2,3-BPG is about the same as the concentration of Hb.

2,3-BPG–Binding Site. Each deoxyhemoglobin tetramer can bind one molecule of 2,3-BPG. The binding site is located between the β-subunits of deoxyhemoglobin, where a cluster of six positively charged side chains interact with the negatively charged 2,3-BPG. Each β-globin chain contributes three positively charged amino acid side chains to the binding site. As shown in the following equation, the binding of 2,3-BPG exclusively to deoxyhemoglobin shifts the equilibrium to the left, favoring oxygen release from Hb.

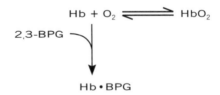

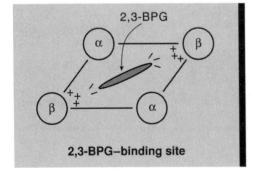

2,3-BPG–binding site

Changes in 2,3-BPG Concentration. The concentration of 2,3-BPG in the RBC can change by as much as 15%–25% in less than 12 hours. An elevation in 2,3-BPG concentration is seen in individuals who live at high altitudes and in patients with disorders in oxygen delivery such as chronic obstructive pulmonary disease (COPD). A decrease in 2,3-BPG concentration occurs in stored blood, resulting in a decreased ability of transfused blood to deliver oxygen to tissues. The decrease can be prevented by storing blood in the presence of inosine, a compound that is converted to 2,3-BPG by the RBC.

FETAL HEMOGLOBIN

The transport of oxygen to the fetus involves diffusion of oxygen from the maternal circulation into the fetal circulation. Fetal hemoglobin (HbF) has a higher affinity for oxygen than HbA, ensuring that there is a net flow of oxygen from mother to fetus (Figure 4-9).

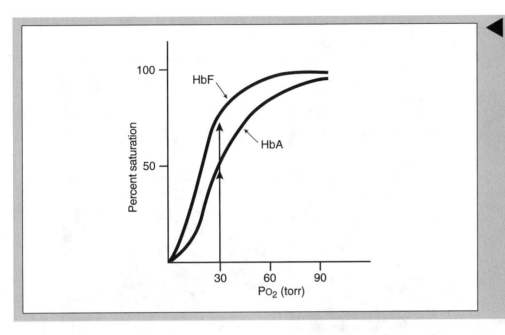

FIGURE 4-9
Oxygen-Binding Curve for Fetal Hemoglo-
bin (HbF) and Adult Hemoglobin (HbA).
HbF has a higher affinity for oxygen than
HbA, as indicated by the shift of the
oxygen-saturation curve to the left. The
arrow illustrates that at a Po_2, where HbA
is about 50% saturated, a significantly
higher percentage of HbF will be oxy-
genated.

The difference in the affinity of HbA and HbF for oxygen is related to the presence of γ-globin chains in HbF. Although the amino acid sequences of the β- and γ-globin chains are highly homologous, they differ slightly in the amino acids that form the binding site for 2,3-BPG. In HbA, the binding site is made up of six positively charged side chains that are contributed by the two β-globin chains. In the γ-chain, one of the basic amino acids has been replaced by a neutral amino acid, thereby reducing the net positive charge in the binding site and resulting in a decreased affinity for 2,3-BPG. Therefore, at the Po_2 found in the capillary bed of the placenta, HbF will be more highly oxygenated than HbA.

TRANSPORT OF CARBON DIOXIDE AND HYDROGEN IONS BY HEMOGLOBIN

In addition to transporting oxygen, Hb transports carbon dioxide and H+ from the tissues to the lungs. Carbon dioxide transport occurs by both direct and indirect mechanisms involving Hb.

Direct Transport: Carbaminohemoglobin

About 15% of the carbon dioxide is transported to the lungs as carbaminohemoglobin, a covalent adduct formed by the binding of carbon dioxide to the amino terminal residues of the α- and β-globin chains. The reaction of carbon dioxide with Hb is described by the following equation:

$$CO_2 + NH_2-Hb \rightleftharpoons {}^-OOC-NH-Hb + H^+$$

This reaction occurs rapidly and does not require an enzyme. The formation of carbaminohemoglobin is favored in the tissue capillaries where the Pco_2 is high. In the lungs, where the Pco_2 is low, the reverse reaction is favored, releasing carbon dioxide in the expired air.

Isohydric Transport: Bicarbonate (HCO_3^-)

Most of the carbon dioxide is transported from the tissues to the lungs as HCO_3^- dissolved in the plasma. The term isohydric indicates that transport occurs with little change in pH, a property that is attributed to the buffering capacity of deoxyhemoglobin. Protons bind to deoxyhemoglobin and are transported to the lungs, where they are released upon oxygenation. The isohydric transport of HCO_3^- involves several reactions (Figure 4-10).

FIGURE 4-10 ▶

Isohydric Transport of Carbon Dioxide. Most of the carbon dioxide generated in peripheral tissues is transported in the plasma as bicarbonate (HCO_3^-) with little change in the pH of the blood. For every HCO_3^- that is formed, a proton (H^+) is also generated, which is picked up by deoxyhemoglobin and taken back to the lungs. When hemoglobin (Hb) becomes oxygenated in the lungs, the proton is released, where it combines with HCO_3^-, forming carbonic acid, which is degraded to carbon dioxide and water.

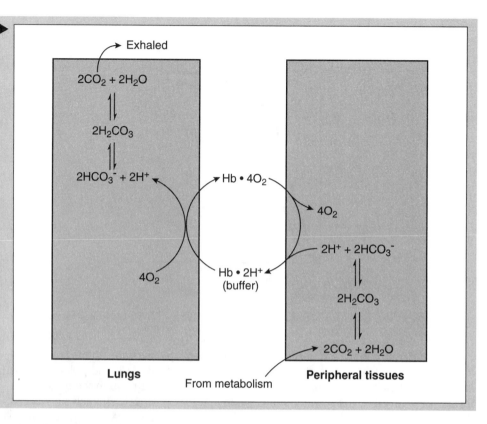

Reactions in the Periphery. In the capillaries of peripheral tissues, carbon dioxide diffuses into the RBC and is hydrated to H_2CO_3. The protons, formed by dissociation of H_2CO_3, are absorbed by deoxyhemoglobin and the HCO_3^- is transferred out of the RBC into the plasma. The transport of HCO_3^- out of the RBC is coupled with the transport of chloride (Cl^-) into the RBC, a process that maintains electrical neutrality.

Reactions in the Lungs. In the lungs, the oxygenation of Hb results in dissociation of protons, which react with HCO_3^-, forming H_2CO_3. The H_2CO_3 is degraded to carbon dioxide and water, which is exhaled. The removal of carbon dioxide allows more HCO_3^- to be transported into the RBC.

INHERITED DEFECTS IN HEMOGLOBIN

Syndromes resulting from defects in Hb structure and function are among the most common known genetic diseases. They are classified in two broad categories: the hemoglobinopathies and the thalassemias.

Hemoglobinopathies

The hemoglobinopathies result from inherited defects, which, in turn, result in structural changes in the Hb molecule. Two of the best characterized are sickle cell hemoglobin (HbS) and hemoglobin C (HbC).

Sickle Cell Hemoglobin. HbS differs from HbA by a single amino acid substitution in the β-globin chain, in which glutamate at position six has been replaced by valine. The altered β-globin chain is designated as $β^s$, and the subunit structure of HbS is designated as $α_2β_2^s$. The replacement of glutamic acid by valine results in a decrease in the negative charge and an altered electrophoretic mobility at alkaline pH, a property that has been exploited in screening for sickle cell carriers. Individuals homozygous for HbS have *sickle cell anemia*, while those who are heterozygous for HbS have *sickle cell trait*, a condition that is usually asymptomatic.

The amino acid substitution in HbS markedly *decreases the solubility of deoxygenated HbS*, although the solubility of oxygenated HbS is indistinguishable from that of

HbA. In the capillaries of peripheral tissues where deoxygenated HbS predominates, aggregates of HbS form fibrous polymers that distort the shape of the RBC (Figure 4-11). The sickle (crescent-shaped) cells are more fragile and have a shorter life span. When a sufficient number of sickle cells form, blood flow through the capillaries may cease, resulting in tissue damage and death. The extent of sickling is increased by any condition that promotes the formation of deoxygenated HbS.

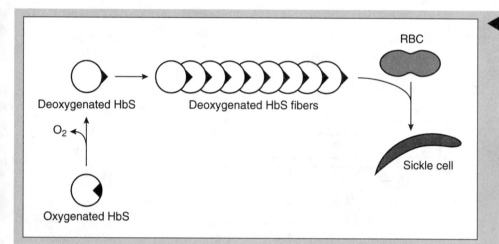

FIGURE 4-11
Polymerization of Hemoglobin S (HbS) and Formation of Sickle Cells. The replacement of glutamate by valine introduces a hydrophobic patch onto the surface of the beta chains of HbS. In the deoxygenated form, the subunits polymerize into rigid fibers that deform the shape of the RBC.

Hemoglobin C. HbC has a single amino acid change at position six in the β-globin chain, where glutamate is replaced by lysine. The deoxygenated form of HbC, like that of HbS, is less soluble than HbA, but it aggregates into microcrystals rather than fibrous polymers. In the homozygous state, known as HbC disease, the HbC crystals increase the fragility of the RBCs, resulting in mild hemolytic anemia.

Thalassemias

The thalassemias are a group of syndromes resulting from the inability to synthesize adequate quantities of normal globin chains. Normally the synthesis of the α- and β-globins is balanced, but in the thalassemias, there is a decrease in the rate of synthesis of either the α- or the β-globin. The globin that is present in excess usually precipitates in the cell, resulting in hemolysis. The thalassemias are characterized clinically by hemolytic anemia.

α-Thalassemias. In the α-thalassemias, the synthesis of α-globin chains is impaired, usually as a result of deletions in the α-globin gene. Disorders in synthesis of α-globin chains decreases the production of both HbF and HbA, resulting in both intrauterine and postnatal disease. In the absence of alpha-chains, the gamma-chains associate in utero forming *Bart's Hb* with a composition of γ_4. Postnatally, the beta-chains associate to form HbH with a composition of β_4. Neither Bart's Hb nor HbH can release oxygen to tissues under normal conditions.

β-Thalassemias. The synthesis of the β-globin chain is impaired in the β-thalassemias. Decreased β-globin synthesis affects the production of Hb only in the postnatal state and can be readily distinguished from α-thalassemia by an increased concentration of HbF ($\alpha_2\gamma_2$) and HbA$_2$ ($\alpha_2\Delta_2$). The synthesis of the β-globin chain is usually decreased as a result of single base changes in the gene. The excess α-globin chains precipitate, leading to membrane damage and lysis of the RBC. *β-Thalassemia major* occurs in individuals with two mutant alleles and is characterized by severe anemia that has to be treated by periodic transfusions throughout life. Cardiomyopathy due to iron overload frequently leads to death. *β-Thalassemia minor* occurs in carriers with only one mutant allele and is characterized by mild anemia.

Hydrops fetalis is an α-thalassemia resulting from total loss of the alpha genes. Neither HbF nor HbA can be synthesized. Death occurs before birth, although the fetus survives for awhile by making HbE that has the zeta rather than the alpha chain ($\zeta_2\varepsilon_2$ and $\zeta_2\gamma_2$).

Detection of Mutant Hemoglobins

Several hundred different types of mutant Hb have been identified by examining patients with clinical symptoms and by electrophoretic screening of normal populations. The

HbA	Val-His-Leu-Thr-Pro-**Glu**-Glu-
HbS	Val-His-Leu-Thr-Pro-**Val**-Glu-
HbC	Val-His-Leu-Thr-Pro-**Lys**-Glu-

mutations that result in differences in the net charge of the globin chain can be detected by electrophoresis (Figure 4-12). Most abnormal forms of Hb have properties that are indistinguishable from those of HbA and have no adverse effect on the individual with the mutation.

FIGURE 4-12 ▶

Electrophoresis of Mutant Hemoglobins (Hb). The relative mobilities of Hb isolated from patients with various hemoglobinopathies from top to bottom are: normal control, sickle cell trait, sickle cell anemia, hemoglobin C (HbC) trait, HbC disease, and normal control. Electrophoresis is performed at pH 8.6 where all the species of Hb migrate toward the positive electrode.

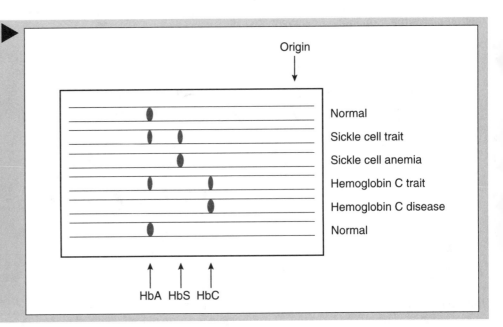

RESOLUTION OF CLINICAL CASE

The patient described in the case at the beginning of the chapter was suspected of having carbon monoxide poisoning. A tentative diagnosis was made on the basis of his unconscious state and the cherry-red discoloration of his skin and nails when he was brought into the emergency room [1]. The diagnosis was confirmed by direct measurement of the HbCO level in the patient's blood, which was 42%. Normally less than 5% of the Hb molecules contain bound carbon monoxide. Values greater than 60% HbCO are lethal. The heart and CNS, with their high metabolic rates, are most susceptible to the toxic effects of carbon monoxide. The binding of carbon monoxide to Hb impairs the ability to deliver oxygen to the tissues. Additionally, it inhibits cellular respiration directly by competing for the oxygen sites on cytochromes. Treatment of carbon monoxide poisoning with either 100% oxygen or 95% oxygen and 5% carbon dioxide for 1–2 hours usually removes carbon monoxide from the body. After 4 hours of treatment with 100% oxygen, the patient's HbCO level decreased to 2.9%. The neurologic status of the patient improved over the next few days, and by the time he was released from the hospital, his condition was considered to be normal.

REVIEW QUESTIONS

Directions: For each of the following questions, choose the **one best** answer.

1. Most of the carbon dioxide generated during metabolism is transported to the lungs as
   - **(A)** a heme iron complex
   - **(B)** dissolved carbon dioxide
   - **(C)** carbonic acid
   - **(D)** carbaminohemoglobin
   - **(E)** bicarbonate

2. Which of the following types of mutant hemoglobins (Hb) would migrate most rapidly toward the positive electrode during electrophoresis at pH 8.6?
   - **(A)** Hb Koln (valine replaced by methionine)
   - **(B)** HbS (glutamate replaced by valine)
   - **(C)** Hb Seattle (alanine replaced by aspartate)
   - **(D)** HbC (glutamate replaced by lysine)
   - **(E)** HbG (proline replaced by leucine)

3. Fetal hemoglobin (HbF) has which of the following characteristics?
   - **(A)** It has a lower affinity for oxygen than HbA
   - **(B)** It has a lower affinity for 2,3-bisphosphoglycerate (2,3-BPG) than HbA
   - **(C)** It has a subunit structure of $\alpha_2\varepsilon_2$
   - **(D)** It has a lower affinity for oxygen than HbA when both are stripped of 2,3-BPG
   - **(E)** It has a higher P_{50} for oxygen than HbA

4. Which of the following conditions facilitates delivery of oxygen to tissues?
   - **(A)** A decrease in H^+ concentration
   - **(B)** A decrease in the P_{CO_2}
   - **(C)** An increase in 2,3-bisphosphoglycerate (2,3-BPG) concentration
   - **(D)** An increase in carbon monoxide concentration
   - **(E)** An increase in pH

5. Which of the following characteristics best describes hemoglobin (Hb) isolated from a person with sickle cell anemia?
   - **(A)** The solubility is decreased by an increase in the P_{O_2}
   - **(B)** The solubility is decreased by a change in pH from 7.2 to 7.4
   - **(C)** The P_{50} for oxygen is less than that for HbA
   - **(D)** The affinity for 2,3-bisphosphoglycerate (2,3-BPG) is greater than that for HbA
   - **(E)** The solubility is decreased by an increase in the P_{CO_2}

ANSWERS AND EXPLANATIONS

1. The answer is E. More than 70% of the carbon dioxide produced by tissues is transported to the lungs as bicarbonate. Smaller amounts of carbon dioxide are transported as carbaminohemoglobin, with the carbon dioxide covalently bound to amino groups on the globin chains. Low concentrations of carbonic acid and dissolved carbon dioxide are also found in the serum, but neither are significant transport forms for carbon dioxide. Carbon dioxide does not bind to heme.

2. The answer is C. The Hb that would move most rapidly toward the positive electrode (the anode) would be the one with the greatest negative charge at pH 8.6. The replacement of alanine, a neutral amino acid, with aspartate, which has a negatively charged side chain, increases the net charge on Hb Seattle. The replacement in Hb Koln and HbG do not alter the charge properties. In both HbS and HbC, there is a reduction in the negative charge by the respective amino acid replacements.

3. The answer is B. HbF has a higher affinity for oxygen than HbA because it does not bind 2,3-BPG as tightly. If both HbS and HbA are stripped of 2,3-BPG, their oxygen-binding curves are indistinguishable. Since the affinity of HbF for oxygen is higher than that of HbA, the P_{50} will be lower. The subunit structure of HbF is $\alpha_2\gamma_2$. The $\alpha_2\epsilon_2$ composition is that of HbE, which is found in early embryogenesis.

4. The answer is C. Since 2,3-BPG binds only to the deoxygenated form of Hb, an increase in its concentration shifts the equilibrium in the direction of oxygen release. An increase in the P_{CO_2}, an increase in H^+ concentration, and a decrease in pH have a similar effect to that of 2,3-BPG on the equilibrium between oxygenated and deoxygenated Hb. An increase in carbon monoxide interferes with oxygen delivery. It competes with oxygen for the heme-binding sites and has an affinity that is more than 200 times greater than oxygen.

5. The answer is E. The solubility of HbS is decreased by any condition that increases the amount of deoxyhemoglobin. An increase in the P_{CO_2} shifts the equilibrium from oxyhemoglobin to deoxyhemoglobin, whereas the equilibrium is shifted toward oxyhemoglobin by an increased P_{O_2} and a decreased proton concentration (increased pH). The affinity of HbS for both oxygen and 2,3-BPG is essentially the same as that for HbA.

REFERENCES

1. Myers RAM, Snyder SK, Linberg S, et al: Value of hyperbaric oxygen in suspected carbon monoxide poisoning. *JAMA* 246:2478–2480, 1981.

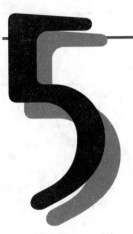

NUTRITION AND METABOLISM

CHAPTER OUTLINE

INTRODUCTION OF CLINICAL CASE

A 72-year-old man was brought to the hospital because of stomach pain. He has lived alone since his wife died 2 years earlier. During the past year, he has been depressed and has rarely left his house. He has had little interest in eating, has lost about 30 lbs, and has become increasingly weak and easily fatigued. The patient indicated that he has had several bruises on his arms and legs and that on two or three occasions he has vomited blood and seen blood in his stools. His diet during the year has consisted mostly of bread, milk, and soups. He described his health as good prior to the last year. Physical examination revealed numerous pinpoint hemorrhages over the arms, legs, and trunk. Laboratory tests showed occult blood in the stools and mild anemia. Gastroscopic examination revealed an ulcer in the stomach [1]. The patient was immediately put on a high-protein diet with vitamin supplementation, and gastric resection was planned. However, the surgery was canceled 2 weeks later because a marked improvement was seen in his condition. He began to engage his doctors and nurses in conversation, seemed to enjoy his meals, and started to gain weight. He began playing cards every day with the patient next-door. The skin hemorrhages decreased, and both the occult blood in the feces and the gastric ulcer disappeared.

INTRODUCTION

Nutrition is the study of the dietary requirements that are necessary to maintain good health. The human body needs a variety of nutrients for growth, reproduction, maintenance of organ structure, and repair of damaged tissues. Various government and private agencies have developed nutritional standards, dietary recommendations, and practical food guides that are designed to promote healthy dietary practices. In the practice of medicine, an understanding of nutrition is essential for both the prevention and treatment of disease.

There are four major types of nutrients: macronutrients, vitamins, minerals, and water. Some are essential; they must be supplied by the diet. Others are considered nonessential because they can be supplied by the body. The macronutrients—carbohydrates, proteins, and lipids—supply energy to the body. Additionally, proteins supply the essential amino acids, lipids supply the essential fatty acids, and carbohydrates supply fiber. Vitamins aid in the utilization of macronutrients and the maintenance of body tissues. Minerals play both structural and functional roles in maintaining homeostasis. Water is the solvent of the body and the transport vehicle for distributing nutrients to the tissues. This chapter focuses on the role nutrients play in maintaining normal body functions. In subsequent chapters, many of these concepts are reinforced by providing examples of their importance in specific aspects of metabolism.

DEFINING A HEALTHY DIET

In the United States, there are currently three types of nutritional guides that are used to promote healthy practices and prevent chronic disease: (1) nutrient standards, (2) dietary recommendations of various health organizations, and (3) practical food guides. Each serves a different purpose.

Nutrient Standards: Recommended Daily Allowances (RDAs)

The RDAs published by the Food and Nutrition Board of the National Research Council provide broad guidelines for the amounts of some well-established nutrients, such as proteins, vitamins, and minerals, which should be consumed daily to maintain normal health [2]. The RDA, an estimate of the amount of specific nutrients required to meet the needs of 95% of the United States population, should be met with a variety of foods. The values given in the RDAs are overestimates, which provide a *margin of safety* for most healthy people. Although the allowances provide for individual variations among most normal people, they do not provide for additional needs that may exist in illness or pathologic disorders.

Key Features of a Healthy Diet
Balance
Variety
Moderation

Dietary Recommendations of Various Health Organizations

Dietary guidelines for promoting health are based on dietary practices that reduce the risk of developing chronic diseases. The dietary guidelines developed by the U.S. Department of Agriculture and the U.S. Department of Health and Human Services are shown in Table 5-1 [3]. The American Heart Association and the American Cancer Society have also issued guidelines for reducing the risk of atherosclerosis and cancer, respectively [4, 5].

Practical Food Guides

A number of food guides have been developed that provide practical information on how to implement sound nutrient standards. For example, the food pyramid is a graphic representation of the elements of a good diet (Figure 5-1). The food group at the base of the pyramid (i.e., breads, cereals, rice, pasta) should be consumed most frequently, while the group at the top of the pyramid (i.e., fats, oils, sweets) should be consumed sparingly. For each food group, the pyramid suggests a range of servings. The lower number of servings is appropriate for individuals requiring about 1600 kilocalories (kcal)/d, while the higher number of servings is for individuals requiring about 2500 kcal/d [6, 7].

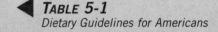

TABLE 5-1
Dietary Guidelines for Americans

Eat a variety of foods.
Maintain a healthy weight.
Choose a diet low in total fat, saturated fat, and cholesterol.
Choose a diet with plenty of vegetables, fruits, and grain products.
Use sugars only in moderation.
Use salt and sodium only in moderation.
If you drink alcoholic beverages, do so in moderation.

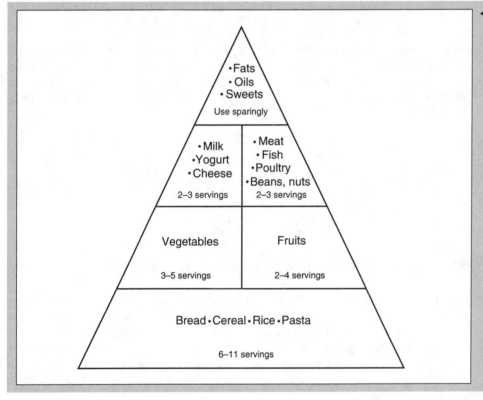

FIGURE 5-1
The Food Pyramid. *The food pyramid indicates the recommended daily servings of various food groups. The levels of the pyramid emphasize the amounts of the different food groups that should be contained in the diet. Foods in one group cannot be substituted for foods in another. Each food group contains some of the nutrients that are needed daily.*

ENERGY REQUIREMENTS

Energy is needed to carry out all of the essential functions of the body. The energy content of foods is expressed in kilocalories and is determined by *direct calorimetry*, a procedure that measures the amount of heat released when food is totally oxidized to carbon dioxide and water in a bomb calorimeter. A kcal is defined as the amount of heat required to raise the temperature of 1 kilogram (kg) of water 1°C. When the amount of nutrients consumed is sufficient to maintain a constant body weight, an individual is said to be in *energy balance*. Insufficient intake results in weight loss, while excessive intake results in weight gain.

Energy Content of Macronutrients	
	kcal/g
Carbohydrate	4.1
Protein	4.1
Fat	9.3
Ethanol	7.1

Daily Energy Requirements

A major portion of energy needed each day is based on the requirement for maintaining normal functions when the body is at rest. This requirement is known as the basal metabolic rate (BMR) or the resting energy expenditure (REE). Additional energy is needed for physical activity and the digestion, absorption, and distribution of nutrients.

Basal Metabolic Rate. The amount of energy required to maintain basic physiologic functions while at rest is influenced by a number of factors. It is directly proportional to the lean body mass, which is defined as the weight after substraction of the fat content, and to body surface area, which can be calculated from height and weight. Adipose tissue has little or no metabolic activity, while tissues such as the liver and kidneys have high metabolic activity. The BMR is higher in men than in women, a reflection of the fact that women have a higher proportion of body fat than men. It is dependent on age, peaking in early childhood and decreasing with increasing age.

An estimate of the BMR in normal individuals can be calculated from the Harris-Benedict equations shown below, where W is weight in kilograms, H is height in centimeters, and A is age in years.

$$\text{Men:} \quad \text{BMR (kcal/hr/kg)} = 66 + (13.7 \times W) + (5 \times H) - (6.8 \times A)$$
$$\text{Women:} \quad \text{BMR (kcal/hr/kg)} = 655 + (9.5 \times W) + (1.8 \times H) - (4.7 \times A)$$

Physical Activity. The energy required to support physical activity is also known as the *energy expenditure of activity (EEA).* The wide variation for individual energy requirements is attributable primarily to the type of exercise involved in the work or recreational activities of the individual. Increased physical activity increases the need for energy (Table 5-2).

TABLE 5-2 ▶
Energy Expenditure of Activity

Type of Activity	Energy Added to BMR (kcal/24 hr)
Sedentary	400–800
Light (office, clerical)	800–1200
Moderate (walking, lifting)	1200–1800
Heavy (construction, athletics)	1800–4500

Note. BMR = basal metabolic rate.

Thermogenic Effect of Feeding. Food intake stimulates metabolism, a property known as the *specific dynamic action* of food. Additional energy is required for the digestion, absorption, and transport of nutrients. An increase in the metabolic rate is observed within an hour after eating. The thermogenic effect varies with the type of nutrient, being maximum with protein, intermediate with carbohydrate, and least with fat. The addition of 10% of the sum of the BMR and the EEA will satisfy the thermogenic effect of feeding.

Factors That Increase the Basal Metabolic Rate

Several factors, some normal and others pathologic, increase the BMR. Additional energy is required by women during *pregnancy* and *lactation*. During the second and third trimesters of pregnancy, an additional 300 kcal/24 hr are required, whereas during lactation, an additional 500 kcal/24 hr are needed. *Injury, sepsis*, and *burns* increase the basal energy requirements by about 30%, 60%, and 100%, respectively, over the BMR predicted by the Harris-Benedict equation.

FUNCTIONS OF THE MACRONUTRIENTS

Energy is provided by the macronutrients—carbohydrate, lipids, and to a lesser extent, protein. Consumption of alcohol can also provide a significant amount of energy. About 40% of the energy that is contained in the energy-containing nutrients is used to synthesize high-energy phosphate compounds, mainly adenosine triphosphate (ATP). The remainder is released into the environment as heat. The recommendations for distributing the calories among the three macronutrients are summarized in Table 5-3 [2]. In addition to supplying energy, each of the macronutrients also has other nutritional functions.

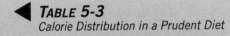
TABLE 5-3
Calorie Distribution in a Prudent Diet

Macronutrients	Percent of Total Calories
Carbohydrate	55%
Protein	15%
Saturated fat	10%
Monosaturated fat	10%
Polyunsaturated fat	10%

Proteins

The major function of dietary protein is to supply essential amino acids for the synthesis of tissue protein and nitrogen for the synthesis of several key compounds, such as neurotransmitters and heme, compounds that play specialized roles in maintaining homeostasis. Ten of the twenty amino acids found in proteins cannot be synthesized by the body in amounts sufficient to support growth, and therefore, they are nutritionally essential. Arginine and histidine are essential only during infancy and early childhood. The remainder of the amino acids can be synthesized in the body from more elemental precursors throughout life. Since there is no storage form for amino acids, the excess arising from dietary protein is either oxidized to produce energy, or it is converted to carbohydrate or lipid.

Essential Amino Acids

Arginine	Valine
Histidine	Threonine
Lysine	Methionine
Leucine	Phenylalanine
Isoleucine	Tryptophan

Fats

There are two essential functions of dietary fat: to provide a vehicle for the absorption of the fat-soluble vitamins and to supply the body with essential fatty acids that cannot be synthesized by humans. The principle function of the essential fatty acids is to act as a precursor for prostaglandins, thromboxanes, and leukotrienes. Dietary lipid also increases the palatability of food and produces a feeling of satiety. Additionally, dietary lipids supply energy and building blocks for membrane assembly, though neither is an essential function, since most lipids can be synthesized from intermediates in carbohydrate and protein metabolism.

Essential Fatty Acids
Linoleic acid
Linolenic acid

Carbohydrates

Most dietary carbohydrate is used as a fuel. It can be degraded immediately as a source of energy, it can be stored as glycogen, or it can be converted to fat for storage. Dietary carbohydrate is of two types, available and unavailable carbohydrate. *Available carbohydrate* is digested, absorbed, and used for energy, while *unavailable carbohydrate* supplies dietary fiber. Fiber is not degraded by the digestive enzymes and does not serve as a source of energy. It is, however, a significant component of the diet. In general, it increases stool bulk and decreases the time that waste material stays in the gastrointestinal tract. Fiber from different sources has different physiochemical properties and often different physiologic effects. Some soluble fibers can be degraded by the bacterial flora in the colon, producing carbon dioxide, methane, and low molecular weight acids.

Fiber and Health
The presence of fiber in the diet has been correlated with a decreased incidence of cardiovascular disease and colon cancer. A healthy diet should contain 25 g–35 g of fiber per day. Excess fiber intake may lower the absorption of mineral nutrients.

VITAMINS

The vitamins are a heterogeneous group of nutrients that are required in small amounts and must be supplied by the diet. They are organic compounds, having molecular weights less than 1000, and they are generally converted by the body to more complex molecules that play key roles in metabolism. The vitamins are usually classified in two major groups, the water-soluble vitamins and the fat-soluble vitamins. The water-soluble vitamins function as precursors for coenzymes, while the fat-soluble vitamins function as coenzymes, hormones, and antioxidants. A balanced and varied diet is the best source of vitamins for a healthy person [8].

Water-Soluble Vitamins

The water-soluble vitamins are vitamin C and the eight vitamins of the B complex: niacin, riboflavin, thiamine, pantothenic acid, pyridoxine, biotin, cobalamin, and folic acid. With the exception of cobalamin, the water-soluble vitamins are not stored and must be provided regularly in the diet. The water-soluble vitamins are usually not toxic since excess amounts are excreted in the urine. The physiologic functions and consequences of a deficiency are summarized in Table 5-4.

TABLE 5-4 ▶

Water-Soluble Vitamins: Functions and Consequences of a Deficiency

Vitamin	Physiologic Function	Deficiency Symptoms
Vitamin C	Reduction of iron and hydroxylation reactions (collagen, catecholamine, carnitine synthesis)	Scurvy
Niacin	Oxidation-reduction reactions (carbohydrate, lipid metabolism)	Pellagra
Riboflavin	Oxidation-reduction reactions (carbohydrate, lipid, amino acid metabolism)	Ariboflavinosis
Thiamine	Oxidative decarboxylation and transketolation reactions (carbohydrate, branched-chain amino acid metabolism)	Beriberi
Pantothenic acid	Acyl group transfer reactions (terminal oxidation of all fuels, lipid metabolism)	Adrenal insufficiency[a]
Pyridoxine	Transamination and decarboxylation reactions (amino acid metabolism)	Irritability, convulsions, and confusion
Biotin	Carboxylation reactions (gluconeogenesis, fatty acid synthesis, branched-chain amino acid metabolism)	Alopecia and dermatitis
Folic acid	One-carbon transfer reactions (purine and pyrimidine synthesis, amino acid interconversions)	Megaloblastic anemia
Cobalamin	Methylation and isomerization reactions (amino acid metabolism)	Pernicious anemia and neurologic effects

[a] Observed only in experimental animals.

Scurvy is a disease caused by vitamin C deficiency; the major symptoms include easy bruising, pinpoint hemorrhages of the skin, soft bleeding gums with loose teeth, swollen joints, and poor wound healing.

Ascorbic Acid (Vitamin C). Vitamin C has two major roles in metabolism. It facilitates the *absorption of iron* by reducing dietary iron to its ferrous state (Fe^{2+}), the form that is transported across the membrane of intestinal cells. Vitamin C also acts as a reducing agent in *hydroxylation reactions*, which are required in the synthesis of collagen, catecholamines, and carnitine. A deficiency in vitamin C causes scurvy. Citrus fruits and fresh vegetables are the best dietary sources of the vitamin. The RDA for vitamin C is 60 mg. More may be required during pregnancy and lactation [8].

Pellagra is a disease caused by niacin deficiency; the major symptoms are the three D's: dermatitis, diarrhea, and dementia.

Niacin (Vitamin B_3). Niacin is the precursor of the oxidized forms of nicotinamide adenine dinucleotide (NAD^+) and nicotinamide-adenine dinucleotide phosphate ($NADP^+$), coenzymes that participate in many *oxidation and reduction reactions* in carbohydrate and lipid metabolism. NAD^+ functions primarily as an oxidizing agent for extracting energy from dietary fuels, while the reduced form of $NADP^+$ (NADPH) serves as a reducing agent in many synthetic reactions in metabolism. A small amount of niacin can be synthesized endogenously from tryptophan, but most is derived from meat, nuts, and grains. Niacin deficiency results in pellagra. The RDA for niacin is expressed in terms of niacin equivalents, where one equivalent is equal to 1 mg of niacin or 60 mg of tryptophan. The RDA for niacin is related to energy expenditure, with 6.6 mg of niacin required per 1000 kcal [8].

Riboflavin (Vitamin B₂). Riboflavin is the precursor for flavin adenine dinucleotide (FAD) and flavin mononucleotide (FMN), coenzymes that are essential for aerobic metabolism. Both participate in *oxidative reactions* of carbohydrate, lipid, and amino acid metabolism. The key enzymes that use FAD are succinate dehydrogenase and fatty acyl CoA dehydrogenase, while the most prominent enzymes using FMN are NADH dehydrogenase and the amino acid oxidases. Good sources of riboflavin are milk products, liver, grains, and vegetables. Riboflavin deficiency is rare, and it is most likely to occur in conjunction with other B vitamin deficiencies. The RDA for riboflavin is related to the total energy needs, with 0.6 mg required per 1000 kcal [3].

Thiamine (Vitamin B₁). The major form of thiamine found in the body is thiamine pyrophosphate (TPP). TPP is used primarily as a coenzyme in reactions that extract energy from glucose or convert excess glucose to fat for storage. Mitochondrial enzymes requiring TTP are pyruvate dehydrogenase, α-ketoglutarate dehydrogenase, and branched-chain α-ketoacid dehydrogenase. All catalyze *oxidative decarboxylation of α-ketoacids*. TPP is also required by transketolase, a key enzyme in the pentose phosphate pathway. Major diseases associated with thiamine deficiency are beriberi and Wernicke-Korsakoff syndrome, which is seen in chronic alcoholism. Good sources of thiamine are unrefined cereal grains and meats. The RDA for thiamine is 0.5 mg/1000 kcal [8].

Pantothenic Acid (Vitamin B₅). Pantothenic acid is converted by the body to coenzyme A (CoA). CoA acts as a universal carrier of acyl groups in metabolic reactions. It is required for the *terminal oxidation* of carbohydrate, lipid, and amino acids, as well as for the synthesis of fatty acids, triglycerides, cholesterol, and steroids. Pantothenic acid is widely distributed in both plant and animal tissues, and there is little evidence of dietary deficiency in humans.

Pyridoxine (Vitamin B₆). Vitamin B₆ refers to pyridoxine, pyridoxal, and pyridoxamine, compounds that are interconvertible by the body. The most important coenzyme derived from vitamin B₆ is pyridoxal phosphate, although pyridoxamine phosphate also participates in some reactions. These coenzymes are involved almost exclusively in *amino acid metabolism*, where they function in numerous transamination, decarboxylation, and racemization reactions. Good sources of pyridoxine are liver, wheat germ, peas, and potatoes. The RDA increases with the amount of protein in the diet. In adults, the RDA is 2.2 mg/100 g of protein. Women taking oral contraceptives also have an increased requirement [3]. Vitamin B₆ deficiency is rare.

Biotin. The function of biotin is to participate in *carboxylation* reactions. Biotin differs from other vitamins in that conversion to the coenzyme form requires only that it be covalently attached to the appropriate enzyme. The attachment of biotin to different carboxylases requires ATP and is catalyzed by an enzyme known as *holoenzyme synthetase*. Biotin-mediated carboxylation reactions are key reactions in gluconeogenesis, fatty acid synthesis, and branched-chain amino acid metabolism. Biotin is widely distributed in natural foods. In plant foods, it is found in a free form, but in animal foods, it is linked to protein, requiring the enzyme *biotinidase* to release it and make it available for use. Biotin is synthesized by intestinal bacteria in amounts that normally meet the daily needs of humans, and a deficiency resulting from inadequate dietary sources is rare. However, deficiency can be induced by the use of broad-spectrum antibiotics over a long period of time, as well as by the excessive consumption of raw eggs. Egg whites contain avidin, a protein that binds biotin very tightly, making it unavailable. Inherited defects in both holoenzyme synthetase and biotinidase also have been reported to result in biotin deficiency.

Folic Acid (Folacin). The coenzyme form of folic acid is *tetrahydrofolate* (THF or TH₄), which acts as a *carrier of one-carbon units* in several reactions of amino acid and nucleotide metabolism. The one-carbon units are donated to THF during the degradation of glycine, serine, histidine, and tryptophan, and they are used in the synthesis of purines, pyrimidines, methionine, and serine. Folic acid is present in many foods, but as much as 50%–90% may be lost during cooking. The RDA for adults is from 180 μg to 200 μg. Additional supplements are required during pregnancy and lactation. Additional folic acid is required during chemotherapy with methotrexate and other folic acid ana-

Ariboflavinosis is a deficiency state associated with riboflavin deficiency; the symptoms are swollen lips, cracks at the corners of the mouth, and a swollen and red tongue. A decline in RBC riboflavin is the earliest biochemical indicator of riboflavin deficiency.

Beriberi is a deficiency state associated with thiamine deficiency; the early symptoms include weight loss, weakness, and anorexia ("dry beriberi"). Symptoms that appear after prolonged deficiency include edema and numerous cardiovascular and neurologic abnormalities ("wet beriberi").

Wernicke-Korsakoff Syndrome
This disorder is observed in chronic alcoholics who are thiamine deficient. The transketolase in these individuals has a greatly reduced affinity for TPP. The symptoms include ataxia, confusion, and paralysis of the ocular muscles, which can be relieved by thiamine administration. If untreated, amnesia develops that is much less responsive to thiamine.

Vitamin B₆ Deficiency
Hyperirritability and convulsive seizures may occur in infants with vitamin B₆ deficiency, while in adults, oily dermatitis and inflammation of the mouth are more commonly seen. Deficiency is most commonly seen in tuberculosis patients being treated with isoniazid and in patients with copper storage disease who are being treated with penicillamine. Both drugs deplete pyridoxine.

Biotin Deficiency
The symptoms are hair loss, dermatitis, and depression, which are reversed by administration of the vitamin.

Antibiotics and Vitamin Deficiencies
Prolonged exposure to antibiotics results in deficiency of vitamin B₁₂, vitamin K, and biotin.

Folic Acid Deficiency
The symptoms are growth failure and megaloblastic anemia, the result of impaired DNA synthesis. Deficiency in the early stages of pregnancy can result in neural tube defects.

logues that interfere with purine and pyrimidine synthesis. Folic acid deficiency is commonly observed in chronic alcoholism and during pregnancy [8].

Cobalamin (Vitamin B$_{12}$). Cobalamin is a complex molecule consisting of a ring structure similar to that of heme but containing a central cobalt atom rather than an iron atom. Cobalamin exists in three forms that differ in the nature of the chemical group attached to cobalt. The cyano derivative, commonly known as cyanocobalamin, is the principal form in commercially available vitamin B$_{12}$. Other forms are methylcobalamin and deoxyadenosylcobalamin. There are only two known reactions in human metabolism that require vitamin B$_{12}$, and both are involved in *amino acid metabolism*. The isomerization of methylmalonyl CoA to succinyl CoA, a key reaction in the catabolism of the branched-chain amino acids, requires deoxyadenosylcobalamin; and the conversion of homocysteine to methionine requires methylcobalamin. In nature, all of the vitamin B$_{12}$ is synthesized by microorganisms. It is found in foods of animal origin but is absent in plant foods. Therefore, strict vegetarians are at risk for vitamin B$_{12}$ deficiency, and their diets should be supplemented with commercial cobalamin or with yeast. Vitamin B$_{12}$ is the only water-soluble vitamin that is stored in significant amounts in the body. The RDA for adults is 400 µg with higher allowances for pregnant and lactating women [3]. The clinical symptoms of vitamin B$_{12}$ deficiency are collectively referred to as pernicious anemia.

Fat-Soluble Vitamins

The fat-soluble vitamins A, D, E, and K are hydrophobic molecules that are assembled from isoprenoid units, the same building blocks that are used to synthesize cholesterol. Because of their hydrophobic nature, they are transported in the blood bound either to lipoproteins or other specific carrier proteins. The fat-soluble vitamins are absorbed from the intestine along with other dietary lipids. Abnormalities in lipid absorption usually result in decreased uptake of all of the fat-soluble vitamins. Large quantities of the fat-soluble vitamins can be stored in the liver and adipose tissue, and toxicity can result from excessive intake of vitamins A and D. Vitamin E and K are considered nontoxic. The fat-soluble vitamins have diverse biologic functions. As a group, they can act as coenzymes, hormones, and antioxidants. The major functions and the deficiency symptoms associated with each of the fat-soluble vitamins are summarized in Table 5-5.

Pernicious Anemia
This anemia results from a defect in the absorption of vitamin B$_{12}$. Intrinsic factor, a protein synthesized in the gastric mucosa and required for vitamin B$_{12}$ absorption is deficient. The RBC morphology is indistinguishable from that seen with folate deficiency.

TABLE 5-5 ▶
Fat-Soluble Vitamins: Functions and Consequences of a Deficiency

Vitamin	Physiologic Function	Deficiency Symptoms
Vitamin A	Vision, reproduction, maintenance, and differentiation of epithelial tissue	Night blindness and hyperkeratosis
Vitamin D	Calcium and phosphate metabolism and maintenance of skeletal integrity	Rickets (children) and osteomalacia (adults)
Vitamin E	Antioxidant	Lipid peroxidation and hemolytic anemia
Vitamin K	Carboxylation of clotting factors	Hemorrhage and bruising

Vitamin A. The primary precursor of vitamin A is β-carotene, the pigment found in yellow vegetables. Beta-carotene can be converted by the body into three forms, *retinol, retinal,* and *retinoic acid,* each having unique biologic functions (Figure 5-2). Retinal is a cofactor for rhodopsin, a protein required for normal vision. Rhodopsin is composed of the protein opsin and 11-*cis* retinal. The initial event in converting light to a nerve impulse is the isomerization of 11-*cis* retinal to the all-*trans* isomer. Lack of vitamin A results in night blindness. Both retinol and retinal act as hormones that regulate the rate at which certain genes are expressed. Retinol is required for the normal reproductive process in both men and women. Lack of vitamin A produces sterility, testicular degeneration, and aborted or malformed offspring. Both retinol and retinoic acid are required for normal growth and differentiation of epithelial tissue. Without vitamin A, epithelial cells become dry and gradually harden to form keratin, a process known as keratinization.

Vitamin A Toxicity
Excessive use of vitamin A can result in joint pain, dry skin, headaches, anorexia, loss of hair, edema, and liver damage. High doses during pregnancy can produce birth defects, such as craniofacial abnormalities, harelip, congenital heart disease, and kidney defects.

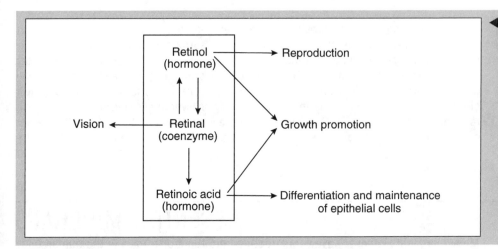

FIGURE 5-2
Forms and Functions of Vitamin A. The three forms of vitamin A correspond to different oxidation states, progressing from an alcohol to an aldehyde to an acid. Retinal acts as a coenzyme in the visual process, and retinol and retinoic acids act as hormones that regulate the rate at which specific genes are transcribed.

Vitamin D. The active form of vitamin D is required for the regulation of *calcium and phosphate metabolism* and the maintenance of skeletal integrity. The exogenous precursors of vitamin D are ergosterol (vitamin D_2), which occurs in plants, and cholecalciferol (vitamin D_3), which occurs in animal tissues. An endogenous precursor of vitamin D_3, 7-dehydrocholesterol, is stored under the skin and converted to vitamin D_3 by ultraviolet irradiation from sunlight. Both vitamins D_2 and D_3 are converted to 1,25-dihydroxy-cholecalciferol, the physiologically active form, by hydroxylation reactions that occur in the liver and kidney (Figure 5-3). The active form of vitamin D stimulates calcium and phosphate absorption from the intestinal lumen, as well as mobilization from bone. A deficiency of vitamin D or inadequate exposure to sunlight results in rickets in children and osteomalacia in adults. The most reliable source of vitamin D is milk that has been fortified. Oily fish and yeast are also good sources.

Vitamin D Toxicity
Symptoms of vitamin D toxicity include weakness, fatigue, headache, nausea, and constipation. Most of the toxic effects are the result of hypercalcemia.

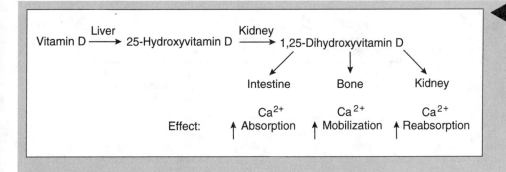

FIGURE 5-3
Activation and Functions of Vitamin D. The conversion of vitamin D_2 and D_3 to the active form requires two hydroxylation reactions, which occur sequentially in the liver and kidney, producing 1,25-dihydroxyvitamin D. The overall effect of vitamin D is to increase the serum level of calcium. This is achieved by stimulating calcium absorption in the intestine, mobilization from bone, and reabsorption by the kidney.

Vitamin E. Vitamin E belongs to a family of compounds known as *tocopherols*. The biologic activity of these compounds is proportional to their ability to act as *antioxidants*, with the most abundant and active species being α-tocopherol. Vitamin E inhibits the peroxidation of polyunsaturated fatty acids and is especially important in preventing hemolysis of red blood cells (RBCs). Vitamin E and selenium act synergistically in protecting against lipid peroxidation. Good dietary sources of vitamin E include corn, soybean, and safflower oils, and a variety of vegetables and fruits. A balanced diet usually provides adequate vitamin E, although supplementation is recommended during pregnancy and lactation. *The requirement for vitamin E increases with an increase in dietary polyunsaturated fatty acids.* Adults normally contain large stores of vitamin E, and signs of a dietary insufficiency are slow to appear. Large doses have been used in a number of clinical situations including malabsorption syndromes, cystic fibrosis, and pancreatic insufficiency. There are relatively few toxic effects associated with vitamin E, although very high doses may interfere with vitamin K metabolism.

Vitamin E Deficiency
The symptoms include hemolytic anemia, psychomotor dysfunction, and myopathy with elevated creatinine in the urine.

Vitamin K. Vitamin K occurs naturally in two forms, phylloquinone, which is found in green plants, and menaquinones, which are produced by microorganisms. It is essential for normal blood clotting. Vitamin K is a cofactor for γ-*glutamate carboxylase*, an enzyme that converts glutamate side chains of prothrombin and other clotting factors to γ-carboxyglutamate. The γ-carboxyglutamate residues act as sites where calcium can form bridges between the clotting factors and the surface of platelets. The accumulation of clotting factors on the surface of platelets markedly enhances the rate of blood clotting. Since vitamin K is synthesized by intestinal bacteria and is also widely distributed in plant and animal foods, a deficiency in adults is rare. Vitamin K deficiency occurs most commonly in fat malabsorption syndromes and in newborns who lack the intestinal bacteria. Concentration of the vitamin is low in both breast milk and cow's milk. The most notable symptoms of vitamin K deficiency are impaired clotting and easy bruising.

ESSENTIAL MINERALS

Many inorganic elements have vital structural and functional roles in the human body. They are frequently classified in two groups: the major minerals that are required in amounts greater than 100 mg/d and the trace elements that are required in amounts less than 100 mg/d.

Major Minerals

The seven minerals most abundant in the human body are calcium, phosphorus, magnesium, sodium, potassium, chloride, and sulfur. The principal functions of each of the major minerals and the deficiency diseases or symptoms associated with each are summarized in Table 5-6. Mineral requirements are usually met by a diet that is adequate in dairy products, whole-grain cereals, legumes, and leafy green vegetables [3].

Calcium and Phosphorus. About 99% of the calcium in the body serves a structural role in bones and teeth where it exists as deposits of calcium phosphate crystals, known as

TABLE 5-6 ▶
Essential Major Minerals: Functions and Consequences of Deficiency

Major Mineral	Physiologic Function	Deficiency Symptoms
Calcium	Calcification of bone, blood clotting, and regulation of nerve, muscle, and hormone function	Tetany, muscle cramps, convulsions, bone fractures, and loss of height and bone mass
Phosphorus	Constituent of bones, teeth, nucleic acids, and ATP; required for energy metabolism	Growth retardation, skeletal deformities, muscle weakness, diminished phagocytic function, and increased hemolysis of RBCs
Magnesium	Cofactor for many enzymes; essential for ATP metabolism, muscle contraction, membrane transport, and nerve transmission	Muscle spasms, tetany, seizures, and deficiency secondary to malabsorption, diarrhea
Sodium	Principal extracellular cation; essential for regulation of plasma volume, acid–base balance, nerve and muscle function; sodium (Na^+), potassium (K^+)-ATPase	Fluid volume depletion and deficiency secondary to vomiting, diarrhea, diuretic abuse, or adrenal insufficiency
Potassium	Principal intracellular cation; nerve and muscle function; Na^+, K^+-ATPase	Muscle weakness, paralysis, and mental confusion; deficiency usually associated with alkalosis
Chloride	Principal extracellular anion; component of gastric fluid; bicarbonate transport in RBCs	Deficiency secondary to vomiting and diarrhea
Sulfur	Connective tissue proteoglycans; bile acid conjugation; detoxification reactions	Unknown

hydroxyapatite. The remaining 1% of the calcium is found mainly in the serum and in the mitochondria of cells. Soluble calcium ions participate in a variety of regulatory mechanisms. Phosphate, a component of cellular ATP and other nucleotides, plays a major role in energy metabolism.

Magnesium. Magnesium is required for normal nerve and muscle function. It is also essential for the metabolism of ATP and acts as a cofactor for more than 300 different enzymes involved in carbohydrate, lipid, protein, and nucleic acid metabolism. It is highly concentrated in the mitochondria of cells. Hypomagnesemia is frequently seen in chronic alcoholism and in patients with abnormalities in fat absorption.

Sodium, Potassium, and Chloride. Sodium, potassium, and chloride are the major dissolved ions in the body fluids. Sodium is found primarily in the extracellular fluid, and potassium in the intracellular fluid, while chloride is found in both. Abnormalities in the extracellular fluid volume are usually caused by increases or decreases in the sodium content. Chloride helps maintain electrical neutrality by acting as counter ions that move across cell membranes to compensate for fluxes in other ions.

Clinical Use of Magnesium Salts
Epsom salt (magnesium sulfate) is used as a laxative, while milk of magnesia and magnesium hydroxide are commonly used as antacids.

Trace Elements

There are a number of elements that are required in small amounts but are essential for normal health and development (Table 5-7). Many of these elements are toxic when consumed in excessive amounts.

◀ **TABLE 5-7**
Trace Elements: Functions and Consequences of Deficiency

Trace Element	Physiologic Function	Deficiency Symptoms
Chromium	Potentiates the effect of insulin	Impaired glucose metabolism
Cobalt	Constituent of vitamin B_{12}	Macrocytic anemia
Copper	Iron absorption and mobilization; oxidative enzymes	Microcytic anemia, depigmentation of skin and hair, connective tissue and skeletal abnormalities
Fluoride	Component of calcified tissues; teeth and bone strength	Dental caries
Iodine	Constituent of thyroid hormones	Cretinism (children) and goiter (adults)
Iron	Oxygen transport and storage; oxidative reactions; electron transport chain	Pallor, fatigue, and microcytic anemia
Manganese	Cofactor for enzymes of glycoprotein and proteoglycan synthesis	Not well defined
Molybdenum	Cofactor for xanthine oxidase, sulfite oxidase, and aldehyde oxidase	Unknown
Selenium	Cofactor for glutathione peroxidase; protects cells against membrane peroxidation	Cardiomyopathy
Zinc	Growth, sexual maturation, fertility, and immune function; cofactor for enzymes in DNA, RNA, and protein synthesis	Hypogonadism, growth failure, impaired wound healing, defects in taste and smell, and loss of appetite

Iron. Most of the iron in the body is found in heme, the cofactor used by hemoglobin and myoglobin for oxygen transport and storage, respectively. Iron is also found in cytochromes and nonheme iron proteins, which participate in oxidative reactions in the cell. Most of the iron is salvaged from heme and reused, making the amount of dietary requirement for iron small. The intestinal absorption of iron is very inefficient but is facilitated by ascorbic acid. Normally, about 10% of the dietary iron is absorbed. Iron is

Iron Deficiency and Hypochromic Microcytic Anemia
A prolonged deficiency of iron or copper results in a type of anemia characterized by small, pale RBCs.

delivered to cells by the plasma protein *transferrin*, and intracellular stores of iron are bound to *ferritin* and *hemosiderin*, an aggregate of ferritin. Iron deficiency is one of the most common nutritional deficiencies in the world, occurring most frequently in infancy and in women who are menstruating, pregnant, or lactating. When iron deficiency occurs in men or in postmenopausal women, bleeding is often the cause of the deficiency. Excessive intake of iron results in iron overload, a condition known as hemochromatosis [8].

Copper. Copper facilitates iron absorption and mobilization. It is also an essential cofactor for cytochrome oxidase and a number of oxidative enzymes that are involved in amino acid metabolism, catecholamine, collagen, elastin, and melanin synthesis. Dietary deficiency of copper is rare but is seen in individuals with *Menke's disease*, a genetic deficiency in copper transport. Copper deficiency has also been seen in children who are fed only cow's milk. The clinical manifestations of copper deficiency include depigmentation of skin and hair, and a type of anemia that is indistinguishable from iron deficiency anemia. Copper toxicity from excessive accumulation of copper is seen in *Wilson's disease*, which results from a genetic deficiency in ceruloplasmin, the plasma protein that transports copper to tissues. Wilson's disease is characterized by low serum levels of copper, high urinary copper, and excessive copper accumulation in the liver, kidney, brain, and eye.

Iodine. Most dietary iodine is taken up by the thyroid gland where it is incorporated into the thyroid hormones, thyroxin and triiodothyronine. The thyroid hormones have an anabolic effect on most tissues, stimulating growth and development. A dietary deficiency of iodine in children results in *cretinism*, a condition characterized by impaired physical and mental development. An iodine deficiency in adults stimulates the proliferation of thyroid epithelial cells, resulting in *goiter*. Paradoxically, goiter can also result from high concentrations of iodine, probably because the incorporation of iodine into the thyroid hormones is blocked by high plasma iodine concentrations.

Zinc. Zinc is a cofactor for more than 100 enzymes and is of particular importance in rapidly growing tissues. The synthesis of DNA, RNA, and protein is inhibited by a deficiency of zinc. Most of the zinc in plasma is bound to albumin and α-macroglobulin, while most of the intracellular zinc is bound to the metal-binding protein metallothioneine.

Manganese. Manganese is required by a number of enzymes that are involved in glycoprotein and proteoglycan biosynthesis. Manganese deficiency has been associated with diabetes, pancreatic insufficiency, and protein-calorie malnutrition. The clinical signs of manganese deficiency are not well defined. Toxicity occurs as an industrial disease in workers who inhale fumes or dust containing manganese. Symptoms of toxicity include psychosis and neuromuscular effects similar to those of Parkinson's disease.

Selenium. Selenium is found in all body tissues except fat. It is an integral component of *glutathione peroxidase*, an enzyme that protects cells and membranes against oxidative damage. The effects of selenium and vitamin E are synergistic, each sparing the need for the other. The selenium content of food varies with the content of soil. In areas of China where the intake is low, a high incidence of *cardiomyopathy* occurs that can be prevented by selenium supplements. Selenium also acts as a structural component found in the protein matrix of teeth.

Chromium. Chromium is an essential component of glucose tolerance factor, a protein that facilitates the binding of insulin to its receptors. Chromium deficiency results in a decreased response to insulin and impaired removal of glucose from the circulation.

RESOLUTION OF CLINICAL CASE

The patient in the case presented at the beginning of the chapter was living alone, eating poorly, and suffering from malnutrition. He was ultimately diagnosed as having scurvy. Many of the symptoms in this case can be attributed to a deficiency in vitamin C. His diet consisted mainly of milk, bread, and soup, which are poor sources of vitamin C. The primary function of vitamin C is to serve as a cofactor in the hydroxylation reactions that are required for the maturation of collagen. Collagen formed in the absence of vitamin C does not form normal cross-linked fibers, resulting in fragile blood vessels that rupture easily. One of the most common characteristics of scurvy is small perifollicular hemorrhages in the skin, like those that were found on the arms, legs, and trunk of this patient. Collagen synthesis is a normal component of wound healing; therefore, it is not surprising that scurvy can present as a gastric ulcer that disappears with vitamin supplementation. The amount of ascorbic acid given to this patient was 1 g daily for 2 weeks, followed by 150 mg daily for a month. Blood tests showed that the serum vitamin C level was within the normal range following this treatment. Mild anemia is seen in about 75% of individuals with scurvy as a result of bleeding. Another factor that may also contribute to anemia is inadequate absorption of iron, which is secondary to the deficiency in vitamin C. The possibility of a vitamin B_{12} deficiency may also contribute to anemia. Morphologic examination of blood cells should help distinguish between these possibilities, since iron deficiency anemia is characterized by RBCs that are small and hypochromic, whereas vitamin B_{12} deficiency results in abnormally large RBCs. The psychologic changes seen in this patient are common in scurvy. A triad of hysteria, depression, and hypochondria is typical; and in older people, it may be confused with a syndrome associated with aging. The psychological response to ascorbic acid in these patients can be dramatic [9].

REVIEW QUESTIONS

Directions: For each of the following questions, choose the **one best** answer.

1. An impaired ability to oxidize carbohydrate and fats is directly related to a deficiency of which of the following vitamins?

   (A) Pyridoxine

   (B) Vitamin D

   (C) Niacin

   (D) Biotin

   (E) Folic acid

2. A decrease in nucleic acid synthesis is directly related to a deficiency in which of the following vitamins?

   (A) Vitamin A

   (B) Folic acid

   (C) Vitamin D

   (D) Vitamin C

   (E) Vitamin K

3. A biotin deficiency is likely to decrease which of the following metabolic processes?

   (A) Pyruvate oxidation

   (B) Fatty acid oxidation

   (C) Cholesterol synthesis

   (D) Fatty acid synthesis

   (E) Glycogen synthesis

4. Which of the following vitamins can cause birth defects when taken in large doses during pregnancy?

   (A) Vitamin B_{12}

   (B) Vitamin C

   (C) Vitamin A

   (D) Folate

   (E) Vitamin E

Directions: The groups of questions below consist of lettered choices followed by several numbered items. For each numbered item, select the appropriate lettered option with which it is most closely associated. Each lettered option may be used once, more than once, or not at all.

Questions 5-10

For each clinical condition listed below, select the vitamin deficiency most likely to be associated with it.

- **(A)** Niacin
- **(B)** Thiamine
- **(C)** Vitamin K
- **(D)** Folic acid
- **(E)** Vitamin B_{12}
- **(F)** Vitamin A
- **(G)** Vitamin D
- **(H)** Vitamin C
- **(I)** Pyridoxine
- **(J)** Vitamin E

5. Pernicious anemia

6. Night blindness

7. Wernicke-Korsakoff syndrome

8. Osteomalacia

9. Hemolytic anemia

10. Pellagra

Questions 11-15

For each clinical condition listed below, select the mineral most likely to be deficient.

- **(A)** Iron
- **(B)** Zinc
- **(C)** Cobalt
- **(D)** Chromium
- **(E)** Manganese
- **(F)** Selenium
- **(G)** Molybdenum
- **(H)** Iodine

11. Hypogonadism

12. Cardiomyopathy

13. Goiter

14. Microcytic anemia

15. Glucose intolerance

ANSWERS AND EXPLANATIONS

1. The answer is C. Niacin is the precursor for NAD+, a coenzyme required for the oxidation of both carbohydrate and fat. Pyridoxine is involved almost exclusively in amino acid metabolism, and folic acid transfers one-carbon units between amino acids and intermediates in purine and pyrimidine synthesis. Biotin participates in synthetic, but not oxidative, pathways of glucose and fatty acid metabolism. A deficiency in vitamin D affects skeletal integrity but has no direct effect on carbohydrate or fat metabolism.

2. The answer is B. Nucleic acid synthesis requires purine and pyrimidine nucleotide building blocks. Folic acid is required for the synthesis of both purines and pyrimidines. A deficiency in vitamins A and D alters the rate at which specific genes in DNA are transcribed but has no effect on the synthesis of nucleic acids. Vitamins K and C are not required for nucleic acid synthesis.

3. The answer is D. Biotin is required for fatty acid synthesis but not for oxidation. Other pathways that are decreased by biotin deficiency are gluconeogenesis and branched-chain amino acid metabolism. Pyruvate oxidation, cholesterol synthesis, and glycogen synthesis are unaffected.

4. The answer is C. When taken during pregnancy, large doses of vitamin A can cause multiple birth defects and malformations in the developing fetus. A deficiency in folate during the early stages of embryogenesis can result in spina bifida. Supplementation with vitamins B_{12}, C, E, and folate is recommended during pregnancy.

5–10. The answers are: 5-E, 6-F, 7-B, 8-G, 9-K, 10-A. Pernicious anemia is associated with vitamin B_{12} deficiency, although the megaloblastic appearance of the RBCs is the same with vitamin B_{12} and folate deficiency. Night blindness results from a deficiency of retinal, one of the forms of vitamin A. Wernicke-Korsakoff syndrome and beriberi are both associated with thiamine deficiency, but Wernicke-Korsakoff syndrome is the form of the deficiency seen in chronic alcoholism. Osteomalacia, a weakening of the bones, is observed in adults with a vitamin D deficiency. A deficiency in vitamin E frequently leads to increased lipid peroxidation, resulting in hemolytic anemia. Pellagra, seen with a niacin deficiency, is characterized by dermatitis, diarrhea, and dementia.

11–15. The answers are: 11-B, 12-F, 13-H, 14-A, 15-D. Zinc is required for normal sexual maturation and fertility. Selenium is required to prevent oxidative damage to cells and membranes. One of the most common consequences of selenium deficiency is cardiomyopathy. Goiter can result from either a deficiency or an excess of iodine. Microcytic anemia can result from either an iron or copper deficiency and is characterized by small pale RBCs. Chromium is required for insulin to function properly. A deficiency in either insulin or chromium can result in an impaired ability to remove glucose from the circulation.

REFERENCES

1. Dewhurst K: A case of scurvy simulating a gastric neoplasm. *Br Med* 2:1148–1150, 1954.
2. Food and Nutrition Board, Commission on Life Sciences, National Research Council: *Recommended Dietary Allowances*, 10th ed. Washington, DC: National Academy Press, 1989.
3. Weinser RL, Morgan SL: *Fundamentals of Clinical Nutrition*. St. Louis, MO: C. V. Mosby, 1993.
4. American Heart Association: Dietary guidelines for healthy American adults. *Circulation* 94:1465–1468, 1986.
5. American Cancer Society: Guidelines on diet, nutrition, and cancer. *Cancer* 41:335–338, 1991.
6. Willet WC: Diet and health: what should we eat? *Science* 294:532–537, 1994.
7. U.S. Department of Health and Human Services: *Surgeon General's Report on Nutrition and Health*. Washington, DC: U. S. Department of Health and Human Services (Publication No. 88-50211), 1988.
8. Williams SR: *Essentials of Nutrition and Diet Therapy*, 5th ed. St. Louis, MO: C. V. Mosby, 1990.
9. Scurvy in an old man. *Nutr Rev* 41:152–154, 1983.

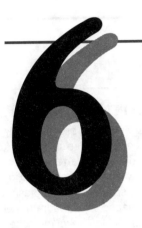

BIOENERGETICS: BASIC PRINCIPLES OF ENERGY METABOLISM

CHAPTER OUTLINE

INTRODUCTION OF CLINICAL CASE

A 15-year-old girl was admitted to the hospital complaining of shortness of breath and leg cramps after walking one block. She complained of low tolerance to exercise since age 7, but her condition worsened when at age 10 muscle weakness developed after exercise. Upon physical examination, her vital signs were normal. There was mild muscle wasting and marked weakness of all muscle groups. Laboratory studies showed normal plasma electrolytes except for bicarbonate, which was reduced. When placed on a treadmill, her pulse rate increased from 80 to 160 in 3 minutes, and her serum lactate level increased fourfold. Electron microscopy of muscle biopsy material revealed abnormal mitochondria, and deposits of glycogen and fat in the muscle cells [1]. She was treated with a variety of vitamins, including thiamine, pyridoxine, biotin, nicotinic acid, and riboflavin, but none affected her serum lactate levels or relieved her symptoms [2]. She was discharged to an outpatient clinic where she was followed routinely. At age 17, she had a serious episode of lactic acidosis and was readmitted to the hospital. Noninvasive analysis of muscle using ^{31}P-NMR techniques showed a creatine phosphate/inorganic phosphate ratio that was sixfold lower than that of a normal person of the same age and sex. Measurement of several mitochondrial enzymes in muscle tissue showed an absence of cytochrome-c reductase activity when incubated with either malate or succinate as oxidizable substrates. The cytochrome-b content of the patient's mitochondria was undetectable. The patient was treated with pharmacologic doses of menadione and ascorbic acid. Within 24 hours of starting treatment, she showed marked improvement. She was able to walk several blocks without stopping. Over the next year, her improvement was maintained. Her blood lactate level remained elevated, although it was not as high as before treatment.

OVERVIEW

Bioenergetics is the study of energy changes that accompany chemical reactions in living organisms. Some reactions are exergonic and release energy, while others are endergonic and require energy. Adenosine triphosphate (ATP) plays a major role in energy-exchange reactions. The synthesis of ATP requires energy, while the hydrolysis of ATP to adenosine diphosphate (ADP) liberates energy that can be used in a variety of endergonic reactions. In mammalian systems, the energy for ATP synthesis is supplied by the oxidation of food. The two major pathways that transform the energy contained in food to high-energy phosphate bonds in ATP are the tricarboxylic acid (TCA) cycle and oxidative phosphorylation; both occur in the mitochondria.

METABOLIC SOURCES OF ENERGY

Animal cells extract energy from their environment by the oxidation of carbohydrate, protein, and fat to carbon dioxide and water. The process by which the energy contained in these macronutrients is converted to high-energy phosphate bonds in ATP occurs in four stages (Figure 6-1).

In the first stage, the macromolecules are hydrolyzed to their building blocks, resulting in a diverse set of molecules including monosaccharides, fatty acids, and amino acids. In the second stage, the building blocks are oxidized by different pathways to a common product, acetyl coenzyme A (acetyl CoA). Most of the energy in the original foods is conserved in the chemical bonds of acetyl CoA, with only a fraction of the total released in the first and second stages. In the third stage, acetyl CoA is oxidized to carbon dioxide by the TCA cycle. Energy is extracted from acetyl CoA by the transfer of electron pairs in the carbon–carbon and carbon–hydrogen bonds to the electron carriers, the oxidized forms of nicotinamide adenine dinucleotide (NAD$^+$) and flavin adenine dinucleotide

Most of the useful energy in foods is stored in the pairs of electrons that make up the chemical bonds.

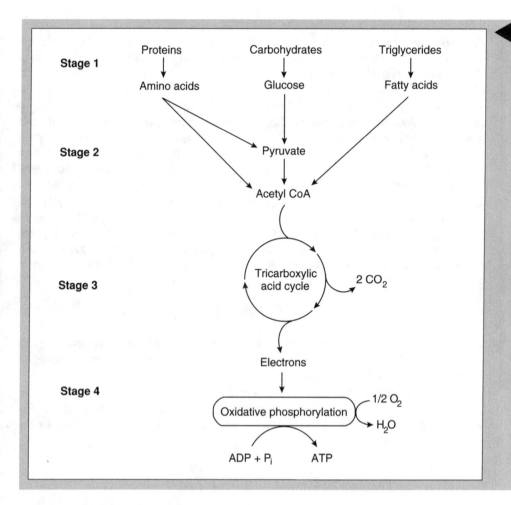

FIGURE 6-1
Overview of Oxidative Energy Metabolism.
The transformation of energy in food to ATP involves diverse pathways that converge at acetyl CoA. A common pathway for the oxidation of acetyl CoA is found in mitochondria.

(FAD), resulting in their reduced forms, NADH and $FADH_2$. In the fourth stage of energy extraction, NADH and $FADH_2$ are oxidized by the electron transport chain, and oxygen, the terminal electron acceptor, is reduced to water. The energy released by this process is used to synthesize ATP.

THERMODYNAMIC PRINCIPLES OF ENERGY METABOLISM

The concepts underlying energy metabolism are based on thermodynamic principles of chemical reactions. Chemical reactions either consume or release energy, depending on the relative energy content of the reactants and products. The concepts of free energy change and coupled reactions are central themes in metabolism.

Free Energy Change (ΔG) of Reactions

The free energy change of a reaction is defined as the portion of the total energy change that is available for doing work. For any reaction, ΔG is equal to the difference in the free energy (G) of the products and the reactants. Mathematically, ΔG can be expressed by the following equation:

$$\Delta G = G_{products} - G_{reactants} = \Delta H - T\Delta S$$

In this equation, ΔH is the change in the heat content or the "inner energy" of the products and reactants, and ΔS is the change in the disorder or randomness of the products and reactants. An increase in ΔS corresponds to an increase in randomness. T is the absolute temperature, expressed in degrees kelvin (°K).

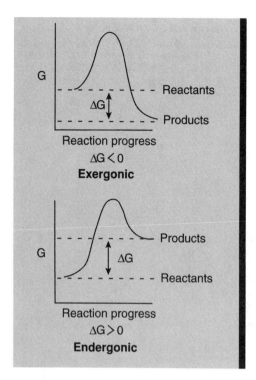

Pathway Independent of ΔG. The ΔG of a reaction is independent of the pathway by which reactants are converted to products. For example, the ΔG for the oxidation of glucose is the same regardless of whether it occurs through a series of enzyme-catalyzed reactions or by combustion in a calorimeter. The ΔG for the reaction is dependent only on the energy content of the reactants and products.

Direction of Reaction Predicted by Sign of ΔG. Reactions can be classified into two groups based on whether the ΔG has a positive or a negative value. Reactions with a negative ΔG are *exergonic reactions* and will proceed spontaneously from a higher to a lower energy state. Reactions with a positive ΔG are *endergonic reactions*, and energy must be supplied for the reaction to proceed from a lower to a higher energy state.

Standard Free Energy Change (ΔG°). The change in free energy that occurs when all of the reactants and products are present at a concentration of 1 M is defined as the standard free energy change of a reaction. The ΔG° for any reaction is a constant and is related to the equilibrium constant (K_{eq}) by the following equation, where R is the gas constant (1.98 kcal/mol · °K), T is the absolute temperature, and $\ln K_{eq}$ is the natural logarithm of the equilibrium constant.

$$\Delta G° = -RT \ln K_{eq}$$

Although the concentrations of reactants and products found in cells are usually much lower than 1 M, the concept of ΔG° is useful for comparing the relative energy changes for different reactions that occur in cells.

Relationship Between ΔG and ΔG°. The value of ΔG is dependent on the actual concentration of reactants and products and may differ significantly from the value of ΔG°. For any reaction A + B ⇌ C + D, the relationship between ΔG and ΔG° is given by the following equation:

$$\Delta G = \Delta G° + RT \ln \frac{[C]\,[D]}{[A]\,[B]}$$

Two conclusions can be made from this equation. First, when ΔG = 0, the reaction is at equilibrium. Second, the magnitude of ΔG (and in some cases the sign) can be changed by altering the concentrations of the reactants and products. An increase in the concentration of reactants or a decrease in the concentration of products lowers the ΔG for the reaction, making it more thermodynamically favorable.

Coupled Reaction Systems

By definition, two reactions are coupled if the product of one reaction is a reactant in the other reaction. Reactions that are coupled are also additive. Cells frequently couple an exergonic reaction with an endergonic reaction to ensure that the endergonic reaction proceeds in the desired direction. Many enzymes that use ATP as a substrate catalyze coupled reactions, in which the energy released by the hydrolysis of ATP is used to drive another reaction that requires energy. For example, all cells are able to carry out the following reaction, in which glucose is converted to glucose-6-phosphate (G6P):

$$\text{Glucose} + P_i \longrightarrow \text{G6P} \qquad \Delta G° = +3.3 \text{ kcal/mol}$$

This reaction has a positive ΔG° and will not proceed in the direction of G6P formation unless energy is added. The function of hexokinase is to couple the hydrolysis of ATP, an exergonic reaction, with the formation of G6P. As shown below, the sum of these two reactions has a negative ΔG° and proceeds in the direction of G6P formation.

$$\text{ATP} + H_2O \longrightarrow \text{ADP} + P_i \qquad \Delta G° = -7.3 \text{ kcal/mol}$$

$$\text{Glucose} + P_i \longrightarrow \text{G6P} + H_2O \qquad \Delta G° = +3.3 \text{ kcal/mol}$$

$$\text{Sum:} \quad \text{Glucose} + \text{ATP} \longrightarrow \text{G6P} + \text{ADP} \qquad \Delta G° = -4.0 \text{ kcal/mol}$$

ROLE OF ATP IN ENERGY METABOLISM

The ATP molecule has two high-energy phosphate bonds that are frequently designated by a squiggle ($\sim$). The most important feature of the ATP molecule in energy-transfer reactions is the energy-rich *anhydride bond* that links the γ- and β-phosphate groups together. The ΔG^o for the hydrolysis of this bond is -7.3 kcal/mol.

ATP as a Universal Carrier of Energy

Most phosphate-containing compounds found in cells either receive their phosphate groups from ATP or donate their phosphate groups to ADP, with the formation of ATP. Some of these compounds have ΔG^o values for hydrolysis that are more negative than that of ATP, while others have values that are less negative than ATP (Table 6-1). The intermediate ΔG^o value for ATP allows it to be an effective carrier of energy between many phosphate-containing compounds. Compounds with a more negative ΔG^o than that of ATP are described as *high-energy phosphates*, and they can transfer their phosphate groups to ADP with the formation of ATP. Conversely, ATP can transfer its phosphate group to compounds having a less negative ΔG^o.

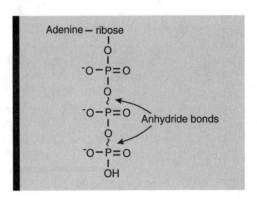

Metabolites	ΔG^o (kcal/mol)
Phosphoenolpyruvate	-14.8
1,3-Bisphosphoglycerate	-11.8
Creatine phosphate	-10.3
Adenosine triphosphate	**-7.3**
Adenosine diphosphate	-6.6
Glucose-1-phosphate	-5.0
Fructose-6-phosphate	-3.8
Adenosine monophosphate	-3.4
Glucose-6-phosphate	-3.3
Glycerol-3-phosphate	-2.2

◀ **TABLE 6-1**
Standard Free Energy of Hydrolysis for Common Phosphate-Containing Metabolites

Synthesis of ATP by Substrate-Level Phosphorylation

The synthesis of ATP by phosphate transfer from a high-energy phosphate donor is defined as substrate-level phosphorylation. The designation distinguishes this pathway of ATP synthesis from the major pathway of oxidative phosphorylation that occurs in mitochondria. There are very few cellular compounds that have enough energy to support substrate-level phosphorylation. The most important ones are phosphoenolpyruvate and 1,3-bisphosphoglycerate, both intermediates in glycolysis, and creatine phosphate, a compound found primarily in muscle, where it serves as a reservoir of high-energy phosphate for ATP synthesis.

Other High-Energy Carriers in Metabolism

Many reactions in metabolism involve the transfer of some chemical group from a high-energy carrier to an acceptor. The bond that links the group to the carrier is a high-energy bond that is cleaved during the transfer, thereby providing the energy required to make the reaction thermodynamically favorable. Examples of commonly transferred groups, their high-energy carriers, and the types of reactions or pathways in which they participate are shown in Table 6-2.

A thermodynamically favorable reaction has a ΔG less than 0.

TABLE 6-2 ▶

High-Energy Carriers of Chemical Groups in Metabolism

Group	High-Energy Carrier	Reaction or Pathway
Phosphate	Adenosine triphosphate	Kinase reactions
Sugars	Uridine diphosphate sugar	Glycogen synthesis
Acetate	Acetyl~CoA	Fatty acid synthesis
Fatty acids	Acyl~CoA	Triglyceride synthesis
Amino acids	Aminoacyl adenylate	Protein synthesis
Carboxyl	Carboxy~biotin	Carboxylation reactions
Methyl	S-adenosylmethionine	Methylation reactions
Sulfate	Phosphoadenosinephosphosulfate	Sulfation reactions

BIOLOGIC OXIDATIONS

Biologic oxidations are central to respiration and energy conservation in cells. Energy is extracted from metabolic fuels by a series of oxidations, in which pairs of electrons (e^-) are transferred from the fuel, through a series of electron carriers, to oxygen. Energy released in these reactions is conserved in the high-energy phosphate bonds of ATP.

Nomenclature and Thermodynamic Principles

Oxidation and reduction reactions involve the transfer of electrons between a donor and an acceptor. *Oxidation* is defined as the *loss of electrons*, with the electron acceptor being the oxidizing agent. Conversely, *reduction* is defined as the gain of electrons, with the electron donor being the reducing agent.

Redox Reactions. Since every oxidation reaction is accompanied by a reduction reaction, each is considered to be a half-reaction. A redox reaction, therefore, consists of *two half-reactions* that are *coupled*. The electrons lost in one half-reaction are used as reactants in the other half-reaction. For example, the oxidation of $FADH_2$ by oxygen involves the following half-reactions:

$$FADH_2 \longrightarrow FAD + 2H^+ + 2e^- \qquad \text{Oxidation reaction}$$

$$\tfrac{1}{2} O_2 + 2H^+ + 2e^- \longrightarrow H_2O \qquad \text{Reduction reaction}$$

$$\text{Sum:} \quad FADH_2 + \tfrac{1}{2} O_2 \longrightarrow FAD + H_2O \qquad \text{Redox reaction}$$

A *redox pair* is defined as the reduced and oxidized forms of a particular compound. In the above reaction, there are two redox pairs, $FAD/FADH_2$ and oxygen/water. By convention redox pairs are written with the oxidized form over the reduced form.

Standard Reduction Potential (E°). By definition, E° is a measure of the tendency of a redox pair to lose electrons. Each redox pair has a characteristic E° with units of volts. *The more negative the standard reduction potential, the greater its tendency to lose electrons.* In a redox reaction, the redox pair with the more negative E° will be the electron donor. Therefore, knowledge of the E° values is useful for predicting the direction in which a redox reaction spontaneously proceeds. The E° values for some common half-reactions are shown in Table 6-3.

Relationship Between ΔE° and ΔG°. For any redox reaction, the change in standard reduction potential (ΔE°) is defined as the $E^\circ_{\text{(electron acceptor)}} - E^\circ_{\text{(electron donor)}}$. The ΔE° can be used to calculate the ΔG° for the reaction. The equation relating these parameters is given below, where n is the number of electrons transferred, and F is the Faraday constant that converts volts into kcal (F = 23 kcal/volt).

$$\Delta G^\circ = nF\Delta E^\circ$$

A reaction with a positive ΔE° will have a negative ΔG°, and under standard conditions, such a reaction proceeds spontaneously in the direction written.

The use of ΔE° to calculate ΔG° can be illustrated with the reaction that describes

TABLE 6-3
Standard Reduction Potentials of Common Redox Pairs

Redox Pair	E° Volts
NAD+/NADH	−0.32
Pyruvate/lactate	−0.19
Oxaloacetate/malate	−0.17
FAD/FADH$_2$	−0.06
Coenzyme Q/coenzyme QH$_2$	+0.10
Fumarate/succinate	+0.13
Cytochrome a (Fe^{3+})/ cytochrome a (Fe^{2+})	+0.29
½ oxygen/water	+0.82

the oxidation of FADH$_2$ by oxygen (discussed above). In this reaction, the electron acceptor is oxygen and the donor is FADH$_2$. Therefore,

$$\Delta E° = E°_{(oxygen)} - E°_{(FADH)} = 0.82 \text{ volt} - (-0.06 \text{ volt}) = +0.88 \text{ volt}$$

Since two electrons are transferred in this reaction, n = 2. Substituting these values into the equation for $\Delta G°$, as shown below, gives a $\Delta G°$ of −40.5 kcal/mol of FADH$_2$ oxidized.

$$\Delta G° = -(2)(23 \text{ kcal/volt})(0.88 \text{ volt}) = -40.5 \text{ kcal}$$

Major Electron Carriers in Metabolism

The oxidation of metabolic fuels involves a large number of dehydrogenases, which require coenzymes that act as electron carriers. The most important coenzymes in oxidative reactions are NAD$^+$, FAD, and flavin mononucleotide (FMN). In contrast, the reduced form of nicotinamide-adenine dinucleotide phosphate (NADPH) is the most important coenzyme in reductive reactions that occur in biosynthetic pathways.

Niacin (nicotinic acid) is the vitamin precursor of NAD$^+$ and NADP$^+$.
Riboflavin is the vitamin precursor of FAD and FMN.

NAD$^+$. Most of the NAD$^+$ and NADH in the cell is found in the mitochondria, where most of the oxidative reactions in metabolism occur. The structures of NAD$^+$ and NADH are shown in Figure 6-2.

Dehydrogenases that use NAD$^+$ catalyze the *transfer of a hydride ion* (two electrons and a proton). Most of the reactions involve the oxidation of a hydroxylated carbon atom to an aldehyde or ketone, as shown in the following equation.

$$\begin{array}{c} O-H \\ | \\ R-C-R + NAD^+ \\ | \\ H \end{array} \longrightarrow \begin{array}{c} O \\ || \\ R-C-R + NADH + H^+ \end{array}$$

Oxidation reactions that are NAD$^+$-dependent also release a proton (H$^+$). Reactions of this type are common in carbohydrate metabolism and in the TCA cycle.

FAD and FMN. Most of the FAD is found in the mitochondria and peroxisomes of cells. FAD-dependent dehydrogenases catalyze the transfer of two hydrogen atoms, usually from adjacent carbon atoms, to FAD resulting in the formation of FADH$_2$ (see Figure 6-2). A typical reaction is shown in the following equation.

$$\begin{array}{c} H \ H \\ | \ \ | \\ R-C-C-R + FAD \\ | \ \ | \\ H \ H \end{array} \longrightarrow \begin{array}{c} R-C=C-R + FADH_2 \\ | \ \ \ \ | \\ H \ \ \ \ H \end{array}$$

NAD$^+$ = nicotinamide−ribose−P−P−ribose−adenine
NADP$^+$ = nicotinamide−ribose−P−P−ribose−adenine P
  |
  P
FAD = flavin−ribose−P−P−ribose−adenine
FMN = flavin−ribose−P

NADPH. NADPH is a universal carrier of reducing equivalents (electrons) for reductive reactions in metabolism. In contrast to NAD$^+$ and NADH, most of the NADPH and its oxidized form, NADP$^+$, are found in the cytoplasm of cells where reductive reactions occur. Most of the NADPH is formed in the pentose phosphate pathway (see Chapter 14).

FIGURE 6-2 ▶

Structures of Nicotinamide and Flavin Adenine Nucleotides. *The reduction of NAD+ to NADH involves the transfer of a hydride ion (H:) from a donor to the nicotinamide ring. The reduction of FAD to FADH₂ involves the addition of two hydrogen atoms (H·) to nitrogen atoms in the flavin ring system.*

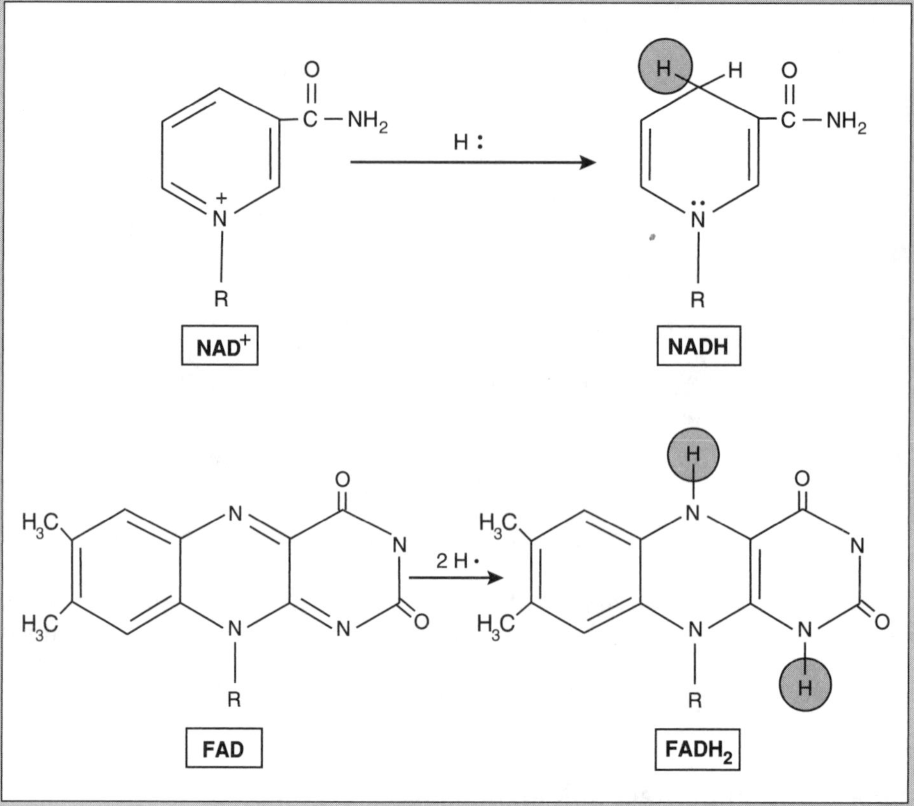

MITOCHONDRIAL COMPARTMENTS

Mitochondria are the subcellular organelles that specialize in oxidative metabolism and ATP synthesis. The number of mitochondria in a cell varies, depending on the function of the cell and its need for ATP. The key structural features of mitochondria are shown in Figure 6-3.

FIGURE 6-3 ▶

Mitochondrial Compartments. *Mitochondria have two membranes, a porous outer membrane and an impermeable inner membrane, which is highly folded into cristae to increase the surface area. The inner membrane of mitochondria has a larger percentage of protein than any other mammalian membrane.*

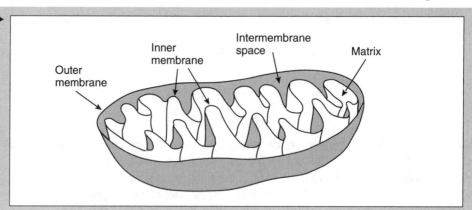

Outer Mitochondrial Membrane (OMM)

The OMM is highly porous and is permeable to most ions and small molecules. It can be easily solubilized with digitonin, a detergent that selectively solubilizes the outer membrane while having no effect on the inner membrane.

Inner Mitochondrial Membrane (IMM)

The IMM is highly impermeable, and the transport of most molecules across the IMM requires either a specific transport protein or a shuttle system. The high degree of folding provides the large surface area needed to accommodate the many functions of the IMM. Embedded in the membrane are many proteins, including transport proteins, several

FAD-dependent dehydrogenases, and all of the enzymes and proteins required for oxidative phosphorylation.

Intermembrane Space

The space between the IMM and the OMM contains two enzymes that play an important role in energy metabolism, adenylate kinase and nucleoside-diphosphate kinase. These enzymes are important for the interconversion of adenine nucleotides. As shown in the following equations, adenylate kinase allows all three forms of adenine nucleotides to be interconverted, while nucleoside-diphosphate kinase allows ATP and ADP to be interconverted with all other nucleoside diphosphates and triphosphates (designated XDP and XTP). Both reactions are reversible, and the direction of the reaction is determined by the relative concentrations of the substrates and products.

$$\text{2 ADP} \xrightleftharpoons{\text{adenylate kinase}} \text{ATP + AMP}$$

$$\text{XTP + ADP} \xrightleftharpoons{\text{nucleoside-diphosphate kinase}} \text{XDP + ATP}$$

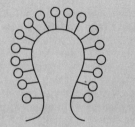

Cristae are the folds in the inner mitochondrial membrane. Electron micrographs show that the matrix side of the membrane is studded with spherical particles, which are attached by stalks to the membrane. The spheres are the ATP synthase that makes most of the cellular ATP.

Mitochondrial Matrix

The matrix contains oxidative enzymes, including pyruvate dehydrogenase, glutamate dehydrogenase, branched-chain amino acid dehydrogenase, the enzymes of the TCA cycle, and the enzymes involved in fatty acid oxidation. Also in the matrix are granules of calcium phosphate.

TRICARBOXYLIC ACID (TCA) CYCLE

The TCA cycle is also known as the citric acid cycle or the Krebs cycle. It is located in the mitochondria, where it is acts as an *integration center* for coordinating various pathways of carbohydrate, lipid, and protein metabolism.

Functions

The TCA cycle is an *amphibolic pathway*, having both oxidative and synthetic functions.

Oxidative Function. The TCA cycle is the terminal furnace for the oxidation of acetyl CoA (Figure 6-4). In the first reaction of the cycle, acetyl CoA brings two carbon atoms into the cycle by condensing with oxaloacetate to form citrate. With one complete turn of the cycle, two carbon atoms are released as carbon dioxide, oxaloacetate is regenerated, and four pairs of electrons are transferred from intermediates to NADH and $FADH_2$.

Synthetic Functions. Several intermediates in the TCA cycle serve as substrates for synthetic pathways. Citrate can be used for fatty acid synthesis; oxaloacetate can be used for the de novo synthesis of glucose; succinyl CoA can be used for heme synthesis; and α-ketoglutarate and oxaloacetate can both be used for the synthesis of several nonessential amino acids.

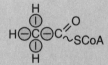

Acetyl CoA

During the oxidation of acetyl CoA, the three pairs of electrons that are circled are transferred to NADH, and one pair is transferred to $FADH_2$.

Anaplerotic Reactions

Since several intermediates in the TCA cycle are used as substrates for synthetic pathways, it is necessary to replenish intermediates so that the cycle can continue to operate. Reactions that replenish intermediates in the TCA cycle are known as anaplerotic reactions. The major anaplerotic reaction is the carboxylation of pyruvate to oxaloacetate, a reaction catalyzed by *pyruvate carboxylase*.

$$\text{Pyruvate} + HCO_3^- + \text{ATP} \xrightarrow[\oplus \text{ acetyl CoA}]{\text{biotin}} \text{oxaloacetate} + \text{ADP} + P_i$$

Biotin acts as a high-energy carrier of the carboxyl group in this reaction. The hydrolysis of ATP supplies the energy needed to drive the reaction in the direction of oxaloacetate formation. Pyruvate carboxylase is allosterically activated by acetyl CoA.

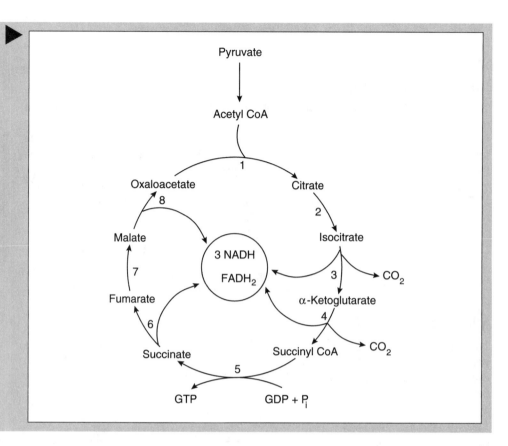

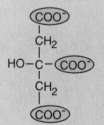

Reactions of the TCA Cycle

The overall reaction catalyzed by the TCA cycle is the sum of the individual reactions and can be represented by the following equation:

$$\text{Acetyl CoA} + 3\ NAD^+ + FAD + GDP + P_i + 2\ H_2O \longrightarrow$$

$$2\ CO_2 + 3\ NADH + FADH_2 + GTP + 2\ H^+ + CoA$$

The first reaction in the cycle is the condensation of oxaloacetate with acetyl CoA, a reaction catalyzed by citrate synthase (see Figure 6-4). The product of this reaction is citrate, a C_6 tricarboxylic acid that is converted to its isomer, isocitrate. The remaining reactions in the cycle are considered in three sequences, each resulting in the transfer of energy.

Conversion of Isocitrate to Succinyl CoA. Isocitrate is converted to succinyl CoA through two sequential oxidative decarboxylation reactions, resulting first in α-ketoglutarate and followed by succinyl CoA (Figure 6-5). In each of these reactions, carbon dioxide is released, and a hydride ion is transferred from the substrate to NADH.

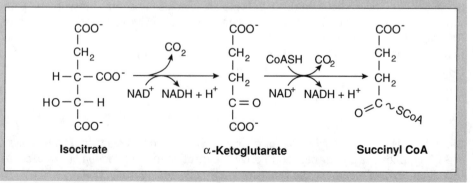

Conversion of Succinyl CoA to Succinate. Succinyl CoA is a thioester, having a ΔG° of hydrolysis equal to −8.0 kcal/mol, which is more than enough energy to drive the synthesis of a high-energy phosphate bond. The hydrolysis of succinyl CoA to succinate is coupled with the synthesis of GTP. This is the only reaction in the TCA cycle that results in the direct synthesis of a high-energy phosphate bond and is classified as a substrate-level phosphorylation reaction. GTP is energetically equivalent to ATP, and the two are interconvertible by nucleoside-diphosphate kinase. These reactions are shown in the following equations.

$$\text{Succinyl}\sim\text{CoA} + \text{GDP} + P_i \xrightleftharpoons{\text{succinyl CoA synthetase}} \text{succinate} + \text{CoA} + \text{GTP}$$

$$\text{GTP} + \text{ADP} \xrightleftharpoons{\text{nucleoside-diphosphate kinase}} \text{ATP} + \text{GDP}$$

Conversion of Succinate to Oxaloacetate. Two energy-transfer reactions occur in the remaining steps of the TCA cycle (Figure 6-6). Succinate is oxidized to fumarate, with the formation of $FADH_2$. Following hydration of fumarate, malate is oxidized to oxaloacetate, with the formation of NADH.

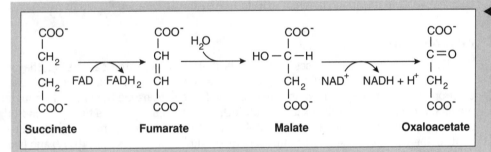

FIGURE 6-6
Conversion of Succinate to Oxaloacetate. *The conversion of succinate to oxaloacetate conserves energy. The oxidation of succinate to fumarate, catalyzed by succinate dehydrogenase, transfers electrons to $FADH_2$. Fumarase catalyzes hydration of fumarate to malate. The oxidation of malate to oxaloacetate, catalyzed by malate dehydrogenase, conserves energy by transferring electrons to NADH.*

Regulation of the TCA Cycle

The rate at which the cycle operates is dependent on the energy state of the cell. When ATP accumulates, indicating an energy-rich environment, the rate of the cycle decreases. Conversely, the accumulation of ADP signals a depletion of ATP, and the rate of the cycle increases. The primary site of regulation is *isocitrate dehydrogenase* (IDH), the enzyme that catalyzes the rate-limiting step in the TCA cycle. Its activity is allosterically inhibited by ATP and activated by ADP. Secondary sites of regulation are α-ketoglutarate dehydrogenase and citrate synthase. Citrate synthase is inhibited by ATP, and α-ketoglutarate dehydrogenase is inhibited by NADH. All three enzymes catalyze reactions that are essentially irreversible under the conditions that exist in the mitochondria.

Vitamin Deficiencies and the TCA Cycle

The cofactors required by the enzymes of the TCA cycle, together with their vitamin precursors, are listed in Table 6-4. A deficiency in any of these vitamins can result in

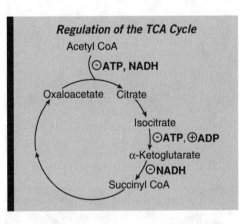

TABLE 6-4
Cofactors and Vitamin Precursors Required by TCA Cycle Enzymes

Enzyme	Prosthetic Group[a]	Coenzyme	Vitamin Precursor
Aconitase	Iron–sulfur centers		
Isocitrate dehydrogenase		NAD+	Niacin
α-Ketoglutarate dehydrogenase	Thiamine pyrophosphate	NAD+ CoA	Thiamine and niacin Pantothenic acid Riboflavin
	FAD Lipoic acid[b]		
Succinyl CoA synthetase	Iron–sulfur centers[b]	CoA	Pantothenic acid
Succinate dehydrogenase	FAD		Riboflavin
Malate dehydrogenase		NAD+	Niacin

[a] Prosthetic groups are tightly bound cofactors that do not dissociate from the enzymes, whereas coenzymes freely dissociate.
[b] Lipoic acid and iron–sulfur centers have no vitamin precursors.

decreased oxidation of acetyl CoA, with lactic acidosis being a common clinical manifestation. A major source of mitochondrial acetyl CoA is pyruvate, which is in equilibrium with lactic acid. Therefore, any condition leading to decreased utilization of pyruvate results in the accumulation of lactic acid.

ELECTRON TRANSPORT AND OXIDATIVE PHOSPHORYLATION

The final step in the oxidation of metabolic fuels is carried out by the electron transport chain (ETC), which oxidizes NADH and $FADH_2$ to NAD^+ and FAD. The electrons are transferred from NADH and $FADH_2$, through a series of electron carriers to molecular oxygen, forming water. The ETC, also known as the respiratory chain, is the major consumer of oxygen in the cell. The energy released by oxidation of NADH and $FADH_2$ is coupled with the phosphorylation of ADP to ATP by the enzyme, ATP synthase.

Electron Carriers

The ETC consists of four classes of cofactors that act as electron carriers: (1) flavin nucleotides, (2) coenzyme Q (CoQ), (3) iron–sulfur centers, and (4) heme. Each of these electron carriers is first reduced and then oxidized as electrons are transported through the chain to oxygen. With the exception of CoQ, all of the cofactors are tightly bound to the integral membrane proteins that catalyze electron transfer reactions. The components of the ETC can be separated into four protein–lipid complexes (I, II, III, IV) and two mobile components (CoQ, cytochrome-c). CoQ transports electrons from complexes I and II to complex III, and cytochrome-c transports electrons from complex III to complex IV (see Figure 6-7).

Flavin Nucleotides. Both FMN and FAD participate in two-electron transfer reactions. FMN is a cofactor for complex I, which oxidizes NADH to NAD^+, with the concomitant reduction of FMN to $FMNH_2$. FAD is the cofactor for complex II, which oxidizes succinate to fumarate, with the formation of $FADH_2$.

Coenzyme Q (CoQ). CoQ, also known as ubiquinone because of its widespread occurrence, is a small lipophilic cofactor that moves freely in the lipid bilayer, collecting electrons from $FMNH_2$ and $FADH_2$ and transferring them to complex III. CoQ transfers two electrons from the flavin nucleotides to complex III, but the transfer, both to and from CoQ, occurs one electron at a time. CoQ is a unique component of the ETC because of its ability to accept electrons from a variety of reactions that produce $FADH_2$.

Iron–Sulfur Centers. Iron–sulfur centers contain iron atoms, which are linked either to organic sulfur or to protein-bound sulfur found in cysteine side chains. The iron–sulfur centers participate in one-electron transfer reactions. Proteins containing iron–sulfur centers are associated with complexes I, II, and III.

Heme. Heme, the prosthetic group of the cytochromes, has a central iron atom that participates in one-electron transfer reactions. In contrast to the heme moiety of myoglobin and hemoglobin, where the heme iron atom must be in the ferrous (Fe^{2+}) state to be active, the heme iron of cytochromes undergoes cyclic reduction and oxidation as a part of its function. The classification of cytochromes (a, b, c) found in the ETC is based on slight structural differences in the heme moiety of these proteins.

Pathway of Electron Transport

The pathway of electron transport through the ETC is shown in Figure 6-7. The electron carriers are arranged in an order that facilitates the sequential transfer of electrons from one component to the next in the chain. The $E^°$ of the components increases progressively from a more negative to a more positive value, with NADH having the most negative reduction potential and oxygen having the most positive. Therefore, each step in the transfer is characterized by a $\Delta E^° > 0$ and a $\Delta G^° < 0$, a condition that promotes the spontaneous flow of electrons from NADH or $FADH_2$ to oxygen.

Coenzyme Q
(oxidized)

2H·

Coenzyme Q
(reduced)

An Iron–Sulfur Center

Complex II (of the ETC) and **succinate dehydrogenase** (of the TCA cycle) are two different names for the same enzyme.

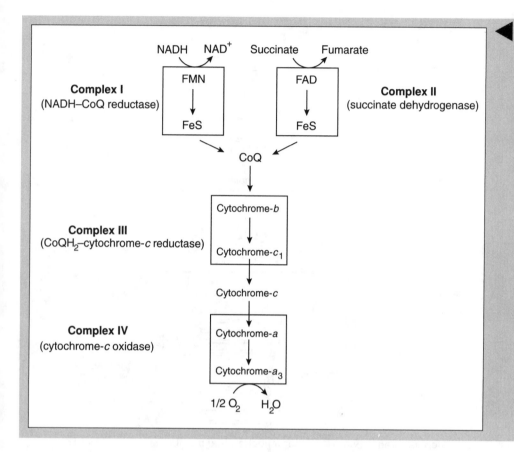

FIGURE 6-7
Electron Transport Chain. The sequence of the electron carriers is shown. The components of the four protein-lipid complexes are shown in boxes. Coenzyme Q collects electrons from both complex I and complex II and transfers them to complex III. Cytochrome-c is mobile in the membrane and transfers electrons from complex III to complex IV. The terminal electron acceptor is molecular oxygen. The reduction of each atom of oxygen to water requires two electrons.

Energy Released by Oxidation of NADH and FADH$_2$

The energy released by the transport of electrons can be calculated from the difference in the standard reduction potentials of the electron acceptor and the electron donor. The energy released by the transfer of electrons from NADH and FADH$_2$ to oxygen is shown below.

$$NADH \qquad \Delta G° = -52.6 \text{ kcal/mol}$$

$$FADH_2 \qquad \Delta G° = -40.5 \text{ kcal/mol}$$

By comparison, the energy required for the synthesis of ATP from ADP and P$_i$ is 7.3 kcal/mol.

Coupling of Oxidation and Phosphorylation

An explanation of how the energy released by the oxidation of NADH and FADH is used for mitochondrial ATP synthesis is provided by the *chemiosmotic theory*. This theory has two basic postulates: (1) As electrons flow through the ETC, the energy released is used to create a H+ gradient (protomotive force) across the inner mitochondrial membrane; and (2) the movement of protons back across the membrane releases energy that can be used to drive the synthesis of ATP.

Forming a H+ Gradient. Complexes I, III, and IV are H+ pumps that transfer H+ from the mitochondrial matrix into the space between the IMM and the OMM (Figure 6-8). The energy required to pump H+ out of the mitochondrial matrix is provided by the transfer of electrons through each of these complexes. The formation of a H+ gradient across the inner mitochondrial membrane can be demonstrated by pH measurements that show an increase in pH (a decrease in H+ concentration) in the matrix of mitochondria that are actively engaged in oxidation.

ATP Synthesis. The synthesis of ATP by mitochondria is catalyzed by *ATP synthase* (also known as complex V). ATP synthase has two major components, F$_o$ and F$_1$. The F$_o$ component spans the inner mitochondrial membrane, forming a channel through which H+ can reenter the matrix. The F$_1$ component protrudes into the matrix and contains the active site where ADP and P$_i$ are condensed to form ATP. *Oligomycin*, a compound that blocks movement of H+ through the F$_o$ channel, inhibits ATP synthesis.

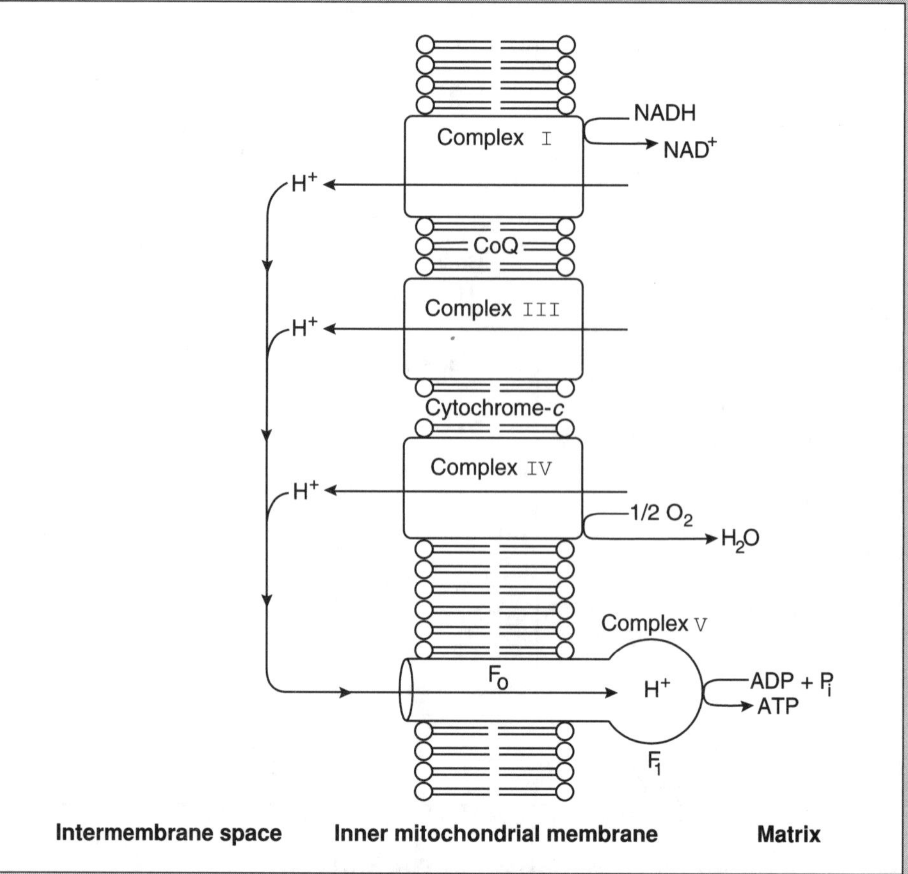

FIGURE 6-8 ▶

Coupling of Oxidation and Phosphorylation. The transfer of two electrons through complexes I, III, and IV releases energy that is used to pump protons (H⁺) from the matrix to the intermembrane space. A total of 10 H⁺ are translocated for each molecule of NADH oxidized. The H⁺ reenter the matrix through the F_o channel of complex V (the ATPase), with a release of energy that is used for ATP synthesis.

P/O Ratio. By definition, the P/O ratio is the number of inorganic phosphate groups incorporated into ATP per atom of molecular oxygen consumed (½ O_2). Substrates that are oxidized with the formation of NADH (pyruvate, malate, isocitrate) have P/O ratios of 3, indicating that the oxidation of NADH by the ETC results in a H⁺ gradient sufficient to support the synthesis of 3 mol of ATP per mole of NADH. The oxidation of substrates that generate $FADH_2$ (succinate, α-glycerol phosphate) have a P/O ratio of 2. The transfer of electrons from $FADH_2$ to oxygen bypasses complex I, one of the H⁺ pumps. (Recent measurements indicate that the P/O ratio of NAD⁺-linked substrates may be closer to 2.5, while that of FAD-linked substrates is closer to 1.5. However, for simplicity, the numbers 3 and 2 are used throughout this book.)

Efficiency. The oxidation of NADH by the ETC has a $\Delta G° = -52.6$ kcal/mol, whereas the synthesis of ATP from ADP and P_i has a $\Delta G° = +7.3$ kcal/mol. Theoretically, 7 mol of ATP could be synthesized by the oxidation of 1 mol of NADH. However, since only 2.5 to 3 mol of ATP are actually formed, the efficiency is between 35% and 40%. Most of the additional energy is released as heat.

INHIBITORS OF MITOCHONDRIAL ATP SYNTHESIS

A large number of compounds inhibit oxidative phosphorylation. These compounds can be divided into three major classes: (1) inhibitors of electron transport, (2) inhibitors of complex V (ATP synthase), and (3) uncouplers of oxidation and phosphorylation.

Site-Specific Inhibitors of Electron Transport

Compounds that block the transport of electrons inhibit ATP synthesis by decreasing the ability of the ETC to establish a H⁺ gradient. A number of drugs and toxins have been shown to be site-specific inhibitors of electron transport (Figure 6-9). For example, cyanide binds to complex III and prevents the transfer of electrons to oxygen, whereas

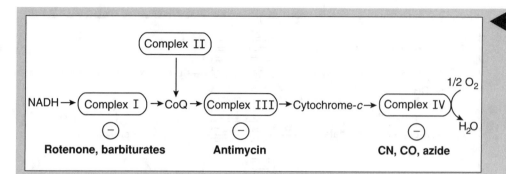

FIGURE 6-9
Site-Specific Inhibitors of Electron Transport. The complexes that bind inhibitors are indicated. Both electron transport and proton pumping are decreased by the binding of an inhibitor to a complex.

rotenone and several barbiturates bind to complex I, preventing the transfer of electrons from NADH to CoQ.

Inhibitors That Bind to ATP Synthase

Some inhibitors of mitochondrial ATP synthesis bind directly to ATP synthase. For example, the antibiotic oligomycin binds to the F_o component of ATP synthase, blocking the return of H^+ to the mitochondrial matrix. Oligomycin also inhibits electron transport, a secondary effect resulting from the difficulty of pumping H^+ uphill against a concentration gradient.

Uncouplers of Oxidative Phosphorylation

Compounds that abolish the H^+ gradient across the IMM inhibit ATP synthesis because of the inability to maintain a H^+ gradient. In contrast, the rate of oxidation is increased by uncouplers. The energy associated with oxidation is released as heat. An example of an uncoupler is dinitrophenol, a lipophilic compound that carries H^+ into the mitochondrial matrix. Dinitrophenol is a weak acid that is protonated at the lower pH of the intermembrane space. However, when it enters the matrix where the pH is higher, the proton dissociates. A naturally occurring uncoupler is thermogenin, a protein found in mitochondria of brown adipose tissue, which plays a key role in thermogenesis. The large blood vessels of newborns are surrounded by brown adipose tissue, where the oxidation of fatty acids releases heat that helps maintain the temperature of circulating blood.

Aspirin is an uncoupler of oxidative phosphorylation, and when taken in large doses, it increases the body temperature.

MITOCHONDRIAL MEMBRANE TRANSPORT SYSTEMS

The IMM contains many transport proteins that allow molecules to be transported into and out of the mitochondrial matrix. The transport systems that are particularly important for oxidative phosphorylation are the shuttle systems for transporting electrons into the matrix and the adenine nucleotide transport protein.

Shuttles for Transporting Electrons into the Mitochondria

Although most NADH is generated in the mitochondrial matrix, a small amount is produced in the cytosol during glycolysis. For glycolysis to continue, NADH must be oxidized back to NAD^+, a process that occurs in mitochondria under aerobic conditions. The IMM, however, is impermeable to NADH, and there is no transport protein for NADH in the membrane. There are, however, two shuttle systems for getting the electrons in NADH into the mitochondria (Figure 6-10).

Shuttle systems are used to move impermeable molecules across membranes. They consist of two enzymes located on opposite sides of a membrane and a transport protein within the membrane. The two enzymes catalyze the same reaction but in opposite directions.

α-Glycerol Phosphate Shuttle. The α-glycerol phosphate shuttle results in the transfer of electrons from cytosolic NADH to mitochondrial $FADH_2$. The key feature of this shuttle is the presence of α-glycerol phosphate dehydrogenase isozymes on both sides of the membrane. The cytosolic isozyme catalyzes the transfer of electrons from NADH to dihydroxyacetone phosphate, producing α-glycerol phosphate, which carries the electrons across the membrane. Once inside the mitochondria, the electrons are transferred from α-glycerol phosphate to $FADH_2$, which can be oxidized by the ETC. Dihydroxyacetone phosphate is transported back to the cytosol to complete the shuttle.

FIGURE 6-10 ▶

Shuttles for Transporting Electrons into Mitochondria. All tissues have shuttles for transporting electrons into the mitochondria. The energy yield from the α-glycerol phosphate shuttle is less than that for the malate–aspartate shuttle.

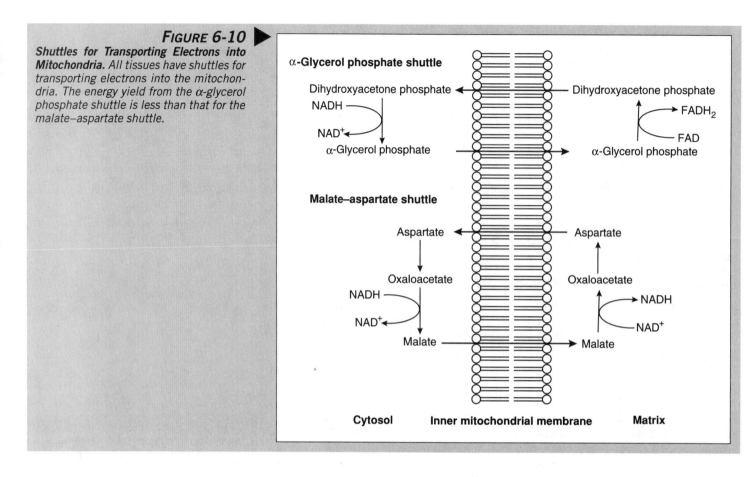

FIGURE 6-10 ▶

Shuttles for Transporting Electrons into Mitochondria. All tissues have shuttles for transporting electrons into the mitochondria. The energy yield from the α-glycerol phosphate shuttle is less than that for the malate–aspartate shuttle.

Malate–Aspartate Shuttle. The malate shuttle effectively transfers electrons from cytosolic NADH to mitochondrial NADH. This shuttle is more complex than the α-glycerol phosphate shuttle because oxaloacetate cannot be transported across the IMM. Therefore, two sets of isozymes operate in this shuttle. The malate dehydrogenase isozymes are responsible for converting cytosolic NADH to mitochondrial NADH. The aspartate aminotransferase isozymes catalyze the reversible interconversion of oxaloacetate and aspartate.

Adenine Nucleotide Transport Protein

The adenine nucleotide transporter exchanges mitochondrial ATP for cytosolic ADP. *Atractyloside*, a toxin found in plants, inhibits the transporter, resulting in a decrease in mitochondrial ADP and an inhibition of mitochondrial ATP synthesis.

COORDINATE REGULATION OF MITOCHONDRIAL PATHWAYS

The major metabolic pathways in mitochondria are fatty acid oxidation, the TCA cycle, and oxidative phosphorylation. Additionally, pyruvate dehydrogenase plays a critical role in the terminal oxidation of carbohydrate. Pyruvate, the end product of glycolysis, is transported into mitochondria where it is converted to acetyl CoA by pyruvate dehydrogenase. This reaction is a major source of substrate for the TCA cycle. The rates for all of these pathways are closely coordinated and are dependent primarily on the availability of oxygen and ADP (Figure 6-11). This phenomenon is known as *respiratory control*.

Anaerobic Conditions

In the absence of an adequate supply of oxygen, the rate of oxidative phosphorylation decreases, and NADH and $FADH_2$ accumulate. The accumulation of NADH, in turn, in-

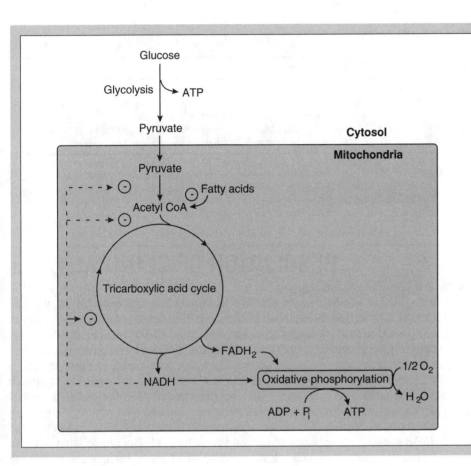

FIGURE 6-11
Coordinate Regulation of Oxidative Metabolism in Mitochondria. When there is an oxygen deficit, the rate of oxidative phosphorylation decreases, and NADH increases. The accumulation of NADH leads to a decreased rate of the TCA cycle and a decreased rate at which acetyl CoA is formed, both from pyruvate and fatty acid oxidation. Under these conditions, the cell becomes more dependent on glycolysis for its ATP.

hibits the TCA cycle, the oxidation of pyruvate to acetyl CoA, and the oxidation of fatty acids. Under these conditions, the cell becomes dependent on anaerobic glycolysis for its supply of ATP.

Aerobic Conditions

In the presence of an adequate supply of oxygen, the rate of oxidative phosphorylation is dependent primarily on the availability of ADP. The concentrations of ADP and ATP are reciprocally related, where an accumulation of ADP is accompanied by a decrease in ATP, and vice versa. Thus, an accumulation of ADP signals the need for ATP synthesis. An increase in ADP increases the rate of the TCA cycle by activating IDH, resulting in increased production of NADH and FADH$_2$, which, in turn, increases the rate of electron transport and ATP synthesis.

CONGENITAL DEFECTS IN OXIDATIVE PHOSPHORYLATION

Mitochondrial DNA (mtDNA) contains genes that code for some of the subunits of all four complexes of the ETC and ATP synthase. The mutation rate of mtDNA is higher than that of nuclear DNA, and most mutations that result in congenital defects in oxidative phosphorylation have been identified in mtDNA. The tissues most affected are tissues that require large amounts of ATP, including skeletal muscle, cardiac tissue, central nervous system, liver, and kidney. Abnormalities in oxidative phosphorylation affect a variety of developmental stages, resulting in phenotypes that are encountered in all age groups. Infants and children usually present with various combinations of symptoms, including seizures, hypotonia, failure to thrive, delay of developmental milestones, abnormalities in eye movement, and stroke-like symptoms [3]. Some of the clinical entities that result from mutations in mtDNA are summarized in Table 6-5. Diagnosis of these diseases involves muscle biopsy and isolation of mitochondria for morphologic, biochemical, and genetic analysis.

*Diseases caused by a defect in mitochondrial DNA are always **inherited maternally**. No affected male transmits the disease, because mitochondria from sperm do not enter the fertilized egg.*

Disease	Clinical Features
LHON	Bilateral loss of central vision, tremor, and ataxia
MERRF disease	Abnormal eye movements, loss of hearing, ataxia, lactic acidosis, ragged red muscle fibers, and progressive dementia
MELAS	Stroke-like episodes, abnormal motor and cognitive development, lactic acidosis, cardiomyopathy, deafness, dementia, and renal disease

Note. LHON = Leber's hereditary optic neuropathy; MERRF = myoclonic epilepsy and ragged-red fiber disease; MELAS = mitochondrial encephalomyopathy, lactic acidosis, and stroke-like episodes.

RESOLUTION OF CLINICAL CASE

The patient presented at the beginning of this chapter had a defect in complex III of the ETC, decreasing her ability to synthesize ATP by oxidative phosphorylation. Most of the ATP in cells is synthesized by oxidative phosphorylation. Since the ETC is defective in this patient, she is dependent on glycolysis for her supply of ATP. The amount of ATP that can be derived from glycolysis is only about 5% of that derived by complete oxidation of glucose. The symptoms of weakness, cramps, and lack of tolerance to exercise can be attributed to decreased ATP synthesis [1]. The low creatine phosphate/P_i ratio found in the patient's muscle cells indicates a low concentration of ATP. The elevated level of serum lactate is due to increased anaerobic glycolysis. The end products of glycolysis are pyruvate and NADH. Since NADH oxidation by the ETC is impaired, NAD^+ is regenerated by the NADH-dependent reduction of pyruvate to lactic acid. The dissociation of lactic acid to lactate releases H^+, which are absorbed by bicarbonate, thereby decreasing the level of serum bicarbonate. The absence of cytochrome-c reductase activity in this patient suggested a defect in complex III, which was confirmed by direct demonstration of a marked decrease in cytochrome-b. The rationale for treating this patient with menadione and ascorbic acid was to provide a shunt for transporting electrons around the defective complex III [2]. Menadione and ascorbic acid are able to carry electrons from CoQ to cytochrome-c. Menadione can transfer electrons from CoQ to ascorbic acid, and ascorbic acid can reduce cytochrome-c. This shunt allows electrons to flow through two of the three complexes that pump H^+ (complexes I and IV), thereby increasing the patient's ability to carry out oxidative phosphorylation. Theoretically, her ATP production would be about two-thirds that found in normal tissue.

REVIEW QUESTIONS

Directions: For each of the following questions, choose the **one best** answer.

1. The standard free energy change (ΔG°) for the hydrolysis of creatine phosphate is -10.3 kcal/mol, and the ΔG° for the hydrolysis of ATP to ADP and P_i is -7.3 kcal/mol. What is the ΔG° for the following reaction?

$$ADP + \text{creatine phosphate} \longrightarrow ATP + \text{creatine}$$

   (A) -10.6 kcal/mol

   (B) $+3.0$ kcal/mol

   (C) $+10.6$ kcal/mol

   (D) -3.0 kcal/mol

   (E) $+7.3$ kcal/mol

2. How many moles of ATP can be formed by the complete mitochondrial oxidation of 1 mol of acetyl CoA to carbon dioxide and water?

   (A) 1 mol

   (B) 3 mol

   (C) 5 mol

   (D) 11 mol

   (E) 12 mol

3. Which of the following effects would result from an exposure of mitochondria to dinitrophenol?

   (A) Decreased rate of the TCA cycle

   (B) Decreased transport of electrons from NADH to oxygen

   (C) Decreased ATP synthesis by oxidative phosphorylation

   (D) Decreased pumping of protons by complexes I, III, and IV

   (E) Decreased oxygen uptake

Directions: The groups of questions below consist of lettered choices followed by several numbered items. For each numbered item, select the appropriate lettered option with which it is most closely associated. Each lettered option may be used once, more than once, or not at all.

Questions 4–6

For each of the steps in the TCA cycle listed below, select the letter in the figure that best describes the step.

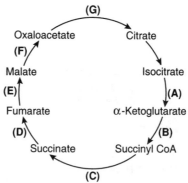

4. The rate-limiting step

5. The step at which substrate-level phosphorylation occurs

6. The step at which FADH$_2$ is produced

Questions 7–10

For each description given below, select the most closely associated compound.

    (A) Aspirin

    (B) Atractyloside

    (C) Cyanide

    (D) Antimycin

    (E) Oligomycin

7. Inhibits ATP synthesis most directly

8. Uncouples oxidation and phosphorylation

9. Inhibits translocation of ADP into the mitochondrial matrix

10. Inhibits the transport of electrons from cytochrome oxidase to oxygen

ANSWERS AND EXPLANATIONS

1. The answer is D. This reaction can be treated as the sum of two half-reactions. In one half-reaction, creatine phosphate is hydrolyzed to creatine and P$_i$ with a $\Delta G°$ of -10.3 kcal/mol. In the second half-reaction, ADP is condensed with P$_i$ to form ATP, which is the reverse of ATP hydrolysis and has a $\Delta G°$ of $+7.3$ kcal/mol. The sum of these half-reactions is -3.0 kcal/mol.

2. The answer is E. The oxidation of 1 mol of acetyl CoA by the TCA cycle results in 2 mol of carbon dioxide, 1 mol of GTP (readily converted to ATP by nucleoside-diphosphate kinase), 3 mol of NADH, and 1 mol of FADH$_2$. The oxidation of NADH results in the reduction of oxygen to water and supports the synthesis of 3 mol of ATP per mol of NADH, while FADH$_2$ supports the synthesis of 2 mol of ATP per mol of FADH$_2$.

3. The answer is C. Dinitrophenol uncouples oxidation and phosphorylation by abolishing the proton gradient across the inner mitochondrial membrane. Dinitrophenol increases the transport of electrons through the electron chain, oxygen uptake, and the pumping of protons by complexes I, III, and IV. Dinitrophenol freely permeates the membrane, carrying H^+ protons from the intermembrane space into the matrix and thus abolishing the H^+ gradient across the membrane.

4–6. The answers are: 4-A, 5-C, 6-D. The rate-limiting step is the oxidative decarboxylation of isocitrate to α-ketoglutarate, catalyzed by isocitrate dehydrogenase. The rate of this reaction is increased by ADP and decreased by ATP. Substrate-level phosphorylation occurs when succinyl CoA is hydrolyzed to succinate. The hydrolysis of the high-energy thioester bond between succinate and CoA is used to drive the synthesis of GTP from GDP and P_i. The oxidation of succinate to fumarate is the only reaction in the TCA cycle that produces $FADH_2$.

7–10. The answers are: 7-E, 8-A, 9-B, 10-C. Oligomycin binds to the F_o subunit of ATP synthase and prevents the movement of electrons through the H^+ channel. Aspirin uncouples oxidation and phosphorylation, accounting for the observation that aspirin overdose is accompanied by a fever. Atractyloside binds to the adenine nucleotide transport protein and inhibits ADP entry into the mitochondria in exchange for ATP. Cyanide binds to cytochrome oxidase and blocks the transport of electrons from cytochrome oxidase to oxygen. Antimycin binds to complex III and inhibits the transfer of electrons from complex III to cytochrome-c.

REFERENCES

1. Kennaway NG, Buist NRM, Darley-Usmar NM, et al: Lactic acidosis and mitochondrial myopathy associated with a deficiency of several components of complex III of the respiratory chain. *Pediatr Res* 18:991–999, 1984.
2. Lactic acidosis and mitochondrial myopathy in a young woman (Editorial Review). *Nutr Rev* 46:157–163, 1988.
3. Shoffner JM, Wallace DC: Oxidative phosphorylation diseases. In *The Metabolic and Molecular Bases of Inherited Disease*, 7th ed. Edited by Scriver CR, Beaudet AL, Sly WS, et al. New York, NY: McGraw-Hill, 1995, pp 1535–1609.

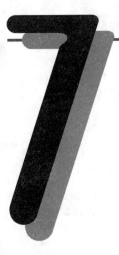

PRINCIPLES AND DESIGN OF METABOLISM

OVERVIEW OF METABOLISM

The word metabolism comes from the Greek word for "change," and it is used to describe the sum of all the chemical reactions that occur in living cells. Although several thousand different enzyme-catalyzed reactions occur simultaneously in cells, both the internal and external environment of the cell remain remarkably constant. The reactions are organized into functional sequences or pathways, where the product of one reaction is the substrate for the next reaction. Any compound that is a part of a pathway is known as a metabolite.

Major Goals of Metabolism

All of the metabolic pathways in cells are organized around two major goals that are necessary for the cell to maintain and replicate itself. The first goal is to extract energy (adenosine triphosphate [ATP]) and reducing power (reduced form of nicotinamide-adenine dinucleotide phosphate [NADPH]) from nutrients that can be used for the synthesis of more complex molecules. The second goal of metabolism is to provide a small set of precursors that can be converted to a diverse group of larger molecules, including proteins, nucleic acids, polysaccharides, and phospholipids.

Types of Metabolic Pathways

The metabolic pathways found in cells can be divided into three major categories: catabolic, anabolic, and amphibolic.

Catabolic Pathways. Catabolic pathways degrade large, complex molecules into smaller compounds by cleaving chemical bonds. These pathways involve oxidative processes and release energy, which can be conserved in the form of ATP, the reduced forms of nicotinamide adenine dinucleotides (NADH and NADPH). Examples of catabolic pathways are glycolysis and fatty acid oxidation.

Anabolic Pathways. Anabolic pathways synthesize larger molecules from smaller intermediates in metabolism by the formation of chemical bonds. Synthetic pathways are reductive processes, which require energy in the form of ATP and reducing power in the form of NADPH or NADH. Examples of anabolic pathways are gluconeogenesis and fatty acid synthesis.

Amphibolic Pathways. A metabolic pathway that functions both as a catabolic and anabolic pathway is defined as an amphibolic pathway. An example is the tricarboxylic acid (TCA) cycle, which oxidizes acetyl coenzyme A (acetyl CoA) to carbon dioxide (CO_2) and water and also includes several intermediates that serve as substrates for synthetic pathways.

Interconversion of Metabolic Fuels

Each dietary fuel has a storage form, a transport or circulating form, and characteristic cellular intermediates that converge with the formation of acetyl CoA (Figure 7-1).

FIGURE 7-1
Interconversion of Metabolic Fuels. Each metabolic fuel has a characteristic storage form, transport form, and low-molecular-weight tissue metabolites. The arrows indicate the interconversions that can occur. Double-headed arrows indicate reversible reactions, and single-headed arrows indicate unidirectional pathways or reactions.

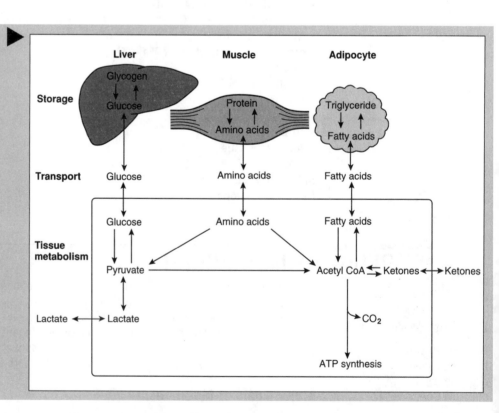

Storage and Transport Forms. The storage forms and the transport forms for each macronutrient are interconvertible. Glucose, fatty acids, and amino acids are transport forms of metabolic fuels that are stored as glycogen, triglyceride, and protein, respectively. The pathways for interconverting the different forms of a fuel provide a mechanism for storing excess dietary fuels following a meal and retrieving fuels between meals. Separate pathways, however, exist for storage and retrieval.

De Novo Synthesis of Transport Forms. All of the transport forms of fuels, except the essential amino acids, can be synthesized from smaller metabolic intermediates that are generated in the cell. The essential amino acids, however, must be supplied by the diet.

There are two transport forms of carbohydrate: *glucose*, which is released from glycogen, and *lactate*, which is derived from glucose. Lactate is formed by the NADH-dependent reduction of pyruvate and released into the blood. Lactate can be removed from the blood by several tissues and either oxidized for ATP production or used for de novo glucose synthesis.

There are two circulating (transport) forms of fat: *fatty acids*, which are released from triglyceride stores, and *ketones*, which are small, soluble derivatives of fatty acids. Ketones can be removed from the circulation by many tissues and used either as a source of energy or as a substrate for membrane lipid synthesis. Ketones are formed only when excess acetyl CoA exits.

Permitted and Nonpermitted Transitions. The transitions among metabolic fuels are frequently described as either permitted and nonpermitted transitions. *Permitted transitions* are: carbohydrate to fat, protein to fat, and protein to carbohydrate. *Nonpermitted transitions* are: fat to protein, carbohydrate to protein, and fat to carbohydrate. Protein cannot be synthesized from either carbohydrate or fat because of the dietary requirement for the essential amino acids. Fat cannot be converted to carbohydrate because the conversion of acetyl CoA (a two-carbon compound) to pyruvate (a three-carbon compound) is an irreversible reaction. There is no enzyme in human tissues that can convert acetyl CoA back to pyruvate or any other three-carbon compound.

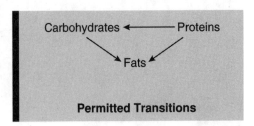

Permitted Transitions

ORGANIZATIONAL THEMES IN METABOLISM

An apparent paradox in metabolism is that thousands of different enzyme-catalyzed reactions occur in cells, yet both the intracellular and extracellular environment of the cell stays remarkably constant. The thousands of reactions are organized into a few functional pathways that are interconnected with one another. The rate at which any particular pathway operates in a cell is very carefully regulated and is also coordinated with the rate at which other pathways operate. There are a few *recurring themes and patterns* that provide a framework for the simplification and organization of metabolism and contribute to homeostasis.

Types of Reactions That Occur in Cells

Although there are thousands of different enzymes, each having a different substrate and product, all can be classified into six groups, based on the type of reaction each catalyzes (see Chapter 3). Certain types of reactions always use the same coenzyme and may occur in many different pathways. For example, CoA is a coenzyme in all reactions that transfer acyl groups. This type of reaction occurs in many pathways, including the TCA cycle, fatty acid oxidation, fatty acid synthesis, phospholipid synthesis, and cholesterol synthesis.

Types of Reactions That Occur in Cells
Oxidation-reduction
Group transfer
Hydrolysis
Nonhydrolytic cleavage
Isomerization
ATP-dependent formation of bonds

Building Blocks for Assembly of Large Molecules

Cells synthesize a diverse group of complex molecules from a small number of simple building blocks. For example, proteins are synthesized from 20 amino acids, the nucleic acids are synthesized from five mononucleotides, heme is synthesized from glycine and succinyl CoA, and cholesterol is synthesized from acetyl CoA.

Connections of Pathways by Branch Points

Many metabolic pathways are connected to one another by a limited number of branch points. Four important branch points are shown in Figure 7-2. *Glucose-6-phosphate* is the substrate for four different enzymes, each initiating different pathways leading to the

FIGURE 7-2

FIGURE 7-2 ▶
Key Branch Points in Metabolism. Metabolic pathways are linked to one another by a few branch points. Metabolites that act as branch points are substrates or products of more than one enzyme. Glucose-6-phosphate, pyruvate, acetyl CoA, and succinyl CoA link together numerous pathways in carbohydrate, lipid, and amino acid metabolism.

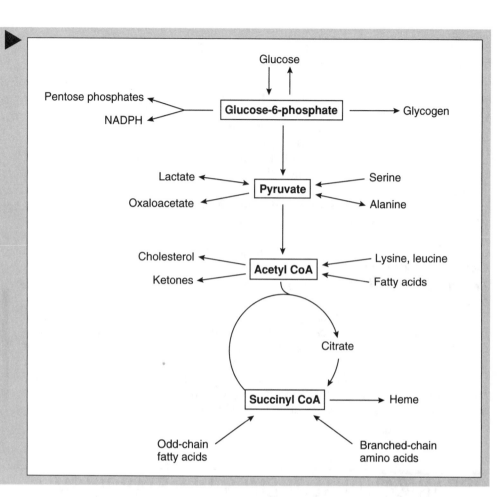

Opposing Pathways in Metabolism
Glycogen synthesis/glycogen degradation
Gluconeogenesis/glycolysis
Triglyceride synthesis/triglyceride degradation
Fatty acid synthesis/fatty acid oxidation
Protein synthesis/protein hydrolysis

production of glucose, glycogen, pyruvate, pentose phosphates and NADPH. Similarly, *pyruvate, acetyl CoA*, and *succinyl CoA* form branch points that connect various other pathways with one another.

Biosynthetic and Degradative Pathways

Pathways that degrade and synthesize metabolic fuels are unidirectional. For example, fatty acid synthesis and fatty acid oxidation are opposing pathways, having no enzymes in common and occurring in different subcellular compartments. Other opposing pathways may occur in the same subcellular compartment and share some of the same enzymes, but there are always some enzymes that are specific for each pathway. For example, glycolysis and gluconeogenesis are opposing pathways that share many of the same enzymes, but each pathway has unique enzymes that catalyze reactions that are irreversible under the conditions found in the cell. Having distinctive synthetic and degradative steps in opposing pathways allows each pathway to operate independently of the other. A futile cycle would exist if uncontrolled synthesis and degradation occurred simultaneously.

Universal Carriers in Catabolic and Anabolic Pathways

Many connections between catabolism and anabolism are provided by carriers of energy and electrons. ATP, a universal carrier of chemical energy, is an end product of catabolic pathways and a substrate for anabolic pathways. Similarly, the nicotinamide adenine dinucleotides (NAD^+ and $NADP^+$) are universal carriers of electrons in metabolism. NAD^+ and $NADP^+$ are oxidizing agents in catabolic pathways, whereas NADPH is a universal reducing agent in biosynthetic reactions (Figure 7-3).

Mechanisms for Regulating Metabolic Pathways

The rates at which metabolic pathways are regulated and coordinated with one another are controlled by allosteric effectors, covalent modification, and induction or repression of enzyme synthesis. All metabolic pathways are regulated by one or more of these mechanisms (see Chapter 8).

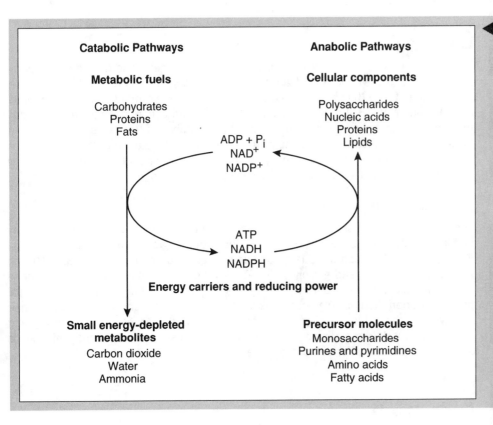

◀ FIGURE 7-3
Integration of Catabolism and Anabolism by Energy Carriers. *The two major branches of metabolism are linked to one another by energy in the form of high-energy phosphate bonds and reducing power. Catabolic pathways degrade large molecules to small metabolites and release energy that is conserved as ATP, NADH, and NADPH. Anabolic pathways synthesize large molecules from small precursor molecules and require ATP, NADPH, and NADH. ADP = adenosine diphosphate; P_i = inorganic phosphate.*

METABOLIC SPECIALIZATION OF MAJOR ORGANS

The metabolic pathways that operate in an organ, tissue, or cell are closely correlated with the function of the cell or tissue. Some metabolic pathways, such as glycolysis and the pentose phosphate pathway, are found in all cells, whereas other pathways may occur to different degrees in various cell types (Table 7-1).

◀ *TABLE 7-1*
Metabolic Profile of Major Organs

Pathway	Liver	Muscle	Brain	Kidney	Adipocyte	RBC
TCA cycle	+++	+++	+++	+++	+	−
Fatty acid oxidation	+++	+++	−	+++	−	−
Ketone synthesis	+++	−	−	−	−	−
Ketone oxidation	−	+++	+++[a]	++	+	−
Pentose phosphate	+++	+	+	+	++	+++
Glucose synthesis	+++	−	−	++[b]	−	−
Fatty acid synthesis	+++	−	−	−	+	−
Lactate synthesis	+	+++[c]	−	+	+	+++
Glycogen metabolism	+++	+++	+/−	+	+	−
Urea synthesis	+++	−	−	−	−	−

[a] Ketones are oxidized only in the fasted state.
[b] Glucose synthesis is maximum during metabolic acidosis when glutamine is being converted to ammonia and α-ketoglutarate.
[c] Lactate is formed under anaerobic conditions that exist during prolonged exercise.

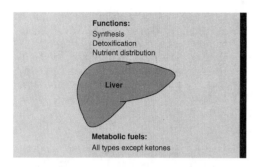

Liver

The major functions of the liver include a variety of synthetic and detoxification pathways. The liver is the major site of glucose, fatty acid, and cholesterol synthesis, and it is the only site of urea, bile acid, and ketone synthesis. These synthetic processes require both ATP and NADPH. The liver has a high content of mitochondria and a high capacity for oxidative metabolism, and it can use all of the metabolic fuels as a source of energy. Most of the *detoxification* functions of the liver involve *hydroxylation* and *conjugation reactions*, which are catalyzed by enzymes of the smooth endoplasmic reticulum. The hydroxylation reactions are dependent on a supply of oxygen.

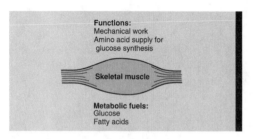

Skeletal Muscle

The major function of skeletal muscle is to perform mechanical work, and the primary metabolic pathways in skeletal muscle are those that degrade fuels for ATP synthesis. *White muscle fibers* can store large amounts of glycogen and are very dependent on glycogen degradation and glycolysis for ATP synthesis. They have fewer mitochondria than red muscle fibers, resulting in a limited capacity to generate ATP by oxidative phosphorylation. *Red muscle fibers* have a high content of mitochondria and derive their energy from the oxidation of glucose, fatty acids, and ketones. During fasting and starvation, muscle protein is degraded, and the carbon skeletons from the amino acids are used as precursors for de novo glucose synthesis.

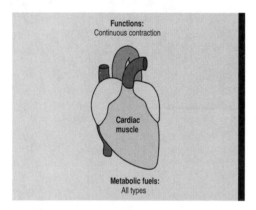

Cardiac Muscle

The heart, in contrast to other muscles, is constantly contracting and requires a constant supply of ATP. It is rich in mitochondria and has a high capacity for oxidation of glucose, pyruvate, lactate, fatty acids, and ketones. The synthetic capacity of the heart is limited.

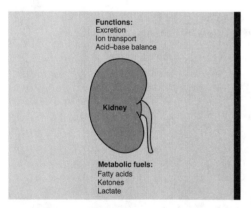

Kidney

The kidney has a number of highly specialized functions including active transport of ions and regulation of acid–base balance. The high rate of active transport requires a large supply of ATP, most of which is derived by the oxidation of fatty acids, lactate, and ketones. The excretion of ammonium ions (NH_4^+) contributes to acid–base balance. Most of the NH_4^+ excreted is derived from the deamination of glutamine, resulting in ammonia, which absorbs a proton (H^+) to form NH_4^+. The carbon skeleton remaining after deamination of glutamine is used for de novo glucose synthesis.

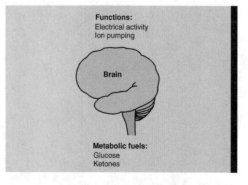

Brain and Nerve

Brain and nerve cells specialize in ion pumping and the generation of electrical signals. A constant supply of ATP is needed for active transport of ions. The major source of ATP is derived from the oxidation of glucose. Fatty acids cannot be oxidized because of the impermeability of the blood–brain barrier. During prolonged fasting and in starvation, some of the ATP can be derived from the oxidation of ketones.

Adipose Tissue

Adipose tissue specializes in the synthesis and degradation of triglycerides. Most of the fatty acids that are stored in triglycerides are from dietary sources, or they are synthesized in the liver from excess glucose and transported to the adipose tissue for storage. The glycerol backbone of triglycerides is derived from dihydroxyacetone phosphate, an intermediate in glycolysis.

Red Blood Cells (RBCs)

The major function of RBCs is to transport oxygen from the lungs to the tissues and to transport carbon dioxide from the tissues to the lungs. The maintenance of the biconcave-disc shape of the RBC requires ATP, which is derived solely from glycolysis. 2,3-Bisphosphoglycerate, the compound that regulates the binding and release of oxygen from hemoglobin, is also derived from glycolysis. The end product of glucose metabolism in the RBC is lactate.

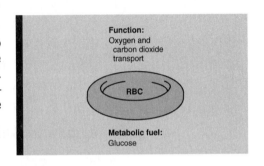

SUBCELLULAR LOCALIZATION OF MAJOR PATHWAYS

Specific pathways usually occur within a particular subcellular compartment, and in some cases, opposing pathways are localized in different subcellular compartments. The localization of a pathway is always determined by the localization of the enzymes in that pathway. The major pathways in metabolism, together with the subcellular compartments that house the pathways, are summarized in Table 7-2. Some pathways have enzymes that are located in more than one cellular compartment. In these instances, the intermediates must be transported back and forth across the membranes that separate the compartments.

◀ **TABLE 7-2**
Subcellular Compartmentation of Major Metabolic Pathways

Cytosol	Mitochondria	Cytosol and Mitochondria	Smooth Endoplasmic Reticulum
Glycolysis	TCA cycle	Gluconeogenesis	Triglyceride synthesis
Pentose phosphate pathway	Ketogenesis	Urea synthesis	Phospholipid synthesis
Fatty acid synthesis	Fatty acid oxidation		Cholesterol synthesis
Nucleotide synthesis	Ketone oxidation		Detoxification reactions
Protein synthesis	Oxidative phosphorylation		

REVIEW QUESTIONS

Directions: For each of the following questions, choose the **one best** answer.

1. Which of the following compounds is an end product of anabolism?
    (A) ATP
    (B) NADH
    (C) NADP+
    (D) Carbon dioxide
    (E) Ammonia

2. Which of the following transitions among metabolic fuels is a nonpermitted transition?
    (A) Carbohydrate to fat
    (B) Protein to fat
    (C) Protein to carbohydrate
    (D) Fat to carbohydrate

Directions: The group of questions below consists of lettered choices followed by several numbered items. For each numbered item, select the appropriate lettered option with which it is most closely associated.

Questions 3–7

For each metabolic function listed below, select the organ, tissue, or cell that is most closely associated with the function. (In this question, each letter can be used only once or not at all.)
    (A) Adipose tissue
    (B) Kidney
    (C) Liver
    (D) Skeletal muscle
    (E) Heart
    (F) Brain
    (G) RBC

3. Urea synthesis

4. Deamination of glutamine

5. 2,3-Bisphosphoglycerate synthesis

6. Glycogen metabolism

7. Fatty acid storage

ANSWERS AND EXPLANATIONS

1. The answer is C. Anabolic pathways use NADPH as a universal reducing agent, resulting in the formation of NADP$^+$. ATP, NADH, carbon dioxide, and ammonia are the products of catabolic pathways.

2. The answer is D. Fat cannot be converted to carbohydrate because acetyl CoA, the tissue metabolite derived from fatty acids, cannot be converted to pyruvate or any other three-carbon intermediate in gluconeogenesis. Protein can be converted to carbohydrate because some of the amino acids are degraded to pyruvate. Both carbohydrate and protein can be degraded to acetyl CoA, the substrate for fatty acid synthesis.

3–7. The answers are: 3-C, 4-B, 5-G, 6-D, 7-A. Urea synthesis only occurs in the liver. The deamination of glutamine is closely associated with the ability of the kidney to regulate acid–base balance. In cases of metabolic acidosis, accelerated deamination of glutamine occurs, resulting in the release of ammonia that can absorb protons and be excreted as ammonium ion. The RBCs synthesize 2,3-bisphosphoglycerate, which regulates the affinity of hemoglobin for oxygen. Glycogen metabolism occurs in both liver and muscle, but since each organ or tissue can be used only once and since urea synthesis occurs only in the liver, the correct associated organ for glycogen metabolism is skeletal muscle. Almost all of the fatty acid storage occurs in the adipose tissue where fatty acids are esterified and stored as triglycerides.

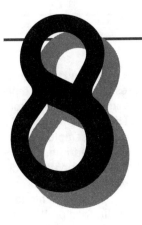

REGULATION OF METABOLISM

INTRODUCTION OF CLINICAL CASE

A 25-year-old woman was on a kayaking trip in Costa Rica when she began to experience mild abdominal pains and watery diarrhea. By the next day, she was vomiting, and the diarrhea was almost continuous. By the time her friends got her to a hospital, she was almost comatose. The diarrhea was a clear liquid resembling rice water, and the patient was losing fluid at a rate of about 800 mL per hour. Her blood pressure was 75/50 (normal 120/80), and her skin turgor was poor and had a shriveled appearance. Laboratory analysis of a blood sample showed metabolic acidosis (pH 7.15) with a bicarbonate level about half the normal value. Microscopic examination of a stool sample showed *Vibrio cholerae* bacteria. Intravenous administration of fluids was started immediately and was continued for 24 hours. She was also given tetracycline. The patient's condition improved rapidly, and her blood pressure returned to normal. By the second day, she was able to take an oral rehydration solution containing glucose, sodium chloride, potassium chloride, and sodium bicarbonate. She began eating solid food on the fifth day. Her condition continued to improve, and on day 12, she was dismissed from the hospital.

OVERVIEW

Homeostasis in living organisms demands that metabolism be carefully controlled. Cells are continually adjusting the rates of metabolic pathways to ensure that adequate energy and building blocks are available for carrying out normal cellular functions. A variety of mechanisms exist within the cell that allow metabolism to proceed in an orderly and balanced fashion. Imposed on the intracellular regulatory mechanisms are hormonal mechanisms that coordinate the metabolic activities between different cells and tissues. In all metabolic pathways, these mechanisms involve a few key enzymes that are the targets of regulation. Each metabolic pathway has at least one regulatory enzyme that may be subject to several different types of regulation.

Regulatory Enzymes

Many human diseases can be traced to abnormalities in metabolic regulation. Examples are diabetes, whooping cough, and many forms of tumors.

The activity of a regulatory enzyme can change in response to small changes in its environment. Enzymes that catalyze the rate-limiting step or the committed step in a pathway are usually the targets of regulation.

Rate-limiting Step. The slowest step in a pathway sets the pace at which the pathway operates. If the conversion of B to C is the slowest reaction in the following sequence, then an increase or decrease in the flow of metabolites through the pathway will occur only if the rate of the reaction catalyzed by enzyme b is increased or decreased.

$$A \longrightarrow B \xrightarrow{\text{Enzyme b}} C \longrightarrow D \longrightarrow E$$

This concept is analogous to a bottleneck in traffic created by funneling four lanes of rush-hour traffic into a two-lane tunnel.

Committed Step. In a branched pathway, the first reaction that is committed to the formation of a particular end product is frequently inhibited by the accumulation of that product. For example, in the following pathway, product E may act as a feedback inhibitor of the enzyme that converts B to C, whereas product G may inhibit the enzyme that converts B to F.

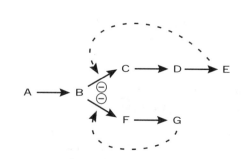

Types of Regulatory Mechanisms

Cells use three major mechanisms to control the activity of key regulatory enzymes: (1) noncovalent interactions, (2) covalent modifications, and (3) changes in abundance of the enzyme. The first two mechanisms alter a preexisting enzyme while the third mechanism involves the synthesis, degradation, or both of an enzyme. The time required for an enzyme to respond to each of these mechanisms differs, ranging from minutes to days. A particular enzyme may be regulated by all three mechanisms.

REGULATION OF ENZYME ACTIVITY BY NONCOVALENT INTERACTIONS

The noncovalent interaction between an enzyme and another molecule in the cell is the most rapid type of regulation, occurring within seconds. The binding of the molecule to the enzyme alters the activity of the enzyme. There are three categories of noncovalent interactions that can alter the rate of enzyme-catalyzed reactions: (1) substrate availability, (2) allosteric regulation, and (3) protein–protein interactions.

> Some regulatory mechanisms are faster than others. **Allosteric regulation** occurs in seconds; **covalent regulation** may require minutes; and **induction of enzyme synthesis** may require hours to days.

Substrate Availability

The simplest type of regulation is mediated by a change in the concentration of the substrate. As long as the concentration of substrate is significantly below that required for saturation, the activity of the enzyme increases or decreases as the substrate concentration varies. The in vivo concentration of most substrates is close to the Michaelis constant (K_m) of the enzyme for that substrate. Most enzymes have substrate saturation curves that are hyperbolic and obey Michaelis-Menten kinetics, indicating that the binding of substrate to one site is not influenced by the binding to other sites. However, regulatory enzymes usually show cooperativity between their substrate-binding sites (Figure 8-1). The cooperativity may be either positive or negative.

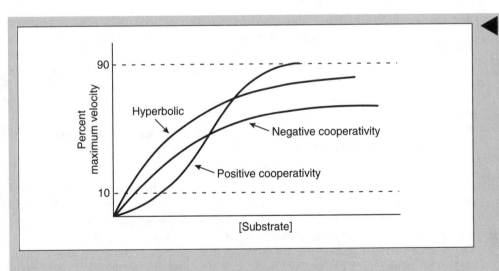

FIGURE 8-1
Comparison of Hyperbolic and Cooperative Substrate Saturation Curves. Hyperbolic kinetics are seen when each site binds substrate independently. Positive cooperativity is observed when binding to one site increases the affinity of subsequent sites for substrate, and negative cooperativity is seen when binding to one site makes it more difficult for binding to occur at other sites. For hyperbolic kinetics, an 81-fold increase in substrate concentration is required to increase the rate from 10% to 90% of the maximum rate, whereas for positive cooperativity, the same effect is achieved with an increase in substrate that is less than 81-fold, and for negative cooperativity, an increase greater than 81-fold is required.

Positive Cooperativity. Enzymes that show positive cooperativity have sigmoidal (S-shaped) substrate saturation curves. The binding of substrate to one site induces a conformational change that increases the catalytic activity at other sites. This property allows an enzyme to respond rapidly to small changes in substrate concentration.

Negative Cooperativity. Enzymes that show negative cooperativity have substrate saturation curves that are desensitized to changes in substrate concentration. The binding of substrate to one site decreases the catalytic activity at subsequent sites.

Allosteric Regulation

The activity of many regulatory enzymes is controlled by the binding of small molecules to sites that are distinct from the active site. These sites are known as allosteric sites, and the molecules that bind to the sites are allosteric effectors. Allosteric effectors usually have little, if any, structural resemblance to the substrate. Allosteric sites may occur on the same subunit as the catalytic site, or there may be a separate regulatory subunit that binds the allosteric effector. In either case, the binding of an allosteric effector results in a conformational change that alters the structure and function of the active site (Figure 8-2). This type of regulation is rapid, usually occurring within seconds.

FIGURE 8-2 ▶
Active and Regulatory Sites of an Allosteric Enzyme. *The binding of an allosteric effector induces a conformational change in the enzyme, which alters the events that occur at the active site. Either the affinity for the substrate or the rate at which substrate is converted to product can be altered by an allosteric effector.*

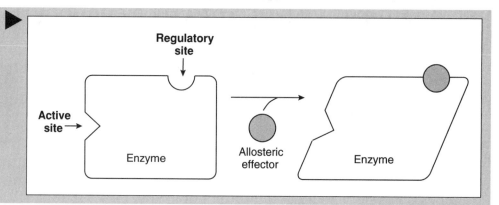

SUBSTRATE SATURATION CURVES

The substrate saturation curves for allosteric enzymes cannot be described by Michaelis-Menten kinetics. The structural changes that occur upon binding of an allosteric effector alter either the K_m of the enzyme for its substrate or the maximum velocity (V_{max}) of the reaction. Effectors that alter the K_m are known as K-type effectors, while those that alter the V_{max} are known as V-type effectors. Allosteric effectors are classified into two major classes, activators and inhibitors.

Allosteric Activators. Allosteric activators increase the reaction rate by either *decreasing the K_m* of the enzyme for its substrate or by *increasing the V_{max}* of the reaction (Figure 8-3). Activators that decrease the K_m produce a shift to the left in the substrate saturation curve, whereas activators that increase the V_{max} produce an upward shift in the plateau of the saturation curve.

> An increase in the affinity of an enzyme for its substrate is reflected by a decrease in K_m.

Allosteric Inhibitors. Allosteric inhibitors decrease the reaction rate by either *increasing the K_m* of the enzyme for its substrate or by *decreasing the V_{max}* of the reaction (see Figure 8-3). Inhibitors that increase the K_m shift the substrate saturation curves to the right, and those that decrease the V_{max} decrease the plateau.

MOLECULES THAT ACT AS ALLOSTERIC EFFECTORS

Molecules that act as allosteric effectors fall into two general categories: (1) end products of metabolic pathways and (2) metabolites that are indicators of the energy status of the cell.

End Products of Pathways. Biosynthetic pathways are frequently inhibited by the accumulation of end products of the pathway, a phenomenon known as *feedback inhibition*. The enzyme that is regulated usually catalyzes the committed step or the rate-limiting step in the pathway. The end product binds to an allosteric site, resulting in a decrease in the activity of the key regulatory enzyme in the pathway.

> Loss of feedback inhibition has been implicated in the pathogenesis of several diseases, including familial hypercholesterolemia, porphyrias, and gout.

Indicators of Energy Status. The intracellular accumulation of adenosine triphosphate (ATP) indicates a high-energy state, whereas the accumulation of adenosine diphosphate (ADP) and adenosine monophosphate (AMP) indicates a low-energy state. The energy charge of a cell is an index of the metabolically available energy and is defined by the following equation:

$$\text{Energy charge} = \frac{[ATP] + \frac{1}{2}[ADP]}{[ATP] + [ADP] + [AMP]}$$

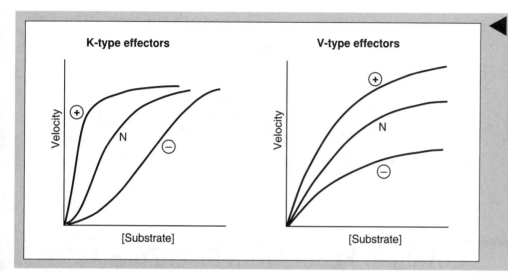

FIGURE 8-3
Substrate Saturation Curves for Allosteric Enzymes. K-type allosteric effectors alter the K_m of the enzyme for the substrate, and they result in a shift in the substrate saturation curves to the left (activators) or to the right (inhibitors). V-type effectors either increase or decrease the V_{max} of the reaction, shifting the curve up or down. N = no allosteric effector present; + = allosteric activator; − = allosteric inhibitor.

Catabolic pathways that lead to ATP synthesis tend to increase the energy charge, whereas anabolic pathways that use ATP tend to decrease the energy charge. However, over time the energy charge remains reasonably constant because as ATP begins to accumulate, it inhibits key enzymes in pathways that lead to further ATP synthesis and activates key enzymes in pathways that use ATP. The accumulation of ADP and AMP have the opposite effect, stimulating catabolic pathways that lead to ATP synthesis and inhibiting anabolic pathways that use ATP. The accumulation of acetyl coenzyme A (acetyl CoA), citrate, and the reduced form of nicotinamide adenine dinucleotide (NADH) may also indicate a high-energy state in the cell. These metabolites, like the adenine nucleotides, are allosteric effectors of several regulatory enzymes (Table 8-1).

TABLE 8-1
Allosteric Regulation by Compounds That Are Indicators of the Energy State of the Cell

Pathway	Enzyme	Activator	Inhibitor
Catabolic pathways			
Glycogen degradation	Glycogen phosphorylase	AMP	ATP
Glucose oxidation	Phosphofructokinase-1	AMP	ATP and citrate
	Pyruvate dehydrogenase		ATP, NADH, and acetyl CoA
	Pyruvate kinase		ATP and acetyl CoA
TCA cycle	Isocitrate dehydrogenase	ADP	ATP
Anabolic pathways			
Gluconeogenesis	Fructose-1,6-bisphosphatase	ATP and citrate	AMP
	Pyruvate carboxylase	Acetyl CoA	
Fatty acid synthesis	Acetyl CoA carboxylase	Citrate	

Note. TCA = tricarboxylic acid.

Protein–Protein Interactions

The activity of an enzyme can be regulated by interaction with other proteins that have no catalytic function. This type of regulation is analogous to allosteric regulation, except, in this case, the allosteric effector is a protein rather than a low-molecular-weight metabolite or an end product of metabolism.

An example of a regulatory protein that alters the activity of several enzymes is *calmodulin*, a small calcium (Ca^{2+})-binding protein that sensitizes several enzymes to changes in the cytosolic concentration of Ca^{2+} (Figure 8-4). Calmodulin has no catalytic activity, but when it binds Ca^{2+}, it undergoes a conformational change that allows it to interact with several cellular enzymes, resulting in an increase in their catalytic activity.

Large differences in Ca^{2+} concentration exist between the exterior and the interior of the cell. The intracellular concentration is normally about $10^{-7}M$, while the extracellular concentration of Ca^{2+} is approximately 5 mM. Intracellular proteins that are activated by Ca^{2+} usually respond to an increase in Ca^{2+} from about $10^{-7}M$ to $10^{-6}M$.

FIGURE 8-4

FIGURE 8-4
Activation of Enzymes by Interaction with the Ca²⁺ -Calmodulin Complex. The binding of Ca²⁺ by calmodulin results in a conformational change that allows the complex to interact with a number of enzymes, resulting in an increase in their catalytic activity.

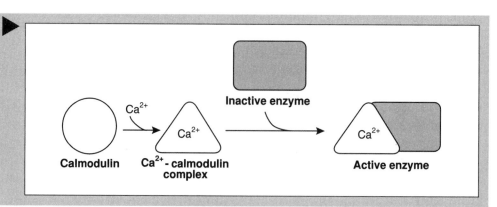

COVALENT REGULATION OF ENZYME ACTIVITY

The activity of an enzyme can also be regulated by covalent modification of its structure. The modification may be either reversible or irreversible, and it is always mediated by another enzyme. The most common reversible modifications that occur in metabolism are the phosphorylation and dephosphorylation of key enzymes in metabolic pathways. Phosphorylation of an enzyme may result in either an increase or decrease in activity. The most common type of irreversible modification is the conversion of inactive enzyme precursors to active enzymes by limited proteolysis. Since covalent modification of one enzyme is mediated by another enzyme, the change in catalytic activity takes longer to occur but persists for a longer period than changes that are mediated by allosteric interactions.

Phosphorylation and Dephosphorylation

A family of protein kinases and protein phosphatases are found in cells that catalyze protein phosphorylation and dephosphorylation, respectively (Figure 8-5). The protein kinases transfer phosphate groups from ATP to a hydroxyl group on the side chain of either *serine, threonine,* or *tyrosine* residues in the target enzyme, forming phosphate esters. Usually, only one serine residue in a protein is recognized by a particular protein kinase. The serine residue that is phosphorylated is surrounded by a specific amino acid sequence, known as the *consensus sequence*. Each protein kinase recognizes a different consensus sequence. The protein phosphatases hydrolyze the phosphate ester linkage, releasing inorganic phosphate and returning the enzyme to its dephosphorylated state.

The addition or removal of a phosphate group results in a change in both the conformation of the enzyme and its kinetic properties. The K_m, V_{max}, or both may be altered, and in some cases, the affinity of the enzyme for an allosteric effector may also be changed. Protein kinases and phosphatases are regulated by hormones that bind to the surface of cells and, through a series of intermediate steps, either increase or decrease the activity as well as the phosphorylation state of their target enzymes. The

Phosphorylation activates pathways that mobilize energy from glycogen and triglyceride stores, and it inactivates pathways that lead to energy storage.

FIGURE 8-5
Covalent Modification by Adding and Removing Phosphate Groups. The properties of a protein can be altered by protein kinase, which transfers a phosphate group from ATP to a specific serine, threonine, or tyrosine side chain. The reaction is reversed by a protein phosphatase, which removes the phosphate by hydrolysis.

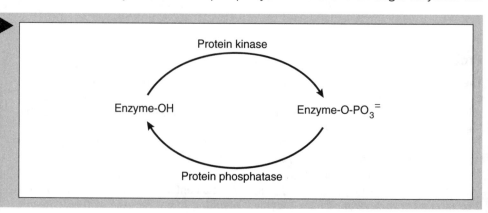

connection between hormonal control and protein phosphorylation provides a mechanism for both the intracellular and intercellular coordination of metabolic pathways (Table 8-2).

Pathway	Key Regulatory Enzyme	Effect of Phosphorylation
Intracellular coordination		
Glycogen degradation	Glycogen phosphorylase	Activation
Glycogen synthesis	Glycogen synthase	Inhibition
Intercellular coordination		
Fatty acid mobilization (adipose tissue)	Hormone-sensitive lipase	Activation
Fatty acid synthesis (liver)	Acetyl CoA carboxylase	Inhibition

Limited Proteolysis

Limited proteolysis is a mechanism used to activate key enzymes and proteins involved in many diverse cellular processes, including digestion of dietary protein, blood clotting, collagen assembly, and peptide hormone activation. In all of these cases, the proteins are synthesized and stored as inactive precursors, known as *zymogens* or *proenzymes*, which are converted to their biologically active forms by the cleavage of one or two specific peptide bonds (Figure 8-6). The proteolysis is accompanied by a conformational change that allows the protein to acquire a new function.

Enzyme Cascades

Enzyme cascades provide mechanisms for the amplification of a small regulatory signal, resulting in a large response. Cascades are generated when one enzyme activates another enzyme. The first enzyme in a cascade is activated by a regulatory signal, and the last enzyme in the cascade catalyzes a reaction directly related to the biologic response (Figure 8-7). The amplification potential is increased by increasing the number of enzymes in the cascade. Two major types of cascades are found in biologic systems, those that are initiated by phosphorylation of an enzyme and those that are initiated by limited proteolysis of an enzyme precursor. Several examples of enzyme cascades are discussed in subsequent chapters, including the phosphorylation cascade involved in glycogen degradation and the cascade of limited proteolysis involved in the digestion of dietary protein.

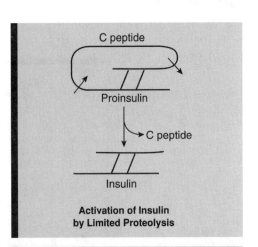

Activation of Insulin by Limited Proteolysis

Hemophilia B results from an inherited deficiency in one of the factors in the blood clotting cascade. Each factor is synthesized as an inactive precursor and is sequentially activated by limited proteolysis. At least eight enzymes are activated in the cascade, resulting in an extremely large amplification.

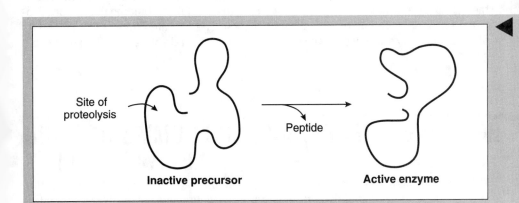

Inactive precursor   **Active enzyme**

Site of proteolysis → ... Peptide

◀ **FIGURE 8-6**
Enzyme Activation by Limited Proteolysis.
The hydrolysis of one or two specific peptide bonds in an inactive enzyme precursor removes a conformational restraint, which allows the enzyme to undergo a conformational change to a form that has catalytic activity.

FIGURE 8-7 ▶
Enzyme Cascades and Amplification of Regulatory Signals. Cascades are formed when one enzyme converts another enzyme to an active form. Each step in the cascade magnifies the effect of the preceding step.

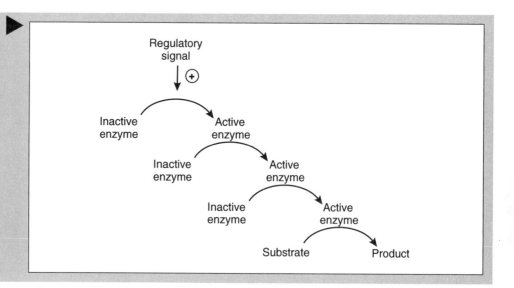

FIGURE 8-7 ▶

Enzyme Cascades and Amplification of Regulatory Signals. *Cascades are formed when one enzyme converts another enzyme to an active form. Each step in the cascade magnifies the effect of the preceding step.*

CHANGES IN ENZYME ABUNDANCE

The rate at which an enzyme-catalyzed reaction occurs is dependent on the amount of enzyme present in the cell. Most enzymes in cells are present at a constant concentration throughout the life of the cell. These enzymes are known as *constitutive enzymes*. In contrast, the concentration of regulatory enzymes that set the pace at which pathways operate may vary significantly, depending on the needs of the cell. Enzymes that increase in concentration are said to be *inducible*.

Inducible Enzymes

Induction of enzyme synthesis always involves increased messenger RNA (mRNA) and protein synthesis. The rate of gene transcription and the synthesis of mRNA is regulated by a group of proteins known as *transcriptional factors*. A period of time extending from hours to days may pass between the initiating signal and the actual change in enzyme concentration.

Regulation of Enzyme Levels

The abundance of an inducible enzyme is subject to hormonal regulation. The effect of the hormones is exerted in the nucleus of the cell where RNA transcription occurs. There, the hormones activate transcriptional factors, either by directly binding to the transcriptional factor or by stimulating its phosphorylation. The activated transcriptional factors bind to regulatory sequences in the DNA and increase the rate of transcription of specific genes.

HORMONES, RECEPTORS, AND COMMUNICATION BETWEEN CELLS

The metabolic activities of different tissues are coordinated by hormones that are synthesized in the endocrine glands and released into the circulation. The hormones act as *chemical signals* or *primary messengers*, which produce a characteristic response in other tissues, known as *target tissues*. The target tissues for a particular hormone have *receptors* that bind the hormone with a high degree of specificity. Hormone receptors can be classified in two major groups based on their subcellular location.

Intracellular Receptors

Lipid-soluble hormones, such as steroid hormones, thyroid hormones, vitamin D, retinol, and retinoic acid, exert their action in the nucleus of cells. These hormones transmit their signal by entering the cell. The receptors for these hormones are transcriptional factors, which are activated by hormone binding. The hormone-receptor complex binds to regulatory elements in the DNA and alters the rate of transcription and mRNA synthesis. An increase in mRNA synthesis is followed by an increase in translation into new protein (Figure 8-8). Hormone-receptor complexes can either induce or repress RNA synthesis, depending on the type of regulatory sequence in the DNA. *Enhancer sequences* result in increased transcription, while *silencer sequences* result in decreased transcription.

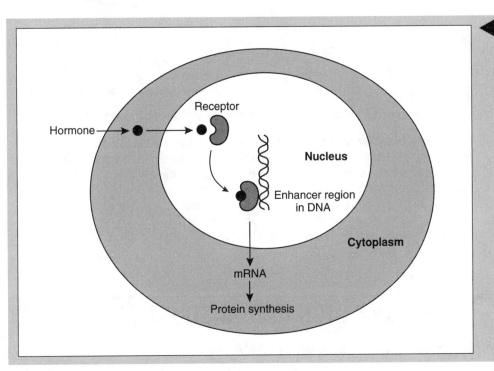

FIGURE 8-8
Hormonal Induction of Enzyme Synthesis.
The hormone-receptor complex binds to an enhancer region in the DNA, resulting in an increase in the rate of transcription of a specific gene. mRNA is translated to protein in the cytosol.

Cell-Surface Receptors

Peptide hormones, catecholamines, and neurotransmitters are water-soluble molecules that cannot cross the plasma membrane of target tissues. They transmit their signal to the inside of the cell by binding to cell-surface receptors. The hormone-receptor complex undergoes a conformational change that triggers the transmission of a signal across the membrane. There are three major classes of cell-surface receptors, which differ from one another in their mechanism of signal transduction across the membrane: (1) ligand-gated receptors, (2) catalytic receptors, and (3) G protein–linked receptors (Figure 8-9).

Ligand-Gated Receptors. Ligand-gated receptors consist of several subunits that form ion channels in the membrane. The ligand is usually a neurotransmitter, which binds to the extracellular surface of the receptor, making the channel selectively permeable to one or more ions. In the absence of a ligand, the channel is closed. The direction in which a particular ion moves is determined by the concentration gradient of that ion across the membrane.

Catalytic Receptors. Catalytic receptors span the plasma membrane and have globular domains on both the extracellular and cytosolic sides of the membrane. The extracellular domain binds a hormone or growth factor, and the cytosolic domain has intrinsic tyrosine kinase activity. The binding of a hormone or growth factor to the extracellular domain results in a conformational change that activates the tyrosine kinase domain. Tyrosine kinase catalyzes the transfer of phosphate from ATP to specific tyrosine side chains in a subset of cellular proteins, resulting in an alteration in their biologic functions.

Valium and librium are antianxiety medications that act on ligand-gated receptors, which open chloride channels in the brain. The ligand that opens the channel is γ-aminobutyric acid (GABA). In the presence of valium or librium, the amount of GABA required to open the channel is decreased.

The insulin receptor is a catalytic receptor with tyrosine kinase activity.

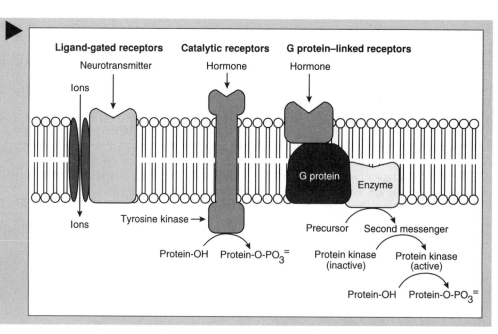

FIGURE 8-9 ▶

Cell-Surface Receptors. *Cell-surface hormone and neurotransmitter receptors use three basic mechanisms for transmitting signals across the plasma membrane: (1) ligand-gated receptors are linked to ion channels in the membrane; (2) catalytic receptors have intrinsic tyrosine kinase activity; and (3) G protein–linked receptors activate a GTP-binding protein, which, in turn, alters the activity of another enzyme that synthesizes second messenger molecules.*

G Protein–Linked Receptors. G protein–linked receptors are homologous integral membrane proteins that always cross the membrane seven times. They have an extracellular domain that binds a specific hormone and a globular domain within the membrane that binds to a G protein. The G protein provides a *communication link* between the hormone receptor and an enzyme that synthesizes second messenger molecules, such as cyclic adenosine monophosphate (cAMP) and diacylglycerol (DAG). Each type of second messenger activates a specific protein kinase that phosphorylates a subset of target proteins, resulting in a change in the biologic activity.

THE cAMP SIGNAL TRANSDUCTION PATHWAY

Synthesis and Degradation of cAMP

The second messenger in the action of many hormones is cAMP. It is synthesized by adenylate cyclase, an integral membrane protein. As shown in the following equation, the synthesis of cAMP is stimulated by some hormones and inhibited by others. The degradation of cAMP is catalyzed by phosphodiesterase, an enzyme that is activated by insulin and inhibited by caffeine and theophylline.

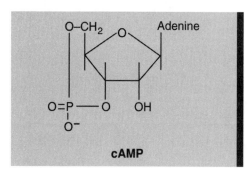

cAMP

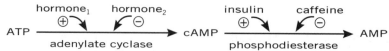

Whether a particular hormone stimulates or inhibits the synthesis of cAMP is determined by the type of G protein that is activated by the binding of a hormone to its receptor. Stimulatory G proteins (G_s) activate adenylate cyclase, while inhibitory G proteins (G_i) inhibit this enzyme.

Activation of Protein Kinase A by cAMP

The best characterized function of cAMP in eukaryotic cells is the activation of protein kinase A. Protein kinase A consists of two types of subunits, catalytic and regulatory (Figure 8-10). In the absence of cAMP, the regulatory and catalytic subunits are associated with one another in a complex that has no catalytic activity. The binding of cAMP to the regulatory subunits leads to dissociation of the complex, resulting in free catalytic subunits that have protein kinase activity. The catalytic subunits transfer phosphate from ATP to the hydroxyl group of specific serine residues in several target proteins and enzymes. When the concentration of cAMP decreases in the cell, the catalytic and regulatory subunits reassociate into the inactive form of protein kinase A.

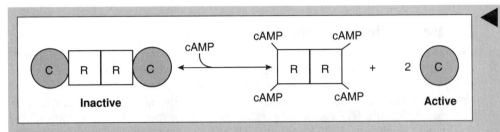

FIGURE 8-10
Activation of Protein Kinase A by cAMP. *The binding of cAMP by the regulatory subunits (R) results in dissociation of free catalytic subunits (C), which are active. The regulatory subunits remain as a dimer. As cAMP decreases and dissociates from the regulatory dimer, the catalytic and regulatory subunits reassociate into the inactive form.*

Family of G Proteins

The G proteins are trimers having α-, β-, and γ-subunits. The G_s and G_i proteins differ only in their α-subunits, having α_s and α_i, respectively. The α-subunits bind both guanosine triphosphate (GTP) and guanosine diphosphate (GDP), and they have intrinsic guanosine triphosphatase (GTPase) activity that slowly hydrolyzes GTP to GDP. The G proteins exist in inactive and active forms (Figure 8-11). The inactive form is the trimer that has GDP bound to the α-subunit. When a hormone binds to its receptor, GDP is displaced by GTP, and the complex dissociates, resulting in a free α-subunit containing GTP. The active forms of the G proteins, the α_s- and α_i-subunits, can associate with adenylate cyclase, stimulating and inhibiting its activity, respectively. The free α-subunits retain their ability to interact with adenylate cyclase only as long as GTP is bound. As GTP is slowly hydrolyzed to GDP, the inactive $\alpha\beta\gamma$ trimer is reformed. Thus, the GTPase activity serves as a "clock" that regulates the length of time that adenylate cyclase is activated or inhibited in response to a specific hormone.

Oncogenes *are mutant genes that code for proteins that stimulate uncontrolled cellular growth and differentiation. The expression of these genes results in cancer. Many of the oncogenes code for proteins that are mutant forms of proteins normally found in signal transduction pathways, such as hormone receptors, G proteins, and protein kinases.*

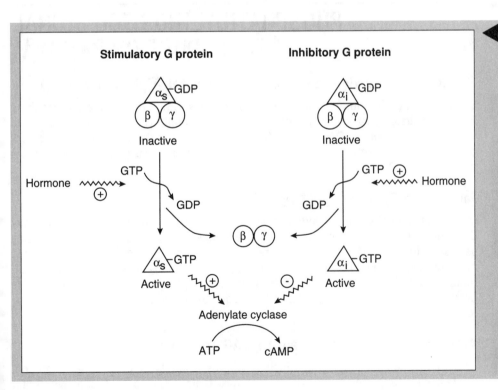

FIGURE 8-11
Active and Inactive Forms of G Proteins. *The G proteins consist of three subunits (α, β, and γ). The stimulatory and inhibitory proteins have distinctive α-subunits. In the inactive forms, GDP is bound to the trimer. The interaction of a hormone causes GTP to displace GDP, resulting in dissociation of the α-subunit with bound GTP. This is the form that interacts with adenylate cyclase, either stimulating or inhibiting the production of cAMP, depending on the type of α-subunit.*

Signal Amplification in the cAMP Pathway

The signal that results from a hormone binding to its receptor is amplified at three steps in the signal transduction pathway: (1) a single hormone-receptor complex can activate many G proteins; (2) each α_s-subunit can interact with adenylate cyclase, producing many molecules of cAMP; and (3) each molecule of cAMP-activated protein kinase can phosphorylate and alter the activity of many molecules of the target protein.

Disease Resulting from Abnormal G Proteins

Several bacterial toxins establish disease by altering the structure and function of G proteins. The best characterized examples are cholera toxin and pertussis toxin, which result in the overproduction of cAMP. *V. cholerae* binds to intestinal epithelial cells and releases a toxin that covalently modifies the α_s-subunit (Figure 8-12). The modification inactivates the GTPase activity, resulting in a permanently active form of the α_s-subunit, which persistently stimulates adenylate cyclase, resulting in an overproduction of cAMP. The increased concentration of cAMP results in a massive efflux of ions and water from the cell. Pertussis toxin, which is synthesized by the bacteria responsible for whooping cough, covalently modifies the α_i-subunit. The modified α_i-subunit does not dissociate from the trimer and, therefore, cannot inhibit adenylate cyclase.

Cholera toxin and pertussis toxin exert their effects by covalently modifying G proteins and altering their function. These toxins transfer the ADP-ribose moiety from NAD^+ to a specific amino acid side chain in the G protein. The structure of NAD^+ can be described as follows: nicotinamide-ribose-P-P-ribose-adenine. The other product of the reaction is nicotinamide-ribose.

FIGURE 8-12 ▶
Effect of Cholera Toxin on the Stimulatory G Protein (G_s). The GTPase activity of the α_s-subunit is inactivated by ADP-ribosylation. GTP cannot be hydrolyzed, and the α_s-subunit is permanently activated, resulting in hyperstimulation of adenylate cyclase.

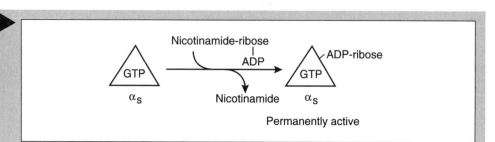

PHOSPHATIDYLINOSITOL SIGNAL TRANSDUCTION PATHWAY

Synthesis of Diacylglycerol (DAG) and Inositol Triphosphate (IP_3)

Some hormones and neurotransmitters activate the enzyme *phospholipase C*, resulting in the conversion of a membrane phospholipid (phosphatidylinositol bisphosphate) to two second messengers, DAG and IP_3 (Figure 8-13). This pathway requires a specific G protein (G_p) that is activated by the hormone-receptor complex, which in turn activates phospholipase C.

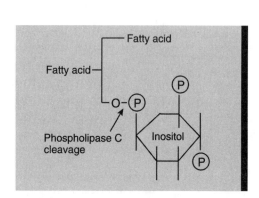

Increase in Cytosolic Ca^{2+} by IP_3

IP_3 binds to receptors on the endoplasmic reticulum (ER), resulting in a rapid release of Ca^{2+} from intracellular stores. The Ca^{2+} activates a number of enzymes, including several different Ca^{2+}-dependent protein kinases. Most of the effects of Ca^{2+} are mediated by calmodulin, although some enzymes, including phospholipase C, are directly activated by Ca^{2+}. IP_3 has a very short half-life, lasting only a few seconds. It is degraded by a series of phosphatases that sequentially remove the phosphate groups, forming inositol.

Activation of Protein Kinase C by DAG and Ca^{2+}

Lithium, a drug used to treat manic depression, inhibits one or more of the phosphatases involved in the metabolism of inositol phosphates to free inositol.

DAG is a very lipophilic molecule, which remains associated with the plasma membrane, where it activates protein kinase C. Protein kinase C also requires Ca^{2+} for activity, but it does not bind Ca^{2+} in the absence of DAG. The binding of DAG increases the affinity of protein kinase C for Ca^{2+}. Protein kinase C catalyzes the phosphorylation of serine and threonine side chains in a number of target proteins, including various membrane pumps and channel proteins.

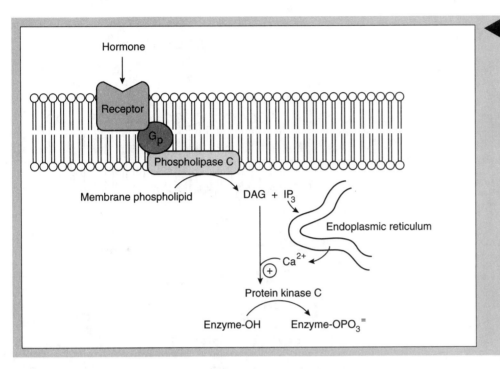

FIGURE 8-13
Phosphatidylinositol Signaling Pathway. Hormones that stimulate the synthesis of diacylglycerol (DAG) and inositol triphosphate (IP_3) use a specific G protein (G_p) as an intermediary in the activation of phospholipase C. Inositol binds to the endoplasmic reticulum, resulting in release of Ca^{2+} into the cytosol. Phospholipase C is activated by Ca^{2+}, and protein kinase C is activated by both DAG and Ca^{2+}.

THE cGMP SIGNAL TRANSDUCTION PATHWAY

The cyclic nucleotide, cyclic guanosine monophosphate (cGMP), is a second messenger that has a unique role in hormone action. Its functions as a second messenger are linked to a number of processes, which work together to lower blood pressure. The biologic effects elicited by cGMP differ in different tissues (Table 8-3).

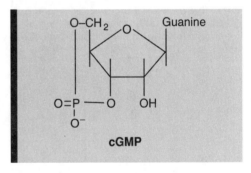

cGMP

Synthesis of cGMP

Guanylate cyclase, the enzyme that catalyzes the conversion of GTP to cGMP, is found in two forms, which have different cellular locations and different mechanisms of activation. One form is located in the plasma membrane and is activated by peptide hormones, whereas the other form is in the cytosol and is activated by nitric oxide (NO) [Figure 8-14].

Hormone-Activated Guanylate Cyclase. The membrane-bound guanylate cyclase is a transmembrane protein that spans the membrane and has globular domains on both the extracellular and cytosolic sides. Its structure and function are analogous to that of catalytic hormone receptors. The extracellular domain binds to *atrial natriuretic factor* (ANF), a family of peptide hormones that regulates cardiovascular function and body fluid homeostasis. The cytosolic domain has guanylate cyclase activity, which is active when the receptor domain is occupied.

ANF is a peptide hormone released into the circulation when increased blood pressure stretches the atrium of the heart. ANF acts on the kidney and vascular smooth muscle to lower the blood pressure.

TABLE 8-3
Effects of cGMP on Various Cells and Tissues

Cell or Tissue Type	Effect
Cardiac muscle	Relaxation
Vascular smooth muscle	Vasodilation
Kidney	Increased excretion of sodium and water
Platelets	Decreased aggregation
Cardiac muscle	Relaxation

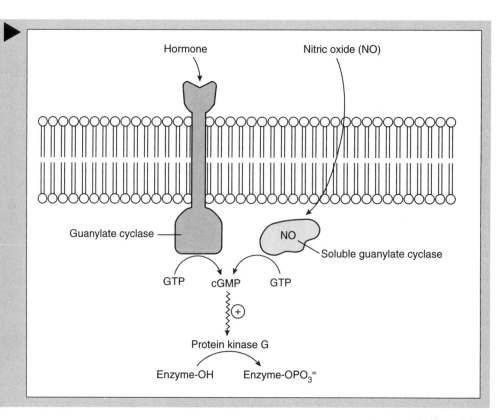

FIGURE 8-14
Synthesis and Effects of cGMP. The membrane-bound form of guanylate cyclase is directly activated by the binding of a hormone to its receptor. The cytosolic form is a different protein, having tightly bound heme, and is activated by nitric oxide (NO) or other nitrogen-containing compounds that give rise to NO. Protein kinase G is activated by cGMP. The allosteric site for cGMP and the catalytic site are on the same protein.

Angina is treated with nitroglycerin, a drug that is slowly converted to NO, resulting in relaxation of cardiac and vascular smooth muscle.

Nitric Oxide-Activated Guanylate Cyclase. The cytosolic form of guanylate cyclase contains heme and is activated by NO, a free radical that is synthesized from arginine. The synthesis of NO is catalyzed by nitric oxide synthase, an enzyme that is activated by Ca^{2+}. NO binds to the heme of guanylate cyclase, thereby stimulating the synthesis of cGMP. NO is permeable to membranes and readily diffuses from one cell into another. Its half-life is short, usually less than 5 seconds, and it is rapidly degraded by nonenzymatic reactions.

cGMP-Dependent Protein Kinase and its Target Proteins

Most of the effects of cGMP are mediated by protein kinase G, an enzyme that has both catalytic and regulatory domains on the same polypeptide chain. In the absence of cGMP, the catalytic domain is inactive. The binding of cGMP induces a conformational change that unmasks the active site and allows the kinase to phosphorylate serine and threonine side chains in its target proteins. Several smooth muscle proteins, including myosin light chain kinase, are phosphorylated by protein kinase G. These proteins are presumably involved in smooth muscle relaxation and vasodilation.

RESOLUTION OF CLINICAL CASE

The patient described at the beginning of this chapter was diagnosed with cholera, an acute infectious disease resulting from ingestion of *V. cholerae* bacteria. The bacteria secrete a toxin that binds to the surface of intestinal mucosal cells, leading to the permanent activation of the G_s protein. The activated G_s protein, in turn, persistently stimulates adenylate cyclase, resulting in the accumulation of high levels of cAMP and the cAMP-dependent phosphorylation of membrane proteins involved in ion transport. The result of these events is the efflux of massive amounts of sodium, chloride, potassium, bicarbonate, and water into the intestinal lumen. The metabolic acidosis seen in this patient resulted from the loss of bicarbonate. The loss of fluid resulted in hypotension, as indicated by the patient's low blood pressure, and was also responsible for the shriveled appearance of the skin. If the fluid loss is as much as 10%–12% of the body weight, loss of consciousness usually occurs. The primary goal of treatment is to restore the extracellular fluid volume and the electrolyte composition to normal. If untreated, the dehydration and electrolyte imbalance can lead to death. Rehydration and correction of the electrolyte balance can be re-established within a few hours. Although tetracycline is usually given, antibiotics are not necessary as long as adequate replacement fluids and electrolytes are continued for 5–6 days. During this time, a volume of fluid equal to 1–2 times the body weight will be lost, resulting both in the clearing of the bacteria from the gastrointestinal tract and in the replacement of damaged epithelial cells [1].

The toxin secreted by *V. cholerae* is a protein having two subunits, A and B. Subunit B binds to a glycolipid (ganglioside G_{M1}) on the plasma membrane of the intestinal cell, thereby facilitating the entry of subunit A into the cell. Subunit A catalyzes the ADP-ribosylation of the G_s protein, resulting in the inability of the α-subunit to hydrolyze GTP. Therefore, the G_s protein is locked into a permanently activated form that stimulates adenylate cyclase as long as the cells live. ADP-ribosylation reactions are catalyzed by a number of bacterial toxins that use NAD as a source of ADP-ribose [2].

REVIEW QUESTIONS

Directions: For each of the following questions, choose the **one best** answer.

1. Which of the following characteristics best describes an allosteric enzyme?

   (A) The substrate saturation curve obeys Michaelis-Menten kinetics

   (B) The affinity for substrate is increased by an allosteric inhibitor

   (C) The substrate saturation curve is shifted to the right by an allosteric inhibitor

   (D) The allosteric site is on a separate subunit from the catalytic site

   (E) The response to increasing substrate concentration is desensitized by positive cooperativity

2. Which of the following descriptions of cAMP is most accurate?

   (A) The synthesis is stimulated by hormones that activate G_i proteins

   (B) It activates protein kinase A by binding to the catalytic subunit

   (C) The concentration is decreased by cholera toxin

   (D) It is degraded by phosphodiesterase

   (E) It is synthesized by a catalytic receptor

3. Which of the following statements about Ca^{2+} is true?

   (A) The concentration in the cytosol is increased by diacylglycerol (DAG)

   (B) It mediates its effects as a second messenger by binding to calmodulin

   (C) Its release from mitochondria is stimulated by inositol triphosphate

   (D) It decreases the affinity of protein kinase C for DAG

   (E) It inhibits the synthesis of nitric oxide (NO)

4. Which of the following statements about cGMP is true?

   (A) The synthesis by membrane-bound guanylate cyclase is stimulated by nitric oxide (NO)

   (B) It is synthesized from GMP

   (C) It activates protein kinase G by binding to a separate regulatory subunit

   (D) The synthesis requires participation of a G protein

   (E) The accumulation leads to relaxation of smooth muscle and vasodilation

5. Which of the following statements about G proteins is true?

   (A) They participate in signal transduction mechanisms of catalytic receptors

   (B) They consist of three identical subunits

   (C) The active form has GTP bound to it

   (D) They are required for the opening of ligand-gated ion channels in the membrane

   (E) They are required to mediate the effects of insulin

ANSWERS AND EXPLANATIONS

1. The answer is C. Allosteric inhibitors either increase the K_m for the substrate (decrease the affinity) or decrease the V_{max} of the reaction. A decrease in K_m always results in a shift in the substrate saturation curves to the right, making C a better answer than D. The allosteric site may be on the same subunit as the catalytic site, or it may be on a separate subunit. Allosteric enzymes do not obey Michaelis-Menten kinetics. Enzymes with negative (not positive) cooperativity are desensitized to increasing substrate concentrations.

2. The answer is D. Phosphodiesterase hydrolyzes cAMP to AMP. Its synthesis is stimulated by hormones that activate G_s proteins. Cholera toxin increases the concentration of cAMP by covalent modification of the α_s-subunit of G_s proteins. This modification permanently locks α_s into its active form, which persistently stimulates adenylate cyclase. Protein kinase A is activated by the binding of cAMP to the regulatory subunits, which results in dissociation of active catalytic subunits. The synthesis of cGMP, but not cAMP, is catalyzed by a catalytic receptor.

3. The answer is B. Most of the effects of Ca^{2+} are mediated by calmodulin. The Ca^{2+}-calmodulin complex binds to a number of enzymes, resulting in an increase in their catalytic activity. Inositol triphosphate binds to receptors on the endoplasmic reticulum, resulting in release of Ca^{2+} into the cytosol. Both Ca^{2+} and DAG are required for maximum activity of protein kinase C. DAG increases the affinity of phospholipase C for Ca^{2+}. The synthesis of NO is stimulated by Ca^{2+}.

4. The answer is E. The primary role of cGMP as a second messenger is to mediate vasodilation, a process that is facilitated by relaxation of vascular smooth muscle. cGMP is synthesized from GTP by two forms of guanylate cyclase, a cytosolic form that is stimulated by NO and a membrane-bound form that is stimulated by atrial natriuretic factor. The cGMP signal transduction pathway does not involve a G protein. Most of the effects of cGMP are mediated by protein kinase G, an enzyme with its cGMP-binding site on the same subunit as the catalytic site.

5. The answer is C. The G proteins are active only when GTP is bound. The hydrolysis of GTP to GDP results in a reversion to its inactive form. The G proteins consist of three nonidentical subunits. G proteins are not involved in signal transduction mechanisms of hormones, like insulin, that use catalytic receptors, and they are not required for the opening of ligand-gated ion channels. These channels can be opened by the direct binding of neurotransmitters to the extracellular domain of the channel proteins.

REFERENCES

1. Holmgren J: Actions of cholera toxin and the prevention and treatment of cholera. *Nature* 292:413–419, 1981.
2. Middlebrook JL, Dorland RB: Bacterial toxins: cellular mechanisms of action. *Microbiol Rev* 48:199–221, 1984.

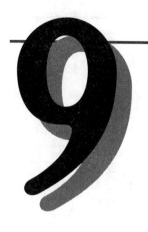

OVERVIEW OF CARBO-HYDRATE METABOLISM: THE IMPORTANCE OF REGULATING BLOOD GLUCOSE LEVELS

CHAPTER OUTLINE

INTRODUCTION OF CLINICAL CASE

A 20-year-old college student was admitted to the emergency room by his roommate, who returned from an early morning class and was unable to awaken him. Several times during the semester he had experienced episodes where he became sweaty and confused, but the symptoms rapidly disappeared after eating. Upon arrival at the emergency room, his blood glucose concentration was 28 mg/dL (normal fasting range: 70–100 mg/dL). He was treated with intravenous glucose and admitted to the hospital for observation. He said that for religious reasons he had never used alcohol, and he denied the use of any drugs or prescribed medications. On the third day of hospitalization, he had another episode before breakfast. His skin became clammy and he was lethargic, but he did not lose consciousness. His blood glucose level dropped to 48 mg/dL but was restored to normal by the oral administration of glucose. Laboratory tests on blood samples taken at the time of admission and during the second episode of hypoglycemia revealed insulin levels that were 297 pM and 215 pM, respectively (normal fasting range: 30–180 pM). C-peptide levels were elevated on both occasions, being 6.2 ng/mL and 4.9 ng/mL, respectively (normal range: 1.0–4.0 ng/mL). All other laboratory values, including numerous assessments of liver and kidney function, were normal. Computed tomography (CT) scans of the body cavity were normal. The patient was dismissed from the hospital and advised to eat small, carbohydrate-rich meals frequently and to come back in 2 months for another examination. He had no further hypoglycemic episodes until 3 days before his next scheduled appointment. As soon as he recognized the symptoms, he ate a bowl of cereal and drank some orange juice, and within an hour, the symptoms disappeared. When he returned to his physician, another extensive examination revealed a small tumor located near the pancreas. The tumor was removed surgically. For the last 3 years he has experienced no symptoms of hypoglycemia.

GLUCOSE: AN OBLIGATE FUEL OF THE CENTRAL NERVOUS SYSTEM AND RED BLOOD CELLS

The *brain* can neither synthesize nor store significant amounts of glucose. Therefore, normal cerebral function requires a continuous supply of glucose. Similarly, the *red blood cell* (*RBC*) has an absolute requirement for glucose. It contains no mitochondria and cannot carry out oxidative metabolism, making it entirely dependent on anaerobic glycolysis to meet its energy needs. In the normal person, several pathways of carbohydrate, lipid, and protein metabolism are regulated coordinately so that glucose is made available to the tissues that depend on it for survival.

At rest, the whole body consumes between 160 and 200 g of glucose per day. The brain is the major consumer, using approximately 120 g of glucose per day. The blood serves as the vehicle for transporting glucose to the brain, but since normal homeostasis requires that blood glucose levels be maintained within a narrow concentration range (70–110 mg/dL), there must be mechanisms for releasing glucose into the blood between meals. The major reservoir of glucose that can be readily mobilized is *liver glycogen*. Although considerably more glycogen is stored in muscle than in liver, muscle is unable to release glucose into the circulation. The amount of glucose held in reserve by the liver can be depleted within a few hours, and if the individual is not fed, the liver begins *de novo synthesis of glucose* (*gluconeogenesis*) in which protein is broken down to provide the carbon precursors, and fatty acids are oxidized to provide the energy needed for glucose synthesis. Following a high carbohydrate meal, the glycogen stores in both liver and muscle are rapidly replenished.

Body Glucose Reserves	
Extracellular glucose	*10 g*
Liver glycogen	*75 g*
Muscle glycogen	*250 g*

INSULIN AND GLUCAGON REGULATE BLOOD GLUCOSE LEVELS

The *liver* is the organ primarily responsible for controlling the concentration of glucose in the blood. It can rapidly take up and release glucose in response to the concentration of circulating glucose, which is regulated by hormonal signals. The two major hormones of glucose metabolism are insulin and glucagon.

Effects of Insulin

Hyperglycemia
Elevated blood glucose

Insulin is an *anabolic hormone* that lowers blood glucose and promotes its storage by stimulating the synthesis of glycogen and fatty acids. Following a high carbohydrate meal, the transient *hyperglycemia*, resulting from digestion and absorption of dietary carbohydrate, stimulates the pancreatic beta cells to release insulin. The major effects of insulin are illustrated in Figure 9-1. The three primary target tissues for insulin are liver, muscle, and adipose tissue.

Liver. Insulin lowers blood glucose levels by stimulating three pathways of glucose utilization in the liver: glycogen synthesis, glycolysis, and fatty acid synthesis. After liver glycogen reserves have been replenished, excess glucose is converted to acetyl coenzyme A (CoA) by the combination of glycolysis and the pyruvate dehydrogenase (PDH) reaction. The acetyl CoA is used for fatty acid synthesis. The fatty acids are converted to triglycerides, packaged into very low-density lipoproteins (VLDLs), and secreted into the circulation.

Muscle. Insulin stimulates the transport of glucose into muscle, where it replenishes glycogen stores that are used exclusively by muscle as a source of energy.

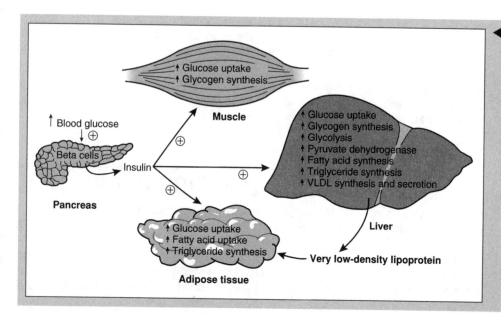

FIGURE 9-1
Role of Insulin in Lowering Blood Glucose Levels. *The release of insulin by the pancreas is a signal indicating elevated blood glucose. Numerous pathways in muscle, adipose tissue, and liver are activated, which result in both the lowering of blood glucose and the conversion of glucose to the storage forms of glycogen and fat.*

Adipose Tissue. In the capillary bed of adipose tissue, insulin stimulates the release of fatty acids from triglyceride-rich lipoproteins (VLDLs and chylomicrons), allowing fatty acids to be taken up by adipocytes. Insulin also stimulates the transport of glucose into adipose tissue, where it is used to synthesize α-glycerol phosphate (αGP), the precursor for the synthesis of triglycerides.

Effects of Glucagon

The role of glucagon is to respond to *hypoglycemia* by promoting the release of glucose into the blood. This is in contrast to insulin, whose primary effect is to prevent *hyperglycemia* by stimulating the uptake and utilization of glucose from the blood. In response to a decrease in the concentration of circulating glucose, the alpha cells of the pancreas release glucagon. The major effects of glucagon are shown in Figure 9-2. The two organs that are primary targets for glucagon are liver and adipose tissue.

Liver. Glucagon activates the pathways of glycogen degradation and gluconeogenesis, both of which contribute to the glucose that is released into the circulation. The major

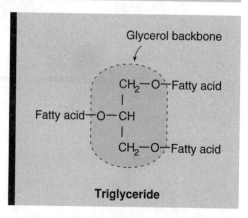

Triglyceride

Hypoglycemia
Low blood glucose

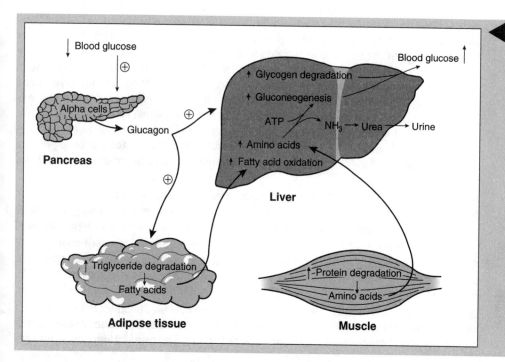

FIGURE 9-2
Role of Glucagon in Increasing Blood Glucose Levels. *The release of glucagon by the pancreas is a signal indicating low blood glucose. Orchestrated metabolic responses in liver, adipose, and muscle result in the restoration of blood glucose to normal values.*

precursors for gluconeogenesis come from the degradation of muscle protein, and the energy (adenosine triphosphate, ATP) for driving glucose synthesis comes from the oxidation of fatty acids.

Adipose Tissue. Glucagon stimulates the release of fatty acids from adipose tissue. The free fatty acids are bound to serum albumin and transported to liver and other tissues, where they are oxidized as a source of energy.

METABOLIC ZONATION IN THE LIVER

All hepatocytes do not have the same complement of enzymes, and consequently there are different functions that are more pronounced in some hepatocytes than in others. The *periportal hepatocytes* that surround the portal vein are enriched in the enzymes of *gluconeogenesis*, whereas the enzymes of *glycolysis* are enriched in the *perivenous hepatocytes* that surround the central vein. This topological separation of metabolic pathways provides a mechanism for cellular specialization that avoids wasteful substrate cycling. Differences in gene expression in the periportal and perivenous zones of the liver are believed to be related to concentration gradients of oxygen, substrates, and hormones in the microcirculation of the liver.

DIABETES MELLITUS: A VEHICLE FOR STUDYING THE INTEGRATION OF METABOLISM

The word "diabetes" is derived from a Greek word meaning "to pass through" or "to siphon," referring to the observation that individuals with diabetes mellitus drink lots of water (polydipsia) and excrete large volumes of urine (polyuria). Metabolically, diabetes can be described as a *multiorgan catabolic response* caused by an insufficiency of insulin.

Metabolic Consequences of Insulin Insufficiency

Some of the consequences that result from either an actual or a functional deficiency of insulin are illustrated in Figure 9-3. If the condition is untreated, *hyperglycemia* develops. Both the overproduction and underutilization of glucose contribute to the hyperglycemia. When the concentration of glucose in the blood exceeds the renal threshold for reabsorption from the glomerular filtrate (> 180 mg/dL), glucose is lost by excretion in the urine. The need to maintain a constant number of solute particles (*osmolality*) results in increased excretion of water as well as glucose, thus accounting for the polyuria and polydipsia. Although the circulating concentration of glucose is elevated and glucose is being excreted in the urine, the tissues that are dependent on insulin for glucose uptake and utilization are experiencing a state of "starvation." The liver responds to the "perceived glucose deprivation" by activating the machinery required for gluconeogenesis. The major organs responding to insulin insufficiency are muscle, adipose tissue, liver, and kidney.

Muscle. Protein is degraded to amino acids, providing carbon skeletons for glucose synthesis. The amino groups are incorporated into urea and excreted in the urine. Muscle wasting leads to *negative nitrogen balance* in which the amount of nitrogen excreted exceeds the dietary intake. Normally, insulin suppresses protein degradation.

Adipose Tissue. Fatty acids are released from triglyceride. The oxidation of fatty acids that are taken up by the liver provides the driving force for glucose synthesis. Normally, the release of fatty acids from adipose triglyceride is suppressed by insulin.

Liver. Amino acids and fatty acids are taken up by the liver and used for the synthesis of glucose. Accelerated oxidation of fatty acids by the liver leads to excess acetyl CoA, which is condensed and conserved by the formation of *ketones*. The primary ketones, acetoace-

Consequences of Ketoacidosis
Decreased blood pH
Depletion of serum bicarbonate
Fruity odor of breath due to acetone

tate and β-hydroxybutyrate, accumulate in the blood and can lead to *ketoacidosis*. When the concentration of ketones in blood exceeds the renal threshold for reabsorption, the excess ketones are excreted in the urine.

Kidney. The ketones are small organic acids that exist as anions at physiologic pH. Therefore, the excretion is accompanied by a cation. To conserve sodium (Na^+) and potassium (K^+), which play a major role in electrolyte balance, the kidney begins to excrete ammonium ions (NH_4^+). In contrast to Na^+ and K^+, NH_4^+ is expendable. Most of the NH_4^+ is derived from glutamine.

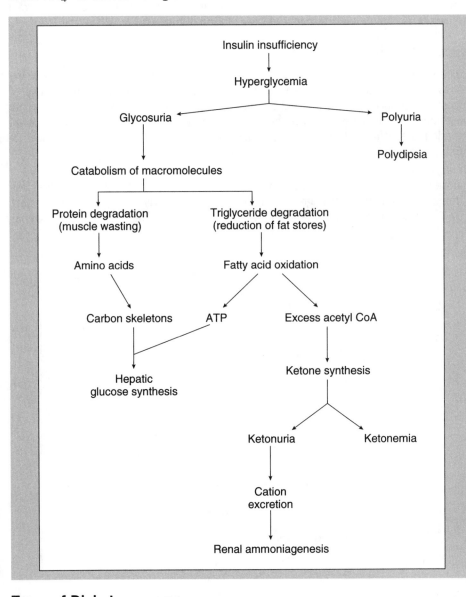

FIGURE 9-3
Metabolic Consequences of Insulin Insufficiency. *Both anabolic pathways (gluconeogenesis) and catabolic pathways (protein degradation, triglyceride hydrolysis, fatty acid oxidation, ketogenesis, and ammoniagenesis) are activated in the absence of insulin.*

Types of Diabetes

There are two major types of diabetes, type I and type II. Type I diabetes, also known as insulin-dependent diabetes or juvenile-onset diabetes, is frequently caused by an auto-immune disorder that destroys the pancreatic beta cells. Type I diabetes is treated by insulin replacement. Type II diabetes, also known as insulin-independent or adult-onset diabetes, is characterized by a resistance to insulin rather than a lack of insulin. Circulating insulin levels are frequently elevated in type II diabetes.

Glucose Tolerance Test

The hallmark of diabetes mellitus is *sustained hyperglycemia*, arising from both over-production and underutilization of glucose. The ability to dispose of blood glucose can be assessed by the glucose tolerance test. Following an overnight fast, 50–100 g of glucose, depending on the size of the individual, are ingested, and plasma glucose levels are determined at 30-minute intervals over a period of 4 hours. The results of a glucose tolerance test are shown in Figure 9-4. The *top panel* shows the response of a normal individual. The plasma glucose concentration peaks between 30 and 60 minutes and then drops off with a slight "overshoot" (*shaded area*) below normal before re-establishing a normal baseline glucose concentration. The "overshoot" of glucose to below normal levels follows a pulse of insulin secretion. A typical glucose tolerance test for a diabetic is shown in the *lower panel* of Figure 9-4. Plasma glucose levels start higher than normal and persist at higher levels throughout the duration of the test.

Glucose Toxicity

The persistence of elevated plasma glucose levels poses a threat to the diabetic. In many tissues, such as nerve, retina, lens, kidney, and small blood vessels, the uptake of glucose is insulin-independent. These same tissues are most susceptible to the chronic complications of diabetes. Two types of reactions, the glycosylation of proteins and polyol formation, are believed to be involved in some of the chronic changes that are seen in both type I and type II diabetes.

Glycosylation of Protein. Glucose is highly reactive with protein. The aldehyde group of glucose reacts easily with amino groups of proteins to form Schiff's base. Schiff's base undergoes an Amadori rearrangement to produce a stable glycosylated protein (Figure 9-5). This reaction is nonenzymatic and is driven by the concentration of glucose. It has

FIGURE 9-4 ▶

Glucose Tolerance Test in a Normal Person and a Diabetic. The key feature of the normal curve is the shaded area *where glucose transiently falls below control level. This overshoot is never seen in diabetics.*

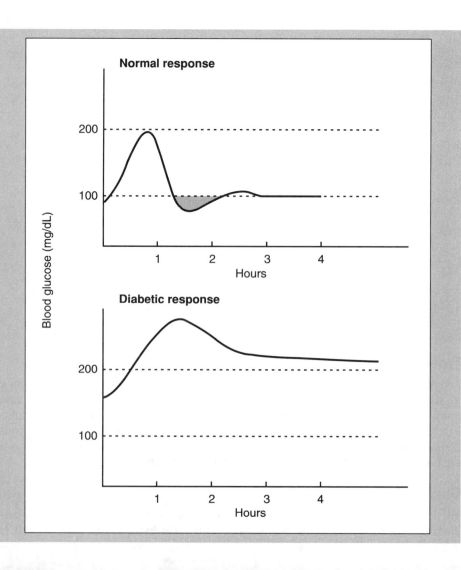

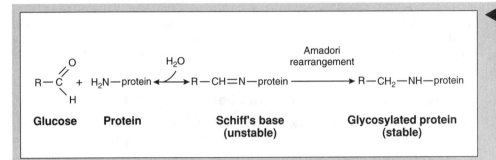

FIGURE 9-5
Formation of Glycosylated Proteins. The formation of glycosylated proteins involves an aldimine (Schiff's base) intermediate that rearranges to form a stable keto-amine. The protein amino groups come from lysine side chains and from the amino-terminal groups.

been suggested that glycosylation of proteins in the lens of the eye, peripheral nerves, and basement membrane of kidneys may be related to some of the pathologic changes that develop in these tissues of diabetics.

Glycosylated Hemoglobin (HbA$_{1c}$). HbA$_{1c}$ is a minor form of normal adult hemoglobin (HbA) with carbohydrate covalently attached to the protein chain. Its formation in the RBC is well documented. Although glycosylation appears to have little, if any, effect on the functional properties of Hb, it is clinically valuable in monitoring long-term control of blood glucose levels in diabetics. Since RBCs have a life span of about 120 days, the content of HbA$_{1c}$ is an indicator of how effectively blood glucose levels have been regulated over the previous 2–3 months. The correlation between blood glucose concentration and the amount of HbA$_{1c}$ is shown in Figure 9-6. Normally, HbA$_{1c}$ constitutes less than 5% of the total Hb. With persistent hyperglycemia, this value can increase up to approximately 15%.

Polyol Formation. Glucose that is taken up by peripheral nerve, lens, renal glomeruli, and seminal vesicles is reduced to sorbitol by the action of aldol reductase. As shown in the following equation, the reduced form of nicotinamide-adenine dinucleotide phosphate (NADPH) reduces the aldehyde group at C-1 of glucose, resulting in sorbitol.

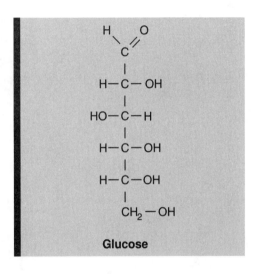

Glucose

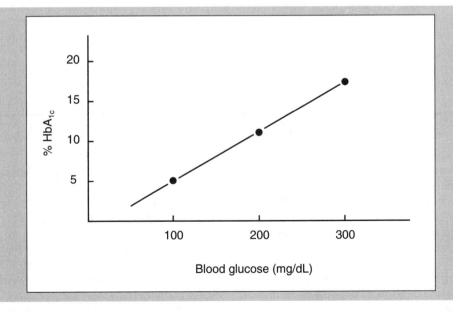

FIGURE 9-6
Variation of Hemoglobin A$_{1c}$ (HbA$_{1c}$) Content with Blood Glucose Levels. A value of 5% HbA$_{1c}$ is typical of nondiabetics with a fasting blood glucose of 90 mg/dL. Levels of HbA$_{1c}$ of 9%–10% correspond to a mean blood glucose of 240 mg/dL [1].

Sorbitol accumulates in the lens and cannot leave the cell, resulting in osmotic shifts that lead to cataracts.

Sorbitol does not diffuse through membranes easily and has been shown to accumulate in the human lens, causing osmotic damage. Both the accumulation of sorbitol and the formation of cataracts in diabetics can be prevented by the use of inhibitors of aldol reductase.

Determination of Glucose Concentration in Body Fluids

The concentration of glucose in fluids such as blood, urine, and cerebrospinal fluid (CSF) can be determined quickly and inexpensively by either the Fehling-Benedict test or the glucose oxidase test.

Fehling-Benedict Test. This test, also known as the reducing sugar test, is the basis for the copper sulfate (Clinitest) tablets that have been widely used to determine the concentration of reducing sugars in urine. The reaction is shown below.

$$\text{Glucose} + 2Cu^{2+} + 5OH^{-} \xrightarrow{\text{tartrate}} Cu_2O + 3H_2O + \text{gluconic acid}$$

The carbonyl group ($\overset{R}{\underset{H}{\diagup}}C=O$) of glucose reduces the Cu^{2+} ion to Cu_2O, a compound having a red color that can be quantitated spectrophotometrically. The presence of tartrate prevents Cu_2O from precipitating out of solution. The major disadvantage of this reaction is that it is *nonspecific*. Any monosaccharide with an unsubstituted carbonyl group gives a positive test. The advantages are that it is inexpensive and can be used on blood, feces, and urine as an initial screening test for reducing sugars. This test is commonly used by nutritionists in carbohydrate balance studies.

Glucose Oxidase Test. The other widely used test for determining blood glucose levels is the enzyme-based glucose oxidase test. The major advantage is that it is highly specific for glucose. Both clinical laboratory tests and commercially available home monitoring kits are based on the glucose oxidase test, which involves the two following coupled enzymatic reactions:

$$\text{Glucose} + O_2 \xrightarrow{\text{glucose oxidase}} \text{gluconic acid} + H_2O_2$$

$$H_2O_2 + \text{dye}_{red} \xrightarrow{\text{peroxidase}} \text{dye}_{ox} + 2H_2O$$

The hydrogen peroxide produced in the first reaction is used to oxidize a colorless dye to a form having a yellow color and can be quantitated spectrophotometrically. Both of the enzymes and all of the substrates required for the reactions have been incorporated into a dipstick that is used in home monitoring kits.

RESOLUTION OF CLINICAL CASE

The patient introduced at the beginning of the chapter is suffering from episodes of hypoglycemia that are caused by elevated insulin levels. Insulin lowers blood glucose and promotes glucose storage by stimulating its conversion to glycogen and lipid. Under normal conditions, the concentration of glucose in blood is maintained within a narrow concentration range by a delicate balance between the opposing actions of insulin and glucagon. Any factor that alters the balance between these two hormones results in a corresponding decrease or increase in blood glucose levels. In this patient, the high insulin levels resulted in hypoglycemia, which led to sweating, lethargy, confusion, and loss of consciousness. The underlying cause of the high insulin levels in this patient was initially puzzling. The observation that both insulin and C-peptide were elevated was a key finding in ruling out an exogenous source of insulin. C-peptide is not present in commercially available insulin. Endogenous insulin, however, is synthesized as proinsulin and subsequently cleaved to insulin and C-peptide. Both fragments are stored in secretory granules and secreted simultaneously from the pancreas. The elimination of exogenous insulin led the physician to search for an endogenous source. The most likely cause was an insulin-producing tumor, but the CT scans initially failed to find a tumor. In view of the uncertainty as to the cause of the elevated insulin, the strategy for treatment was to minimize the potential for hypoglycemic attacks by eating small, frequent meals that are rich in carbohydrates. This is a commonly used approach to managing hypoglycemia in many patients, regardless of the cause. The source of the insulin was identified 2 months later when a tumor was found and surgically removed.

REVIEW QUESTIONS

Directions: For each of the following questions, choose the **one best** answer.

Questions 1–5

Jane, a 27-year-old woman who is an insulin-dependent diabetic, went on a weekend cross-country ski trip and forgot to pack her insulin.

1. Analysis of a blood sample taken when Jane returned home most likely revealed
    - **(A)** unchanged levels of hemoglobin A_{1c} (HbA_{1c})
    - **(B)** no detectable ketones
    - **(C)** below normal levels of blood glucose
    - **(D)** below normal levels of glucagon
    - **(E)** below normal levels of fatty acids

2. Which of the following metabolic alterations are likely to have occurred over the weekend?
    - **(A)** Decreased gluconeogenesis
    - **(B)** Increased oxidation of fatty acids by the liver
    - **(C)** Decreased breakdown of skeletal muscle protein
    - **(D)** Increased oxidation of fatty acids by RBCs

3. Analysis of a urine sample would likely show
    - **(A)** a negative Fehling-Benedict test
    - **(B)** a negative glucose oxidase test
    - **(C)** a positive test for urea
    - **(D)** a negative test for β-hydroxybutyrate

4. Which of the following results would be most likely if the patient had a glucose tolerance test after an overnight fast?
    - **(A)** A glucose concentration less than 100 mg/dL at zero time
    - **(B)** An "overshoot" in the decline of blood glucose occurring at 4 hours
    - **(C)** A glucose concentration less than 100 mg/dL at 4 hours
    - **(D)** A peak in glucose occurring between 1 and 2 hours

5. Which of the following cell types demonstrates insulin-dependent uptake of glucose?
    - **(A)** Brain
    - **(B)** Kidney
    - **(C)** Muscle
    - **(D)** Liver

ANSWERS AND EXPLANATIONS

1. The answer is A. The level of HbA_{1c} would not be expected to change significantly over 2–3 days. Detectable increases in HbA_{1c} that are observed in uncontrolled diabetes represent the cumulative effect over weeks and months. Triglyceride hydrolysis and increased release of fatty acids from adipose are enhanced due to the absence of insulin. Uncontrolled fatty acid oxidation by the liver may lead to excess acetyl CoA and increased ketone synthesis. Both glucagon and blood glucose levels will be elevated.

2. The answer is B. Increased oxidation of fatty acids by the liver is secondary to insulin deficiency. RBCs have no mitochondria and cannot oxidize fatty acids. Both skeletal muscle protein degradation and increased gluconeogenesis are occurring.

3. The answer is C. The level of urea in the urine will be slightly elevated because amino acids are beginning to be used for glucose synthesis. The presence of glucose in the urine will give a positive Fehling-Benedict (reducing sugar) test and a positive glucose oxidase test. The presence of ketones would be indicated by a positive test for β-hydroxybutyrate.

4. The answer is D. Following an oral glucose load, the blood glucose usually increases to above 200 mg/dL and peaks between 1 and 2 hours. The absence of an "overshoot" of blood glucose to below the baseline values is a key characteristic of the glucose tolerance test in a diabetic. Typically, blood glucose levels are greater than 100 mg/dL after an overnight fast. After 4 hours the blood glucose concentration still has not returned to the basal level.

5. The answer is C. Muscle and adipose tissue are the two tissues that show a marked dependence on insulin for glucose uptake.

REFERENCES

1. Nathan DM: *Glycosylated Hemoglobin: A Measure of Control*. Medfield, MA: Corning Medical, 1984, p 11.

10 DIGESTION AND ABSORPTION OF CARBOHYDRATES

INTRODUCTION OF CLINICAL CASE

Tim was born at full term after a normal pregnancy and delivery. He was breast-fed and in good health until 3 months of age, when he developed diarrhea and vomiting and had a temperature of 103.5°F. He was admitted to the hospital with a diagnosis of gastroenteritis. At the time of admission, he was dehydrated, his abdomen was bloated, and his stools were frothy. The stool pH was 5.0 and contained volatile acids and a reducing sugar that was identified as lactose. Urine analysis revealed the presence of lactose. He was treated for dehydration by intravenous administration of electrolytes and glucose. After 24 hours, the vomiting and diarrhea ceased, the stools contained no volatile acids or reducing sugars, and his urine was free of lactose. He was released from the hospital and placed on a formula that substituted sucrose for lactose. He was re-examined by his physician 4 weeks later and was given a lactose tolerance test. Following ingestion of lactose, the level of hydrogen (H_2) gas in the breath did not increase significantly over the next 6 hours; his stools were firm and contained no lactose. He was placed on a formula containing cow's milk and experienced no further difficulties.

CARBOHYDRATE CHEMISTRY AND NOMENCLATURE

Almost all of the clinically important carbohydrate metabolism involves five simple monosaccharides. All of the dietary disaccharides and complex carbohydrates are made up of one or more of these monosaccharides.

Monosaccharide Structure

The most commonly occurring monosaccharides in human biology are glucose, galactose, mannose, fructose, and ribose (Figure 10-1). All of these compounds are polyols that have a carbonyl group ($>C=O$). Glucose, galactose, mannose, and fructose are *hexoses*, and ribose is a *pentose*. The most important monosaccharide is glucose. All of the other monosaccharides in Figure 10-1 are structurally related to glucose and can be derived from glucose.

FIGURE 10-1 ▶

Structures of Common Carbohydrates. Glucose, galactose, and mannose are epimers, differing only in the configuration around a single carbon atom. Glucose and fructose are isomers that differ in the position of the carbonyl group.

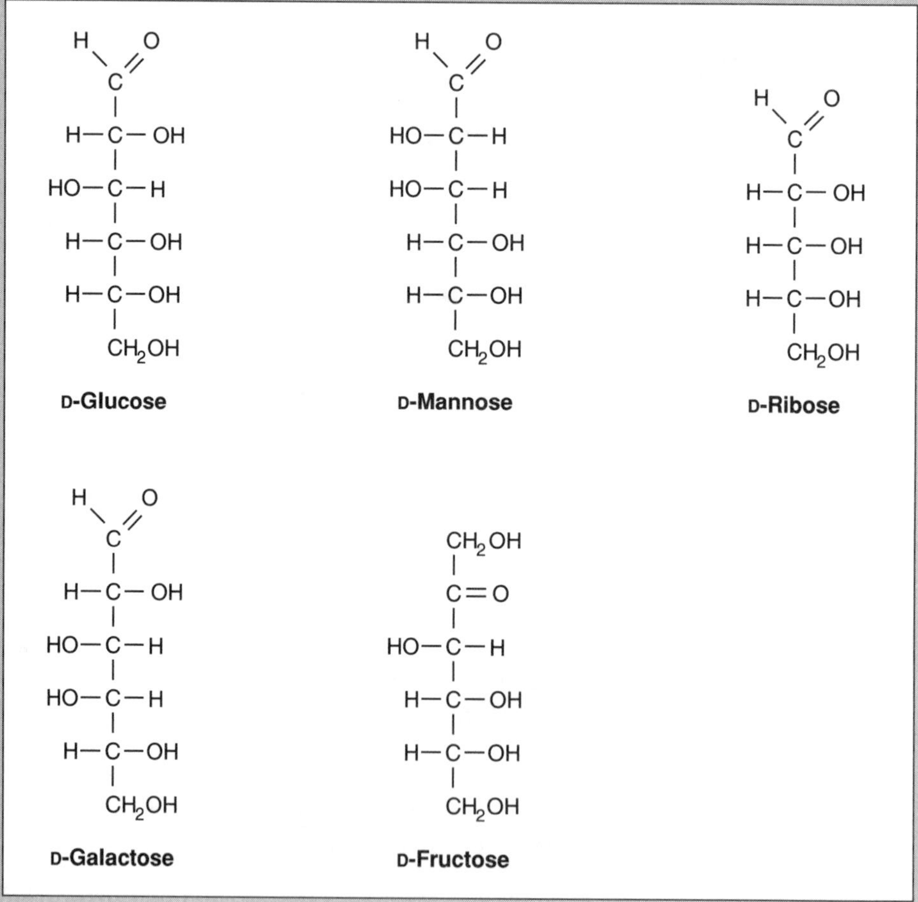

D-Glucose

D-Mannose

D-Ribose

D-Galactose

D-Fructose

Definitions and Nomenclature

The student who knows the structure of glucose and the definitions that follow will have the essential structural information for most of the biologically important monosaccharides.

Anomeric Carbon. The carbonyl carbon ($>C=O$) is known as the anomeric carbon. As shown in Figure 10-1, the anomeric carbon of glucose, galactose, and mannose at C-1 is an aldehyde and is the basis for classifying these sugars as *aldoses*. For fructose, the anomeric carbon at C-2 is a ketone, making fructose a *ketose*. The most reactive carbon in all of these sugars is the anomeric carbon; it always participates in the formation of cyclic forms of the monosaccharides, and it is always involved in the bond that joins monosaccharides together to produce disaccharides or larger polymers.

Penultimate Carbon. The chiral carbon most distant from the anomeric carbon is known as the penultimate carbon. For glucose and other hexoses, the penultimate carbon is C-5. For ribose, it is C-4. As shown below, the penultimate carbon is important in distinguishing D and L forms of sugars.

D and L Configurations. The designation of either D or L refers to the dextro or levo configurations around the penultimate carbon atom. L-Glucose is the mirror image of D-glucose with the hydroxyl group at C-5 on the left. Most of the *biologically important monosaccharides* are of the *D configuration*.

Epimer. Monosaccharides that differ from one another in the configuration around a single carbon atom are known as epimers. For example, galactose is the 4-epimer of glucose.

Cyclic Forms of Monosaccharides

The most stable form of monosaccharides in aqueous solutions is cyclic rather than an open chain structure. As shown in Figure 10-2, glucose can exist in two cyclic forms, α-D-glucose and β-D-glucose. These forms result from reaction of the hydroxyl group on C-5 with the anomeric carbon at C-1. The carbonyl oxygen on C-1 of the straight chain structure becomes a hydroxyl group that can exist in two possible configurations (written either down or up on the anomeric carbon), forming α-D-glucose and β-D-glucose, respectively. The most stable form of glucose is β-D-glucose, comprising more than 99% of the glucose in solution. Fructose has its anomeric carbon at C-2 and, therefore, forms a five-member ring structure. The cyclic structures shown in Figure 10-2 are known as *Haworth projections*. The substituents attached to the ring are drawn either above or below the plane of the ring. The rules for placing a substituent above or below the ring are as follows: (1) the —CH$_2$OH group attached to the penultimate carbon is always up; (2) groups on the anomeric carbon may be either up or down; (3) for all other carbons, groups on the left in the straight chain form are up, and groups on the right are down.

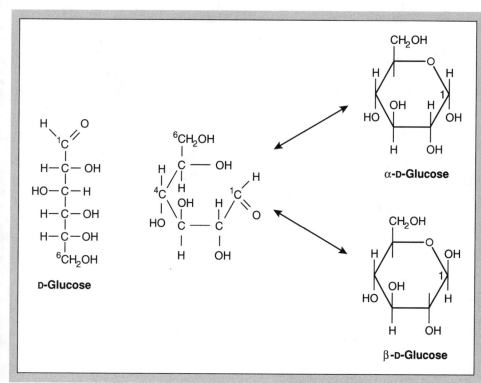

◀ **FIGURE 10-2**
Cyclic Structures of Glucose. *The oxygen in the ring structure is contributed by the hydroxyl group on C-5.*

Glycosidic Bond
The glycosidic bond joins the anomeric carbon of one sugar with a hydroxyl group from a second sugar. The configuration of the anomeric carbon is designated either α or β.

α-(1,4)

β-(1,4)

SOURCES OF DIETARY CARBOHYDRATE

Although dietary carbohydrates are not essential, their metabolism provides the most important source of energy, and restriction of carbohydrate in the diet to less than about 0.5 g/kg body wt/d is likely to result in excessive breakdown of muscle protein, ketosis, cation depletion, and dehydration.

The major foods from which carbohydrates are obtained are potatoes, corn, rice, bread, and yams. Although some monosaccharides are found in natural foods, most dietary carbohydrate is ingested as disaccharides and complex carbohydrates.

Monosaccharides

The three monosaccharides important to human nutrition are glucose, fructose, and galactose. Glucose is a moderately sweet sugar that is found naturally in only a few foods, such as corn syrup. Fructose, the sweetest of the monosaccharides, is found in fruits and honey. Galactose is not found free in foods but is produced by digestion of lactose.

Disaccharides

Four important disaccharides arise from dietary sources (Figure 10-3). Each consists of two simple sugars that are linked by a *glycosidic bond*, connecting the anomeric carbon of one sugar with a hydroxyl group of the second sugar. Most disaccharides are reducing sugars and will result in a positive Fehling-Benedict test because one of the anomeric carbons in the disaccharide has an unsubstituted hydroxyl group that is in equilibrium with the open chain form of that monosaccharide.

FIGURE 10-3 ▶
Structures of Common Disaccharides. *The numerical description of a glycosidic bond defines the carbon atoms that connect the two sugars. The sugar contributing the anomeric carbon is written first.*

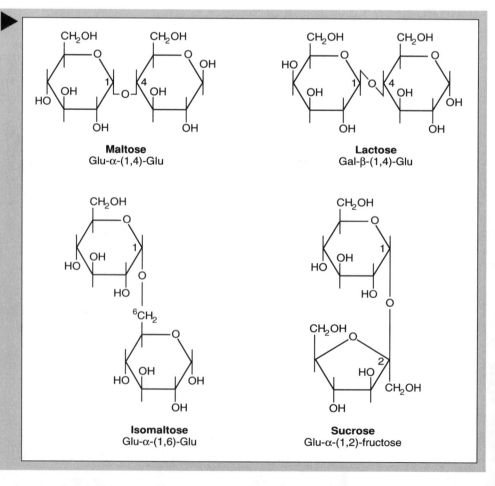

Maltose
Glu-α-(1,4)-Glu

Lactose
Gal-β-(1,4)-Glu

Isomaltose
Glu-α-(1,6)-Glu

Sucrose
Glu-α-(1,2)-fructose

Maltose occurs in commercial malt products and is produced as an intermediate in the digestion of starch and glycogen. It consists of two glucose molecules that are linked by an α-(1,4) glycosidic bond.

Isomaltose arises from the digestion of starch and glycogen. It consists of two glucose molecules linked by an α-(1,6) glycosidic bond. Since the anomeric carbon in both maltose and isomaltose is donated by α-D-glucose, these disaccharides are known as *α-glucosides*.

Lactose is the major carbohydrate found in milk. It is composed of galactose and glucose that are linked by a β-(1,4) glycosidic linkage. The anomeric carbon of the bond comes from β-D-galactose, making lactose a β-*galactoside*.

Sucrose, also known as "table sugar," is the most common disaccharide. It is made commercially from sugar cane and beets and can be found in molasses and many processed foods. Sucrose often contributes 30%–40% of the total calories in the American diet. Sucrose consists of glucose and fructose linked by an α-(1,2) glycosidic bond. The linkage in sucrose involves the anomeric carbons of both monosaccharides, making sucrose a nonreducing sugar.

Complex Carbohydrates

Polysaccharides, containing many monosaccharide units, are known as complex carbohydrates. The most common complex carbohydrates are starch, glycogen, and dietary fiber.

Starch is the plant storage form of glucose. It consists of two polysaccharides, amylose, and amylopectin, whose structures are shown in Figure 10-4. *Amylose* is a linear polymer of glucose units linked by α-(1,4) glycosidic bonds. *Amylopectin* is a branched polymer having both α-(1,4) and α-(1,6) glycosidic bonds. The branch points in amylopectin are created by α-(1,6) bonds and occur at intervals of 25–30 glucose units.

Glycogen is the animal storage form of glucose. Its structure is similar to amylopectin except that it is more highly branched, having α-(1,6) linkages at intervals of about 10–12 glucose units.

Fiber, also known as "unavailable carbohydrate," cannot be digested by humans because the appropriate enzymes are not present in the gastrointestinal tract. Although there is no

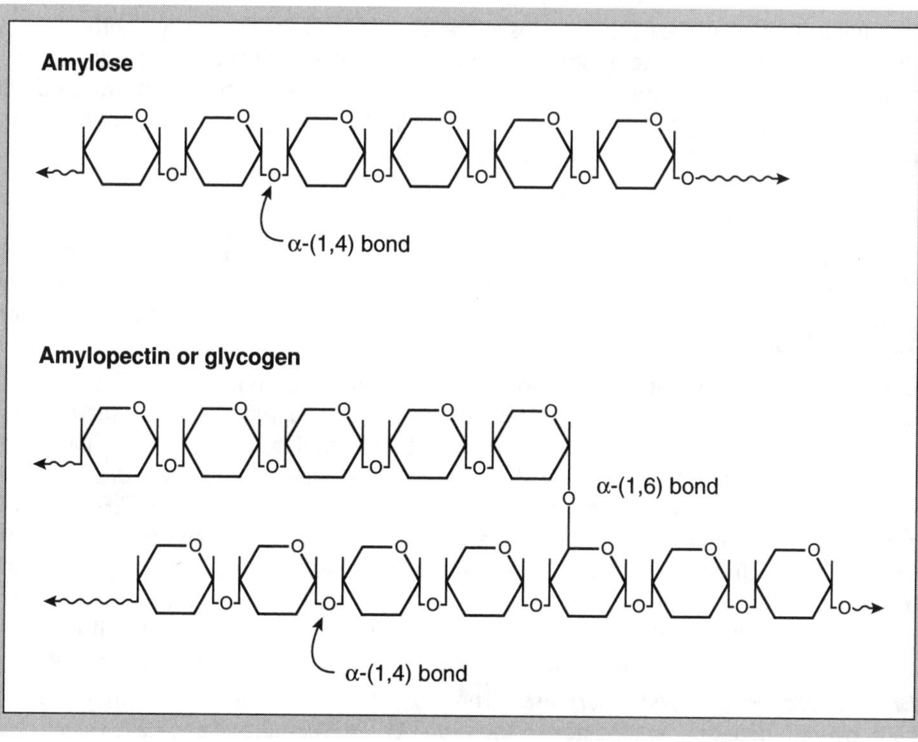

FIGURE 10-4

Structure of Starch. Amylose contains only α-(1,4) bonds. Amylose and glycogen contain both α-(1,4) and α-(1,6) bonds. Glycogen is more highly branched than amylopectin and contains more α-(1,6) linkages.

known metabolic requirement for fiber, there is ample evidence that a high-fiber diet is associated with reduced incidence of a number of diseases. The recommended fiber content of the diet is between 20 and 35 g/d. There are two major classes of fiber, cellulose and noncellulose. *Cellulose* is present in unrefined cereals. It increases the bulk of stools and decreases transit time. *Noncellulose* fiber consists of pectins (fruits), gums (oats and dried beans), and lignin (pulpy part of plants). These fibers bind a number of small organic compounds, including carcinogens, cholesterol, and bile acids, thereby reducing plasma cholesterol. Pectins and gums slow the rate of gastric emptying and retard the rate of digestion and absorption of many nutrients. This effect is beneficial to diabetics because it can attenuate the rise in blood glucose following a carbohydrate-rich meal.

> A high-fiber diet has been correlated with decreased incidence of the following:
> 1. Cardiovascular disease
> 2. Colon cancer
> 3. Diverticulosis
> 4. Diabetes

DIGESTION OF CARBOHYDRATE

Monosaccharides need no digestion prior to absorption, whereas disaccharides and polysaccharides must be hydrolyzed to simple sugars before they can be absorbed. The major sites of carbohydrate digestion are the mouth and the small intestine. Most of the intestinal digestion occurs in the jejunum.

Oral Cavity: Salivary α-Amylase

Digestion of amylose, amylopectin, and glycogen starts in the mouth where salivary α-*amylase* begins to degrade starch. Alpha-amylase is an *endoglycosidase* that catalyzes the random hydrolysis of internal α-(1,4) glycosidic bonds. It is maximally active at neutral pH and requires chloride for activity. It *cannot* catalyze the cleavage of α-(1,6) bonds found at the branch points. The products of the salivary α-amylase reaction are shown in the equation below.

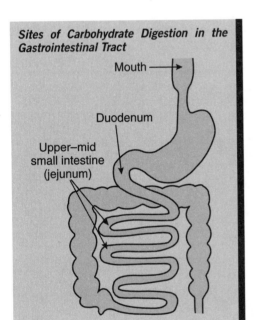

Sites of Carbohydrate Digestion in the Gastrointestinal Tract

Mouth

Duodenum

Upper–mid small intestine (jejunum)

$$\begin{array}{c} \text{Amylose} \\ \text{Amylopectin} \\ \text{Glycogen} \end{array} + H_2O \xrightarrow[\substack{pH\ 7.0 \\ Cl^-}]{\alpha\text{-amylase}} \text{maltose} + \text{maltriose} + \text{dextrins}$$

The major product is dextrin, an oligosaccharide with an average chain length of 8–10 glucose residues and containing all of the α-(1,6) glycosidic bonds. Small amounts of maltose and maltriose are formed. As the partially digested *chyme* moves into the stomach, the action of α-amylase is completely stopped by the acidic environment. Virtually no carbohydrate digestion occurs in the stomach.

Small Intestine

There are two phases of intestinal digestion. The first phase occurs in the lumen and is also known as the hormonal or pancreatic phase. The second phase occurs in the brush border membrane and involves the action of a number of integral membrane proteins with disaccharidase activity.

Luminal Phase: Pancreatic α-Amylase. The movement of partially digested chyme into the small intestine stimulates mucosal cells of the *duodenum* to release *secretin* and *cholecystokinin (CCK)*, two peptide hormones that stimulate the exocrine pancreas to release its secretions into the intestinal lumen. As shown in Figure 10-5, secretin stimulates the release of pancreatic juice, which is slightly alkaline (pH 7.6–7.9) and enriched in bicarbonate (HCO_3^-). Its major function is to neutralize the acidic chyme from the stomach. CCK stimulates the release of digestive enzymes, including pancreatic α-amylase, whose function is to degrade dextrins further, resulting in a mixture of maltose, isomaltose, and alpha–limit dextrins. The limit dextrins are small oligosaccharides containing 3–5 glucose units and all of the α-(1,6) branch-point linkages.

Brush Border Phase: Disaccharidases. The enzymes responsible for the final phase of carbohydrate digestion are located in the brush border membrane and have their active sites extending into the lumen. The enzymes are protected from degradation by a mucus

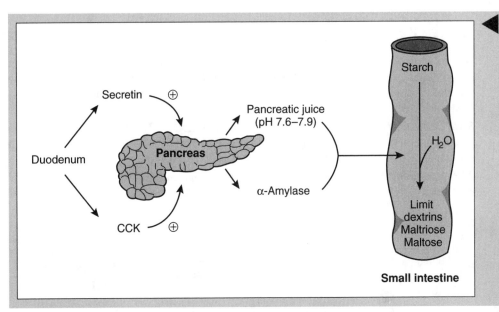

FIGURE 10-5
Role of Secretin and Cholecystokinin (CCK) in Carbohydrate Metabolism. Both hormones are secreted by the duodenum and carried via the blood to the pancreas, where secretin stimulates release of pancreatic juice and CCK stimulates the release of α-amylase into the small intestine.

coat known as the *glycocalix.* The enzymes and the reactions they catalyze are summarized in Table 10-1.

All of the enzymes in the brush border membrane are disaccharidases except dextrinase, which hydrolyzes the α-(1,6) bonds at the branch points of the limit dextrins. Isomaltase/sucrase is a bifunctional enzyme, having one domain with isomaltase activity and another with sucrase activity on the same polypeptide.

Trehalose is a rare disaccharide found in young mushrooms where it makes up about 1.5% of their weight. Trehalase deficiency exists in 10%–15% of the Greenland Inuit population, resulting in varying degrees of intestinal disturbances following ingestion of edible mushrooms [1].

TABLE 10-1
Summary of Carbohydrate Digestion in the Gastrointestinal Tract

Site	Enzyme	Substrate	Major Products
Mouth	Salivary amylase	Starch	Dextrins
Stomach	None	None	None
Small intestine			
Lumen	Pancreatic amylase	Dextrins	Alpha-limit dextrins Maltriose Maltose
Brush border	Maltase	Maltose	Glucose
	Isomaltase	Isomaltose	Glucose
	Trehalase	Trehalose	Glucose
	Sucrase	Sucrose	Glucose and fructose
	Lactase	Lactose	Glucose and galactose
	Dextrinase	Alpha-limit dextrins	Glucose, maltose, and maltriose

ABSORPTION OF MONOSACCHARIDES

Monosaccharides are absorbed from the small intestine into the portal blood, which goes directly to the liver. Absorption across the intestinal epithelial cells involves movement across two membranes, the *apical membrane* on the luminal side and the *basolateral membrane* on the serosal side of the cell. The process of absorption appears to be tightly coupled with digestion since little, if any, monosaccharide leaks back out into the lumen. Three kinetic properties of glucose absorption indicate that the process is *carrier-mediated.* It shows (1) monosaccharide specificity, (2) saturation kinetics, and (3) inhibition by structural analogs of the monosaccharide. In general, glucose and galactose are transported by the same proteins. The absorption of pentoses and fructose is not well understood, although it is likely they move down a concentration gradient across membranes by both simple diffusion and facilitated diffusion.

Transport Across Apical Membrane

The net transport of glucose from the intestinal lumen into the epithelial cell is sodium (Na^+)-dependent and occurs against a concentration gradient. Two transport proteins are involved, a sodium-dependent glucose transporter (SGLT) and the adenosine triphosphate (ATP)-dependent Na^+/K^+ pump (Figure 10-6).

SGLT cotransports Na^+ and glucose in the same direction. The energy for transporting glucose against a concentration gradient is provided by the movement of Na^+ from a high extracellular concentration to a low intracellular concentration.

ATP-dependent Na^+/K^+ pump maintains the Na^+ gradient across the membrane by expelling Na^+ from the cell in exchange for K^+. The energy for pumping Na^+ back out of

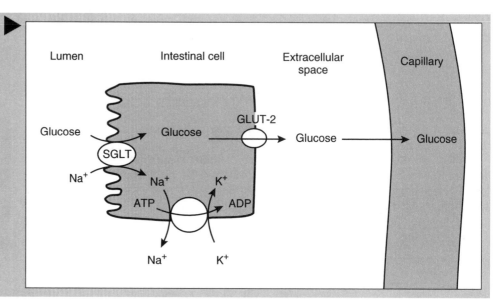

FIGURE 10-6

Absorption of Glucose from Intestinal Lumen into Portal Circulation. Glucose concentration in the intestinal cell is greater than that of both the lumen and the extracellular space. The energy for transport into the intestinal cell is derived from the cotransport of Na^+, which moves down a gradient from about 140 mM to 30 mM. Transport of glucose across the basolateral membrane is driven by the higher intracellular concentration. The energy for expelling Na^+ from the cell is provided by ATP and the Na^+/K^+-ATPase. SGLT = sodium-dependent glucose transporter; GLUT-2 = glucose transporter type 2.

the cell is provided by the hydrolysis of ATP. *Ouabain*, a potent and specific inhibitor of the ATP-dependent Na^+/K^+ pump, is also an inhibitor of glucose transport.

Transport Across Basolateral Membrane

The transport of glucose from the cytosol of the epithelial cell into the portal circulation requires a Na^+-independent glucose transporter known as *GLUT-2* (Figure 10-6). The driving force for glucose transport across the basolateral membrane is provided by the concentration of glucose, which is higher inside the intestinal cell than in the extracellular space.

Transport of Glucose from Blood into Other Cells

A family of closely related proteins, the *GLUT family*, transports glucose across cell membranes. With the exception of SGLT, the GLUT transporters are Na^+-independent and participate in facilitated diffusion of glucose with glucose moving down a concentration gradient. A low concentration of glucose is maintained inside the cell by the rapid conversion of glucose to glucose-6-phosphate (G6P). Members of the GLUT family differ in their kinetic properties, cell and tissue distribution, and response to insulin. The properties of a particular transporter appear to correlate well with the overall role that glucose metabolism plays in a particular cell or tissue. The Na^+-independent transporters are inhibited by *cytochalasin B*.

Brain and red blood cell (RBC) membranes are enriched in *GLUT-1*. These transporters bind glucose with a high affinity and are always saturated at physiologic concentrations of glucose, thus ensuring a constant supply of glucose to these cells.

Liver and pancreatic beta cells have *GLUT-2* as their predominant transporter. GLUT-2 has a low affinity and high capacity for glucose transport. These transporters are not saturated under physiologic conditions. Therefore, the rate of glucose transport increases as the extracellular concentration of glucose increases.

Skeletal muscle, heart, and fat cells are enriched in *GLUT-4*, which is sensitive to insulin. Under basal conditions, spare GLUT-4 transporters are stored in the Golgi. When insulin binds to the surface of these cells, spare transporters are moved from the trans-Golgi into the plasma membrane, where they increase the rate of glucose uptake.

ABNORMALITIES IN CARBOHYDRATE DIGESTION AND ABSORPTION

Any condition that results in impaired ability to digest and absorb carbohydrate may result in bacterial fermentation in the large intestine (Figure 10-7) with the production of H_2 and carbon dioxide (CO_2) gases and low molecular weight acids that are osmotically active. Abdominal cramps and flatulence result from the accumulation of gases, and the osmotically active products draw water from the intestinal cells into the lumen, resulting in diarrhea and dehydration.

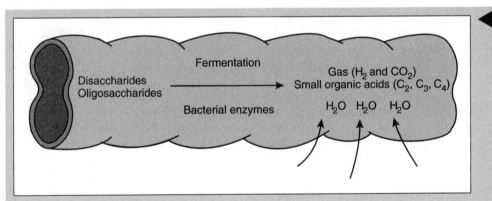

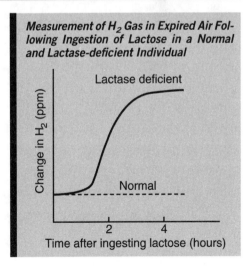

FIGURE 10-7
Microbial Fermentation of Glucose in the Colon. *Undigested carbohydrate can be degraded to a mixture of acetic, propionic, and butyric acids with the release of gases (predominantly H_2). Differences in the intestinal flora can result in large variations in severity of symptoms in individuals with disaccharidase deficiency [1].*

Genetic deficiencies in most of the disaccharidases have been described, resulting in the symptoms described above [1]. *Lactase deficiency* is the most common with the frequency varying widely among different age and ethnic groups. It can also occur secondary to diseases that damage the intestinal mucosa. With such diseases, some lactose may be absorbed without hydrolysis and excreted in the urine. Lactase is more sensitive to mucosal damage than maltase and sucrase. The diagnosis of lactase deficiency can be made by performing an intestinal biopsy and directly assaying the tissue for lactase. A less invasive and more reliable method is the *hydrogen breath test* [2], which measures the presence of H_2 gas in the expired air following oral administration of a "lactose cocktail." The symptoms disappear after changing to a lactose-free diet.

Measurement of H_2 Gas in Expired Air Following Ingestion of Lactose in a Normal and Lactase-deficient Individual

RESOLUTION OF CLINICAL CASE

The physical symptoms, together with analysis of stools and urine, suggest that this patient was experiencing lactose intolerance. A genetic deficiency in lactase can be eliminated as a cause since prior to this episode the patient had been successfully breast-feeding for 3 months. The temporary lactase deficiency was secondary to gastroenteritis. The fact that some lactose appeared in the urine is indicative of damaged mucosal cells. Normally, disaccharides are not absorbed. Most of the lactose is fermented by colonic bacteria, producing H_2, CO_2, and small organic acids, accounting for the low pH of the stools. The diarrhea and dehydration are secondary to the osmotic activity of the acids. Substitution of sucrose for lactose with no adverse consequences is consistent with the observation that lactase is more severely affected by membrane damage than sucrase. A normal lactose tolerance test 4 weeks later indicates that the damaged mucosal cells have been repaired and provides the basis for either returning the patient to breast-feeding or placing him on a formula containing cow's milk.

REVIEW QUESTIONS

Directions: For each of the following questions, choose the **one best** answer.

1. The disaccharide shown below has which of the following characteristics?

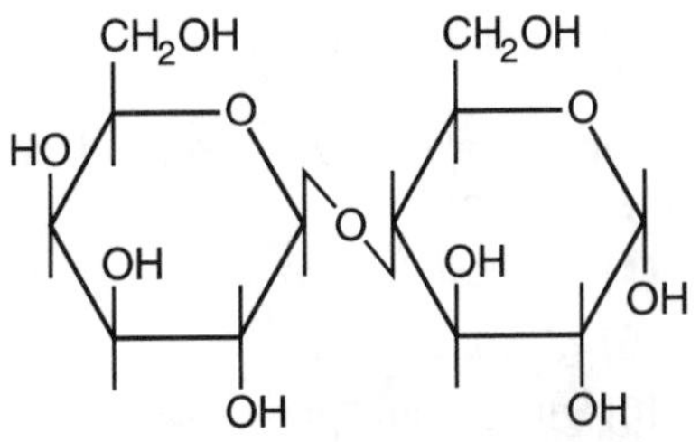

(A) It is found in high concentrations in fruits

(B) It gives a negative reducing sugar test

(C) It contains an α-(1,4) glycosidic bond

(D) It is hydrolyzed in the intestine to glucose and galactose

(E) It is cleaved by sucrase

2. The monosaccharides shown below are both

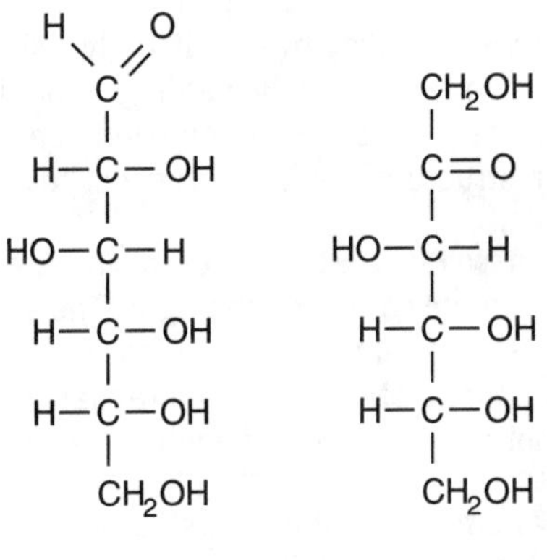

(A) aldoses

(B) epimers

(C) D-monosaccharides

(D) ketoses

(E) enantiomers

3. The linkage between glucose residues at branch points in starch is

(A) α-(1,6)

(B) β-(1,4)

(C) α-(1,4)

(D) α-(1,2)

(E) β-(1,6)

4. A patient has a deficiency in sucrase, resulting from the inability to synthesize the enzyme rather than from an alteration in the enzyme structure. Which of the following dietary sources of carbohydrate would you recommend for meeting the energy needs of this patient?

   (A) Table sugar

   (B) Amylose

   (C) Glycogen

   (D) Amylopectin

   (E) Limit dextrin

5. Following a meal of pizza, coke, and ice cream, the major monosaccharides absorbed into the blood are

   (A) fructose

   (B) glucose

   (C) glucose and galactose

   (D) glucose and fructose

   (E) galactose, glucose, and fructose

ANSWERS AND EXPLANATIONS

1. The answer is D. Lactose is found in milk and some milk products. It is hydrolyzed by lactase to galactose and glucose. Sucrase has no effect on lactose. The two monosaccharides are linked by a β-(1,4) glycosidic bond. Lactose is a reducing sugar and gives a positive reaction in the Fehling-Benedict test. Any aldehyde gives a positive reducing sugar test, and since the anomeric carbon of glucose is in equilibrium with the open chain structure, C-1 is an unsubstituted aldehyde.

2. The answer is C. Both structures have a D configuration with the hydroxyl group of the penultimate carbon on the right. The structures are glucose (*left*) and fructose (*right*). Glucose is an aldose and fructose is a ketose. They are not epimers since they differ in their configuration around more than one carbon. They are not enantiomers since they are not mirror images of each other.

3. The answer is A. Starch has no beta-type linkages. All the bonds in starch are either α-(1,4) or α-(1,6) with the latter being found only at the branch points.

4. The answer is B. Since isomaltase and sucrase activities are located on the same protein, this patient would be deficient in both enzymes and could not hydrolyze sucrose or isomaltose. Since isomaltose is one of the products of glycogen and amylopectin degradation, these carbohydrates should be eliminated from the diet. Amylose contains only α-(1,4) glycosidic bonds and is the only carbohydrate listed that can be used as a source of energy by this individual. Since one of the products of limit dextrin degradation is isomaltose, this should be eliminated from the diet.

5. The answer is E. The pizza dough contains starch and milk, the coke contains sucrose, and ice cream contains both lactose and sucrose. The monosaccharides generated by intestinal hydrolysis of these foods are glucose, galactose, and fructose, all of which are absorbed into the portal circulation.

REFERENCES

1. Semenza G, Auricchio S: Small intestinal disaccharidases. In *The Metabolic and Molecular Bases of Inherited Disease*, 7th ed. Edited by Scriver CR, Beaudet AL, Sly WS, et al. New York, NY: McGraw-Hill, 1995, pp 4451–4471.
2. Perman JA, Barr RG, Watkins JB: Sucrose malabsorption in children: non-invasive diagnosis by interval breath hydrogen determination. *J Pediatr* 1978, 93:17.

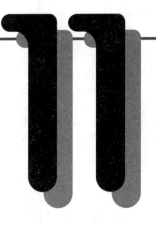

GLYCOLYSIS: THE CENTRAL PATHWAY OF GLUCOSE DEGRADATION

INTRODUCTION OF CLINICAL CASE

Angie, a 15-year-old girl, was admitted to the hospital because of recurrent episodes of pallor, jaundice, and an ulcer on her left leg. Diagnosis of hemolytic anemia had been made at the age of 3 months, and she had been transfused several times since the diagnosis. Physical examination showed jaundice, skeletal growth retardation, and enlargement of the spleen. An analysis of blood showed low hemoglobin content, low RBC count, and elevated reticulocyte count. Morphologic analysis revealed a mixed population of RBCs containing some irregularly contracted cells with irregular surface projections. The life span of the RBCs was found to be severely shortened. Both total and indirect serum bilirubin levels were markedly elevated. Fecal urobilinogen excretion was increased. Biochemical analysis of RBC metabolites showed elevated levels of 2,3-

bisphosphoglycerate (2,3-BPG) and reduced levels of ATP. A splenectomy was per formed; the spleen showed congestion and the presence of hemosiderin granules. Fol lowing splenectomy, there was improvement in both the clinical and hematologi symptoms. An increase in hemoglobin concentration as well as in the number of RBC and reticulocytes was observed. The biochemical composition of the RBCs did no change significantly after splenectomy.

GLYCOLYSIS: DEFINITION AND FUNCTION

Glycolysis, also known as the Embden-Myerhof pathway, is the central pathway o carbohydrate metabolism and occurs in the cytosol of all cells (Figure 11-1). The pathway consists of ten sequential reactions that convert glucose to two molecules o

FIGURE 11-1 ▶

The Pathway of Glycolysis. *Reactions indicated by double-headed arrows (↔) are reversible. Three reactions in the pathway are essentially irreversible under cellular conditions (→), and the reverse of these actions requires a different enzyme.*

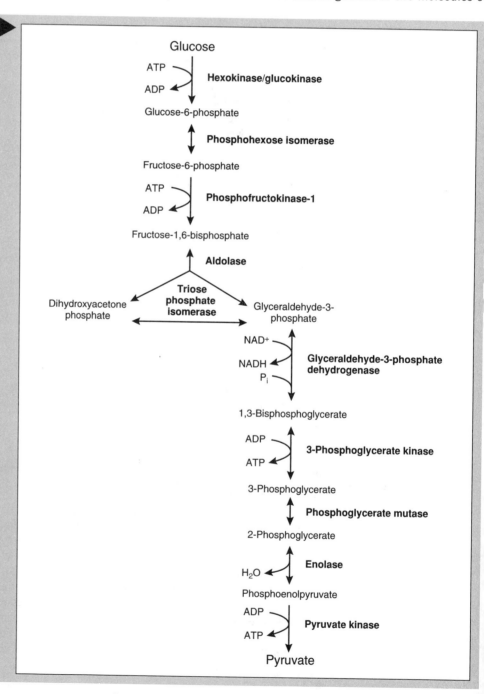

pyruvate. Additionally, two molecules of ATP are formed from adenosine diphosphate (ADP) and inorganic phosphate (P_i), and two molecules of NADH are formed from oxidized nicotinamide-adenine dinucleotide (NAD^+). All of the intermediates in the pathway are phosphorylated, which ensures that they will stay inside the cell. The two major functions of glycolysis are: (1) to provide energy for the cell in the form of ATP, and (2) to generate intermediates that may be used as starting points for other pathways. The primary role of glycolysis, however, may vary in different cells and tissues, as described below.

RBCs depend entirely on glycolysis for ATP synthesis. They have no mitochondria and cannot synthesize ATP by the oxidative pathways that are available to most cells.

Skeletal muscle uses glycolysis to generate ATP for muscle contraction. Although other oxidative pathways for generating ATP are present in muscle, glycolysis is the major pathway under conditions of oxygen deprivation.

Adipose tissue specializes in the storage and mobilization of triglyceride. One of the major functions of glycolysis in adipocytes is to provide dihydroxyacetone phosphate (DHAP), the precursor of the glycerol backbone of triglycerides.

Liver derives most of its energy from noncarbohydrate sources. The role of glycolysis in liver depends on the nutritional state of the organism. In the well-fed state, dietary carbohydrate is stored either as glycogen or as fat. The pyruvate resulting from glycolysis may be used to generate precursors for fatty acid synthesis. These energy-storage pathways are stimulated by insulin. In the fasting state, pyruvate and other low molecular precursors are used for the de novo synthesis of glucose. This process is stimulated by glucagon, and it requires all of the enzymes in the glycolytic pathway that catalyze reversible reactions.

ENTRY AND TRAPPING OF GLUCOSE IN CELLS

The entry of glucose into cells is carrier-mediated by integral membrane transporters that move glucose down a concentration gradient into the cell. Once inside the cell the glucose is rapidly phosphorylated to glucose-6-phosphate (G6P). This ensures that the concentration gradient across the plasma membrane is maintained and that glucose does not leak back out of the cell (Figure 11-2). The ATP-dependent phosphorylation of glucose is catalyzed by *glucokinase* in liver and by *hexokinase* in muscle and other tissues. This reaction is exergonic ($\Delta G^o = -4.0$ kcal/mol), and under the conditions that prevail within the cell, it is essentially irreversible.

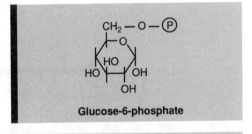

Glucose-6-phosphate

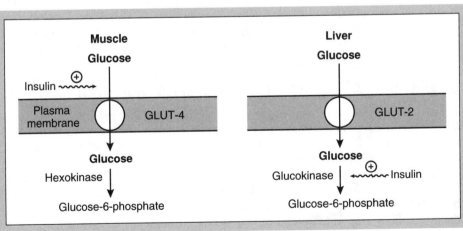

◀ **FIGURE 11-2**
Entry and Trapping of Glucose in Muscle and Liver Cells. The effect of insulin on the uptake of glucose is indicated by an arrow *($\sim\!\!\sim\!\!\sim\!\!\rightarrow$). In muscle, the rate of movement of glucose across the plasma membrane is increased, whereas in liver, the rate of the glucokinase reaction is increased.*

The net transport of glucose across the plasma membrane of both muscle and liver is enhanced by insulin. In muscle, insulin increases the number of glucose transporters (GLUT-4) in the plasma membrane but has no effect on hexokinase activity. In liver, insulin increases the synthesis of glucokinase, but the GLUT-2 transporters are unaffected.

A comparison of the properties of hexokinase and glucokinase is shown in Table 11-1. The most important functional differences in these enzymes are their kinetic and regulatory properties.

Effects of Insulin on Glucose Uptake in Muscle

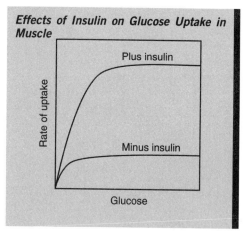

Hexokinase has a high affinity for glucose ($K_m < 0.1$ mM) and is saturated at physiologic concentrations of glucose. The enzyme is also strongly inhibited by its product, G6P, a property that prevents the production of G6P in excess of the amount needed by the cell. Hexokinase is constitutively expressed in cells.

Glucokinase has a low affinity for glucose ($K_m \cong 10$ mM) and is not inhibited by G6P. The high K_m of glucokinase contributes to the ability of the liver to lower blood glucose levels following a meal. The GLUT-2 transporter in liver also has a high K_m. The synthesis of glucokinase is induced by insulin.

TABLE 11-1 ▶
Properties of Glucokinase and Hexokinase

	Glucokinase	Hexokinase
Kinetic parameters		
K_m	High (10 mM)	Low (<100 μM)
V_{max}	High	Low
Tissue distribution	Liver	Most tissues
	Pancreatic beta cells	
Regulation		
Short-term	Activity responds to changes in glucose concentration	Inhibited by glucose-6-phosphate
Long-term	Synthesis induced by insulin	Constitutive

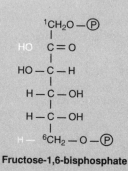

Fructose-1,6-bisphosphate

Dihydroxyacetone phosphate

Glyceraldehyde-3-phosphate

STAGES OF GLYCOLYSIS

Based on whether ATP is used or synthesized, the reactions in glycolysis can be divided into two major stages. Stage 1 requires the investment of two molecules of ATP to convert glucose to two molecules of glyceraldehyde-3-phosphate (G3P). Stage 2 converts two molecules of G3P to two molecules of pyruvate with the formation of four molecules of ATP. Energy is conserved in stage 2 by using high-energy phosphate bonds of glycolytic intermediates to drive the synthesis of ATP.

Stage 1: Utilization of ATP (Conversion of Glucose to G3P)

The pathway in Figure 11-1 starts with the conversion of glucose to G6P by *glucokinase/hexokinase*, as described above. This is the first reaction that requires ATP. G6P is converted rapidly to fructose-6-phosphate (F6P) by the action of *phosphohexose isomerase*, an enzyme that interconverts aldoses and ketoses by shifting the position of the carbonyl group from C-1 to C-2.

The second ATP-requiring step in the pathway converts F6P to fructose-1,6-bisphosphate (F1,6P$_2$). The reaction, catalyzed by *phosphofructokinase-1 (PFK-1)*, is the rate-limiting step in the pathway. It is also an irreversible step with a $\Delta G^\circ = -3.4$ kcal/mol. The presence of phosphate groups on each end of F1,6P$_2$ sets the stage for cleavage of the six-carbon (C$_6$) intermediate into two three-carbon (C$_3$) metabolites, each containing a phosphate group. Acting as a pair of metabolic scissors, *aldolase* cleaves F1,6P$_2$ between C-3 and C-4, generating DHAP and G3P. These two C$_3$ intermediates can be interconverted by the action of *phosphotriose isomerase*, allowing both to be further metabolized by a common pathway.

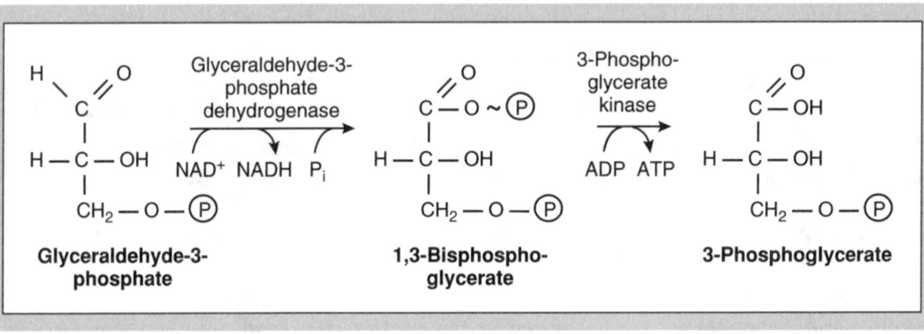

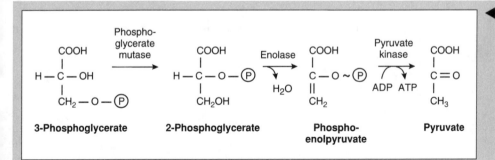

FIGURE 11-3
The First ATP-Generating Sequence in Glycolysis. The reaction catalyzed by glyceraldehyde-3-phosphate dehydrogenase produces a mixed anhydride formed from a carboxylic acid and phosphoric acid. In this reaction, the phosphate group is transferred to ADP with the formation of ATP. The energy released by cleavage of the mixed anhydride is used to form the anhydride linkage between ADP and P_i.

Stage 2: Generation of ATP (Conversion of G3P to Pyruvate)

In the second stage of glycolysis, intermediates containing high-energy phosphate groups are used to drive the synthesis of ATP. This process is known as *substrate-level phosphorylation*, a term that distinguishes it from oxidative phosphorylation, which is the major pathway of ATP production in most cells.

In two sequential reactions, G3P is converted to 3-phosphoglycerate (3-PG) with the production of ATP (Figure 11-3). The first reaction, catalyzed by *G3PD*, is complex and involves the oxidation of C-1 from an aldehyde to an acid with the concomitant reduction of NAD+ to NADH. Following the oxidation, a mixed anhydride is formed between the carboxyl group and P_i. The significance of this reaction is that anhydride bonds have enough energy to drive the synthesis of ATP. In the following reaction, *3-phosphoglycerate kinase* catalyzes the transfer of the phosphate at C-1 to ADP, producing ATP and 3-PG.

The overall function of the last three reactions in glycolysis is to convert 3-PG into another high-energy compound that can be used for ATP synthesis (Figure 11-4). *Phosphoglycerate mutase* catalyzes the transfer of phosphate from C-3 to C-2, forming 2-phosphoglycerate (2-PG). The dehydration of 2-PG to phosphoenolpyruvate (PEP) is catalyzed by *enolase*. The phosphate bond in PEP is a high-energy bond with a ΔG° of hydrolysis of -14.8 kcal/mol. In the final step of glycolysis, *pyruvate kinase* couples the hydrolysis of PEP with the synthesis of ATP, a reaction requiring energy ($\Delta G^\circ = +7.3$ kcal/mol). The enol form of pyruvate is unstable and spontaneously rearranges to pyruvate. The overall reaction catalyzed by pyruvate kinase is essentially irreversible, having a ΔG° of -7.5 kcal/mol.

High-Energy Intermediates in Glycolysis
A compound with a bond containing enough energy to drive the synthesis of ATP (7.3 kcal/mol) is arbitrarily defined as a "high-energy" compound, and the bond is designated by $\sim$. Only two intermediates in glycolysis have high-energy bonds.

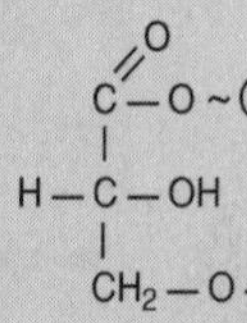

1,3-Bisphosphoglycerate
$\Delta G^\circ = -11.8$ kcal/mol

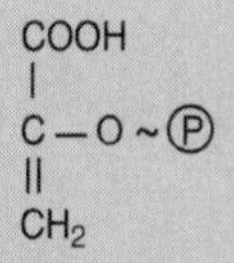

Phosphoenolpyruvate
$\Delta G^\circ = -14.8$ kcal/mol

FIGURE 11-4
The Second ATP-Generating Sequence in Glycolysis. The movement of the phosphate group from C-3 to C-2 is followed by dehydration, resulting in phosphoenolpyruvate (PEP). The phosphate bond in PEP contains the energy required for ATP synthesis. In the reaction catalyzed by pyruvate kinase, the phosphate is transferred from phosphoenolpyruvate to ADP with the formation of ATP.

AEROBIC VS. ANAEROBIC GLYCOLYSIS

Under aerobic conditions where there is an adequate supply of oxygen to tissues, the overall reaction for the glycolytic pathway can be described as follows:

$$\text{Glucose} + 2\ NAD^+ + 2\ P_i + 2\ ADP \longrightarrow 2\ \text{pyruvate} + 2\ NADH + 2\ H^+ + 2\ ATP$$

The reducing equivalents in NADH can be shuttled into the mitochondria with the regeneration of cytosolic NAD+, a requirement for the continuation of glycolysis. However, under anaerobic conditions such as exist in RBCs (having no mitochondria) or in rapidly contracting skeletal muscle experiencing an oxygen debt, the regeneration of cytosolic NAD+ must rely on an extramitochondrial mechanism. Under these conditions, pyruvate is reduced to lactate in an NADH-dependent reaction catalyzed by LDH. As shown below, the product of anaerobic glycolysis is lactate; there is no net production of NADH.

$$\text{Glucose} + 2\ P_i + 2\ ADP \longrightarrow 2\ \text{lactate} + 2\ ATP$$

Under anaerobic conditions, cytosolic NAD+ is regenerated by reducing pyruvate to lactate, a reversible reaction catalyzed by LDH.

REGULATION OF GLYCOLYSIS

The primary site of regulation of glycolysis is PFK-1, the enzyme catalyzing the rate-limiting step in the pathway. Secondary sites of regulation are the first and last steps in the pathway. The activity of hexokinase/glucokinase controls the rate at which glucose enters the pathway, and pyruvate kinase controls the rate at which the product leaves the pathway (Figure 11-5).

FIGURE 11-5 ▶
Sites of Regulation in Glycolysis. The enzymes catalyzing the three irreversible reactions (⟳) are sites of regulation. Separate arrows pointing in different directions indicate that a different enzyme is required to reverse the reaction. The slowest enzyme in the sequence, phosphofructokinase-1, is the major site of regulation. The initial enzyme, hexokinase/glucokinase, and the last enzyme, pyruvate kinase, are secondary sites of regulation. G6P = glucose-6-phosphate; F6P = fructose-6-phosphate; F1,6P$_2$ = fructose-1,6-bisphosphate; F2,6P$_2$ = fructose-2,6-bisphosphate; DHAP = dihydroxyacetone phosphate; G3P = glyceraldehyde-3-phosphate; 1,3-BPG = 1,3-bisphosphoglycerate; 3-PG = 3-phosphoglycerate; 2-PG = 2-phosphoglycerate; and PEP = phosphoenolpyruvate.

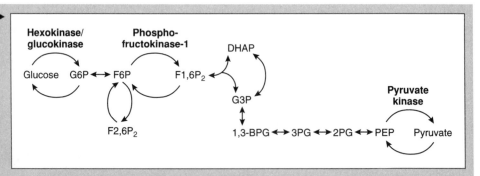

In addition to being regulated at these three steps, the rate of glycolysis is dependent on the *availability of substrate* and the *oxidation/reduction state* of the cell. A supply of glucose, ADP, P$_i$, and NAD+ is required. Since glycolysis is an oxidative process, it is controlled, at least in part, by the ratios of NAD+/NADH and pyruvate/lactate. These ratios, in turn, depend on the respiratory chain and the availability of oxygen. The elevation of either NADH or lactate indicates that oxygen is limited, a condition that leads to reduced mitochondrial oxidative phosphorylation and increased dependence of the cell on glycolysis for its ATP production. The relationship between the rate of glycolysis and the oxidation/reduction state of the cell, as measured by the NADH/NAD$^+$ and lactate/pyruvate ratios, is known as the *Pasteur effect*.

Regulation of PFK-1

The key regulatory features of PFK-1 are summarized in Table 11-2. Activators include AMP and fructose-2,6-bisphosphate (F2,6P$_2$) with adenosine monophosphate (AMP) being the primary activator in muscle and F2,6P$_2$ the most important in liver. ATP and citrate are inhibitors in both tissues. Each of the allosteric effectors alters the activity of PFK-1 by either increasing or decreasing the apparent K_m of the enzyme for F6P (Figure 11-6). There is little, if any, effect on the V$_{max}$. Subtle variations in the allosteric effectors of PFK-1 are found in different tissues, and these variations reflect different roles that glycolysis plays in a particular tissue.

◀ **TABLE 11-2**
Properties of Key Regulatory Enzymes in Glycolysis

Enzyme	Type of Regulation	Effect
Phosphofructokinase-1	Allosteric	Activated by AMP and fructose-2,6-bisphosphate (F2,6P$_2$)^a
		Inhibited by ATP and citrate
Pyruvate kinase	Allosteric	Activated by F1,6P$_2$
		Inhibited by ATP and alanine
	Covalent^a	Inhibited by phosphorylation
Hexokinase	Allosteric	Inhibited by glucose-6-phosphate^b
Glucokinase^a	Gene transcription	Induced by insulin

^{a} Effects are liver-specific.
^{b} Accumulates when ATP is high.

Muscle. In muscle, where the primary role of glycolysis is to supply energy for contraction, the most important allosteric effectors are AMP and ATP. Elevated concentrations of AMP indicate a decreased energy status of the cell and signal the need for activation of PFK-1 and accelerated glycolysis. Conversely, when the concentration of ATP is elevated, the rate of glycolysis and the activity of PFK-1 are diminished.

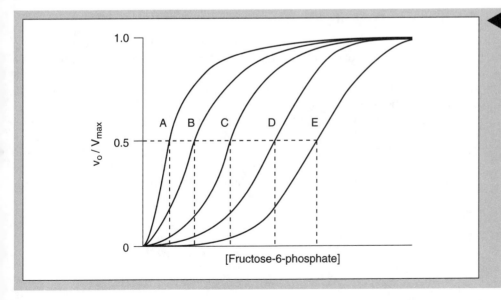

◀ **FIGURE 11-6**
Allosteric Activation and Inhibition of Phosphofructokinase-1. *Curve C is the substrate saturation curve for fructose-6-phosphate (F6P) in the absence of allosteric effector molecules. The ratio v_o/V_{max} is the fraction of the maximum velocity observed at any substrate concentration. The K_m is the concentration of substrate required for half-maximum velocity. Curves A and B illustrate the effect of fructose-2,6-bisphosphate (F2,6P$_2$) and AMP, respectively, in decreasing the apparent K_m for F6P, while curve E shows the effect of ATP or citrate in increasing the apparent K_m for F6P. Curve D represents the ability of F2,6P$_2$ to overcome the inhibition by ATP.*

Liver. The function of glycolysis in liver depends on the level of blood glucose. When there is an abundance of glucose, and insulin is elevated, the pathway is used to provide substrates for fatty acid synthesis. When, however, there is a deficit of blood glucose, and glucagon is elevated, the reversible portion of the pathway is used for the de novo synthesis of glucose. Therefore, to avoid a futile cycle of glucose synthesis and degradation, it is important to coordinate the opposing pathways of glycolysis and gluconeogenesis. The coordinate control of these opposing pathways (Figure 11-7) is achieved by the concentration of F2,6P$_2$, which accelerates glycolysis and inhibits gluconeogenesis (Figure 11-8). The intracellular concentration of F2,6P$_2$ is, in turn, hormonally regulated by the levels of insulin and glucagon in the blood.

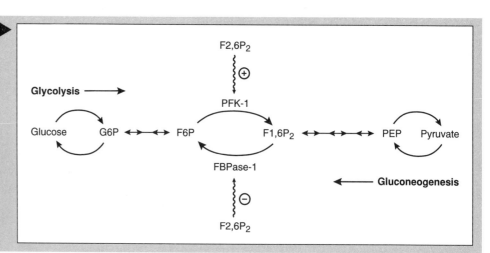

FIGURE 11-7

Coordinate Regulation of Hepatic Glycolysis and Gluconeogenesis by Fructose-2,6-bisphosphate (F2,6P$_2$). In the opposing pathways of glycolysis and gluconeogenesis, the direction in which intermediates move is regulated reciprocally at each of the three irreversible steps. F2,6P$_2$ activates the rate-limiting enzyme (phosphofructokinase-1) in glycolysis, whereas F2,6P$_2$ inhibits the corresponding enzyme (FBPase-1) in the opposing pathway. G6P = glucose-6-phosphate; F6P = fructose-6-phosphate; PEP = phosphoenolpyruvate; and FBPase-1 = fructose bisphosphatase-1.

Hormonal Regulation of Intracellular Concentrations of F2,6P$_2$

The F2,6P$_2$ concentration is increased by insulin and decreased by glucagon. In uncontrolled diabetes, the F2,6P$_2$ concentration is lower than normal.

The mechanism by which F2,6P$_2$ increases the activity of PFK-1 is complex and involves an alteration in a number of the kinetic parameters. In the presence of F2,6P$_2$: (1) the apparent K_m for F6P is decreased, making it a better substrate; (2) the activation constant (K_a) for AMP is decreased, making it a more powerful activator; and (3) the inhibition constant (K_i) for ATP is increased, making it a less effective inhibitor.

The intracellular concentration of F2,6P$_2$ is increased by insulin and decreased by glucagon. Thus, in a well-fed state when blood glucose and insulin are transiently increased, the synthesis of F2,6P$_2$ is stimulated, PFK-1 activity is increased, and the rate of glycolysis is increased. Conversely, in a fasting state when blood glucose is lower and glucagon is elevated, the F2,6P$_2$ is degraded, and the activity of PFK-1 and the rate of glycolysis are decreased.

Regulation of Pyruvate Kinase

The activity of pyruvate kinase is controlled by a number of allosteric effectors. F1,6P$_2$, an intermediate in glycolysis, allosterically activates pyruvate kinase. Functioning as a pacing mechanism, this ensures that excess intermediates proximal to pyruvate do not accumulate. ATP, acetyl coenzyme A (acetyl CoA), and alanine, on the other hand, allosterically inhibit pyruvate kinase.

The isozyme of pyruvate kinase found in the liver is inhibited by cyclic adenosine monophosphate (cAMP)–dependent phosphorylation (Figure 11-8). Thus, elevated glucagon leads to decreased pyruvate kinase activity, whereas elevated insulin leads to increased activity. Insulin both decreases the concentration of hepatic cAMP and activates the protein phosphatase that dephosphorylates the enzyme.

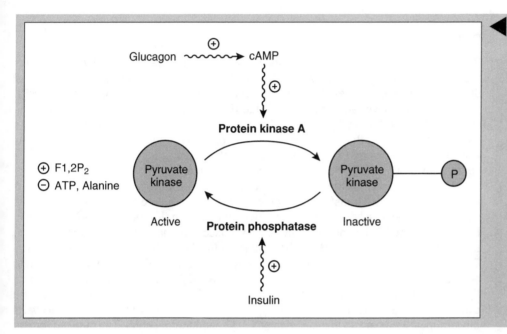

◀ **FIGURE 11-8**
Regulation of Hepatic Pyruvate Kinase Activity. The interconversion of the phosphorylated and dephosphorylated forms of pyruvate kinase is regulated by the ratio of insulin to glucagon. The more active, dephosphorylated form is also regulated allosterically. $F1,2P_2$ = fructose-1,2-bisphosphate.

Regulation of Hexokinase and Glucokinase

Hexokinase, the isozyme found in most tissues, is allosterically inhibited by G6P. Glucokinase is present only in liver and pancreatic beta cells. In these cells, the concentration of glucose is never high enough to saturate the enzyme. Therefore, the activity of glucokinase increases or decreases as the concentration of glucose fluctuates.

Dietary fructose stimulates glucokinase activity and increases glucose uptake by the liver. Liver contains a protein that can either inhibit or stimulate the activity of glucokinase. When the protein binds F6P, it inhibits glucokinase, but this inhibition is reversed by F1P. Liver takes up dietary fructose and converts it to F1P, thereby enhancing the activity of glucokinase and promoting further uptake of glucose.

PYRUVATE DEHYDROGENASE: THE ENZYME THAT LINKS GLYCOLYSIS WITH THE TCA CYCLE

Only a small portion of the energy contained in the glucose molecule is extracted by glycolysis. Approximately 90% of the biologically available energy in the molecule remains in pyruvate. Following transport into the mitochondria, additional energy can be captured by the oxidation of pyruvate to carbon dioxide (CO_2) and water (H_2O), a process requiring pyruvate dehydrogenase (PDH) and the TCA cycle.

PDH catalyzes an *oxidative decarboxylation* reaction in which the carboxyl group of pyruvate is released as CO_2. The remaining C_2 fragment is oxidized to acetate and transferred to CoA, forming acetyl CoA.

$$CH_3-\overset{\overset{\text{O}}{\|}}{C}-COOH + \text{CoA-SH} + NAD^+ \longrightarrow CH_3-\overset{\overset{\text{O}}{\|}}{C}\sim S-\text{CoA} + CO_2 + NADH + H^+$$

Pyruvate   **Acetyl CoA**

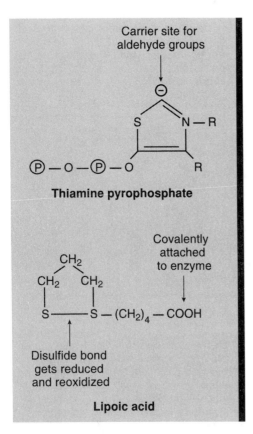

Thiamine pyrophosphate

Carrier site for
aldehyde groups

Lipoic acid

Covalently
attached
to enzyme

Disulfide bond
gets reduced
and reoxidized

PDH Complex

PDH is a *multienzyme complex* consisting of three enzymes that use five coenzymes (Table 11-3). Two of the coenzymes (CoA-SH and NAD⁺) readily associate with and dissociate from the complex. The other three coenzymes (thiamine pyrophosphate [TPP], lipoic acid, and flavin adenine dinucleotide [FAD]) remain tightly associated with the complex through the catalytic cycle. Multiple copies of each of the three enzymes are found in the complex, the number of copies varying with the enzyme source. The complex also contains a specific PDH kinase and phosphatase that regulate the activity of the complex by a phosphorylation/dephosphorylation cycle.

The arrangement of the enzymes in a multienzyme complex provides an efficient mechanism for direct transfer of the product of one reaction to the next enzyme in the sequence without dissociating and mixing with the surrounding medium. As illustrated in Figure 11-9, the PDH complex catalyzes five consecutive reactions. In the first reaction, pyruvate is decarboxylated by E_1. TPP, which is tightly bound to E_1, acts as a carrier of the C_2 fragment. The next two reactions are catalyzed by E_2. The C_2 fragment is oxidized to acetate with the concomitant reduction of lipoic acid. Acetate is then transferred from lipoic acid to CoA and released from the enzyme. The remaining reactions regenerate oxidized lipoic acid so that the catalytic cycle can continue. The E_3 subunit converts dihydrolipoic acid back to lipoic acid in an FAD-dependent reaction. The reduced form of FAD (FADH₂) remains tightly bound to E_3, and is converted back to FAD by the transfer of electrons to NAD⁺ and the subsequent release of NADH from the enzyme complex.

TABLE 11-3 ▶

Components of the Pyruvate Dehydrogenase (PDH) Complex

Enzymes	Cofactors	Role in Overall Reaction of PDH Complex
E_1 (pyruvate dehydrogenase)	Thiamine pyrophosphate	Decarboxylation
E_2 (dihydrolipoyl transacetylase)	Lipoic acid CoA-SH	Oxidation Acyl transfer
E_3 (dihydrolipoyl dehydrogenase)	FAD NAD⁺	Regeneration of lipoic acid
PDH kinase		Phosphorylation and inactivation of E_1
PDH phosphatase		Dephosphorylation and activation of E_1

FIGURE 11-9 ▶

The Function of the Pyruvate Dehydrogenase Complex. The decarboxylation is catalyzed by E_1. The aldehyde attached to E_1–thiamine pyrophosphate is oxidized by E_2-bound lipoic acid prior to transfer to CoA-SH. The reduced form of lipoic acid (Lip) is oxidized by E_3 to complete the catalytic cycle.

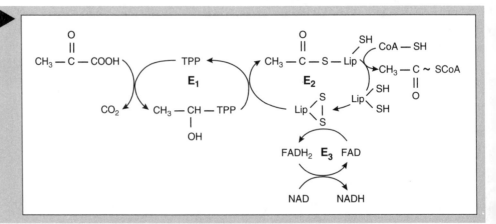

Regulation of PDH Activity

Closely correlated with the energy status of the cell, the activity of PDH is regulated both allosterically and by covalent modification (Figure 11-10). PDH is allosterically inhibited by acetyl CoA, NADH, and ATP, metabolites that signal a high-energy state of the cell. The PDH complex from mammalian tissues is inhibited also by phosphorylation of the E_1 subunit. PDH kinase is activated by acetyl CoA, NADH, and ATP, thereby providing a second mechanism that ensures minimal activity of PDH when the energy state of the cell is high. The dephosphorylation (and activation) of E_1 by PDH phosphatase is stimulated by insulin.

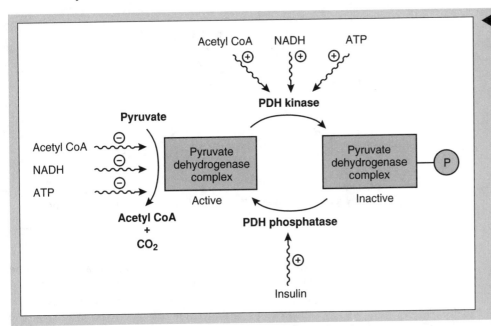

◀ **FIGURE 11-10**
Regulation of Pyruvate Dehydrogenase (PDH) Activity. *The decarboxylation of pyruvate to acetyl CoA is inhibited (⊖) by acetyl CoA, NADH, and ATP. These same metabolites also stimulate (⊕) the conversion of PDH to an inactive phosphorylated form.*

The regulation of PDH plays an important role in conserving glucose and sparing protein during periods of fasting or starvation. The PDH reaction controls the rate at which carbohydrate and many amino acid carbon skeletons are converted to acetyl CoA and are terminally oxidized by the TCA cycle. The products resulting from fatty acid oxidation (e.g., acetyl CoA, NADH, ATP) inhibit PDH, thereby conserving glucose and protein. This is especially important both because glucose is an obligatory fuel for some tissues and because there is no protein that serves as an energy-storage form of amino acids.

During fasting and starvation, PDH activity is inhibited. This helps conserve glucose for brain, CNS, and RBCs. It also spares proteins from being degraded.

Other Multienzyme Complexes Analogous to PDH

Two other important enzymes in metabolism are both structurally and functionally analogous to PDH: *α-ketoglutarate dehydrogenase* (in the TCA cycle), and *branched-chain α-keto acid dehydrogenase* (in the catabolism of branched-chain amino acids). All three structures are multienzyme complexes located in the mitochondrial matrix, and all three catalyze the oxidative decarboxylation of α-keto acids. All three complexes have E_1, E_2, and E_3 subunits and require TPP, lipoic acid, CoA, FAD, and NAD^+ for activity. The E_3 subunit is identical in all three enzyme complexes.

OTHER METABOLIC FATES OF PYRUVATE

Pyruvate occupies a position at one of the major crossroads of carbohydrate, lipid, and protein metabolism (Figure 11-11). Four major products are derived directly from pyruvate: lactate, alanine, acetyl CoA, and oxaloacetate. Pyruvate is converted to lactate and alanine in reversible reactions that occur in the cytosol of cells. The equilibrium between

METABOLISM

Lactic Acidosis and PDH Deficiency
Lactic acidosis arising from a deficiency in PDH activity may be either an acquired or inherited condition. An acquired PDH deficiency is often seen in chronic alcoholism and is most often associated with a thiamine deficiency. Exposure to arsenite and mercurials can also inactivate PDH and lead to lactic acidosis.

these metabolites can be rapidly adjusted in accordance with simple laws of mass action. Thus, any condition that leads to elevated pyruvate will be accompanied by an elevation in blood lactate; and in some cases, alanine will also be elevated.

FIGURE 11-11
Central Role of Pyruvate in Metabolism. *Reactions and pathways that are reversible are indicated by double-headed arrows (↔).*

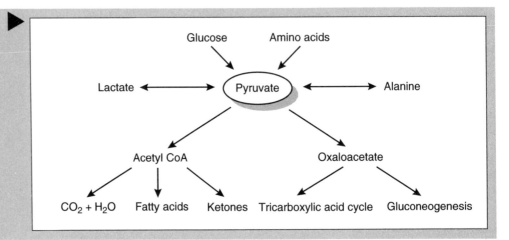

And the Point Is . . .
Enzymes that catalyze irreversible reactions in metabolism are frequently key regulatory enzymes in pathways.

Both irreversible, the reactions for the conversion of pyruvate to acetyl CoA and oxaloacetate occur in the mitochondria and are highly regulated. The acetyl CoA derived from pyruvate can be used for generating energy (e.g., oxidation by the TCA cycle), for energy storage (e.g., fatty acid and ketone synthesis), or for cholesterol synthesis. The oxaloacetate derived from pyruvate can be used either for replenishing intermediates in the TCA cycle or for gluconeogenesis.

Reduction of Pyruvate to Lactate

The conversion of pyruvate to lactate occurs only under anaerobic conditions. This reaction is catalyzed by *lactate dehydrogenase* (LDH) and requires NADH as a source of reducing power.

$$\underset{\text{O}}{\overset{\text{O}}{\text{CH}_3-\overset{\|}{\text{C}}-\text{COOH}}} + \text{NADH} + \text{H}^+ \xrightleftharpoons{\text{LDH}} \underset{\text{OH}}{\overset{\text{OH}}{\text{CH}_3-\overset{|}{\text{CH}}-\text{COOH}}} + \text{NAD}^+$$

Most of the lactate found in blood is produced either by RBCs or by rapidly contracting skeletal muscle that depends on glycogen stores and glycolysis for much of its energy. The content of mitochondria in rapidly contracting muscle ("white muscle fibers") is considerably lower than that in slower contracting muscle ("red muscle fibers"), which derives most of its energy from oxidative phosphorylation.

Lactate, a dead-end product, has no other metabolic fate than to be converted back to pyruvate. Most of the circulating lactate in blood is extracted either by the liver where it is oxidized back to pyruvate, or by cardiac muscle. In cardiac muscle, the pyruvate can be converted to acetyl CoA and used by the TCA cycle as a fuel. In the liver, the pyruvate can be used as a substrate for gluconeogenesis.

The distribution of LDH isozymes differs significantly in skeletal muscle and cardiac muscle. The kinetic properties of the major form in skeletal muscle (M_4) favor the reduction of pyruvate to lactate, while the properties of the major form in cardiac muscle (H_4) favor the oxidation of lactate to pyruvate.

Transamination of Pyruvate to Alanine

The reaction that interconverts pyruvate and alanine is catalyzed by *alanine aminotransferase* (ALT). The carbon skeletons of pyruvate and alanine differ only by the substitution of an α-amino group for the carbonyl oxygen.

$$\text{Pyruvate } + \text{ glutamate } \underset{}{\overset{\text{ALT}}{\rightleftharpoons}} \text{ alanine } + \text{ }\alpha - \text{ketoglutarate}$$

Although the reaction is reversible, it usually operates in the direction of glutamate synthesis. Under normal conditions, only a small amount of the total pyruvate is transaminated to alanine. However, a defect in any of the pathways of pyruvate utilization may lead to an accumulation of alanine in the blood. Similarly, any condition that leads to the accumulation of glutamate will also shift the equilibrium toward alanine synthesis.

> *Elevated Serum Alanine*
> *The accumulation of either pyruvate (in deficiencies of PDH or pyruvate carboxylase) or glutamate (secondary to hyperammonemia and defects in the enzymes of the urea cycle) shifts the equilibrium of the ALT reaction and leads to increased production of alanine.*

Carboxylation of Pyruvate to Oxaloacetate

The reaction catalyzed by *pyruvate carboxylase* has two major functions: (1) it is the major reaction for replenishing intermediates in the TCA cycle that may have been removed and used in other biosynthetic pathways; and (2) it is the first step in the pathway of gluconeogenesis. The enzyme, pyruvate carboxylase, is located in the mitochondrial matrix and has an absolute requirement for acetyl CoA as an allosteric effector (see Chapter 13).

ENERGY YIELD FROM THE COMPLETE OXIDATION OF GLUCOSE

Starting in the cytosol, glucose oxidation results in 2 mols each of pyruvate, NADH, and ATP. Each mol of NADH generated during glycolysis can result in either 2 or 3 mols of ATP. The yield depends on the shuttle system used to transport the electrons in NADH into the mitochondria (see Chapter 6). Use of the malate shuttle results in a maximum of 3 mols of ATP per mol of NADH, whereas use of the α-glycerol phosphate shuttle results in a maximum of 2 mols of ATP per mol of NADH. Additionally, each mol of pyruvate can be transported into the mitochondria and completely oxidized to CO_2 and H_2O by reactions involving PDH, the TCA cycle, and the pathway of oxidative phosphorylation. The oxidation of each mol of pyruvate can result in a maximum of 15 mols of ATP. The enzymes involved in generating ATP (or guanosine triphosphate [GTP]) from glucose are summarized in Table 11-4. Thus, under aerobic conditions, the complete oxidation of one mol of glucose can result in 36–38 mols of ATP.

RESOLUTION OF CLINICAL CASE

Inherited deficiencies of several RBC enzymes, including most of the enzymes of glycolysis, are recognized causes of hemolysis in infants. The RBC depends on glycolysis as its sole source of ATP, and much of the ATP generated in glycolysis is needed to maintain sodium/potassium–adenosine triphosphatase (Na+/K+-ATPase) activity and ion pumps in the RBC membrane. Alterations in ion pumps can lead to changes in RBC shape, leading to excessive cell destruction and anemia. In this patient, the early symptoms suggesting hemolytic anemia were pallor, jaundice, low hemoglobin, low RBC count, and elevated reticulocyte count. Persistence of hemolysis beyond the newborn period often indicates an underlying inherited enzyme defect. Jaundice, elevated bilirubin, and increased urobilinogen excretion in the feces all result from excessive degradation of heme [1].

Although biochemical analysis of RBC metabolites can be helpful in tentatively identifying the defective enzyme, definitive diagnosis requires demonstration of specific enzyme abnormalities. In this patient, all of the glycolytic enzymes were slightly elevated above the normal level except pyruvate kinase, which was less than 10% of the normal range. Defects in pyruvate kinase in RBCs generally result in elevated concentrations of 2,3-BPG and decreased concentrations of ATP. Additionally, NAD+ concentration may also be decreased, since the conversion of niacin to NAD+ requires ATP. Accumulation of intermediates behind the block, especially 2,3-BPG and 3-PG, is commonly seen with pyruvate kinase deficiency, and changes in the 2,3-BPG/ATP ratio is a useful diagnostic parameter [2].

Pyruvate kinase deficiency is the most common of the enzyme deficiencies in glycolysis, leading to hemolytic anemia. It is inherited as an autosomal recessive disorder. RBC transfusions may be required in infancy and early childhood to maintain sufficient levels of hemoglobin. Splenectomy may be of value in severely affected cases but appears to be of little value in less severe cases.

TABLE 11-4 ▶
Energy Obtained from Complete Oxidation of Glucose

Pathway	Enzyme	Product	Method of Energy Generation	ATP/Glucose
(Cytosol) Glycolysis				
	• Glyceraldehyde-3-phosphate dehydrogenase	2 NADH	Oxidative phosphorylation	4–6[a]
	• Phosphoglycerate kinase	2 ATP	Substrate-level phosphorylation	2
	• Pyruvate kinase	2 ATP	Substrate-level phosphorylation	2
ATP produced/glucose				8–10[a]
ATP consumed/glucose (hexokinase and PFK)				−2
Net ATP produced/glucose				6–8[a]
(Mitochondria) Pyruvate Dehydrogenase and the Tricarboxylic Acid Cycle				
	• Pyruvate dehydrogenase	2 NADH	Oxidative phosphorylation	6
	• Isocitrate dehydrogenase	2 NADH	Oxidative phosphorylation	6
	• α-Ketoglutarate dehydrogenase	2 NADH	Oxidative phosphorylation	6
	• Succinate thiokinase	2 GTP	Substrate-level phosphorylation	2
	• Succinate dehydrogenase	2 $FADH_2$	Oxidative phosphorylation	4
	• Malate dehydrogenase	2 NADH	Oxidative phosphorylation	6
Net ATP produced/glucose				30
Total ATP per glucose (aerobic oxidation)				36–38[a]
Total ATP per glucose (anaerobic oxidation) = 2 (reactions in glycolysis)				

[a] Transfer of electrons in cytosolic NADH via malate shuttle produces mitochondrial NADH and three molecules of ATP, whereas transfer via α-glycerol-phosphate shuttle produces $FADH_2$ and two molecules of ATP.

REVIEW QUESTIONS

Directions: For each of the following questions, choose the **one best** answer.

1. A total deficiency in which of the following enzymes would most directly compromise the ability of RBCs to pump Na+ out of the cell?

    (A) Enolase

    (B) Pyruvate carboxylase

    (C) 3-Phosphoglycerate kinase

    (D) Phosphoglycerate mutase

    (E) Lactate dehydrogenase

2. The oxidation of glucose to pyruvate would be compromised by a deficiency in which of the following vitamins?

    (A) Thiamine

    (B) Riboflavin

    (C) Niacin

    (D) Biotin

    (E) Pantothenic acid

3. Which of the following pairs of enzymes in glycolysis is allosterically regulated in skeletal muscle?

    (A) Glucokinase and phosphofructokinase-1 (PFK-1)

    (B) Hexokinase and aldolase

    (C) PFK-1 and 3-phosphoglycerate kinase

    (D) Pyruvate kinase and lactate dehydrogenase (LDH)

    (E) Hexokinase and pyruvate kinase

4. Pyruvate kinase has which of the following characteristics?

    (A) It is activated by phosphorylation

    (B) It is dependent on thiamin pyrophosphate

    (C) It is located in mitochondria

    (D) It inhibited by ATP

    (E) It is the rate-limiting enzyme in glycolysis

5. Pyruvate dehydrogenase (PDH) activity is

    (A) activated by cAMP-dependent phosphorylation

    (B) allosterically activated by a high ratio of NADH/NAD+

    (C) activated under conditions of accelerated fatty acid oxidation

    (D) decreased by an elevated insulin/glucagon ratio

    (E) inhibited by the action of an NADH-activated kinase

6. The effect of selected allosteric effectors on phosphofructokinase-1 (PFK-1) is shown in the graph below.

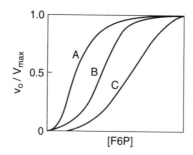

All of the curves were generated in the presence of a constant concentration of ATP. *Curve B* shows the activity of PFK-1 in the absence of any allosteric effectors. *Curves A and C* were generated in the presence of an allosteric effector. Which one of the following conclusions can be made from the data presented?

- **(A)** The allosteric effector in *curve A* increases the K_m for fructose-6-phosphate (F6P)
- **(B)** The effect of AMP on the kinetic properties of the enzyme is described by *curve C*
- **(C)** The effect of citrate on the V_{max} can be described by *curve A*
- **(D)** The allosteric effector in *curve C* increases the K_m for ATP
- **(E)** The effect of fructose-2,6-bisphosphate (F2,6P$_2$) can be described by *curve A*

ANSWERS AND EXPLANATIONS

1. The answer is C. Pumping Na$^+$ requires ATP, and 3-phosphoglycerate kinase catalyzes one of the two steps in glycolysis where ATP is produced by substrate-level phosphorylation. The other enzyme in glycolysis that is directly involved in ATP production is pyruvate kinase.

2. The answer is C. The oxidation of glyceraldehyde-3-phosphate to 1,3-bisphosphoglycerate is the only step in glycolysis requiring a coenzyme. The vitamin precursor for NAD$^+$ is niacin. All of the vitamins listed except biotin are precursors of coenzymes required for the oxidation of pyruvate to CO_2 and H_2O. Biotin is required only in carboxylation reactions.

3. The answer is E. Hexokinase, PFK-1, and pyruvate kinase are allosterically regulated in skeletal muscle. Glucokinase is not present in skeletal muscle. Aldolase, 3-phosphoglycerate kinase, and LDH are all present in skeletal muscle. They catalyze reversible reactions that are regulated only by the availability of substrate.

4. The answer is D. Pyruvate kinase, a cytosolic enzyme, is allosterically inhibited by ATP and covalently inhibited by cAMP-dependent phosphorylation. It requires ADP as a cosubstrate but has no vitamin or cofactor requirements. The rate-limiting step in glycolysis is catalyzed by phosphofructokinase-1.

5. The answer is E. The activity of this enzyme is inhibited by phosphorylation. The kinase responsible for phosphorylation is a part of the multienzyme complex and is activated by NADH, acetyl CoA, and ATP. The PDH phosphatase, which removes the phosphate group and activates PDH, is stimulated by insulin. Additionally, the dephosphorylated form of the enzyme is allosterically inhibited by NADH, acetyl CoA, and ATP.

6. The answer is E. The variable substrate in all of these reactions is F6P, and *curves A and C* illustrate the effect of allosteric effectors on the K_m for F6P. The K_m is defined as the concentration of substrate required to obtain half-maximal velocity. Activators, such as AMP and F2,6P$_2$, decrease the K_m and shift the curve to the left. Inhibitors (such as citrate) increase the K_m and shift the curve to the right. None of the effectors shown alter the V_{max}.

REFERENCES

1. Tanaka KR, Paglia DE: Pyruvate kinase deficiency and other enzymopathies of the erythrocyte. In *The Metabolic Basis of Inherited Disease*, 7th ed. Edited by Scriver CR, Beaudet AL, Sly WS, et al. New York, NY: McGraw-Hill, 1955, pp 3485–3499.
2. Gilman PA: Hemolysis in the newborn infant resulting from deficiencies of red blood cell enzymes: diagnosis and management. *J Pediatr* 84(5):625–634, 1984.

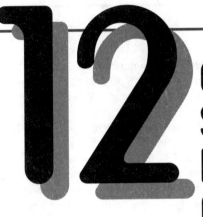

GLYCOGEN METABOLISM: STORAGE AND MOBILIZATION OF GLUCOSE

INTRODUCTION OF CLINICAL CASE

A 6-month-old infant girl was referred to the hospital because of an abdominal fullness. First noticed by her mother when the infant was 1 month of age, the fullness continued to increase. She was born at full term after an uncomplicated pregnancy; there were no neonatal complications. She had one sibling who had experienced no medical problems. Both parents were in good health. When the infant was about 6 weeks of age, her mother noticed that she was irritable and not feeding well through the night. When she awoke in the morning, her skin frequently felt clammy, and she was often listless. However, after feeding she seemed more playful and alert. Prior to coming to the hospital, she had been fasted overnight. Upon arrival, laboratory studies revealed a blood glucose of 28 mg/dL (normal = 70–110 mg/dL) and low blood pH (7.28). Sequential analysis of blood glucose levels over several hours showed that the development of hypoglycemia was associated with elevated plasma lactic acid and mild acidosis. Glucagon levels were elevated, and insulin levels were lower than normal. Plasma lipids and uric acid were markedly elevated. A liver biopsy demonstrated increased staining for fat and carbohydrate deposits. Enzymatic analysis of liver tissue showed less than 5% of the normal glucose-6-phosphatase (G6Pase) activity. Frequent feedings were initiated during the day, and oral glucose was administered overnight by a nasogastric drip. Two days later, the infant was released from the hospital with instructions to the parents to continue the newly established feeding protocol. Evaluation 6 months later showed an acceleration in growth rate and a decrease in plasma lipids, lactic acid, and uric acid.

OVERVIEW

Glycogen is the storage form of glucose in mammalian tissues. Although present in almost all cells, it is most abundant in liver and muscle tissue. The concentration of glycogen is greater in liver than in muscle tissue. However, because muscle tissue comprises a larger mass, its total capacity for storage is three to four times that of liver. The synthesis and degradation of glycogen occur via different pathways, thereby allowing each pathway to operate independently of the other. The rate at which these opposing pathways occur is coordinately regulated by a variety of allosteric and hormonal mechanisms.

GLYCOGEN STRUCTURE

Glycogen is found in the cytosol of cells. In muscle, glycogen is stored as spherical granules known as beta particles that can contain up to 60,000 glucose residues. Liver contains large rosette-like granules of glycogen called alpha particles that are aggregates of beta particles. All of the enzymes and regulatory proteins required for glycogen synthesis and degradation are associated with the glycogen particles.

The structure of glycogen is represented in Figure 12-1. It is highly branched with branching occurring at an average frequency of every ten glucose residues. Branching increases the solubility of glycogen and increases the rate at which glucose can be stored and retrieved from the glycogen particle. Each glycogen molecule has a protein, *glycogenin*, covalently linked to the polysaccharide. The linear glycogen chains consist of glucose molecules linked together by *α-(1,4) glycosidic bonds*. At each of the branch points, two glucose molecules are linked together by *α-(1,6) glycosidic bonds*. The ends of the branches are known as the *nonreducing ends* of the glycogen particle, the sites where both synthesis and degradation occur.

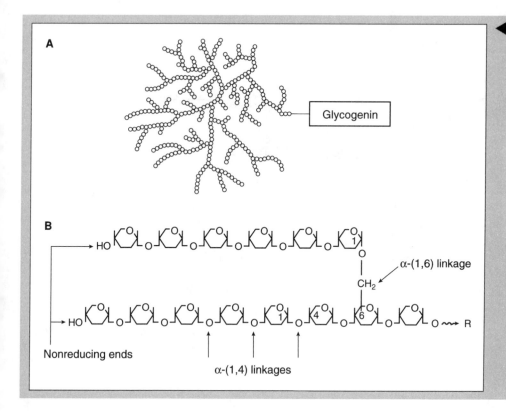

Glycogen Structure. *(A)* Glycogen particle. *At the core of the glycogen molecule, the C-1 of the initial glucose is covalently linked to the hydroxyl group of a specific tyrosine side chain of glycogenin. The frequency of branching is higher in the interior than near the ends of the branches. (B) Structure of two outer branches of glycogen. The remainder of the glycogen molecule is represented by R. The nonreducing ends have a free hydroxyl group on C-4 of the terminal glucose. This is the site to which additional glucose units can be added. When glycogen is degraded, the glucose at the end of the branches is released as glucose-1-phosphate. All of the C-1 hydroxyl groups in the glycogen are involved in glycosidic bonds.*

FUNCTION OF GLYCOGEN

The functional role of glycogen differs considerably from tissue to tissue. For example, in the brain, glycogen provides an emergency supply of glucose that can be used during periods of hypoglycemia or hypoxia. In cardiac muscle, glycogen is mobilized for energy when a heavy work load is imposed. The most striking difference in the functional role of glycogen, however, is seen in liver and skeletal muscle.

Liver glycogen acts as a buffer for regulating blood glucose levels between meals. Following a meal, excess glucose is removed from the portal circulation and stored as glycogen. Conversely, between meals, blood glucose levels are maintained within the normal range by release of glucose from liver glycogen.

Muscle glycogen acts as a store of glucose that can be rapidly mobilized to provide fuel for anaerobic glycolysis. Muscle cannot release glucose into the blood because of the absence of G6Pase. Therefore, muscle glycogen stores are used exclusively by muscle.

Glycogen Content of Liver and Muscle
The amount of glycogen found in tissues varies considerably with the nutritional and physiologic state. Following a meal, glycogen may constitute as much as 6%–8% of the wet weight of liver of a resting individual. Under the same conditions, approximately 1% of the wet weight of muscle may be attributed to glycogen. After 12–15 hours of fasting, liver becomes almost totally depleted of glycogen. Muscle glycogen is depleted only after prolonged strenuous exercise.

GLYCOGEN SYNTHESIS

An overview of the pathway by which blood glucose is converted to glycogen is shown in Figure 12-2. Glucose-6-phosphate (G6P) is an important branch point in carbohydrate metabolism, serving as substrate for several enzymes that initiate different pathways. The pathway by which G6P is converted to glycogen consists of four types of reactions: (1) conversion of G6P to glucose-1-phosphate (G1P), (2) activation of G1P via the formation of uridine diphosphate glucose (UDP~glucose), (3) elongation of glycogen chains, and (4) creation of branch points that can be further elongated.

FIGURE 12-2 ▶

Conversion of Blood Glucose to Glycogen. *Transport of glucose across the plasma membrane is followed by conversion to glucose-6-phosphate. Transport is facilitated by glucose transporter type 4 (GLUT-4) in muscle and glucose transporter type 2 (GLUT-2) in liver. Isomerization to fructose-6-phosphate initiates the pathway of glycolysis, whereas oxidation to 6-phosphogluconate begins the pentose phosphate pathway. The conversion to glucose-1-phosphate and the formation of uridine diphosphate ~glucose (UDP~glucose) set the stage for glycogen synthesis, a process involving elongation of a partially degraded glycogen molecule, creation of branch points, and elongation of the branch points.*

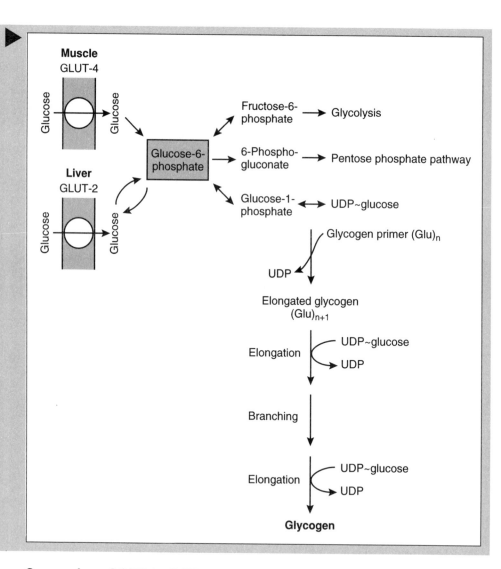

Conversion of G6P to G1P

The reaction directing G6P into the pathway of glycogen metabolism is catalyzed by *phosphoglucomutase*. As shown below, this reaction results in the internal transfer of phosphate from C-6 to C-1 of glucose, producing G1P. The reaction is reversible and is important in both the conversion of glucose to glycogen for storage and the mobilization of glucose from glycogen stores (see Figure 12-2).

$$\text{G6P} \underset{}{\overset{\text{phosphoglucomutase}}{\rightleftharpoons}} \text{G1P} \qquad \text{Glycogen}$$

Formation of UDP~Glucose (Activated Glucose)

UDP~glucose is the activated form of glucose commonly used in the formation of glycosidic bonds. The high-energy bond between C-1 of glucose and the nucleotide provides the energy required for linking one sugar to another. UDP~glucose is formed from G1P and uridine triphosphate (UTP) in a reaction catalyzed by *UDP~glucose pyrophosphorylase*. The other product of the reaction is pyrophosphate (PP$_i$). As shown below, the formation of UDP~glucose is a reversible reaction with a $\Delta G^o = +1.6$ kcal/mol. However, this reaction is made essentially irreversible by the hydrolysis of PP$_i$ in a highly exergonic reaction ($\Delta G^o = -6.6$ kcal/mol) catalyzed by pyrophosphatase.

Structure of UDP~Glucose

(structure diagram showing CH$_2$OH, HO, OH, OH groups, O–P=O, O–P=O, Uridine)

$$\text{G1P} + \text{uridine-P}\sim\text{P}\sim\text{P} \rightleftharpoons \text{UDP}\sim\text{glucose} + \text{PP}_i \qquad \Delta G^\circ = +1.6 \text{ kcal/mol}$$

$$\text{PP}_i + \text{H}_2\text{O} \longrightarrow 2\text{P}_i \qquad\qquad\qquad \Delta G^\circ = -6.6 \text{ kcal/mol}$$

$$\text{G1P} + \text{uridine-P}\sim\text{P}\sim\text{P} + \text{H}_2\text{O} \longrightarrow \text{UDP}\sim\text{glucose} + 2\text{P}_i \qquad \Delta G^\circ = -5.0 \text{ kcal/mol}$$

Elongation and Branching Reactions

The primary reaction in glycogen synthesis is the formation of α-(1,4) glycosidic bonds. In this reaction, glucose is transferred from UDP~glucose to the nonreducing end of a partially degraded glycogen molecule (Figure 12-3). This elongation reaction is catalyzed by *glycogen synthase* and is repeated until the chain has been extended to 11–15 glucose residues from the branch point. When the chain reaches this length, the affinity for glycogen synthase is markedly reduced and further elongation ceases. The *branching enzyme* then transfers an oligosaccharide containing 6–7 glucose residues from the end of the chain to the C-6 of a glucose residue in the interior of the chain. This two-step reaction consists of the cleavage of an α-(1,4) bond followed by the formation of an α-(1,6) bond. The branching enzyme is also known as α-(1,4)→α-(1,6)-glucan transferase.

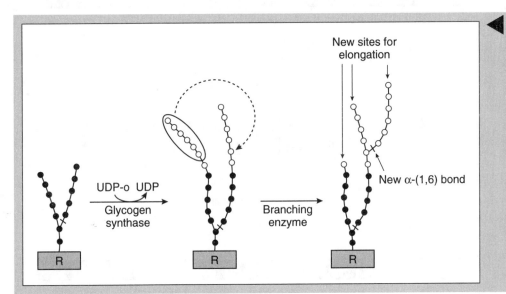

FIGURE 12-3
Schematic Representation of Glycogen Elongation and Branching. Elongation involves α-(1,4) glycosidic bond formation. Glucose (o) is transferred from uridine diphosphate~glucose (UDP~glucose) [UDP-o] to the nonreducing ends of glycogen chains. When the chain extends to 11–15 glucose residues from the nearest branch point, branching occurs. A block of 6–7 glucose residues is moved from the end of one chain to another chain or to an internal position of the same chain. The C-1 of the oligosaccharide is attached to the C-6 of the acceptor glucose. The branching enzyme catalyzes an α-(1,4)→α-(1,6)-glucan transfer. New sites for elongation by glycogen synthase are created. The new α-(1,6) bonds are indicated as 0-|-0. All other bonds are α-(1,4).

Attachment of Glucose to Glycogenin

The primer for glycogen synthesis is the protein glycogenin. Each glycogen molecule is attached to glycogenin through a glycosidic bond formed between the C-1 of glucose and a specific tyrosine side chain of the protein. The addition of the first eight glucose residues to glycogenin occurs in an autocatalytic reaction catalyzed by an active domain on the glycogenin molecule. UDP~glucose is the glucose donor in these reactions. Further elongation and branching are carried out by glycogen synthase and the branching enzyme. Since each glycogen molecule is covalently attached to glycogenin, the number of glycogen particles in a particular cell is determined by the availability of glycogenin.

Regulation of Glycogen Synthase

Glycogen synthase exists in two forms, an *active dephosphorylated* form and an *inactive phosphorylated* form. The phosphorylation requires ATP and produces adenosine diphosphate (ADP). As shown below, inactivation of glycogen synthase is achieved by the phosphorylation of a single serine residue.

Glycogen synthase serine	+ ATP ⟶	Glycogen synthase serine	+ ADP
	Active		**Inactive**
OH		O—PO₃⁼	

The interconversion of these two forms of glycogen synthase is shown in Figure 12-4. The phosphorylation and dephosphorylation reactions are catalyzed by *protein* kinase A and *protein phosphatase-1*, respectively. Glucagon and epinephrine increase the cellular concentration of cAMP, an event that leads to phosphorylation and inactivation of glycogen synthase. In liver, both of these hormones elevate cAMP, whereas in muscle, epinephrine is primarily responsible. Conversely, dephosphorylation and activation of glycogen synthase is stimulated by insulin. Insulin activates protein phosphatase-1 and also reduces cellular cAMP levels.

FIGURE 12-4
Covalent Regulation of Glycogen Synthase Activity. Glycogen synthase is phosphorylated and inactivated by cAMP-dependent protein kinase and by hormones that generate cAMP as a second messenger. Protein phosphatase-1 hydrolyzes the phosphate and returns the enzyme to its active form. The binding of insulin to receptors on the plasma membrane results in the activation of protein phosphatase. The intracellular second messenger for insulin is not known.

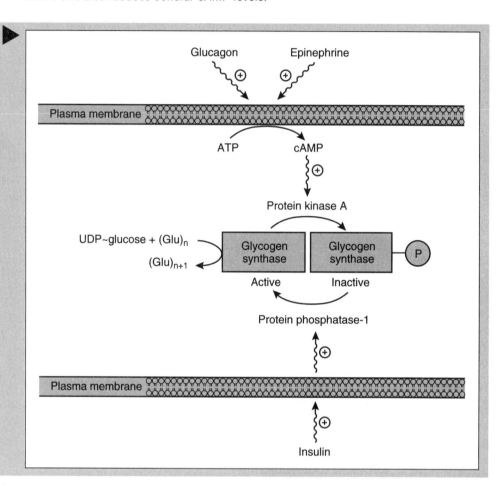

In addition to the covalent regulation by reversible phosphorylation and dephosphorylation, glycogen synthase is also regulated allosterically by G6P. The phosphorylated form of glycogen synthase that is normally inactive can be allosterically activated by the accumulation of G6P in the cell.

GLYCOGEN DEGRADATION

The mobilization of glucose from glycogen stores consists of two types of reactions: the nonreducing ends of the chains are shortened by phosphorolysis, and the branch points are disassembled.

Shortening the Glycogen Chains

The primary step in glycogen degradation is the cleavage of α-(1,4) glycosidic bonds, a reaction catalyzed by *glycogen phosphorylase*. This reaction adds inorganic phosphate (P_i), rather than H_2O, across the glycosidic bond, resulting in the release of G1P from the nonreducing ends (Figure 12-5). Phosphorylase contains covalently bound pyridoxal phosphate, a cofactor that contributes to catalysis by acting as a proton donor. This function is highly unusual for pyridoxal phosphate. All other enzymes known to require this cofactor use it in reactions involving amino acids.

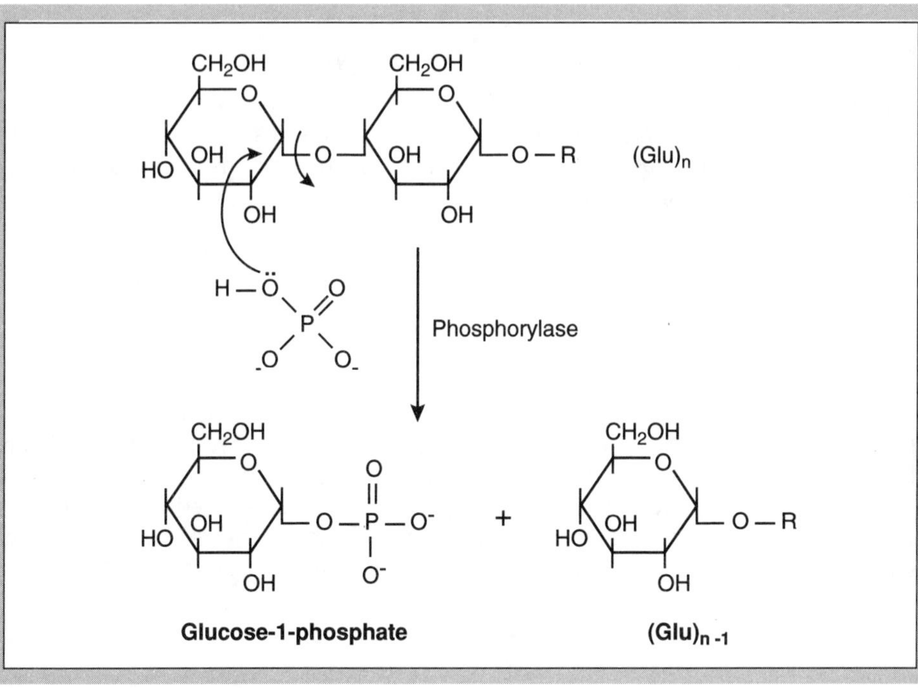

◀ FIGURE 12-5
Glycogen Phosphorylase Reaction. *An outer portion of a glycogen chain is shown, with the remainder of the glycogen molecule being designated as R. Inorganic phosphate attacks C-1 of the terminal glucose residue, resulting in release of glucose-1-phosphate. The oxygen in the glycosidic bond that is cleaved remains on the shortened glycogen chain.*

Removal of Branch Points

The phosphorylase reaction is repeated until the distance from the branch point is four glucose residues (Figure 12-6). The *debranching enzyme* then begins to take apart the branch points. This enzyme is a multifunctional protein containing two catalytic activities, α-(1,4)$\rightarrow\alpha$-(1,4)-glucan transferase and α-(1,6)-glucosidase.

Trisaccharide Transfer. In the first reaction, catalyzed by α-(1,4)$\rightarrow\alpha$-(1,4)-glucan transferase, a trisaccharide is transferred from one shortened chain to another, leaving a single glucose residue attached in α-(1,6) linkage and creating a longer chain that can be further degraded by phosphorylase. This reaction involves cleavage of one α-(1,4) bond and the formation of a new α-(1,4) bond.

Removal of Glucose at Branch Point. Hydrolysis of remaining glucose residue at the branch point is catalyzed by α-(1,6)-glucosidase. The only glucose residues in glycogen released as free glucose are those linked via α-(1,6) bonds at the branch points.

Frequency of Branching in Glycogen
The amount of free glucose released by total enzymatic hydrolysis of glycogen can be used as a measure of the frequency of branching. Only those glucose units that occupy the branch-point positions in glycogen are released as free glucose. All others are released as G1P.

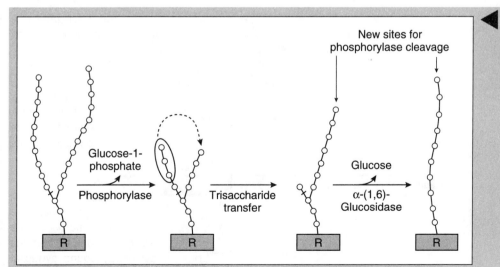

◀ FIGURE 12-6
Schematic Representation of Glycogen Degradation. *Glycogen phosphorylase sequentially removes glucose-1-phosphate from the nonreducing ends of the chains until it gets within four glucose residues of a branch point. The debranching enzyme then transfers a trisaccharide to the end of another chain, a reaction catalyzed by α-(1,4)$\rightarrow\alpha$-(1,4)-glucan transferase. The single glucose remaining at the branch point is removed by the hydrolytic action of α-(1,6)-glucosidase. The α-(1,6) bonds are indicated by 0—0. All others are α-(1,4) bonds.*

Covalent Regulation of Glycogen Phosphorylase

Glycogen phosphorylase exists in two forms, an *active phosphorylated* form (phosphorylase$_a$) and an *inactive dephosphorylated* form (phosphorylase$_b$). As shown below, the conversion of phosphorylase$_b$ to phosphorylase$_a$ occurs by the transfer of phosphate from ATP to a single serine side chain of the enzyme.

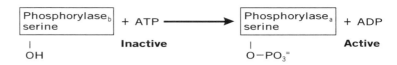

The activation of glycogen phosphorylase involves a cascade of reactions initiated by an increase in cellular cAMP (Figure 12-7). The cascade involves several sequential phosphorylation reactions, ending with the phosphorylation and activation of glycogen phosphorylase. The interconversion of phosphorylase a and b is catalyzed by *phosphorylase kinase* and *protein phosphatase-1*. Phosphorylase kinase is activated by hormones that elevate cAMP, whereas protein phosphatase-1 is activated by insulin.

FIGURE 12-7
Covalent Regulation of Glycogen Phosphorylase. Adenylate cyclase is activated by the binding of glucagon or epinephrine to the cell, resulting in cAMP formation. Protein kinase A is allosterically activated by cAMP. Protein kinase A catalyzes the phosphorylation and activation of phosphorylase kinase, an enzyme specifically associated with the glycogen particle. Active phosphorylase kinase then phosphorylates and activates glycogen phosphorylase, resulting in increased glycogen degradation. These effects are reversed by insulin.

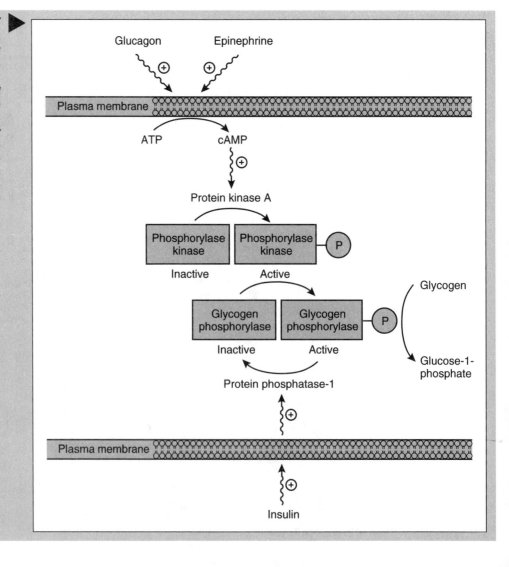

Allosteric Regulation of Glycogen Phosphorylase

The activity of glycogen phosphorylase is sensitive to a number of allosteric effectors, most of which are indicators of the energy state of the cell (Table 12-1). Muscle phosphorylase$_b$ is especially sensitive to the energy state of the cell. It is allosterically activated by the accumulation of AMP, a signal that the energy state of the cell is low. The effect of AMP is reversed by the accumulation of ATP, G6P, and creatine phosphate, metabolites that signal a high-energy state. The activity of the liver phosphorylase isozyme is not affected by AMP. Conversely, the activity of liver phosphorylase$_a$ is inhibited by the accumulation of glucose in the cell, while the muscle isozyme is unaffected by glucose.

	Phosphorylase$_a$	Phosphorylase$_b$	Phosphorylase Kinase^c
Adenosine monophosphate		Activation^b	
Adenosine triphosphate		Inhibition	
Glucose-6-phosphate		Inhibition	
Creatine phosphate	Inhibition^a		
Glucose	Inhibition^b		
Calcium			Activation

^{a} Only with the muscle isozyme.
^{b} Only with the liver isozyme.
^{c} The phosphorylated (covalently inactive) form.

◀ **TABLE 12-1**
Allosteric Effectors of Glycogen Degradation

Synchronization of Muscle Contraction and Glycogen Degradation

Phosphorylase kinase can be allosterically *activated by Ca^{2+}* in a mechanism that is independent of cAMP and phosphorylation (Figure 12-8). This mechanism is of particular importance in muscle, where contraction is initiated by the release of Ca^{2+} from the sarcoplasmic reticulum, because it allows glycogen degradation to be synchronized with contraction. Phosphorylase kinase is a complex enzyme having four types of subunits, α, β, γ, and Δ. The Δ subunit is calmodulin, a calcium-binding protein that sensitizes a number of enzymes to small changes in the cellular concentration of calcium.

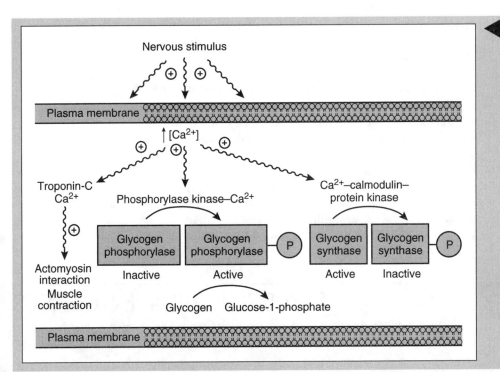

◀ **FIGURE 12-8**
Synchronization of Muscle Contraction and Glycogen Degradation. Muscle contraction is stimulated by an increase in cytosolic [Ca^{2+}], and the subsequent binding of calcium to troponin-C of the thin filament initiates contraction. Phosphorylase kinase is allosterically activated by Ca^{2+}, allowing glycogen phosphorylase to be phosphorylated and activated independent of cAMP. Glycogen synthase can be phosphorylated by several protein kinases, including a calcium-calmodulin–dependent protein kinase. Each kinase results in decreased glycogen synthesis.

COORDINATE REGULATION OF GLYCOGEN METABOLISM

In general, conditions that promote glycogen synthesis inhibit glycogen degradation, and vice versa. Some of these conditions and their effects are summarized in Table 12-2. The primary targets of regulation are glycogen synthase and glycogen phosphorylase, the enzymes catalyzing the rate-limiting step in glycogen synthesis and degradation, respectively. The activities of the enzymes are affected in opposite directions by several interrelated factors including the nutritional state and a number of hormones.

TABLE 12-2 ▶

Conditions Affecting Glycogen Synthesis and Degradation

	Glycogen Synthesis	Glycogen Degradation
Well-fed state	Increased	Decreased
Fasting	Decreased	Increased
Hyperglycemia	Increased	Decreased
Hypoglycemia	Decreased	Increased
Elevated		
Insulin	Increased	Decreased
Glucagon	Decreased	Increased
Epinephrine	Decreased	Increased
Cyclic adenosine monophosphate	Decreased	Increased
Enzyme phosphorylation		
Glycogen synthase	Decreased	. . .
Glycogen phosphorylase	. . .	Increased

A summary of four factors that contribute to the integrated control of these opposing pathways is outlined below.

Hormonal Signals. The same hormonal signals are used to control synthesis as well as degradation of glycogen. An elevation in serum *insulin* signals a well-fed state and promotes glucose storage by activation of glycogen synthesis and inhibition of glycogen degradation. An elevation in serum *glucagon* or *epinephrine* signals the need for glucose release and promotes glucose mobilization by activating glycogen degradation and inhibiting glycogen synthesis.

Cellular cAMP Levels. The cellular concentration of cAMP is regulated by hormonal signals. *Insulin* decreases cAMP levels by activating cAMP phosphodiesterase, the enzyme that degrades cAMP. In liver, both *glucagon* and *epinephrine* elevate cAMP by activation of adenylate cyclase. In muscle, epinephrine is primarily responsible for increasing cellular cAMP. Protein kinase A is activated by cAMP.

Protein Kinases. The rate-limiting enzymes in the pathways of both synthesis and degradation of glycogen are phosphorylated as a result of elevated cellular cAMP, producing opposite effects on their activities. Phosphorylation activates glycogen phosphorylase but inactivates glycogen synthase.

Protein Phosphatase-1. The effects of protein kinases on glycogen metabolism are reversed by protein phosphatase-1. The removal of phosphate groups from phosphorylase kinase, glycogen phosphorylase, and glycogen synthase is catalyzed by protein phosphatase-1, an enzyme that is *activated by insulin*. Dephosphorylation activates glycogen synthase but inactivates glycogen phosphorylase and phosphorylase kinase.

GLYCOGEN STORAGE DISEASES

There are a number of genetic diseases resulting from a deficiency in a specific enzyme involved in glycogen metabolism. These diseases are characterized by the accumulation of either normal or abnormal glycogen. The abnormal forms of glycogen either have short outer chains or have long unbranched chains. Some of the more common forms of these diseases and their characteristics are summarized in Table 12-3.

◀ **TABLE 12-3**
Glycogen Storage Diseases

Type	Name	Enzyme Deficiency	Characteristics
I	von Gierke's disease[a]	Glucose-6-phosphatase (G6Pase)	Glycogen accumulation in liver and kidney; lactic acidemia, hypoglycemia, hyperuricemia, hyperlipidemia; ketosis; normal glycogen structure
II	Pompe's disease	Lysosomal α-(1,4)-glucosidase	Glycogen accumulation in lysosomes; early death; normal blood glucose; normal glycogen structure; frequently heart is main organ involved
III	Cori's disease, Forbes' disease	Debranching enzyme	Abnormal glycogen, having short outer chains; hypoglycemia
IV	Andersen's disease	Branching enzyme	Abnormal glycogen, having long unbranched chains; early death due to cardiac or liver failure
V	McArdle's disease	Muscle glycogen phosphorylase	Abnormally high content of muscle glycogen; weakness, cramping, and decreased serum lactate after exercise; normal glycogen structure
VI	Hers' disease	Liver glycogen phosphorylase	Abnormally high content of liver glycogen; mild hypoglycemia and ketosis; normal glycogen structure

[a] Different subtypes associated with deficiency in different subunits of G6Pase.

RESOLUTION OF CLINICAL CASE

This patient is suffering from type I glycogen storage disease [1]. The abdominal fullness is the result of hepatomegaly arising from the accumulation of glycogen in the liver. Lethargy, irritability, and clammy skin are characteristic symptoms of hypoglycemia, a finding confirmed by the low fasting level of blood glucose. The elevation of glucagon normally stimulates both glycogen degradation and gluconeogenesis. Both pathways lead to the production of G6P, the immediate precursor of free glucose. In this case, the patient is unable to release glucose into the circulation because of a deficiency in G6Pase. The low blood pH is associated with elevated lactic acid that is released from the RBCs and skeletal muscle. Under normal conditions, lactic acid is extracted by the liver and used for gluconeogenesis; however, in this patient, it backs up and accumulates in the blood as a result of the inability to complete gluconeogenesis. Elevated uric acid is caused by both decreased excretion and increased production. The excretion of uric acid is competitively inhibited by lactic acid, and the increased production of uric acid arises from accelerated degradation of adenine nucleotides. Hyperlipidemia is associated with low insulin and elevated glucagon. Low insulin levels result in decreased lipoprotein lipase activity and accumulation of serum lipids, while elevated glucagon leads to increased release of free fatty acids from adipose tissue. Most of the symptoms of type I glycogen storage disease are relieved by the maintenance of normal blood glucose levels, achieved by frequent feedings of a high-carbohydrate diet.

REVIEW QUESTIONS

Directions: For each of the following questions, choose the **one best** answer.

1. Debranching of glycogen requires which of the following enzymes?

    (A) Uridine diphosphate glucose pyrophosphorylase

    (B) Glycogen phosphorylase

    (C) α-(1,4)→α-(1,4)-glucan transferase

    (D) Phosphoglucomutase

    (E) α-(1,4)→α-(1,6)-glucan transferase

2. The complete degradation of glycogen results in which of the following actions?

    (A) Release of glucose-1-phosphate (G1P) from the branch points

    (B) Release of more glucose than G1P

    (C) Fewer phosphorolysis reactions than hydrolysis reactions

    (D) Release of glucose from the nonreducing ends of glycogen

    (E) A ratio of G1P to glucose that is approximately 10:1

3. Muscle glycogen cannot release glucose into the blood for which of the following reasons?

    (A) Muscle plasma membranes contain no glucose transporters

    (B) Muscle contains no glucose-6-phosphatase (G6Pase)

    (C) Muscle contains no α-(1,6)-glucosidase

    (D) Muscle contains no phosphoglucomutase

    (E) Muscle contains no α-(1,4)→α(1,4)-glucan transferase

4. Insulin has which of the following effects on glycogen metabolism?

    (A) Glycogen synthase and phosphorylase are dephosphorylated by protein phosphatase-1.

    (B) Glycogen phosphorylase is activated, and glycogen synthase is inactivated

    (C) Net synthesis is increased in liver and decreased in muscle

    (D) cAMP phosphodiesterase is inactivated, and protein kinase A is activated

    (E) Phosphorylase kinase is activated, and glycogen phosphorylase is inactivated

5. Glycogen synthesis is an efficient mechanism for energy storage when excess glucose is available. The efficiency of storage can be estimated by comparing the number of ATP molecules that can be obtained from the complete oxidation of glucose with the number of ATP molecules required to convert glucose-6-phosphate (G6P) to glycogen and back to G6P. Which of the following most accurately describes the efficiency of glycogen storage?

    (A) <10%

    (B) 30%

    (C) 50%

    (D) 80%

    (E) >95%

ANSWERS AND EXPLANATIONS

1. The answer is C. Alpha-(1,4)→α-(1,4)-glucan transferase transfers a trisaccharide fragment from one shortened chain to another via sequential cleavage and formation of α-(1,4) glycosidic bonds. The α-(1,4)→α-(1,6)-glucan transferase catalyzes the formation of branch points. The other three enzymes have nothing to do with either branching or debranching.

2. The answer is E. The average frequency of branching is about ten. G1P is released from the nonreducing ends by phosphorolysis, and glucose is released from the branch points as free glucose by hydrolysis.

3. The answer is B. Muscle glycogen is degraded to G1P and subsequently converted to G6P and glucose through the actions of phosphoglucomutase and G6Pase, respectively. Free glucose is then transported across the plasma membrane by GLUT transport proteins. Muscle contains both phosphoglucomutase and glucose transporters but does not contain G6Pase. Muscle also contains α-(1,4)→α-(1,4)-glucan transferase and α-(1,6)-glucosidase, which are debranching enzymes.

4. The answer is A. Insulin stimulates glycogen synthesis and inhibits glycogen degradation by activating protein phosphatase-1, the enzyme that catalyzes the dephosphorylation of glycogen synthase, glycogen phosphorylase, and phosphorylase kinase. The effect of dephosphorylation is to activate glycogen synthase and inactivate both phosphorylase kinase and phosphorylase. Insulin also activates cAMP phosphodiesterase, resulting in a decrease in cellular cAMP. Since protein kinase A is allosterically activated by cAMP, its activity decreases in response to insulin.

5. The answer is E. The conversion of G6P to glycogen requires the expenditure of one ATP (UTP is energetically equivalent to ATP); and the total oxidation of G6P via glycolysis, the citric acid cycle, and oxidative phosphorylation results in a maximum of 36–38 ATP. Therefore, the efficiency of glycogen storage is approximately 97%.

REFERENCES

1. Chen Y-T, Burchell A: Glycogen storage diseases. In *Metabolic and Molecular Bases of Inherited Diseases*, 7th ed. Edited by Scriver CR, Beaudet AL, Sly WS, et al. New York, NY: McGraw-Hill, 1995, pp 935–948.

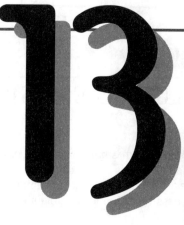

GLUCONEOGENESIS: THE DE NOVO SYNTHESIS OF GLUCOSE AND ITS ROLE IN PREVENTING HYPOGLYCEMIA

CHAPTER OUTLINE

INTRODUCTION OF CLINICAL CASE

A 48-year-old man was admitted to the emergency room in a coma. A friend had found him unconscious and was unable to rouse him. Upon his arrival at the hospital, his breathing was deep and loud, and his breath smelled of alcohol. According to his friend, he had lost his job about 6 months ago and had seemed withdrawn and depressed since then. The man was living alone, eating poorly, and seldom returned phone calls. His friend found him in the early evening when he dropped by to ask the man to dinner. There were several empty whiskey bottles and beer cans scattered around the house. Analysis of a blood sample showed an alcohol level of 86 mmol/L (about 0.4%). Blood glucose was 39 mg/dL, lactate was about tenfold above normal levels, and blood pH was 7.2 (normal 7.4). Hemodialysis was started immediately. His blood alcohol level fell rapidly, and he gained consciousness within a few hours. Following dialysis, administration of intravenous glucose was started to correct the hypoglycemia. He responded well and was released from the hospital 2 days later.

PHYSIOLOGIC SIGNIFICANCE OF GLUCONEOGENESIS

Definition and Overview

Gluconeogenesis is defined as the *synthesis of glucose from small noncarbohydrate sources*. As shown in Figure 13-1, gluconeogenesis and glycolysis are opposing pathways that share many of the same enzymes. However, there are four enzymes that are unique to gluconeogenesis. These enzymes are required to bypass the three irreversible steps in glycolysis.

FIGURE 13-1 ▶

Overview of Gluconeogenesis and Glycolysis. The pathway of gluconeogenesis includes the reverse of seven of the reactions in glycolysis (↔). Four are unique to gluconeogenesis and are required to bypass the three irreversible reactions in glycolysis. The first bypass in gluconeogenesis consists of the two steps catalyzed by pyruvate carboxylase and phosphoenolpyruvate carboxykinase (PEPCK). The second and third bypasses are catalyzed by fructose-bisphosphatase-1 (FBPase-1) and glucose-6-phosphatase (G6Pase), respectively.

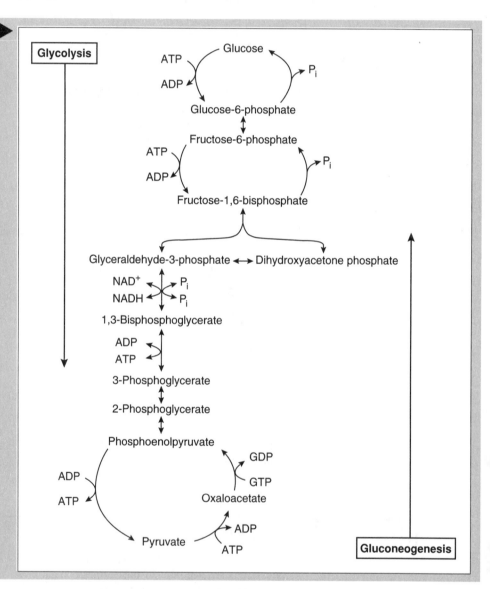

Importance in Preventing Hypoglycemia

The major function of gluconeogenesis is to provide a source of blood glucose that can augment the role of glycogen in preventing hypoglycemia.

Fasting Hypoglycemia. The de novo synthesis of glucose is important during periods of fasting. The daily glucose requirement for an adult is 160–200 g, most of which is consumed by the brain. The liver contains a limited reserve (about 75 g), which can supply glucose to other tissues for a few hours. Synthesis of glucose from protein and

Consequences of Hypoglycemia
If the concentration of blood glucose drops to 40 mg/dL and persists at this concentration or less for more than 30 minutes, damage to the central nervous system is likely to occur.

other noncarbohydrate sources begins and is released into the blood before the supply of glycogen is completely exhausted.

Hypoglycemia in the Neonate. Transient hypoglycemia is frequently seen in normal full-term neonates [1]. The fetus receives glucose from the maternal circulation by facilitated diffusion across the placental membrane. During the last few weeks of gestation, the fetal liver accumulates 10–12 g of glycogen, an amount sufficient to meet the metabolic needs of the newborn for about 12 hours. The neonatal brain is almost entirely dependent on glucose. At birth, the supply of glucose from the maternal circulation stops, and blood glucose concentration of the newborn decreases over the next 1–2 hours. The release of glucagon and epinephrine in response to the low blood glucose results in the activation of glycogen degradation, followed by gluconeogenesis a few hours later.

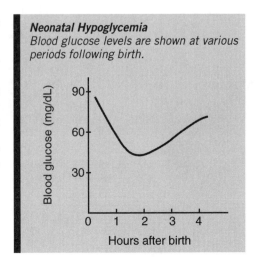

Neonatal Hypoglycemia
Blood glucose levels are shown at various periods following birth.

GENERAL FEATURES OF GLUCONEOGENESIS

Tissues That Synthesize Glucose

Both *liver* and *kidney* contain all of the enzymes required for gluconeogenesis. However, about 80% of the blood glucose derived from gluconeogenesis is made by the liver. Skeletal muscle can convert small gluconeogenic precursors to glucose-6-phosphate (G6P) but cannot release glucose into the blood due to the absence of glucose-6-phosphatase (G6Pase). The G6P can be used to replenish muscle glycogen stores.

Subcellular Localization of Enzymes

The first step in gluconeogenesis occurs in the mitochondria where pyruvate carboxylase catalyzes the conversion of pyruvate to oxaloacetate. The final step in the pathway occurs in the endoplasmic reticulum (ER) where G6P is hydrolyzed to glucose by G6Pase. All of the intervening steps occur in the cytosolic fraction of the cell.

Oxaloacetate Is Transported to the Cytosol by the Malate Shuttle

The inner mitochondrial membrane is impermeable to oxaloacetate. However, malate can be transported in either direction by a transporter located in the membrane. The malate shuttle consists of the transport protein and two *malate dehydrogenase isozymes* that are located on opposite sides of the membrane. Oxaloacetate is first reduced to malate, and after being transported to the cytosol, the malate is oxidized back to oxaloacetate. Malate also acts as a carrier of reducing equivalents across the mitochondrial membrane. The reduced form of nicotinamide adenine dinucleotide (NADH) formed by the oxidation of malate to oxaloacetate in the cytosol can be used in gluconeogenesis.

Energetics

The synthesis of glucose from two molecules of pyruvate requires both energy and reducing power. The energy is supplied by the hydrolysis of four molecules of adenosine triphosphate (ATP) and two molecules of guanosine triphosphate (GTP), while the reducing power is provided by two molecules of NADH. The products of gluconeogenesis include four molecules of adenosine diphosphate (ADP), two molecules of guanosine diphosphate (GDP), six molecules of inorganic phosphate (P_i), and two molecules of oxidized nicotinamide adenine dinucleotide (NAD^+).

Liver and Kidney Are the Glucogenic Organs
The capacity for glucose synthesis is almost identical in the liver and kidney. The weight of the liver exceeds the combined weight of the kidneys by about fourfold, accounting for the major contribution this tissue makes to newly synthesized blood glucose.

Shuttle Systems
The movement of molecules across impermeable membranes frequently uses shuttle systems. All shuttle systems consist of isozymes that are located on opposite sides of the membrane, where they catalyze the same reaction, but they catalyze it in different directions in the two cellular compartments. The malate shuttle is used to move both oxaloacetate and reducing equivalents (hydrogen atoms) across the inner mitochondrial membrane.

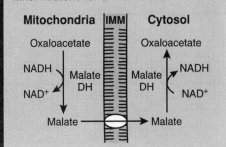

$$2 \text{ Pyruvate} + 4 \text{ ATP} + 2 \text{ GTP} + 2 \text{ NADH} + 2 \text{ H}^+ \longrightarrow$$
$$\text{glucose} + 4 \text{ ADP} + 2 \text{ GDP} + 6 \text{ P}_i + 2 \text{ NAD}^+$$

The presence in gluconeogenesis of unique enzymes that bypass the irreversible reactions in glycolysis allows both of these opposing pathways to be energetically favorable. The overall pathway for gluconeogenesis has a $\Delta G^o = -9$ kcal/mol, while the pathway of glycolysis has a $\Delta G^o = -20$ kcal/mol.

Steps Requiring ATP (or GTP). Three reactions in gluconeogenesis require nucleoside triphosphates: (1) the conversion of pyruvate to oxaloacetate by *pyruvate carboxylase*; (2) the conversion of oxaloacetate to phosphoenolpyruvate (PEP) by *phosphoenolpyruvate carboxykinase* (*PEPCK*); and (3) the conversion of 3-phosphoglycerate (3-PG) to 1,3-bisphosphoglycerate (1,3-BPG) by *3-phosphoglycerate kinase*, an enzyme used in both glycolysis and gluconeogenesis.

Step Requiring NADH. The reduction of 1,3-BPG to glyceraldehyde-3-phosphate (G3P) by *glyceraldehyde-3-phosphate dehydrogenase* (G3PD) is the only reaction in gluconeogenesis requiring NADH. This reaction is reversible and the enzyme participates in both gluconeogenesis and glycolysis.

Fatty Acid Oxidation Promotes Gluconeogenesis

Defects in Fatty Acid Oxidation
The requirement of fatty acid oxidation for gluconeogenesis is underscored by the observation that genetic defects in several enzymes of fatty acid oxidation result in hypoglycemia.

Acetyl coenzyme A (acetyl CoA) and NADH, derived from fatty acid oxidation, have three positive effects on gluconeogenesis. (1) Oxidation of acetyl CoA by the citric acid cycle generates fuel for oxidative phosphorylation and ATP synthesis. (2) Acetyl CoA and NADH are powerful inhibitors of pyruvate dehydrogenase (PDH), thereby increasing the amount of pyruvate available for gluconeogenesis. (3) Acetyl CoA is an essential allosteric activator of the first step in gluconeogenesis.

PRECURSORS FOR GLUCONEOGENESIS

Any cellular compound that can be converted to an *intermediate in glycolysis or the tricarboxylic acid (TCA) cycle* can be used as a substrate for gluconeogenesis. Lactate and alanine are converted to pyruvate, glycerol is converted to dihydroxyacetone phosphate (DHAP), and most of the glucogenic amino acids are degraded to intermediates in the TCA cycle. Most of the precursors for glucose synthesis are supplied by extrahepatic tissues and transported to the liver by *interorgan substrate cycles*.

Adipose Tissue Supplies Glycerol

Lipolysis in adipose tissue degrades triglyceride to free fatty acids and glycerol. Glycerol diffuses out of the adipocyte into the circulation and is extracted by the liver (Figure 13-2). The presence of *glycerol kinase* in liver converts it to glycerol-3-phosphate, which is subsequently oxidized to DHAP in an NAD^+-dependent reaction catalyzed by *glycerol-3-phosphate dehydrogenase*.

FIGURE 13-2
Glycerol from Adipose Tissue Is a Substrate for Gluconeogenesis. About 30% of the blood glucose in the fasted state is derived from glycerol. Glycerol-3-phosphate is required for triglyceride synthesis in the adipocyte, but these cells cannot recycle glycerol because adipocytes do not contain glycerol kinase. The presence of glycerol kinase in liver glycerol traps glycerol in the liver by converting it to glycerol-3-phosphate. The carbon skeleton from glycerol enters the pathway of gluconeogenesis as dihydroxyacetone phosphate (DHAP).

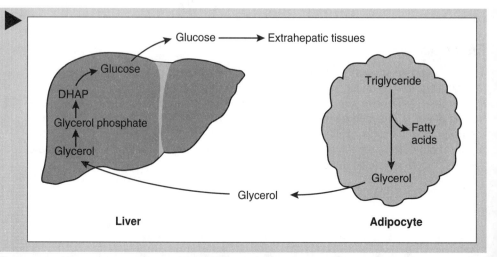

Red Blood Cells (RBCs) and Skeletal Muscle Supply Lactate

The *Cori cycle* is an interorgan cycle between skeletal muscle (or RBCs) and liver that exchanges lactate for glucose (Figure 13-3).

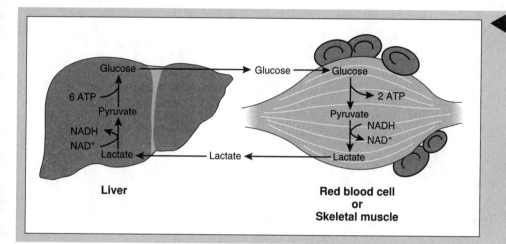

Liver

Red blood cell or Skeletal muscle

FIGURE 13-3
The Cori Cycle. *Lactate is the product of glycolysis in the RBC and anaerobic skeletal muscle. Some of the lactate is converted back to glucose by the liver and released into the blood for use by glucose-dependent tissues. The recycling of lactate by the Cori cycle is an expensive process. Six molecules of ATP are required to synthesize glucose from lactate, whereas only two molecules of ATP are derived from anaerobic glycolysis.*

Lactate, produced in extrahepatic tissues by anaerobic glycolysis, is released into the circulation and can be extracted by the liver where it is oxidized to pyruvate and used for the synthesis of glucose. The newly formed glucose can be released into the circulation and used by muscle and the RBC to generate energy. The key enzymes that facilitate the movement of lactate to be recycled for glucose synthesis are the *lactate dehydrogenase (LDH) isozymes.*

Muscle Supplies Alanine

Some of the pyruvate resulting from glycolysis in skeletal muscle is transaminated to alanine by the reaction shown below.

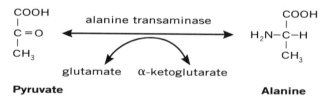

Pyruvate   **Alanine**

The immediate donor of the amino groups in this reaction is glutamate, although most of it originated with valine, isoleucine, and leucine. (The metabolism of these branched-chain amino acids will be discussed in a later chapter.) Alanine, formed by the above reaction, carries amino groups from skeletal muscle to liver where they can be converted to urea. The *alanine cycle* exchanges alanine and glucose between skeletal muscle and liver (Figure 13-4). After release from muscle, alanine is taken up by liver and transaminated back to pyruvate. The pyruvate is used to synthesize glucose, which can be returned to skeletal muscle, completing the cycle.

FIGURE 13-4

The Alanine Cycle. *Alanine is the most important amino acid for hepatic gluconeogenesis. Most of the alanine that leaves skeletal muscle comes from the transamination of pyruvate and provides a nontoxic mechanism for transporting ammonia (NH₃) from muscle. The NH₃ gets incorporated into urea and excreted, and the pyruvate is converted to glucose via gluconeogenesis. Muscle is unable to synthesize urea.*

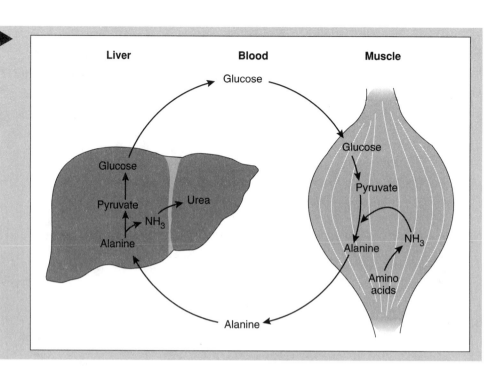

Glucogenic Amino Acids Provide Carbon Skeletons for Glucose Synthesis

The catabolism of glucogenic amino acids results in the net production of pyruvate or oxaloacetate. Oxaloacetate is an intermediate in both gluconeogenesis and the TCA cycle. Therefore, amino acids that are degraded to other intermediates in the TCA cycle (α-ketoglutarate, succinyl CoA, and fumarate) can also be converted to oxaloacetate.

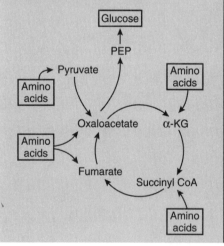

Muscle Supplies Other Glucogenic Amino Acids

Alanine is the predominant amino acid released from muscle during fasting. Many other amino acids are partially degraded, and their products can be used for glucose synthesis. Amino acids can be classified as *glucogenic* or *ketogenic*, depending on whether their degradation products are used for the synthesis of glucose or ketones (Table 13-1). Some amino acids are both glucogenic and ketogenic. Glucogenic amino acids are degraded to either pyruvate or intermediates in the citric acid cycle (TCA cycle). The degradation of *all amino acids except lysine and leucine* provides products that can be used for glucose synthesis.

Glucogenic	Ketogenic	Glucogenic and Ketogenic
Glycine	Leucine	Threonine
Serine	Lysine	Isoleucine
Valine		Phenylalanine
Histidine		Tyrosine
Arginine		Tryptophan
Cysteine		
Proline		
Alanine		
Glutamate		
Glutamine		
Aspartate		
Asparagine		
Methionine		

ENZYMES AND REACTIONS UNIQUE TO GLUCONEOGENESIS

Pyruvate Carboxylase

The reaction catalyzed by pyruvate carboxylase is shown below. Biotin is covalently attached to the enzyme, functioning as a transient carrier of the carboxyl group from bicarbonate (HCO_3^-) to pyruvate.

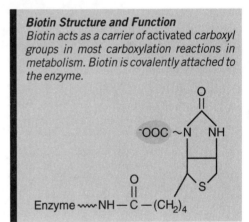

Biotin Structure and Function
Biotin acts as a carrier of activated carboxyl groups in most carboxylation reactions in metabolism. Biotin is covalently attached to the enzyme.

$$\text{Pyruvate} \quad \begin{array}{c} COOH \\ | \\ C=O \\ | \\ CH_3 \end{array} + HCO_3^- + ATP \xrightarrow[\substack{\oplus \\ \text{acetyl CoA}}]{\text{biotin}} \begin{array}{c} COOH \\ | \\ C=O \\ | \\ CH_2 \\ | \\ COOH \end{array} + ADP + P_i \quad \text{Oxaloacetate}$$

The attachment of the carboxyl group to biotin requires input of energy from ATP. Most of this energy is conserved in the newly formed C–C bond of oxaloacetate. Accumulation of acetyl CoA in the mitochondria is a signal that stimulates oxaloacetate synthesis. In addition to being the first reaction in gluconeogenesis, this reaction is also the major reaction for replenishing intermediates in the citric acid cycle.

Phosphoenolpyruvate Carboxykinase (PEPCK)

After translocation to the cytosol, oxaloacetate is converted to PEP by the action of PEPCK.

$$\text{Oxaloacetate} \quad \begin{array}{c} COOH \\ | \\ C=O \\ | \\ CH_2 \\ | \\ COOH \end{array} + GTP \longrightarrow \begin{array}{c} COOH \\ | \\ C-O\sim OPO_3^= \\ || \\ CH_2 \end{array} + GDP + CO_2 \quad \text{Phosphoenolpyruvate}$$

The carbon dioxide (CO_2) released in this reaction is the same carboxyl group that was added to pyruvate in the preceding reaction. The formation of the high-energy enolphosphate bond in PEP requires more energy than is available from the hydrolysis of GTP. Additional energy for formation comes from the cleavage of the C–C bond in oxaloacetate that releases CO_2.

The *sum of the pyruvate carboxylase and PEPCK reactions*, resulting in the conversion of pyruvate to PEP, is shown below.

$$Pyruvate + CO_2 + ATP \longrightarrow oxaloacetate + ADP + P_i$$

$$Oxaloacetate + GTP \longrightarrow PEP + GDP + P_i + CO_2$$

Sum: $Pyruvate + ATP + GTP \longrightarrow PEP + ADP + GDP + P_i \quad \Delta G° = 0.2 \text{ kcal/mol}$

Thus, for every molecule of pyruvate that is converted to PEP, the expenditure of two high-energy bonds is required. Under standard conditions, the overall reaction is reversible with a $\Delta G°$ of $+0.2$ kcal/mol. However, under the conditions that exist in the cell, where the concentration of PEP is extremely low, the ΔG for the reaction is -6 kcal/mol, and the equilibrium strongly favors PEP synthesis.

Fructose Bisphosphatase-1 (FBPase-1)

The hydrolysis of fructose-1,6-bisphosphate ($F1,6P_2$) to fructose-6-phosphate (F6P) is catalyzed by FBPase-1. This reaction bypasses the irreversible reaction of glycolysis that is catalyzed by phosphofructokinase-1 (PFK-1).

$$F1,6P_2 + H_2O \longrightarrow F6P + P_i$$

This reaction is irreversible under the conditions that exist in the cell. FBPase-1 is found in liver, kidney, and skeletal muscle but is absent in adipose tissue.

Glucose-6-Phosphatase (G6Pase)

The final reaction in gluconeogenesis bypasses the irreversible reaction in glycolysis catalyzed by glucokinase (in liver) and hexokinase (in kidney).

$$G6P + H_2O \longrightarrow glucose + P_i$$

G6Pase is located in the ER and consists of five subunits. Three of the subunits transport substrate and products of the reaction across the ER membrane (Figure 13-5). Glucose is released into the lumen of the ER and is transported across the ER membrane by a type 7 transporter (GLUT-7), a transporter that is related to but distinct from the type 2 transporter (GLUT-2) in the plasma membrane of liver cells. G6Pase is found in liver, kidney, and intestine but is absent from skeletal muscle and brain.

FIGURE 13-5 ▶

Glucose-6-Phosphatase System. The catalytic subunit of the G6Pase system is located inside the lumen of the endoplasmic reticulum (ER). A total of five proteins is required for activity. The G6Pase is the catalytic subunit; SP is a calcium (Ca^{2+})-binding regulatory protein; T_1 transports glucose-6-phosphate (G6P) from the cytosol into the lumen of the ER; T_2 transports phosphate from the lumen to the cytosol; T_3 (GLUT-7) transports glucose from the lumen into the cytosol. Deficiencies in each of these subunits have been identified as variants of glycogen storage disease type I.

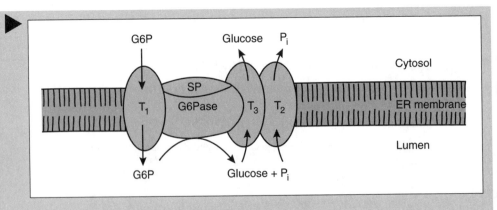

COORDINATE REGULATION OF GLUCONEOGENESIS AND GLYCOLYSIS

The regulation of gluconeogenesis and glycolysis are closely coordinated. Most of the conditions that activate gluconeogenesis inhibit glycolysis and vice versa, as shown in Figure 13-6. The targets of regulation are the enzyme pairs that catalyze opposing reactions at the irreversible steps in these pathways. Coordinate regulation of the opposing enzymes prevents loss of energy by futile cycling of ATP. The direction in which substrate flows through each of these substrate cycles is dependent on the relative activity of the two opposing enzymes at that site. The types of regulatory mechanisms that coordinate the rates of gluconeogenesis and glycolysis include allosteric effects, short-term hormonal effects mediated by phosphorylation and dephosphorylation, and adaptive effects mediated by induction and repression of enzyme synthesis.

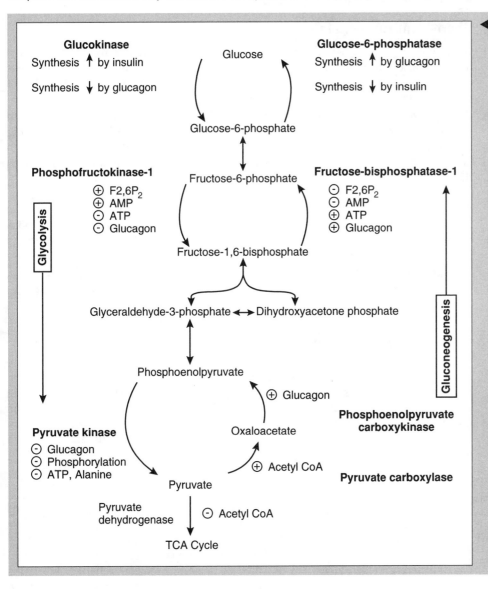

FIGURE 13-6

Coordinate Regulation of Glycolysis and Gluconeogenesis. *The level of fructose-2,6-bisphosphate (F2,6P$_2$) is the most important allosteric effector for controlling the rates of gluconeogenesis and glycolysis at the second substrate cycle. Its concentration is low in the fasted state and high in the well-fed state. Acetyl CoA is an important allosteric effector at the first substrate cycle, where it activates pyruvate carboxylase and inhibits the further oxidation of pyruvate. Glucokinase and glucose-6-phosphatase, the opposing enzymes at the third substrate cycle, both have a high K$_m$ for their substrates and are probably not saturated under physiologic conditions.*

Allosteric Effects

The most rapid change in the relative rates of glycolysis and gluconeogenesis is mediated by allosteric effectors. Two of the substrate cycles are particularly sensitive to allosteric regulation.

Interconversion of Pyruvate and PEP. The major allosteric effectors at this substrate cycle are acetyl CoA, ATP, and alanine. The conversion of pyruvate to oxaloacetate by *pyruvate carboxylase* is *activated by acetyl CoA*. The accumulation of acetyl CoA also inhibits PDH, thereby conserving pyruvate for gluconeogenesis. *Pyruvate kinase*, the opposing enzyme in glycolysis, is *inhibited by ATP and alanine*, which are substrates for gluconeogenesis.

Interconversion of F6P and F1,6P$_2$. The activity of *FBPase-1* is *inhibited by adenosine monophosphate (AMP) and F2,6P$_2$*. In the opposing pathway, *PFK-1* is *activated by AMP and F2,6P$_2$*. In the coordinate regulation of this substrate cycle, AMP serves as an indicator of the energy state of the cell, while F2,6P$_2$ is an index of the glucagon:insulin ratio in the blood.

Short-Term Hormonal Effects

Glucagon and insulin coordinate gluconeogenesis and glycolysis by influencing the intracellular *cyclic AMP (cAMP) concentration* in liver. Epinephrine can also increase cAMP in liver. The increase in cAMP that is elicited by glucagon influences the rates of gluconeogenesis and glycolysis in two ways.

F2,6P$_2$ Content of the Liver Is Decreased. F2,6P$_2$ is both an inhibitor of FBPase-1 and an activator of PFK-1. Therefore, a decrease in the concentration of F2,6P$_2$ relieves these effects, resulting in an increase in the rate of gluconeogenesis and a decrease in the rate of glycolysis. The only known function of F2,6P$_2$ is to direct the flow of intermediates through these opposing pathways.

The effect of glucagon and epinephrine on F2,6P$_2$ concentration is mediated by cAMP-dependent phosphorylation of the *bifunctional enzyme*. This enzyme has two domains: the PFK-2 domain synthesizes F2,6P$_2$, and the FBPase-2 domain degrades F2,6P$_2$. Only one domain is active at any time. When the bifunctional enzyme is phosphorylated, the FBPase-2 domain is active.

Pyruvate Kinase Is Inhibited. The cAMP-dependent phosphorylation of pyruvate kinase inhibits the conversion of PEP to pyruvate, thereby making more PEP available for gluconeogenesis.

Induction and Repression of Enzyme Synthesis

The above mechanisms of allosteric and covalent regulation mediate rapid responses to changes in the level of blood glucose. Under conditions of prolonged fasting or starvation the increase in circulating levels of *glucagon, epinephrine,* and *cortisol* result in changes in the absolute amounts of several enzymes involved in gluconeogenesis and glycolysis. During prolonged fasting, synthesis of key gluconeogenic enzymes is induced while synthesis of key glycolytic enzymes is repressed. These changes are reversed by carbohydrate feeding.

Bifunctional Enzyme and Cellular Levels of F2,6P$_2$

RESOLUTION OF CLINICAL CASE

The patient was diagnosed with a coma resulting from excessive intake of alcohol. Alcohol-induced hypoglycemia results from an inhibition of gluconeogenesis under conditions where glycogen stores are depleted because of poor eating habits. Alcohol is metabolized mainly in the liver by two NAD$^+$-dependent enzymes, alcohol dehydrogenase and aldehyde dehydrogenase. The presence of large quantities of alcohol in the cell makes a heavy demand on the limited supply of NAD$^+$. The metabolism of ethanol significantly increases the intracellular ratio of NADH:NAD$^+$ and alters the equilibrium of other reactions that require NAD$^+$. The reactions catalyzed by LDH, malate dehydrogenase, and glycerol-3-phosphate dehydrogenase are impaired by the decreased availability of NAD$^+$. The low blood pH is associated with accumulation of lactic acid, a weak acid that is deprotonated to lactate at physiologic pH. In addition to inhibitory effects of alcohol on gluconeogenesis, depletion of NAD$^+$ also inhibits fatty acid oxidation. Many of the toxic effects of alcohol are due to acetaldehyde, the product of the alcohol dehydrogenase reaction. Acetaldehyde reacts covalently with proteins and nucleic acids, altering their structure and function. Ethanol also interpolates into membranes, altering membrane function. Treatment of alcohol-induced hypoglycemia routinely involves administering glucose intravenously to restore normal blood glucose levels. Hemodialysis is used only in cases of extreme alcohol levels. Above 0.3%, most people become comatose, and at alcohol levels greater than 0.4%, death from respiratory failure is common.

Oxidation of Alcohol
Two systems are found in liver for oxidizing ethanol. About 90% is normally oxidized by alcohol and aldehyde dehydrogenases. The microsomal ethanol oxidizing system (MEOS) is a cytochrome P-450 enzyme that can be induced by alcohol.

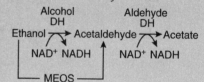

REVIEW QUESTIONS

Directions: For each of the following questions, choose the **one best** answer.

1. A deficiency in which of the following vitamins would markedly compromise the ability to convert glycerol to glucose?

    (A) Pyridoxine

    (B) Thiamine

    (C) Riboflavin

    (D) Biotin

    (E) Niacin

2. Which pair of enzymes listed below is unique to gluconeogenesis?

    (A) Pyruvate carboxylase and phosphofructokinase-1

    (B) Phosphoenolpyruvate carboxykinase (PEPCK) and pyruvate carboxylase

    (C) Pyruvate kinase and PEPCK

    (D) 3-Phosphoglycerate kinase and pyruvate carboxylase

    (E) Fructose-bisphosphatase-1 (FBPase-1) and pyruvate dehydrogenase (PDH)

3. Which set of amino acids listed below can serve as precursors for gluconeogenesis?

    (A) Alanine, glutamate, and leucine

    (B) Serine, lysine, and isoleucine

    (C) Glycine, alanine, and valine

    (D) Glutamine, phenylalanine, and leucine

    (E) Lysine, methionine, and aspartate

4. Which of the following compounds is an allosteric activator of pyruvate carboxylase?

    (A) Biotin

    (B) Acetyl CoA

    (C) ATP

    (D) Fructose-1,6-bisphosphate ($F1,6P_2$)

    (E) Alanine

5. Which of the following effects occurs in liver in response to elevated blood glucagon levels?

    (A) Decreased cAMP content

    (B) Decreased fructose-2,6-bisphosphate ($F2,6P_2$) content

    (C) Decreased fructose-bisphosphatase-1 (FBPase-1) activity

    (D) Increased phosphofructokinase-1 (PFK-1) activity

    (E) Increased pyruvate kinase activity

6. A deficiency in which of the following proteins would most likely result in lactic acidosis and hypoglycemia?

    (A) Glucokinase

    (B) Pyruvate kinase

    (C) Fructose-bisphosphatase-1 (FBPase-1)

    (D) Phosphofructokinase-1

    (E) Hexokinase

ANSWERS AND EXPLANATIONS

1. **The answer is E.** The only reaction involved in converting glycerol to glucose that requires a vitamin-derived cofactor is the NAD^+-dependent oxidation of glycerol-3-phosphate to dihydroxyacetone phosphate. Niacin is the vitamin precursor for NAD^+. Pyridoxine is the vitamin precursor for pyridoxal phosphate, a cofactor for transaminases, and the conversion of alanine to glucose would be impaired by a deficiency in this vitamin. Thiamine and riboflavin are the vitamin precursors for thiamine pyrophosphate and flavin adenine dinucleotide, respectively. Neither of these coenzymes is required for gluconeogenesis. Biotin is required for the carboxylation of pyruvate to oxaloacetate.

2. **The answer is B.** The four enzymes that are unique to gluconeogenesis are pyruvate carboxylase, PEPCK, FBPase-1, and glucose-6-phosphatase. Pyruvate kinase is unique to glycolysis. PDH is not an enzyme of either glycolysis or gluconeogenesis but is required to convert the end product of glycolysis (pyruvate) to acetyl CoA.

3. **The answer is C.** Leucine and lysine are the only two amino acids that are strictly ketogenic and cannot serve as precursors for glucose synthesis. Phenylalanine and isoleucine are both glucogenic and ketogenic. Alanine, glutamate, serine, glycine, valine, glutamine, methionine, and aspartate are strictly glucogenic.

4. **The answer is B.** Acetyl CoA is an essential allosteric activator for pyruvate carboxylase reaction. Biotin and ATP are also required for this reaction, but neither is an allosteric activator. Biotin is the coenzyme that acts as a carrier of carboxyl groups in the transfer from bicarbonate to pyruvate, and ATP supplies the energy for driving the reaction. Pyruvate kinase is activated by $F1,6P_2$ and inhibited by alanine, but neither of these compounds alters the activity of pyruvate carboxylase.

5. **The answer is B.** Glucagon binding to liver cells results in increased concentrations of cAMP. The degradation of $F2,6P_2$ by FBPase-2 is enhanced by cAMP-dependent phosphorylation of the bifunctional enzyme. FBPase-1 activity is increased and PFK-1 activity is decreased by lowering the concentration of $F2,6P_2$. The activity of pyruvate kinase is decreased by cAMP-dependent phosphorylation that occurs in response to elevated blood glucagon.

6. **The answer is C.** A deficiency in FBPase-1 results in the accumulation of intermediates in gluconeogenesis behind the block. The precursors lactate and alanine also accumulate. All of the other enzymes participate in glycolysis, and a deficiency in any one of these would be expected to decrease lactic acid production.

REFERENCES

1. Glew RH, Peters SP: *Clinical Studies in Medical Biochemistry*. New York, NY: Oxford University Press, 1987, pp 69–77.
2. Lieber CS: Biochemical and molecular basis of alcohol-induced injury to liver and other tissues. *N Engl J Med 319*:1639, 1988.

14 PENTOSE PHOSPHATE PATHWAY: GENERATION OF NADPH AND PENTOSES

CHAPTER OUTLINE

INTRODUCTION OF CLINICAL CASE

A 21-year-old male medical student was brought to the hospital with a temperature of 105°F. A native of Algeria, he arrived in the United States a month earlier as an exchange student. Shortly after arriving, he began having severe headaches and a backache. The day before he was admitted to the hospital, he was vomiting and experiencing periodic fever and chills that lasted for about an hour. The emergency room physician suspected malaria and ordered thin and thick blood-smear analysis. The analysis showed RBCs infected with the malarial parasite. Treatment with primaquine was started immediately. Four days later, the patient noticed that his urine was almost black. A complete blood analysis showed a low RBC count and an elevated reticulocyte count. The RBCs contained Heinz bodies. Hemoglobin (Hb) levels were low, and serum bilirubin levels were elevated. A few days later, the patient began to feel better, and most of his symptoms had disappeared. The color of his urine was normal, and a blood analysis showed a decrease in reticulocyte count and an increase in Hb and RBCs. He was released from the hospital with a list of drugs to avoid.

OVERVIEW

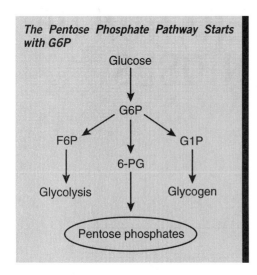

The Pentose Phosphate Pathway Starts with G6P

Glucose → G6P

G6P → F6P → Glycolysis

G6P → 6-PG → Pentose phosphates

G6P → G1P → Glycogen

The pentose phosphate pathway, also known as the *hexose monophosphate shunt*, provides an alternative pathway for the oxidation of glucose. In most tissues, 80%–90% of glucose oxidation occurs by glycolysis, and the remaining 10%–20% is oxidized by the pentose phosphate pathway. Occurring at the point where the two pathways diverge, glucose-6-phosphate (G6P) is an intermediate in both the pentose phosphate pathway and glycolysis. The initial step that commits G6P to pentose synthesis is the oxidation to 6-phosphogluconate (6-PG).

Functions

The pentose phosphate pathway has two major functions in cells.

Nicotinamide-Adenine Dinucleotide Phosphate (NADPH) Production. The major source of NADPH is the pentose phosphate pathway. NADPH is the carrier of reducing power required for most biosynthetic processes. It is also important in preventing oxygen insult to the RBC, and it participates in the bactericidal function of neutrophils.

Ribose Synthesis. The pentoses required for nucleotide and nucleic acids are synthesized by the pentose phosphate pathway. Additionally, a variety of aldoses and ketoses having chain lengths of C_3, C_4, C_5, C_6, and C_7 can be reversibly interconverted by this pathway.

Characteristics

The pentose phosphate pathway is anaerobic, neither using nor requiring oxygen for continued oxidation of glucose. No adenosine triphosphate (ATP) is consumed or generated in the pathway. The pathway is found in all cells, although the enzymes in the pathway are more enriched in some tissues than others.

Tissue Distribution. Tissues most enriched in enzymes of the pentose phosphate pathway are those that have the greatest demand for NADPH. Biosynthetic pathways that depend on NADPH include fatty acid synthesis (liver, adipose, lactating mammary gland), cholesterol and bile acid synthesis (liver), steroid hormone synthesis (adrenal cortex, ovaries, testes), and cytochrome P-450–dependent detoxification reactions (liver). Additionally, many blood cells have a high demand for NADPH to support specialized functions. RBCs require NADPH for maintaining glutathione in its reduced state, whereas neutrophils use NADPH for generating superoxide. All of the enzymes of the pentose phosphate pathway are found in the cytosol.

Oxidative and Nonoxidative Phases. The steps in the pentose phosphate pathway can be divided into two groups of reactions (Figure 14-1). The initial three reactions constitute the oxidative phase of the pathway where all of the NADPH is produced. This phase of the pathway is irreversible. The nonoxidative phase generates ribose-5-phosphate for nucleotide synthesis and converts excess pentoses back to G6P so that it can be recycled. This phase of the pathway consists of a series of reversible reactions that are in equilibrium with intermediates in glycolysis. Fructose-6-phosphate (F6P) and glyceraldehyde-3-phosphate (G3P) are common intermediates in both pathways.

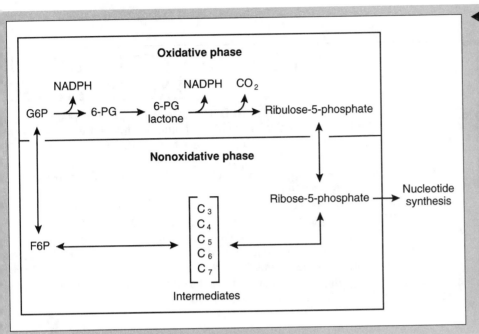

FIGURE 14-1
Overview of the Pentose Phosphate Pathway. The first three steps constitute the oxidative phase and are irreversible. The remaining reactions make up the nonoxidative phase, and all are reversible, allowing a back-up mechanism for ribose-5-phosphate synthesis in cases of a glucose-6-phosphate dehydrogenase deficiency. G6P = glucose-6-phosphate; 6-PG = 6-phosphogluconate; F6P = fructose-6-phosphate.

Regulation

The first step in the pathway, catalyzed by *glucose-6-phosphate dehydrogenase (G6PD)*, is also the rate-limiting step in the pathway. The activity of this enzyme is regulated by *product inhibition*. An increase in the concentration of NADPH decreases the activity of G6PD, an effect that coordinates the production of NADPH with its demand.

KEY ENZYMES IN THE PRODUCTION OF NADPH

The oxidation of G6P to 6-PG is catalyzed by G6PD. The oxidation occurs on C-1, with the hydride ion being transferred to the oxidized form of nicotinamide-adenine dinucleotide phosphate (NADP+), as shown in Figure 14-2. The products of the reaction are NADPH and the cyclic lactone form of 6-PG, which is rapidly converted to the straight chain form by *lactonase*. The second NADPH-producing step is catalyzed by *6-phosphogluconate dehydrogenase*. In this reaction the C-3 is oxidized to a ketone, and the carboxyl group at C-1 is released as carbon dioxide (CO_2).

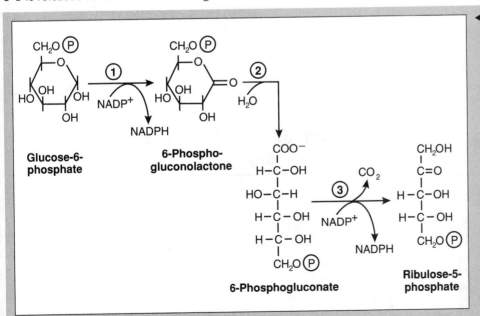

FIGURE 14-2
The NADPH-Producing Reactions. The first and third reactions result in NADPH formation. The lactone formed in the first reaction must be hydrolyzed to the straight chain form of 6-phosphogluconate before the next reaction can occur. The enzymes involved are: (1) glucose-6-phosphate dehydrogenase; (2) lactonase; and (3) 6-phosphogluconate dehydrogenase.

G6PD Deficiency

This is the most common genetic enzymopathy known. Several hundred variants of this enzyme have been identified, and most are caused by single-point mutations in the gene. Many of the variants show abnormal enzyme kinetics or instability of the enzyme. It is particularly prevalent among individuals of Mediterranean, Asian, and African descent.

Wernicke-Korsakoff Syndrome

This is an inherited disease resulting from a change in the structure of transketolase that increases the K_m for TPP by about tenfold. Other enzymes requiring TPP are not affected. Symptoms appear when a person has a chronic thiamine deficiency and often appear in alcoholics whose diets are likely to be deficient in thiamine. Symptoms include loss of memory, weakness, and partial paralysis.

KEY ENZYMES FOR RECYCLING EXCESS PENTOSES

In tissues that use large quantities of NADPH, most of the pentose phosphates are recycled to G6P by the nonoxidative phase of the pathway. This phase of the pathway begins with the conversion of ribulose-5-phosphate to two other C_5 monosaccharides, xylulose-5-phosphate and ribose-5-phosphate (Figure 14-3).

The form of pentoses required for nucleotide synthesis is ribose-5-phosphate. Excess C_5 monosaccharides then undergo a series of transfer and rearrangement reactions that effectively convert three C_5 monosaccharides to two molecules of F6P and one molecule of G3P, intermediates in glycolysis that can be used to resynthesize G6P (Figure 14-4). The two key enzymes that allow the C_5 monosaccharides to equilibrate with intermediates in glycolysis are *transketolase* and *transaldolase*. Both enzymes transfer fragments from a ketose donor to an aldose acceptor. They differ in that transketolase transfers C_2 fragments, whereas transaldolase transfers C_3 fragments. Transketolase requires *thiamine pyrophosphate* (TPP) for catalytic activity.

FIGURE 14-3 ▶

Interconversion of Pentose Phosphates. Ribulose-5-phosphate is converted to a mixture of xylulose-5-phosphate and ribose-5-phosphate. Isomerization alters the position of the carbonyl group from C-2 to C-1, resulting in ribose-5-phosphate. Changing the configuration around C-3 by epimerization produces xylulose-5-phosphate.

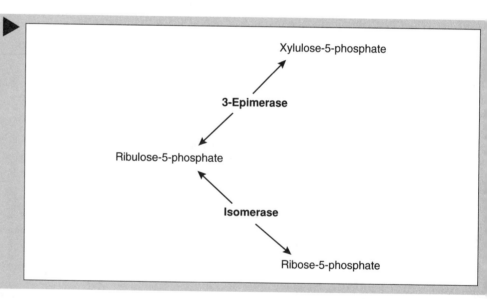

FIGURE 14-4 ▶

Transketolase and Transaldolase Reactions. Transketolase and transaldolase can convert C_5 intermediates in the pentose phosphate pathway to intermediates in glycolysis. In the first reaction, C_5 is used for both ribose-5-phosphate and xylulose-5-phosphate, C_3 is glyceraldehyde-3-phosphate, and C_7 is sedoheptulose-7-phosphate. In the second reaction, C_6 is fructose-6-phosphate and C_4 is erythrose-4-phosphate. In the third reaction, C_5 is xylulose-5-phosphate.

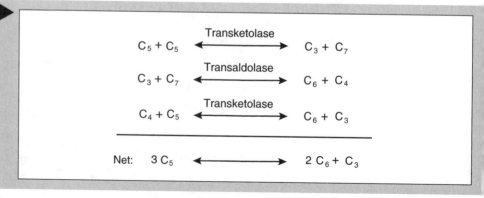

The three sequential reactions catalyzed by transketolase, transaldolase, and transketolase result in the overall reaction shown below.

$$\text{Ribose-5-phosphate} + 2 \text{ xylulose-5-phosphate} \rightleftharpoons$$
$$2 \text{ fructose-6-phosphate} + \text{glyceraldehyde-3-phosphate}$$

Clinical Assessment of Thiamine Deficiency
The most common method for assessing thiamine status uses RBC lysates for measuring the activity of transketolase and its enhancement by the addition of exogenous TPP.

ROLE OF NADPH IN THE RBC

The enzymes in the oxidative phase of the pentose phosphate pathway are particularly enriched in the RBC, where NADPH is essential for *protection from oxidative damage*. Because of the high concentration of Hb, the RBC is exposed to large amounts of molecular oxygen. Some of the oxygen is converted to *superoxide and hydrogen peroxide*, strong oxidizing agents that can cause irreversible damage to the cell. Glutathione, a strong reducing agent, protects against oxidative damage by reducing hydrogen peroxide to water. The role of NADPH is to maintain the concentration of reduced glutathione (GSH) at a concentration of about 5 mM in the RBC.

Drugs Associated with Hemolysis [1]
*Hemolysis is frequently observed in individuals after ingestion of the following drugs: **aspirin, sulfonamides,** and **nitrofurans.***

Production of Superoxide in the RBC

Hb-bound oxygen can be oxidized to superoxide in a nonenzymatic reaction that occurs spontaneously at a rate of up to 1% per hour. As shown in the following equation, an electron from the heme-iron atom is transferred to oxygen, resulting in the formation of *methemoglobin (metHb)* and *superoxide*.

$$\text{Hb-Fe}^{2+} \cdot O_2 \longrightarrow \text{Hb-Fe}^{3+} + O_2^-$$

Both products of this reaction have potentially deleterious effects. *MetHb cannot bind oxygen* and, if uncorrected, can compromise the delivery of oxygen. Superoxide is converted, both spontaneously and enzymatically, to hydrogen peroxide. Both oxygen metabolites are toxic to the cell and can lead to *peroxidation of membrane lipids followed by cell lysis and anemia*. In addition to the spontaneous and continuous formation of superoxide described above, the rate of superoxide production can be greatly enhanced by the ingestion of a large number of antimicrobial drugs. Under normal conditions, a battery of corrective enzymes in the RBC prevents these detrimental effects by reducing metHb back to functional Hb and converting superoxide and hydrogen peroxide to nontoxic molecules.

Detoxification of Superoxide Anion and Hydrogen Peroxide

The sequential action of three enzymes in the RBC maintains the concentrations of superoxide anion and hydrogen peroxide at low levels. These enzymes are superoxide dismutase (SOD), glutathione peroxidase, and glutathione reductase. The role of the pentose phosphate pathway and NADPH in this series of reactions is shown in Figure 14-5.

Metabolic Basis for Dietary Selenium Requirement
Selenium is required for glutathione peroxidase activity. It is found in the active site where it replaces the sulfur atom of a cysteine side chain.

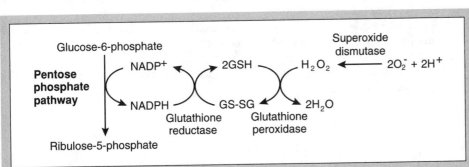

◀ **FIGURE 14-5**
Detoxification of Superoxide and Hydrogen Peroxide in the RBC. *Glutathione is a tripeptide containing a —SH group that acts as the reductant in the glutathione peroxidase reaction. RBCs also contain some catalase (not shown) that converts hydrogen peroxide to water and molecular oxygen. GS-SG is the oxidized form of glutathione.*

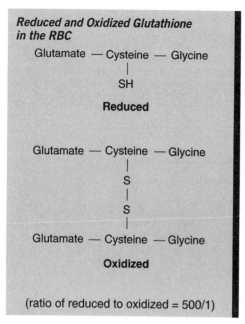

Reduced and Oxidized Glutathione in the RBC

Glutamate — Cysteine — Glycine
|
SH

Reduced

Glutamate — Cysteine — Glycine
|
S
|
S
|
Glutamate — Cysteine — Glycine

Oxidized

(ratio of reduced to oxidized = 500/1)

Superoxide is converted to hydrogen peroxide by the action of *SOD*, an enzyme found in all cells. *Glutathione peroxidase* catalyzes the reduction of hydrogen peroxide to water in a reaction that requires two molecules of GSH. The oxidized glutathione produced in the reaction is reduced back to GSH by NADPH-dependent *glutathione reductase*.

G6PD Deficiency and Hemolytic Anemia

The NADPH required for detoxification of hydrogen peroxide in the RBC is generated almost entirely by the oxidative phase of the pentose phosphate pathway. Therefore, a deficiency in G6PD can drastically impair NADPH production. Individuals homozygous for a G6P mutation are clearly at risk for RBC lysis and anemia. Under most conditions, heterozygotes are asymptomatic. However, exposure to drugs or other compounds that stimulate the production of superoxide and hydrogen peroxide may precipitate an oxidative crisis, resulting in hemolytic anemia.

Reduction of MetHb to Hb

The major mechanism for reducing metHb to functional Hb requires *metHb reductase*, an enzyme complex that contains cytochrome-b_5 and a flavoprotein, cytochrome-b_5 reductase. As shown in the following reaction, these two proteins and their cofactors form an electron transport chain that transfers electrons from NADPH to the heme iron of Hb.

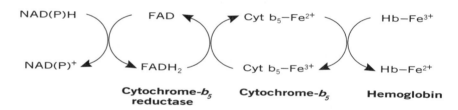

NAD(P)H — FAD — Cyt b_5—Fe^{2+} — Hb—Fe^{3+}

NAD(P)$^+$ — FADH$_2$ — Cyt b_5—Fe^{3+} — Hb—Fe^{2+}

Cytochrome-b_5 reductase · · · **Cytochrome-b_5** · · · **Hemoglobin**

Hereditary Methemoglobinemia
This is a condition caused by a deficiency in cytochrome-b_5 reductase. If metHb makes up 10%–15% of the total Hb, the individual appears "cyanotic" (having a visible blue color) but has no other symptoms.

The NADH is supplied by the glyceraldehyde-3-phosphate dehydrogenase (G3PD) reaction in glycolysis, whereas NADPH is supplied by the pentose phosphate pathway. A genetic deficiency in cytochrome-b_5 reductase results in *methemoglobinemia*.

ROLE OF NADPH IN PHAGOCYTIC CELLS

Neutrophils and other phagocytic cells use *toxic oxygen metabolites to kill bacteria* that have been engulfed by the cell. If a suspension of resting neutrophils is presented with bacteria, phagocytosis is accompanied by a rapid uptake of oxygen, known as the *oxygen burst*. This response is mediated by the binding of bacteria to specific receptors. The rapid uptake of oxygen is used to generate superoxide. The reduction of oxygen to superoxide is catalyzed by *NADPH oxidase* (Figure 14-6). Hydrogen peroxide and hypochlorous acid are produced in sequential reactions catalyzed by *SOD* and *myeloperoxidase (MPO)*, respectively.

A genetic deficiency in NADPH oxidase results in *chronic granulomatous disease*. Granular lesions in the skin and lymph nodes contain microorganisms that have been ingested but not killed. Infectious episodes can be fatal, and treatment may require weeks to months of antibiotics to clear infections. A deficiency in G6PD has similar clinical consequences [2].

Oxygen Burst Associated with Phagocytosis by Neutrophils

O$_2$ uptake / O$_2^-$ production

Oxygen burst

Time

Exposure of neutrophils to bacteria

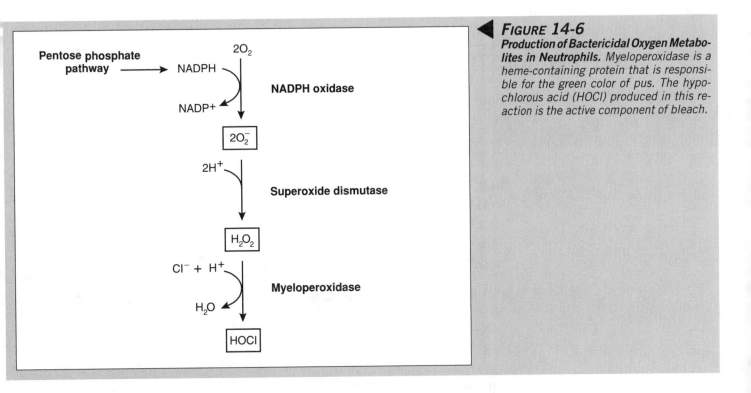

FIGURE 14-6
Production of Bactericidal Oxygen Metabolites in Neutrophils. Myeloperoxidase is a heme-containing protein that is responsible for the green color of pus. The hypochlorous acid (HOCl) produced in this reaction is the active component of bleach.

RESOLUTION OF CLINICAL CASE

The patient described at the beginning of the chapter was deficient in G6PD. When RBC hemolysates were directly assayed for this enzyme, the level of activity found was only 10% of the normal activity for age- and sex-matched controls. Therefore, the ability to generate NADPH was impaired. Using primaquine to treat this patient's malaria resulted in accelerated production of superoxide and hydrogen peroxide. The inability to maintain adequate levels of reduced glutathione to protect the cell membranes from peroxidation precipitated an oxidative crisis that resulted in hemolytic anemia. The presence of Heinz bodies in RBCs usually indicates an oxidative crisis. These inclusions contain aggregates of Hb that have precipitated out of solution because of disulfide-bond formation between Hb molecules and possibly other proteins. GSH normally acts as a sulfhydryl buffer in maintaining cysteine side chains of proteins in their reduced form. Cell lysis releases Hb. The increase in bilirubin results from increased catabolism of heme. Some of the Hb is excreted, resulting in the dark color of the urine. Under normal circumstances, the low level of G6PD activity in this patient's cells was apparently able to generate enough NADPH to maintain sufficient GSH for normal cellular functions. However, treatment with primaquine exacerbated the deficiency by imposing additional demands for GSH that could not be met because of the low level of G6PD [3].

REVIEW QUESTIONS

Directions: For each of the following questions, choose the **one best** answer.

1. The respiratory burst of the neutrophils is associated with which one of the following actions?

    (A) Increased use of oxygen by mitochondria

    (B) Exocytosis

    (C) Formation of superoxide

    (D) Decreased utilization of NADPH

    (E) Decreased hydrogen peroxide synthesis

2. A deficiency in which of the following enzymes in the RBC is most likely to result in hemolytic anemia?

    (A) Glucose-6-phosphatase (G6Pase)

    (B) NADPH oxidase

    (C) Myeloperoxidase (MPO)

    (D) Transketolase

    (E) Glucose-6-phosphate dehydrogenase (G6PD)

3. Which of the following sources of reducing equivalents is most important for steroid hormone synthesis?

    (A) Glycolysis

    (B) Tricarboxylic acid (TCA) cycle

    (C) Pentose phosphate pathway

    (D) Fatty acid oxidation

    (E) Malate shuttle

4. Which of the following enzymes is *directly* involved in the synthesis of hypochlorous acid in the neutrophil?

    (A) Glucose-6-phosphate dehydrogenase (G6PD)

    (B) Myeloperoxidase (MPO)

    (C) NADPH oxidase

    (D) Superoxide dismutase (SOD)

    (E) Glutathione peroxidase

5. Glucose-6-phosphate dehydrogenase (G6PD) is

    (A) inhibited by NADPH

    (B) inhibited by NADH

    (C) inhibited by ATP

    (D) activated by fructose-2,6-bisphosphate

    (E) activated by AMP

6. The activity of which of the following enzymes would be decreased by a thiamine deficiency?

    (A) Glucose-6-phosphate dehydrogenase (G6PD)

    (B) Transaldolase

    (C) Transketolase

    (D) Pentose phosphate isomerase

    (E) Lactonase

ANSWERS AND EXPLANATIONS

1. **The answer is C.** The respiratory burst is associated with superoxide synthesis catalyzed by NADPH oxidase. This enzyme is associated with the plasma membrane and is not found in the mitochondria. The reaction is associated with increased utilization of NADPH. The superoxide produced is a substrate for superoxide dismutase and leads to increased synthesis of hydrogen peroxide.

2. **The answer is E.** NADPH helps prevent lysis by maintaining normal levels of reduced glutathione (GSH). One of the enzymes that generates NADPH is G6PD. G6Pase, an enzyme in gluconeogenesis, is not found in the RBC. NADPH oxidase and MPO are not present in the RBC. They are found in neutrophils, where they are used in the synthesis of superoxide and hypochlorous acid, respectively. Both compounds are used to kill ingested microorganisms. Transketolase is a part of the pentose phosphate pathway but does not generate NADPH. It is required for recycling excess pentoses.

3. **The answer is C.** The synthesis of steroids requires NADPH, which is produced almost exclusively by the pentose phosphate pathway. Glycolysis, the TCA cycle, and fatty acid oxidation produce NADH, not NADPH. The malate shuttle transfers reducing equivalents in NADH (not NADPH) across the inner mitochondrial membrane.

4. **The answer is B.** MPO catalyzes the formation of hypochlorous acid from hydrogen peroxide and chloride ion. NADPH oxidase, SOD, and G6PD are indirectly involved in the synthesis of hypochlorous acid. NADPH oxidase is required for the synthesis of superoxide anion, the immediate precursor of hydrogen peroxide. This reaction also requires NADPH, which is generated in the G6PD reaction. SOD converts superoxide into hydrogen peroxide, the immediate precursor of hypochlorous acid. Glutathione peroxidase neither directly nor indirectly contributes to the synthesis of hypochlorous acid.

5. **The answer is A.** G6PD is the rate-limiting enzyme in the pentose phosphate pathway. Its activity is regulated by the accumulation of NADPH but not by NADH. The other compounds listed act as allosteric effectors of other enzymes in carbohydrate metabolism but have no effect on the activity of G6PD.

6. **The answer is C.** Transketolase requires thiamine pyrophosphate for activity. All of the enzymes listed are a part of the pentose phosphate pathway. The only two vitamins that serve as precursors for coenzymes used in this pathway are niacin and thiamine. G6PD and 6-phosphogluconate dehydrogenase both require $NADP^+$, a coenzyme derived from niacin. Transaldolase, pentose phosphate isomerase, and lactonase require no coenzyme.

REFERENCES

1. Luzzatto L, Mehta A: Glucose-6-phosphate dehydrogenase deficiency. In *Metabolic Basis of Inherited Disease*, 7th ed. Edited by Scriver CR, Beaudet AL, Sly WS, et al. New York, NY: McGraw-Hill, 1995, pp 3378–3385.
2. Forehand JR, Nauseef WM, Curnette JT, et al: Inherited disorders of phagocyte killing. In *Metabolic and Molecular Bases of Inherited Disease*, 7th ed. Edited by Scriver CR, Beaudet AL, Sly WS, et al. New York, NY: McGraw-Hill, 1995, pp 3995–4014.
3. Schwarz V: *A Clinical Companion to Biochemical Studies*. San Francisco, CA: W. H. Freeman, 1978, pp 21–26.

15

INTERCONVERSION OF MONOSACCHARIDES: GALACTOSE, FRUCTOSE, GLUCURONIC ACID, AND AMINO SUGARS

CHAPTER OUTLINE

INTRODUCTION OF CLINICAL CASE

A 7-lb, 8-oz male infant was born to healthy parents as a result of an uncomplicated delivery. The infant was breastfed, but on the third day after delivery, he vomited several times, developed diarrhea, and resisted feeding. By day 5, jaundice was apparent, and enlargement of the liver was observed. By day 10, clouding of the lens was noted, the liver continued to enlarge, and the jaundice was more pronounced. No blood group incompatibility could be demonstrated. Analysis of urine showed a positive reducing sugar test and a negative glucose oxidase test. Blood analysis showed normal hemoglobin levels but elevated levels of liver transaminases, reducing sugars, and bilirubin. Most of the bilirubin was unconjugated. Breastfeeding was discontinued on day 10, and intravenous glucose was started. Within 2 days, the diarrhea and vomiting had subsided, and a negative reducing sugar test on urine was obtained. At 2 weeks of age, the infant was discharged from the hospital with specific feeding instructions. He was seen by his physician 1 month later. The jaundice had disappeared, his liver had returned to normal size, and all of the urine and blood tests were normal.

OVERVIEW

The interconversion of hexoses is important in a number of minor pathways of metabolism. Dietary galactose and fructose can be efficiently converted into compounds that are intermediates in the pathways of glycogen synthesis and glycolysis. In the lactating mammary gland, the interconversion of glucose and galactose plays a special role in the synthesis of lactose. Uridine diphosphate (UDP)–glucuronic acid is required for the synthesis of proteoglycans and the detoxification of several relatively insoluble compounds. The synthesis of glycolipids, proteoglycans, and glycoproteins requires a number of amino sugars, all of which are derived from intermediates in carbohydrate metabolism.

GALACTOSE METABOLISM

Most dietary galactose is derived from lactose, the major disaccharide in human and bovine milk. Hydrolysis by lactase in the small intestine results in a mixture of galactose and glucose. Following absorption, galactose is delivered to the liver by the portal circulation where it is assimilated into the pathways of glycolysis, gluconeogenesis, and glycogen synthesis.

Key Enzymes for Galactose Assimilation

Dietary galactose is metabolized in the liver. The assimilation of galactose into the pathways of glucose metabolism is shown in Figure 15-1 and requires three unique enzymes.

Galactokinase. Upon entering the cell, galactose is converted to galactose-1-phosphate (Gal-1-P) by galactokinase. This reaction prevents galactose from reentering the circulation.

FIGURE 15-1 ▶
Assimilation of Galactose into Pathways of Glucose Metabolism. Dietary fructose can be converted to blood glucose or to glycogen or can be oxidized via glycolysis to pyruvate.

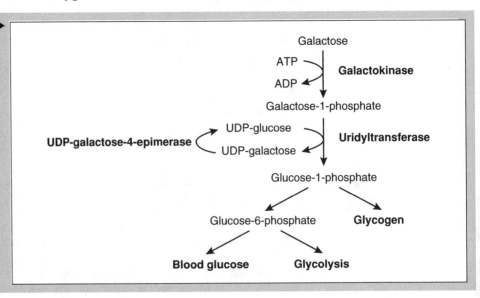

Gal-1-P Uridyltransferase. Gal-1-P is converted to UDP-galactose in an exchange reaction catalyzed by Gal-1-P uridyltransferase. As shown in the following equation, this reaction requires UDP-glucose. The glucose-1-phosphate (G1P) moiety of UDP-glucose is exchanged for Gal-1-P, resulting in UDP-galactose and G1P.

$$Gal\text{-}1\text{-}PO_3^= + \underbrace{\begin{array}{c} O \\ \| \\ Glu\text{-}1\text{-}P\text{-}O\text{-}P\text{-}O\text{-}Uridine \\ | \\ O \end{array}}_{\textbf{UDP-glucose}} \begin{array}{c} O \\ \| \\ \text{-}P\text{-}O\text{-}Uridine \\ | \\ O \end{array} \longleftrightarrow \underbrace{\begin{array}{c} O \\ \| \\ Gal\text{-}1\text{-}P\text{-}O\text{-}P\text{-}O\text{-}Uridine \\ | \\ O \end{array}}_{\textbf{UDP-galactose}} + Glu\text{-}1\text{-}PO_3^=$$

This reaction requires only a catalytic amount of UDP-glucose because in the next reaction it is regenerated by the epimerization of UDP-galactose.

UDP-Galactose-4-Epimerase. UDP-galactose and UDP-glucose can be interconverted by UDP-galactose-4-epimerase in an internal oxidation-reduction reaction. The hydroxyl group attached to C-4 of galactose is first oxidized to a keto group and then reduced back to a hydroxyl group with the opposite configuration. During each catalytic cycle, the oxidized form of nicotinamide adenine dinucleotide (NAD^+), which is tightly bound to epimerase, is first reduced to NADH, and then NADH is oxidized to NAD^+. The intermediates of this reaction never leave the surface of the enzyme. Internal oxidation-reduction reactions are commonly used in the epimerization of hydroxyl groups.

Galactosemia

The accumulation of galactose in the blood results from the inability of the liver to convert dietary galactose into compounds that can enter the pathways of glucose metabolism. The most common cause is a *deficiency in Gal-1-P uridyltransferase*, resulting in the accumulation of Gal-1-P in the cell and galactose in the blood. Symptoms of galactosemia include diarrhea and vomiting when milk is consumed, an enlarged liver, jaundice, and cataracts. The accumulation of galactose in the blood is accompanied by an increased uptake in the lens, where it is reduced to *galactitol*. As shown in the following equation, NADPH is required in reactions catalyzed by *aldol reductase*. This enzyme is nonspecific and catalyzes the reduction of many aldoses to the corresponding alcohol [1].

$$R\text{-}(CHOH)_n\text{-}\overset{\displaystyle O}{\underset{\displaystyle H}{C}} + NADPH \xrightarrow{\textbf{aldol reductase}} R\text{-}(CHOH)_n\text{-}CH_2OH + NADP^+$$

Heterozygotes for Gal-1-P uridyltransferase deficiency frequently are asymptomatic unless continually challenged by a high galactose diet. Diagnosis can be made by directly assaying for Gal-1-P uridyltransferase activity in red blood cells (RBCs).

A rarer form of galactosemia results from a *galactokinase deficiency*. Individuals with galactokinase deficiency have to maintain a galactose-free diet throughout their lives.

Lactose Synthesis

Lactose (galactose–glucose) is the major sugar in human milk and is synthesized by the lactating mammary gland. The synthesis of lactose requires UDP-galactose as the "activated" galactose (Gal) donor and glucose (Glu) as the acceptor. In the following equation, the synthesis does not depend on a source of dietary galactose. It can be synthesized totally from glucose. The UDP-galactose can be derived from the epimerization of UDP-glucose. *Lactose synthase* catalyzes the formation of a β-(1,4) galactosidic linkage between the C-1 of galactose and the C-4 of glucose.

$$\text{UDP-Glu} \xrightarrow[\text{4-epimerase}]{} \text{UDP-Gal} \xrightarrow[\underset{\text{Glucose}}{}]{\text{lactose synthase}} \underset{\text{(lactose)}}{\text{Gal-β-(1,4)-Glu}}$$

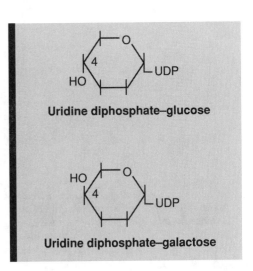

Uridine diphosphate–glucose

Uridine diphosphate–galactose

Galactitol and Cataract Formation
Galactitol is a dead end product that cannot be further metabolized. In galactosemics, it becomes trapped in the lens and nerve cells. Unlike galactose, it cannot pass across the membrane. Its formation depletes NADPH and reduces glutathione levels, which leads to cataract formation.

α-Lactalbumin and Lactose Synthesis
*α-Lactalbumin has no catalytic activity, but it alters the specificity of galactosyltransferase. In the absence of α-lactalbumin, the preferred acceptor for galactose is N-acetylglucosamine. In the presence of α-lactalbumin, the galactosyltransferase has a much higher affinity for glucose than for N-acetylglucosamine, thereby shifting the synthesis from glycoprotein to lactose. During pregnancy, synthesis of α-lactalbumin is inhibited by **progesterone**. After birth, its synthesis is stimulated by **prolactin**.*

Lactose synthase is composed of two subunits, *galactosyltransferase* and *α-lactalbumin*. Galactosyltransferase is a constitutive enzyme that is always present in the mammary gland, but α-lactalbumin synthesis occurs only during lactation. In the absence of α-lactalbumin, galactosyltransferase participates in glycoprotein synthesis with protein-bound *N*-acetylglucosamine serving as the acceptor for galactose. However, in the presence of α-lactalbumin, the acceptor for galactose is glucose.

FRUCTOSE METABOLISM

Most dietary fructose is consumed as sucrose (table sugar). It is also present in honey and fruits where it is responsible for their sweet taste. Under normal conditions, most of the metabolism of fructose occurs in the *liver*, with a small amount occurring in the *kidney*. Fructose metabolism involves cleavage into two 3-carbon fragments followed by condensation into fructose-1,6-bisphosphate (F1,6P$_2$).

Key Enzymes

The assimilation of dietary fructose into the pathways of glucose metabolism, shown in Figure 15-2, requires three unique enzymes that are found in the liver and the kidney.

FIGURE 15-2
Assimilation of Fructose into Pathways of Glucose Metabolism. Dietary fructose can be converted to blood glucose or to glycogen or can be oxidized via glycolysis to pyruvate.

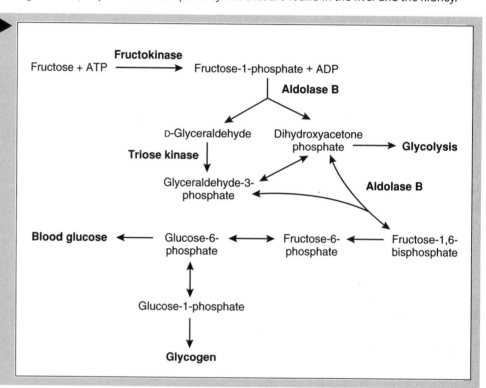

Fructokinase. The metabolism of fructose starts by adenosine triphosphate (ATP)–dependent phosphorylation to yield fructose-1-phosphate (F1P). This reaction is catalyzed by fructokinase, which is specific for fructose.

Aldolase B. Aldolase B (also known as F1P aldolase) cleaves F1P between C-3 and C-4, producing dihydroxyacetone phosphate (DHAP) and glyceraldehyde. Aldolase B also cleaves F1,6P$_2$ and participates in glycolysis in the liver. Aldolase B is different from aldolase A, which is found in muscle and cleaves only F1,6P$_2$.

Triose Kinase. Triose kinase catalyzes the ATP-dependent phosphorylation of glyceraldehyde to G3P. Through the action of the above three enzymes, dietary fructose can be converted into three-carbon compounds that are intermediates in glycolysis. They can be used as a source of fuel by continuing through the glycolytic pathway or for the synthesis of blood glucose or glycogen.

Synergistic Effect of Fructose on Glucose Metabolism

Fructose stimulates the uptake of glucose by the liver by increasing the affinity of glucokinase for glucose. This effect is mediated by an inhibitory protein that can bind either F6P or F1P. When F6P is bound, the protein associates with glucokinase and lowers its affinity for glucose. This effect is reversed by F1P.

Toxicity of Fructose

The formation of F1P by the liver is much more rapid than its rate of cleavage by aldolase B, thereby resulting in a transient accumulation of F1P in liver [2]. The accumulation of F1P stimulates changes in several other metabolites that can lead to toxic effects.

Lactic Acidemia. Lactate is formed several times faster from fructose than from glucose. When the fructose load is particularly high, it may stimulate lactic acidemia. This is attributed to two factors: (1) the assimilation of fructose into the pathway of glycolysis bypasses the rate-limiting step in glycolysis, and (2) F1P can allosterically activate pyruvate kinase.

Hyperuricemia. The administration of large quantities of fructose results in elevated levels of uric acid in blood and urine and may lead to gout. This effect can be attributed to increased degradation of adenine nucleotides by the liver. Normally, the degradation of adenine nucleotides is inhibited by inorganic phosphate (P_i). However, the accumulation of F1P can deplete the levels of P_i in the liver, resulting in accelerated degradation of adenine nucleotides and production of uric acid. The excretion of uric acid is also inhibited by lactate.

Defects in Fructose Metabolism

Two genetic diseases can result from enzyme deficiencies in the pathway of fructose assimilation. Treatment requires dietary restriction of fructose, sucrose, and sorbitol.

Hereditary Fructose Intolerance. Hereditary fructose intolerance (HFI) results from a deficiency in aldolase B. The accumulation of F1P leads to a depletion of intracellular phosphate, a disruption of oxidative phosphorylation, and inhibition of other cellular processes that are energy dependent. Ingestion of fructose typically results in hypoglycemia even though there are glycogen stores in the liver. F1P inhibits glycogen phosphorylase and phosphoglucomutase, resulting in impaired glycogen degradation. Other symptoms include vomiting, jaundice, hepatomegaly, and liver failure.

Essential Fructosuria. Essential fructosuria results from a deficiency in fructokinase and is characterized by the excretion of fructose in the urine. In general, this condition is benign. The increased concentration of fructose in the blood allows it to be converted to F6P and metabolized by extrahepatic tissues. This reaction does not occur under normal conditions because hexokinase has a low affinity for fructose.

Fructose Requirement by Sperm

Sperm use fructose as their major source of energy when they are present in the seminal fluid. Cells of the seminal vesicles convert glucose to fructose and release it into the semen. Fructose synthesis requires two enzymes that constitute the *sorbitol (polyol) pathway.* The reactions involved are shown below:

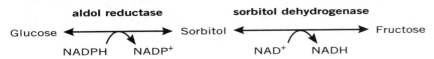

In the first reaction, the aldehyde at C-1 of glucose is reduced, producing sorbitol. The hydroxyl group at C-2 of sorbitol is then oxidized, producing fructose. Both of these enzymes are also found in the liver where they allow dietary sorbitol to be metabolized. Aldol reductase is found in many tissues.

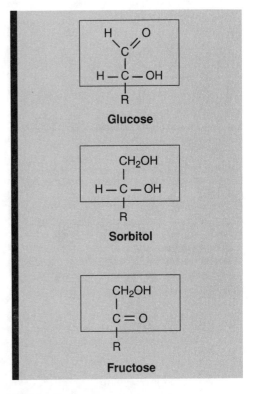

Inheritance Patterns of Fructose Intolerance
Both HFI and essential fructosuria are inherited as autosomal recessive traits.

Glucose

Sorbitol

Fructose

GLUCURONIC ACID METABOLISM

Almost all glucuronic acid metabolism occurs at the nucleoside diphosphate level. The synthesis of glucuronic acid starts with UDP-glucose, and all the pathways that require glucuronic acid use UDP–glucuronic acid as the "active" carrier. An overview of the metabolic functions of glucuronic acid is shown in Figure 15-3.

FIGURE 15-3 ▶
Overview of UDP–Glucuronic Acid Synthesis and Utilization. Glucuronic acid is used in a variety of detoxification reactions. Highly insoluble compounds that are toxic, if allowed to accumulate, are made soluble and excreted as glucuronides.

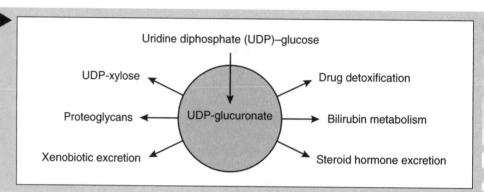

Synthesis

The synthesis of UDP–glucuronic acid involves the oxidation of glucose at C-6, a reaction catalyzed by *UDP–glucose dehydrogenase.* The reaction, shown in the following equation, is a two-step oxidation in which the hydroxyl group is first oxidized to an aldehyde and then to a carboxyl group.

Utilization

Most of the UDP–glucuronic acid pool is used either for the synthesis of proteoglycans or in detoxification reactions. In all cases, the transfer of glucuronic acid from the activated carrier to the acceptor is catalyzed by *UDP-glucuronyltransferase*, a generic name for a family of enzymes. Each enzyme is specific for a different acceptor.

Proteoglycan Synthesis. Proteoglycan synthesis requires both UDP–glucuronic acid and UDP-xylose. Xylose is a five-carbon monosaccharide that links the carbohydrate polymer to the protein core of proteoglycans. UDP-xylose is formed by decarboxylation of UDP–glucuronic acid.

Conjugation Reactions. Conjugation reactions are used to make highly insoluble compounds sufficiently soluble for excretion. Most conjugation reactions occur in the liver. Many hydrophobic compounds, such as bilirubin, steroid hormones, xenobiotics, phenobarbital, zidovudine (AZT), and other drugs, are excreted as *glucuronides.* The hydrophobic molecules have one or more hydroxyl groups that become linked to glucuronic acid through an *O*-glycosidic bond. A typical conjugation reaction is shown below.

Glucuronide

UDP-Glucuronyltransferases and Drug Tolerance
These enzymes are used to increase the solubility of many drugs so they can be more easily excreted. Exposure to a drug frequently induces the synthesis of the transferase specific for that drug, thereby enhancing excretion and promoting tolerance.

$$\text{R-OH} + \text{UDP-glucuronate} \xrightarrow{\textbf{UDP-glucuronyltransferase}} \text{R-O-glucuronide} + \text{UDP}$$
(insoluble)   (soluble)

AMINO SUGARS AND THEIR PRECURSORS

Amino sugars are found in structural macromolecules such as glycoproteins, proteoglycans, and some sphingolipids. The three most common amino sugars found in macromolecules are the two modified hexoses, *N-acetylglucosamine* and *N-acetylgalactosamine*, and a nine-carbon sugar, *N-acetylneuraminic acid* (also known as sialic acid). The amino groups in these compounds are usually linked to an acetyl group via an amide linkage.

The synthesis of *N*-acetylglucosamine and *N*-acetylgalactosamine requires three precursors that are common intermediates in ubiquitous pathways: the carbon skeleton is provided by F6P; the amino group is supplied by the side chain of glutamine; and the acetyl group is donated by acetyl CoA. The "activated" forms required for synthesis of glycoproteins and proteoglycans are UDP~*N*-acetylglucosamine and UDP~*N*-acetylgalactosamine. The synthesis of *N*-acetylneuraminic acid requires three additional carbons that are supplied by *phosphoenolpyruvate*. The activated form of this amino sugar is cytidine monophosphate (CMP)~*N*-acetylneuraminic acid.

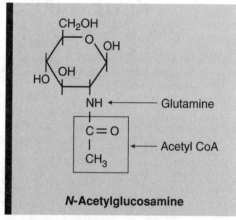

N-Acetylglucosamine

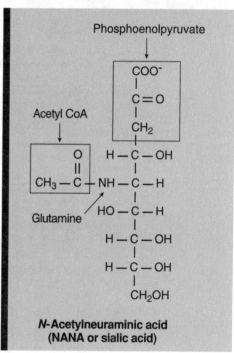

**N-Acetylneuraminic acid
(NANA or sialic acid)**

RESOLUTION OF CLINICAL CASE

The infant was diagnosed as having hereditary galactosemia. A tentative diagnosis was made on the basis of his resistance to breastfeeding and a urine analysis that was positive for reducing sugars but negative for glucose. Chromatographic analysis identified the reducing sugar as galactose. The diagnosis was confirmed by assaying lysates of RBCs for Gal-1-P uridyltransferase and finding less than 5% of the normal activity. The presence of elevated liver transaminases in the serum suggested liver damage with release of cellular contents. The accumulation of Gal-1-P in the cells led to hepatomegaly and cell lysis. Galactose accumulated in the blood and entered the lens, where it was reduced to galactitol. The lens has a high concentration of aldol reductase, which reduces galactose to galactitol in an NADPH-dependent reaction. The accumulation of galactitol coupled with the depletion of NADPH and reduced glutathione levels led to cataract formation. The normal level of hemoglobin suggested that the elevated serum bilirubin was not due to hemolysis. It appeared more likely that the elevated bilirubin and the associated jaundice resulted from the inability of the liver to handle normal amounts of bilirubin. This was consistent with the observation that most of the bilirubin was unconjugated; the conjugation reaction occurs exclusively in the liver. As long as this patient stays on a galactose-free diet, he is expected to develop normally.

REVIEW QUESTIONS

Directions: For each of the following questions, choose the **one best** answer.

1. A pregnant woman is deficient in galactose-1-phosphate uridyltransferase and cannot handle dietary galactose. She plans to breastfeed her child and is assured that she will be able to synthesize lactose. Which of the following enzymes makes this possible?

   (A) Uridine diphosphate (UDP)–glucose dehydrogenase

   (B) N-acetylgalactosamine transferase

   (C) UDP-galactose-4-epimerase

   (D) Triose kinase

   (E) Galactokinase

2. Hereditary fructose intolerance results from a genetic deficiency in which of the following enzymes?

   (A) Fructokinase

   (B) Aldolase A

   (C) Triose kinase

   (D) Aldolase B

   (E) Fructose bisphosphatase-1

3. The synthesis of "activated" N-acetylneuraminic acid but not "activated" N-acetyl-glucosamine requires which of the following precursors?

   (A) Acetyl CoA

   (B) Phosphoenolpyruvate

   (C) Glutamine

   (D) Uridine triphosphate (UTP)

   (E) Pyruvate

4. The synthesis of uridine diphosphate (UDP)–glucuronic acid requires which of the following precursors?

   (A) NADP+

   (B) FAD

   (C) UDP-galactose

   (D) UDP-xylose

   (E) NAD+

5. The reaction catalyzed by aldol reductase

   (A) reduces galactitol to galactose

   (B) uses NADH as a reducing agent

   (C) converts sorbitol to fructose in the seminal vesicles

   (D) reduces glucose to sorbitol in the lens

   (E) occurs only in the liver, seminal vesicles, and lens

ANSWERS AND EXPLANATIONS

1. The answer is C. The synthesis of lactose requires UDP-galactose as a substrate. Although the woman described in the question cannot synthesize UDP-galactose from dietary galactose, UDP-glucose can be converted to UDP-galactose by UDP-galactose-4-epimerase.

2. The answer is D. Aldolase B cleaves fructose-1-phosphate (F1P) to dihydroxyacetone phosphate and glyceraldehyde. Aldolase A is found in muscle, where it cleaves fructose-1,6-bisphosphate, but it has no effect on F1P. A deficiency in fructokinase results in essential fructosuria.

3. The answer is B. *N*-acetylneuraminic acid is a nine-carbon amino sugar in which three of the carbons are derived from phosphoenolpyruvate. The synthesis of both *N*-acetylglucosamine and *N*-acetylneuraminic acid requires acetyl CoA and glutamine as precursors. Synthesis of "activated" *N*-acetylglucosamine requires UTP, while synthesis of "activated" *N*-acetylneuraminic acid requires cytidine triphosphate. Pyruvate is not required for the synthesis of either of these amino sugars.

4. The answer is E. UDP-glucose is oxidized to UDP–glucuronic acid in a reaction that requires 2 mol of NAD$^+$ for each mole of UDP–glucuronic acid formed. The reaction is catalyzed by UDP–glucose dehydrogenase.

5. The answer is D. Aldol reductase is found in many tissues where it catalyzes the reduction of aldoses to the corresponding alcohol (glucose is reduced to sorbitol, and galactose is reduced to galactitol). The reaction requires NADPH as a reducing agent. The enzyme required to synthesize fructose from sorbitol is sorbitol dehydrogenase, and this enzyme is found only in liver and seminal vesicles.

REFERENCES

1. Segal S, Berry GT: Disorders of galactose metabolism. In *Metabolic and Molecular Bases of Inherited Disease*, 7th ed. Edited by Scriver CR, Beaudet AL, Sly WS, et al. New York, NY: McGraw-Hill, 1995, pp 967–990.
2. Gitzelmann R, Steinmann B, Vander Berghe G: Disorders of fructose metabolism. In *Metabolic and Molecular Bases of Inherited Disease*, 7th ed. Edited by Scriver CR, Beaudet AL, Sly WS, et al. New York, NY: McGraw-Hill, 1995, pp 905–925.

16 GLYCOPROTEINS AND PROTEOGLYCANS

CHAPTER OUTLINE

INTRODUCTION OF CLINICAL CASE

When 2-year-old Kevin was taken to his pediatrician for a routine checkup, his physician noticed that his facial features were coarse. Since this symptom is observed with many lysosomal enzyme disorders, a urine analysis for oligosaccharides was ordered, but the analysis showed no abnormalities. Six months later, his mother brought him in again because of a "constant runny nose" and small, "pebbly," ivory-colored skin lesions on his back and upper arms. She was also concerned that he might have difficulty hearing. A family history revealed that Kevin had a maternal uncle who was mentally retarded and had coarse facial features. On this occasion, both blood and urine analyses revealed the presence of high levels of heparan sulfate and dermatan sulfate. No corneal clouding was observed. Enzyme analysis of fibroblasts showed iduronate sulfatase to be less than 5% of normal activity. By the age of 6, Kevin was suffering from stiff joints, severe loss of hearing, and hepatomegaly. His condition continued to degenerate, and by age 12, he showed profound loss of function. He had difficulty swallowing, could not hold objects, and could no longer walk. He died at age 15 of cardiac failure, resulting from valvular dysfunction.

OVERVIEW

Glycoproteins and proteoglycans are macromolecules that contain covalently linked carbohydrate and protein; they are usually distinguished on the basis of the relative proportion of carbohydrate and protein. *Glycoproteins* usually contain considerably more protein than carbohydrate with the carbohydrate occurring in short, branched chains containing 15–20 monosaccharides. *Proteoglycans* contain more than 95% carbohydrate, and the carbohydrate chains, known as *glycosaminoglycans (GAGs)*, are long linear polymers containing hundreds of monosaccharides. They consist of repeating disaccharide units that usually contain an amino sugar, either *N*-acetylglucosamine (GlcNAc) or *N*-acetylgalactosamine (GalNAc), and a uronic acid, either glucuronic or iduronic acid. The amino sugar is usually sulfated, and in many cases the uronic acid also contains sulfate esters.

GLYCOPROTEINS

The occurrence of glycoproteins in nature is widely distributed. They are found in mucus, lysosomes, extracellular matrix, and embedded in membranes. Most of the serum proteins are glycoproteins with the notable exception of albumin. Many enzymes, structural proteins, hormones, immunoglobulins, antigens, receptors, and transport proteins have covalently linked oligosaccharide chains. In many cases, the precise role of the carbohydrate is not entirely clear. Some of the functions that have been attributed to the oligosaccharide component of these proteins include: (1) information for targeting macromolecules to specific destinations, (2) mediators of interactions between cells, (3) embryonic development and differentiation, (4) cell migration, and (5) blood group determinants.

Carbohydrate–Protein Linkages

The oligosaccharide chains are attached to the protein through either *N*-glycosidic or *O*-glycosidic bonds.

N-*Glycosidic Bonds.* *N*-Glycosidic bonds are formed between the amide group of an *asparagine* side chain and the anomeric carbon of *GlcNAc*. The enzyme that catalyzes the formation of the *N*-glycosidic bond recognizes asparagine (Asn) residues in the protein having the sequence Asn-X-Thr or Asn-X-Ser, where X can be any amino acid. This sequence is necessary but insufficient for defining glycosylation sites. Some asparagine residues with this sequence do not become glycosylated.

O-*Glycosidic Bonds.* *O*-Glycosidic bonds are formed between the side chain hydroxyl group of either *serine or threonine* and the anomeric carbon of either *GalNAc or xylose*. In collagen, there is a special type of *O*-glycosidic linkage in which galactose is attached to the hydroxyl group of hydroxylysine. The carbohydrate attached to collagen is always the Gal–Glu disaccharide.

N-Linked Oligosaccharide Synthesis

The core region of all *N*-linked oligosaccharide chains is synthesized on a lipid carrier, *dolichol phosphate*, and subsequently transferred to the appropriate asparagine residue of the acceptor protein. Diverse classes of *N*-linked glycoproteins are created by modification of the core oligosaccharide. Modification reactions start in the endoplasmic reticulum (ER) and proceed as the protein moves through the Golgi.

Synthesis of Core Oligosaccharide. The assembly of the core oligosaccharide on the lipid carrier occurs in the ER (Figure 16-1). The oligosaccharide is composed of 14 monosaccharides (two GlcNAc, nine mannose, three glucose residues).

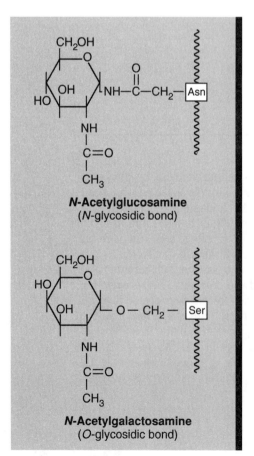

N-Acetylglucosamine
(*N*-glycosidic bond)

N-Acetylgalactosamine
(*O*-glycosidic bond)

Man—Man
Man—Man   Man
Glu—Glu—Glu—Man—Man—Man   Man—GlcNAc————GlcNAc—O—P—O—P—O—Dolichol

FIGURE 16-1
Structure of Core Oligosaccharide. The two N-acetylglucosamine (GlcNAc) residues and the first five mannose (Man) groups are donated by UDP-GlcNAc and GDP-mannose. The remaining mannose residues and all of the glucose (Glu) residues are donated by dolichol phosphate–mannose and dolichol phosphate–glucose.

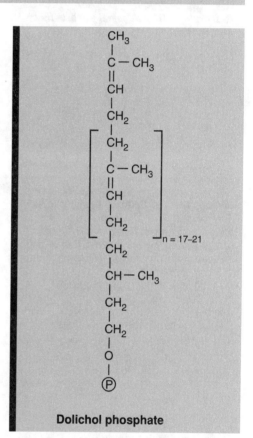

Dolichol phosphate

Synthesis of the core oligosaccharide requires two types of high-energy donors of monosaccharides, *nucleotide sugars* (uridine diphosphate [UDP]–GlcNAc; guanosine diphosphate [GDP]–mannose) and *dolichol phosphate sugars* (dolichol phosphate–mannose; dolichol phosphate–glucose).

Oligosaccharide Modification. After transfer of the core oligosaccharide to an acceptor protein, the oligosaccharide is modified by a number of processing reactions. The ends of the chains are trimmed and extended in different ways to generate two major classes of *N*-linked glycoproteins: *high mannose* and *complex* (Figure 16-2). All mature *N*-linked glycoproteins contain five of the original monosaccharides.

Addition of Zip Codes. By mechanisms that are not completely understood, *proteins are sorted within the Golgi and sent to their specific destinations.* The sorting process for lysosomal acid hydrolases is the best understood of the targeting mechanisms. The presence of *mannose-6-phosphate* in the oligosaccharide chain of an enzyme ensures that it is incorporated into lysosomes. The phosphorylation of mannose requires the sequential action of two enzymes (Figure 16-3). Proteins containing mannose-6-phosphate bind to receptors in the Golgi, and vesicles containing these proteins pinch off and subsequently fuse with lysosomes. The acidic pH of the lysosome allows the acid hydrolases to dissociate from the membrane. A deficiency in *N*-acetylglucosaminylphosphotransferase results in the inability to phosphorylate mannose and leads to *I-cell disease.*

O-Linked Oligosaccharide Synthesis. The synthesis of *O*-linked glycoproteins is strikingly different from that of *N*-linked glycoproteins. Dolichol-linked intermediates are not involved, and there is no preassembly of the oligosaccharide. Oligosaccharide addition starts in the *Golgi* with the addition of either *GalNAc or xylose* to a serine or threonine side chain of the protein. Additional sugars are added one at a time to produce a mature oligosaccharide, ranging from two to twelve monosaccharides in length. The high-energy sugar donors for *O*-linked oligosaccharide synthesis are all nucleotide-linked monosaccharides.

I-Cell Disease
This disease results from a breakdown in the targeting mechanism that normally ensures that acid hydrolases are sent to lysosomes. The term "I-cell" comes from the observation that large "inclusion bodies" are found in the cytosol. These inclusions are lysosomes that are engorged with undegraded GAGs. A deficiency in N-acetylglucosaminylphosphotransferase results in the inability to form mannose-6-phosphate on the oligosaccharide side chains of enzymes that are normally destined for lysosomes. Active lysosomal enzymes are synthesized, but they are secreted into the blood.

FIGURE 16-2 ▶

Structures of the Major Types of N-linked Glycoproteins. *Processing of the core oligosaccharide gives rise to two major classes of oligosaccharides. Both may be found on the same protein at different positions. High-mannose oligosaccharides have no new sugars added in the Golgi. Complex oligosaccharides may have several different sugars added, including N-acetylglucosamine (GlcNAc), galactose (Gal), sialic (NANA), and fucose (Fuc). Man = mannose; Asn = asparagine.*

FIGURE 16-3 ▶

Adding the Zip Code to Lysosomal Acid Hydrolases. *The phosphorylation of specific mannose residues of the N-linked oligosaccharide serves as the signal that sends acid hydrolases to lysosomes. Addition of phosphate requires two enzymes: N-acetylglucosaminylphosphotransferase adds N-acetylglucosamine phosphate to the number 6 position of mannose; N-acetylglucosaminylphosphoglycosidase is required for removal of GlcNAc, leaving mannose-6-phosphate.*

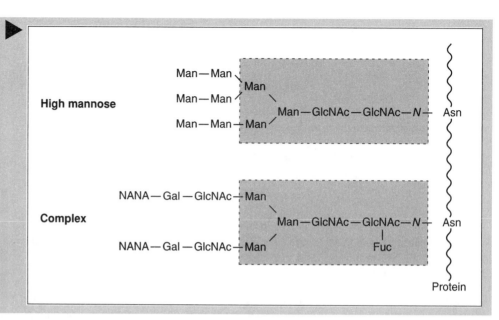

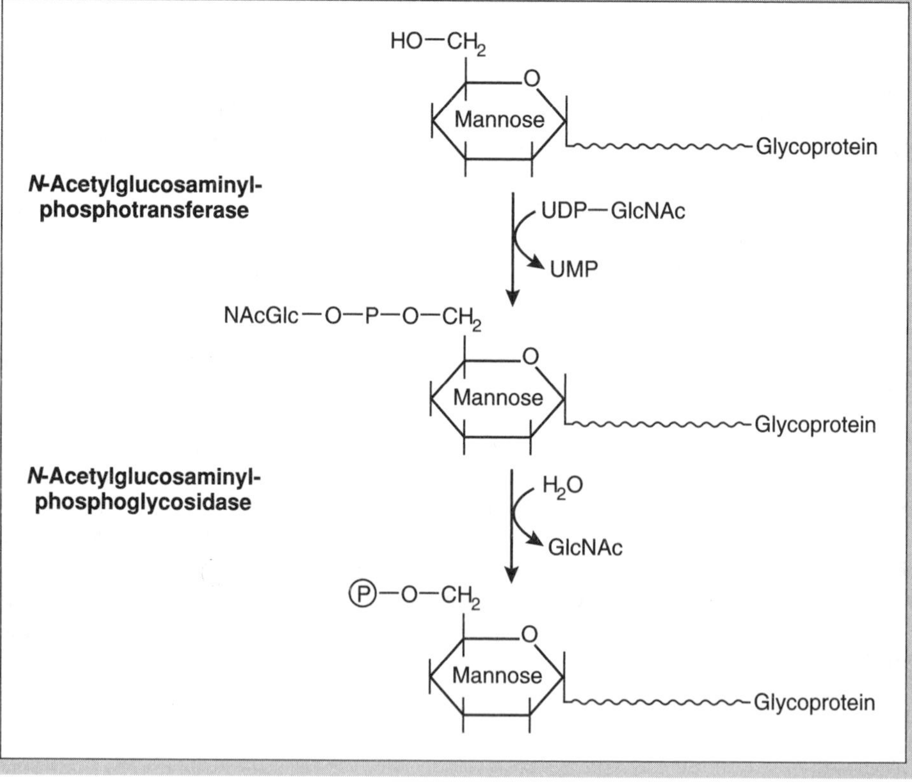

BLOOD GROUP ANTIGENS

A clinically important group of *O-linked oligosaccharides* is the blood group substances. The external surface of the red blood cell (RBC) contains hundreds of antigens that have been classified into more than a dozen genetically distinct blood group systems. The major ones are the A, B, and O antigens that comprise the ABO blood group.

Structural Basis of ABO Specificity

Blood group specificity is determined by a few key monosaccharides that are located near the nonreducing end of the *O*-linked carbohydrate chain (Figure 16-4). The O antigen is an oligosaccharide that is a precursor for both the A and B antigens; it is found in all individuals. The A and B antigens differ by a single monosaccharide at one of the nonreducing ends of an *O*-linked oligosaccharide chain. The A antigen has GalNAc at the end of a chain, while the B antigen has galactose in the corresponding position.

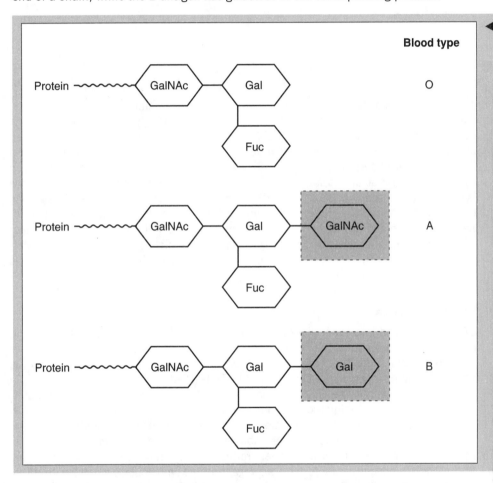

Blood type

◀ **FIGURE 16-4**
Blood Group Determinants of the ABO System. *The blood type is determined in part by the monosaccharide found at the nonreducing end of the oligosaccharide chain (shaded blocks). Fucose (Fuc) is structurally derived from 6-deoxygalactose. GalNAc = N-acetylgalactosamine; Gal = galactose.*

Correlation Between Blood Types, Enzymes, and Antibodies

The formation of type A antigen requires *N-acetylgalactoaminyltransferase*, while the formation of type B antigen requires *galactosyltransferase*. The synthesis of the precursor oligosaccharide (O antigen) requires neither of these enzymes. Thus, A, B, and O blood types can be correlated with the complement of glycosyltransferases that are expressed in the cell. Additionally, blood types can be correlated with the kind of antibodies in the serum. For example, individuals with type A antigen on their RBCs have antibodies against antigen B in their serum, and vise versa. Individuals with both A and B antigens on their RBCs contain neither anti-A nor anti-B antibodies in their serum. Type O individuals have neither A nor B antigens on their RBCs and have both anti-A and anti-B in their serum. In blood transfusions, where packed RBCs are transfused, type O individuals are considered to be universal donors. These relationships are summarized in Table 16-1.

Universal Donors
Universal donors have O type blood. Their RBCs have neither A nor B antigens on their surface. Therefore, these cells are not agglutinated by antibodies to antigen A or B, and it is safe to transfuse individuals having type A, B, AB, or O with RBCs from a type O donor. However, the serum from type O donors has antibodies to both A and B antigens and cannot be used.

TABLE 16-1 ▶

Correlation Between Blood Types, Enzymes, and Antibodies

Blood Type	Antigen on RBC	Glycosyltransferase Present	Antibodies in Serum
Type A	A	N-acetylgalactosaminyltransferase	Anti-B
Type B	B	Galactosyltransferase	Anti-A
Type AB	A and B	Both	Neither
Type O	O[a]	Neither	Anti-A and anti-B

[a] Also known as the H antigen

PROTEOGLYCANS AND GAGs

Typical Repeating Disaccharide Found in Glycosaminoglycans

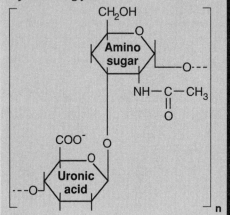

Silicon Cross-links in Proteoglycan Complexes

Silicon (Si) is found with a frequency of about one atom per 100 monosaccharide residues. R and R' are two different GAGs.

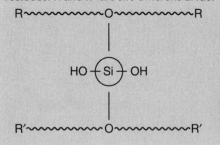

The major components of the *extracellular space* in mammalian tissues are proteoglycans and the fibrous proteins, collagen and elastin. Proteoglycans are found in high concentrations in cartilage, synovial fluid, vitreous humor, and skin. They are composed of GAG chains, hundreds of residues in length, that are tethered to a core protein by a linkage tetrasaccharide (Figure 16-5). The GAGs contain *repeating disaccharides*, in which one sugar is an amino sugar and the other, usually, a uronic acid. The disaccharide is negatively charged as a result of a carboxyl group on the uronic acids or sulfate groups on the amino sugar. The long linear carbohydrate polymers have a high density of *negative charge* and are *highly hydrated* with associated water comprising more than 50% of their weight. GAGs and proteoglycans can associate in highly organized complexes in the extracellular matrix, where they form a viscous *gel-like matrix* in which cells are embedded to form tissues.

Classes of GAGs

GAGs are grouped into five major classes on the basis of their characteristic repeating disaccharide unit. Some of the groups have subclasses that reflect differences in the site and extent of sulfation. The characteristic disaccharide composition for each of the GAGs and the tissue distribution are summarized in Table 16-2.

Hyaluronic acid is the only GAG that is not linked to a core protein. Other distinguishing features of hyaluronic acid are: (1) it is not sulfated, and (2) it is found in microorganisms as well as higher species. The primary function of hyaluronic acid is as a lubricant and shock absorber in the umbilical cord. *Chondroitin sulfate* is the most abundant of the GAGs. In cartilage, chondroitin sulfate, keratan sulfate, and hyaluronic acid associate noncovalently to form *aggregan*, a macromolecular complex with a molecular weight of 10^8 daltons or more. The properties of aggregan make it ideally suited for its role as a shock absorber and lubricant in resisting compression between bones. *Keratan sulfate* is unique in that it is the only GAG that contains neither glucuronic nor iduronic acid.

Heparin and *heparan sulfate* have the same repeating disaccharide but differ in their functions and localization. Heparin is an intracellular molecule, a feature that distinguishes it from the other GAGs. It is found in granules of mast cells that line the arteries of lungs, liver, spleen, and muscle. When released into the circulation, it acts as an anticoagulant. Heparan sulfate is found in the basement membranes and as a part of cell surfaces, where it plays a structural role. The names, however, are misleading; heparin is more highly sulfated than heparan sulfate. *Dermatan sulfate* is found primarily in the skin, heart vessels, and blood vessels. It contains more iduronic acid than glucuronic acid.

Synthesis of Proteoglycans

With the exception of hyaluronic acid, all of the GAGs are linked to a core protein by an *O*-glycosidic bond. Following the addition of the linkage tetrasaccharide, the GAG is assembled by the sequential addition of monosaccharides. The enzymes for transferring the sugars from high-energy nucleotide donors to the growing chain are all located in the Golgi membrane. The synthesis can be described as occurring in three parts: formation of a linkage tetrasaccharide, addition of the GAG chain, and modification of the GAG chain.

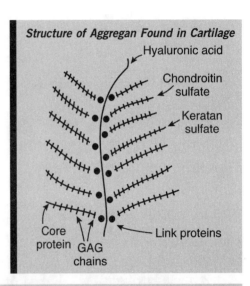

Structure of Aggrecan Found in Cartilage

—Serine —O—Xylose—Galactose —Galactose — Glucuronic — $\left[\begin{array}{cc}\text{Amino} & \text{Uronic} \\ \text{sugar} & \text{acid}\end{array}\right]_n$
                                          acid

| Protein | → | Linkage tetrasaccharide | ↔ | Gluco-saminoglycan | → |

▶ **FIGURE 16-5**

Structural Features of Proteoglycans. *The glycosaminoglycan (GAG) is tethered to the protein by a tetrasaccharide. The synthesis of all proteoglycans starts with the addition of xylose, galactose, galactose, and glucuronic acid to the protein. Diverse classes of proteoglycans are generated by the alternate addition of amino sugars and uronic acids to the linkage oligosaccharide. Different proteoglycans can be distinguished from one another by: (1) the composition of the repeating disaccharide, (2) the type of linkage between the components of the disaccharide, and (3) the type of linkages that exist between disaccharides.*

▶ **TABLE 16-2**

Composition and Distribution of Glycosaminoglycans

	Disaccharide		Tissue Distribution
	Uronic Acid	**Amino Sugar**	
Hyaluronic acid	Glucuronate	GlcNAc	Connective tissue, cartilage, synovial fluid, vitreous humor, and umbilical cord
Chondroitin sulfate	Glucuronate and iduronate	GalNAc-SO$_4$=	Cartilage, cornea, arteries, skin, and bones
Dermatan sulfate	Glucuronate and iduronate sulfate	GalNAc-SO$_4$=	Skin, blood vessels, and heart valves
Keratan sulfate	Galactose sulfate[a]	GlcNAc-SO$_4$=	Cartilage, intervertebral discs, and cornea
Heparan sulfate	Glucuronate and iduronate sulfate	GlcNAc-SO$_4$=	Cell surfaces, lungs, and blood vessels
Heparin	Glucuronate and iduronate sulfate	GlcNAc-SO$_4$=	Mast cells (lung, liver, skin)

Note. GlcNAc = *N*-acetylglucosamine; GalNAc = *N*-acetylgalactosamine.
[a] Galactose found instead of either glucuronate or iduronate.

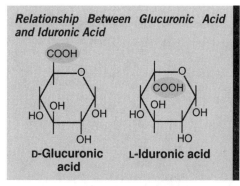

Relationship Between Glucuronic Acid and Iduronic Acid

D-Glucuronic acid

L-Iduronic acid

3'-Phosphoadenosine-5'-Phosphosulfate: The Activated Donor of Sulfate in Biologic Sulfation Reactions

Phosphoadenosinephosphosulfate (PAPS)

Two types of *modification reactions* occur after the GAG chain has been formed. *Epimerization* of glucuronic acid residues results in the formation of iduronic acid. The epimerase alters the configuration of the carboxyl group around C-5 of glucuronic acid residues. *Sulfation* of all the amino sugars and some of the iduronic acids occurs in a reaction that requires 3'-phosphoadenosine-5'phosphosulfate (PAPS), the high-energy donor of sulfate. The factors that determine which monosaccharides are sulfated and which are epimerized are not well understood.

Degradation of Proteoglycans

Proteoglycans are taken up from the extracellular matrix by the invagination of the cell membrane surrounding the GAGs or proteoglycans, thereby producing intracellular vacuoles. The vacuoles then fuse with lysosomes, and degradation is achieved within the lysosome by the action of a family of acid hydrolases. In adult tissues, the turnover of glycoproteoglycans is relatively slow, having half-lives ranging from days to weeks. Degradation of GAGs requires the concerted action of several specific *endoglycosidases, exoglycosidases, and sulfatases.*

Deficiencies in all of the enzymes required for GAG degradation have been reported, resulting in a family of inherited diseases known as the *mucopolysaccharidoses* (e.g., MPS I, MPS II, and so on) [Table 16-3]. These diseases are progressive and frequently result in severe musculoskeletal deformities. The inheritance is autosomal recessive, except for Hunter's syndrome, which is X-linked. The mucopolysaccharidoses are characterized by the accumulation of GAGs in various tissues and the excretion of partially degraded oligosaccharides in urine. The chemical nature of the excreted product is useful in predicting the specific enzyme deficiency. Confirmation can be made by directly assaying fibroblasts for the enzyme. Prenatal diagnosis is possible for all of the mucopolysaccharidoses.

TABLE 16-3
The Mucopolysaccharidoses: Biochemical and Clinical Characteristics

Type	Enzyme Defect	Urinary Metabolites	Clinical Findings
MPS I H: Hurler's syndrome	α-L-Iduronidase	Dermatan sulfate and heparan sulfate	Skeletal deformities, mental retardation, and corneal clouding
MPS II: Hunter's syndrome	Iduronate sulfatase	Dermatan sulfate and heparan sulfate	Skeletal deformities, mental retardation, and deafness
MPS III: Sanfilippo's syndrome, type A	Heparan sulfatase	Heparan sulfate	Mental retardation and mild skeletal changes
Sanfilippo's syndrome, type B	α-N-Acetylglucosaminidase	Heparan sulfate	Mental retardation and mild skeletal changes
MPS IV: Morquio's syndrome, type A	N-Acetylgalactosamine-6-sulfatase	Keratan sulfate	Severe skeletal deformities and corneal clouding
Morquio's syndrome, type B	β-Galactosidase	Keratan sulfate	Severe skeletal deformities
MPS VII: Sly's syndrome	β-D-Glucuronidase	Dermatan sulfate and heparan sulfate	Mental retardation

RESOLUTION OF CLINICAL CASE

Kevin was diagnosed with Hunter's syndrome (also known as MPS II) on the basis of enzyme analysis that showed less than 5% of the normal iduronate sulfatase activity. In the enzyme assay, radiolabeled dermatan sulfate is added to extracts of fibroblasts or leukocytes, and the release of [^{35}S]sulfate is measured over a period of time. The GAGs that accumulate with this deficiency are heparan and dermatan sulfates. Both GAGs contain iduronate sulfate. Typical symptoms of Hunter's syndrome include coarse facial features, short stature, skeletal deformities, stiffness of joints, mental retardation, and skin lesions [1], all of which affected Kevin at some time during the progression of his disease. In most patients, persistent nasal discharge, chronic ear infections, and progressive loss of hearing occur as well. The usual cause of death is either obstructive airway disease or cardiovascular disease. There are severe and mild forms of Hunter's. In the mild form, individuals can live into late adulthood with little impairment of intelligence. There is no specific therapy for Hunter's syndrome. Management consists of supportive care and management of complications. Hunter's syndrome is the only one of the mucopolysaccharidoses that has been shown to have an X-linked inheritance pattern.

REVIEW QUESTIONS

Directions: For each of the following questions, choose the **one best** answer.

1. The oligosaccharide chains of enzymes targeted for lysosomes contain which of the following substances?

    (A) Fucose

    (B) *N*-Acetylgalactosamine (GalNAc)

    (C) Mannose-6-phosphate

    (D) *N*-Acetylglucosamine-6-phosphate

    (E) Sialic acid

2. Glycosaminoglycans (GAGs) have which of the following characteristics?

    (A) They are positively charged

    (B) They contain branched oligosaccharide chains

    (C) They rarely contain sulfate groups

    (D) They contain repeating disaccharides

    (E) They span the plasma membrane of cells

3. In individuals with I-cell disease, which of the following findings would be expected?

    (A) Oligosaccharides cannot be added to asparagine residues of acceptor proteins

    (B) Lysosomal enzymes are found in the serum

    (C) *N*-Acetylglucosaminylphosphoglycosidase is deficient

    (D) Large inclusion bodies are found in the extracellular matrix

    (E) Enzymes are incorrectly targeted to mitochondria

4. UDP–glucuronic acid is required for the synthesis of

    (A) *N*-linked glycoproteins

    (B) keratan sulfate

    (C) *O*-linked glycoproteins

    (D) hyaluronic acid

    (E) bilirubin

5. Dolichol is best described by which of the following statements?

    (A) It is required for the synthesis of *O*-linked oligosaccharides

    (B) It is a carrier for *N*-acetylglucosamine (GlcNAc) in glycoprotein synthesis

    (C) It is required in the synthesis of *N*-linked glycoproteins

    (D) It is a carrier of sialic acid in glycoprotein synthesis

    (E) It is synthesized from intermediates in glycolysis

ANSWERS AND EXPLANATIONS

1. The answer is C. Mannose-6-phosphate is recognized by a specific membrane-bound receptor in the Golgi where sorting occurs. The first step in phosphorylation of mannose residues is the covalent attachment of *N*-acetylglucosamine-6-phosphate to the mannose, but this does not target the protein to lysosomes. The GalNAc has to be removed, leaving only phosphate attached to the mannose before sorting can occur. Fucose and sialic acid are added to complex oligosaccharides in the Golgi, where both serve as signals to stop further monosaccharide addition. GalNAc is found in *O*-linked oligosaccharides and has nothing to do with lysosomal targeting.

2. The answer is D. Each GAG contains its own characteristic repeating disaccharide. These molecules are highly negatively charged because of the presence of sulfate and carboxyl groups. GAGs are found in the extracellular matrix. The only exception to this is heparin, which is located in granules of mast cells.

3. The answer is B. The absence of mannose-6-phosphate results in a sorting error that allows acid hydrolases to be secreted into the serum but has little effect on the catalytic activity of these enzymes. Synthesis of the core oligosaccharide and transfer to asparagine occur normally. The deficient enzyme in I-cell disease is *N*-acetylglucosaminylphosphotransferase, not *N*-acetylglucosaminylphosphoglycosidase. The first of these enzymes catalyzes the addition of *N*-acetylglucosamine-phosphate to mannose, and the second enzyme catalyzes the hydrolysis of *N*-acetylglucosamine, leaving the phosphate group attached to mannose. Inclusion bodies found in the cytosol are lysosomes that are filled with unhydrolyzed proteoglycans.

4. The answer is D. UDP–glucuronic acid is required for the synthesis of all glycosaminoglycans except keratan sulfate. It is not required for either *N*- or *O*-linked glycoprotein synthesis. The iduronic acid found in heparan, keratan, and chondroitin sulfates also has its origin in UDP–glucuronic acid. After the polysaccharide chain has been synthesized, some glucuronate residues are epimerized to iduronate. UDP–glucuronic acid is not required for bilirubin synthesis, although it is used to increase its solubility.

5. The answer is C. Dolichol is a special lipid that plays two roles in the synthesis of *N*-linked glycoprotein synthesis: (1) the core oligosaccharide is assembled on a dolichol phosphate carrier, and (2) dolichol phosphate is an activated donor of glucose and mannose residues. The activated carriers for GlcNAc and sialic acid are UDP-GlcNAc and cytidine monophosphate (CMP)–sialic acid, respectively. Dolichol is synthesized by polymerization of isoprenoid intermediates. These intermediates are derived from acetyl coenzyme A and are also used as intermediates in cholesterol synthesis. Dolichol plays no role in *O*-linked oligosaccharide synthesis.

REFERENCES

1. Neufeld EF, Muenzer J: The mucopolysaccharidoses. In *Metabolic and Molecular Bases of Inherited Disease*, 7th ed. Edited by Scriver CR, Beaudet AL, Sly WS, et al. New York, NY: McGraw-Hill, 1995, pp 2473–2474.

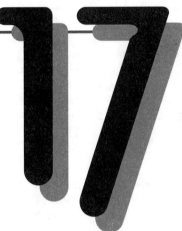

CONNECTIONS BETWEEN METABOLIC PATHWAYS

CHAPTER OUTLINE

INTRODUCTION

The preceding chapters introduced the major pathways of carbohydrate metabolism, with the primary focus on the physiologic function of each pathway and the mechanisms by which the pathways are regulated. The beginning or the end of most of these pathways can be traced to glucose, the major monosaccharide derived from dietary sources. Additionally, there are feeder pathways that convert galactose and fructose to intermediates in the pathways of glucose metabolism. The goal of the current chapter is to integrate the pathways of carbohydrate metabolism into a broader context of physiology with specific emphasis on: (1) how the major pathways of carbohydrate metabolism are integrated with one another and (2) how carbohydrate metabolism is integrated with the major pathways of lipid metabolism.

BRANCH POINTS THAT CONNECT THE PATHWAYS OF CARBOHYDRATE METABOLISM

Glycolysis is the central pathway of carbohydrate metabolism, common to all living cells. It starts with glucose, proceeds through several intermediates, and ends with pyruvate. In some tissues, the primary function of glycolysis is to generate adenosine triphosphate (ATP), while in others, the major purpose is to provide intermediates that serve as branch points or intersections where other metabolic pathways meet, begin, or end. Major intersections in glycolysis are occupied by glucose-6-phosphate (G6P) and pyruvate. Minor intersections are occupied by fructose-6-phosphate (F6P) and the triose phosphates, glyceraldehyde-3-phosphate (G3P) and dihydroxyacetone phosphate (DHAP). Most of the pathways of carbohydrate metabolism are connected by one of these compounds, as shown in Figure 17-1.

Glucose-6-Phosphate (G6P)

The uptake of glucose by a cell is followed by its rapid conversion to G6P, a compound that sits at the crossroads of several pathways of carbohydrate metabolism. G6P is a common precursor for intermediates in glycolysis, glycogenesis, glycogenolysis, the pentose phosphate pathway, and gluconeogenesis.

Fructose-6-Phosphate (F6P). The conversion of G6P to F6P is the first step that directs G6P along the pathway of glycolysis, leading to pyruvate. In most cells, F6P is converted primarily to pyruvate, although a small fraction is used as a precursor for the synthesis of the amino sugars, *N*-acetylglucosamine (GlcNAc) and *N*-acetylgalactosamine (GalNAc).

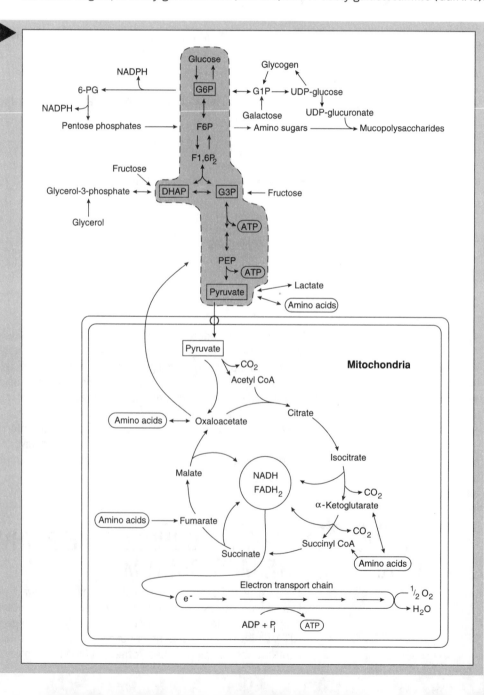

FIGURE 17-1

Connections Between the Pathways of Carbohydrate Metabolism. *The intermediates in glycolysis are shaded. Glucose-6-phosphate is a major intersection that connects glycogen metabolism, pentose phosphate synthesis, and gluconeogenesis with glycolysis, all occurring in the cytosol. Complete oxidation of glucose requires that pyruvate enter the mitochondria and be converted to acetyl CoA before terminal oxidation by the citric acid cycle can occur. The citric acid cycle also provides a major mechanism for integrating amino acid metabolism with carbohydrate metabolism. Most of the amino acids can be degraded to some intermediate in the cycle, and these intermediates get converted to oxaloacetate, an intermediate that is shared by the citric acid cycle and the pathway of gluconeogenesis. 6-PG = 6-phosphogluconate; G6P = glucose-6-phosphate; G1P = glucose-1-phosphate; UDP-glucose = uridine diphosphate–glucose; UDP-glucuronate = uridine diphosphate–glucuronate; F6P = fructose-6-phosphate; F1,6P$_2$ = fructose-1,6-bisphosphate; ATP = adenosine triphosphate; G3P = glyceraldehyde-3-phosphate; DHAP = dihydroxyacetone phosphate; PEP = phosphoenolpyruvate; NADPH = reduced form of nicotinamide-adenine dinucleotide phosphate; NADH = reduced form of nicotinamide adenine dinucleotide; FADH$_2$ = reduced form of flavin adenine dinucleotide; ADP = adenosine diphosphate; P$_i$ = inorganic phosphate.*

The amino sugars are major building blocks for the mucopolysaccharides that form the ground substance of connective tissue.

Glucose-1-Phosphate (G1P). The isomerization of G6P to G1P forms an intersection where glycolysis and glycogen metabolism merge. G1P is a common intermediate in both glycogenesis and glycogenolysis. Additionally, galactose gains entry into the pathways of glucose metabolism by being converted to G1P. Uridine diphosphate–glucose (UDP-glucose), a key intermediate in glycogenesis, can be oxidized to uridine diphosphate–glucuronic acid (UDP-glucuronic acid), forming a minor branch point that feeds into the pathway of mucopolysaccharide synthesis.

6-Phosphogluconate (6-PG). The oxidation of G6P to 6-PG initiates the pentose phosphate pathway, which produces almost all of the cellular NADPH and pentose phosphates. If the demand for NADPH exceeds the demand for pentose phosphates, the excess intermediates reenter the pathway of glycolysis by being converted to F6P.

Glucose. The hydrolysis of G6P to glucose is the final step in the pathway of gluconeogenesis. This pathway converts a diverse set of low-molecular-weight precursors, including lactate, glycerol, and most of the amino acids, to glucose. All of the intermediates in gluconeogenesis are also intermediates in glycolysis, and all of the enzymes in glycolysis that catalyze reversible reactions work in reverse in gluconeogenesis. Lactate enters the pathway by being converted to pyruvate, and glycerol enters by being converted to DHAP. Some amino acids enter gluconeogenesis by conversion to pyruvate, while others are converted to various intermediates in the citric acid cycle, also called the tricarboxylic acid (TCA) or Krebs cycle. These intermediates exit the cycle as oxaloacetate, which is translocated into the cytosol and converted to phosphoenolpyruvate (PEP). Clearly, the citric acid cycle is of major importance in integrating gluconeogenesis with the pathways of amino acid catabolism.

Pyruvate

Pyruvate is a pivotal intersection in metabolism where several pathways of carbohydrate and amino acid metabolism merge. It is a common precursor for several compounds that are intermediates in various metabolic pathways. These compounds include oxaloacetate, acetyl coenzyme A (acetyl CoA), lactate, and several amino acids. All of these compounds, except lactate, link one or more metabolic pathways together. Some of the linkages occur in mitochondria, while others occur in the cytosol.

Oxaloacetate. The mitochondrial carboxylation of pyruvate produces oxaloacetate, a compound that has several metabolic fates. It can condense with acetyl CoA to form citrate, the intermediate that allows acetyl CoA to be oxidized to carbon dioxide by the citric acid cycle. Alternatively, oxaloacetate can be translocated from the mitochondria to the cytosol where it is converted to PEP, an intermediate in gluconeogenesis. And finally, oxaloacetate can be used in the synthesis of a few nonessential amino acids.

Acetyl CoA. The decarboxylation of pyruvate produces acetyl CoA, a compound that forms a bridge linking glycolysis with the citric acid cycle. This reaction occurs in the mitochondria and is essential in cells and tissues that derive most of their energy from the oxidation of glucose to carbon dioxide and water. Most of the energy contained in the acetyl CoA molecule is found in the electron pairs that form the C–H and C–C bonds of the molecule. During the oxidation of acetyl CoA by the citric acid cycle, the energy-rich electron pairs are transferred to NADH and $FADH_2$. The energy that is transiently stored in NADH and $FADH_2$ is subsequently released by transfer of the electrons through the electron transport chain and used to drive the synthesis of ATP.

Lactate. The reduction of pyruvate to lactate occurs in cells that have a limited capacity for oxidative metabolism, either because they contain few mitochondria, or because they are experiencing an oxygen deficit. Under these conditions, the cell or tissue becomes almost totally dependent on anaerobic glycolysis for ATP synthesis. The reduction of pyruvate to lactate allows the oxidized form of nicotinamide adenine dinucleotide (NAD^+) to be regenerated, a condition that must be met if anaerobic glycolysis is to continue. Lactate is a dead-end compound that can only be converted back to pyruvate.

Amino Acids. Pyruvate can serve as the precursor for several nonessential amino acids, thereby forming an intersection between glycolysis and amino acid metabolism. Most of the amino acids that can be degraded to pyruvate for use in gluconeogenesis can also be synthesized from pyruvate.

Triose Phosphates

The triose phosphates, DHAP and G3P both serve as minor, but important, branch points in carbohydrate metabolism. Fructose gains entry into the pathways of glucose metabolism by being converted to DHAP and G3P.

BRANCH POINTS THAT CONNECT CARBOHYDRATE METABOLISM WITH LIPID METABOLISM

Three intermediates in metabolism form important branch points or intersections that connect the major pathways of carbohydrate and lipid metabolism. These intermediates are: (1) acetyl CoA, a compound formed in the mitochondria from the oxidation of either pyruvate or fatty acids; (2) citrate, an intermediate in the citric acid cycle; and (3) glycerol-3-phosphate, a compound formed by the reduction of DHAP. Additionally, the conversion of pyruvate to oxaloacetate plays a critical role in oxidative metabolism by replenishing intermediates in the citric acid cycle. These interrelationships are illustrated in Figure 17-2.

Acetyl CoA

Acetyl CoA is a common product resulting from the mitochondrial oxidation of metabolic fuels. Pyruvate, fatty acids, and many of the amino acids derived from protein can be oxidized to acetyl CoA. The fate of acetyl CoA is determined largely by the energy status of the cell or tissue. If energy is needed, acetyl CoA is further oxidized by the citric acid cycle. If hepatic fatty acid oxidation produces acetyl CoA faster than it is used by the citric acid cycle, the excess is converted to ketones that can be transported to extrahepatic tissues and used as fuel. If there is excess dietary carbohydrate, the pyruvate produced by glycolysis is converted to acetyl CoA, and the acetyl CoA is used for fatty acid synthesis.

Citrate

Citrate links carbohydrate metabolism with fatty acid and cholesterol synthesis by serving as a carrier of acetyl CoA groups from the mitochondrial matrix to the cytosol. The pyruvate derived from excess dietary carbohydrate is converted to acetyl CoA in the mitochondrial matrix. However, the pathways of lipid synthesis from acetyl CoA occur in the cytosol. Since acetyl CoA is unable to cross the inner mitochondrial membrane, it condenses with oxaloacetate, forming citrate, which is readily transported across the membrane and cleaved, releasing acetyl CoA in the cytosolic compartment.

Glycerol-3-Phosphate

The reduction of DHAP produces glycerol-3-phosphate, an intermediate that links glycolysis with triglyceride and phospholipid synthesis. The glycerol backbone of both triglycerides and phospholipids is dependent on a source of glucose and the pathway of glycolysis. Glycerol, resulting from triglyceride hydrolysis in adipose tissue, is converted to glycerol-3-phosphate by the liver and used as a substrate for glucose synthesis.

Oxaloacetate

One of the characteristics of all metabolic cycles is that the intermediates get regenerated with each turn of the cycle. However, if intermediates are removed from the cycle, it will eventually cease to operate. There are a number of synthetic pathways that use intermediates in the citric acid cycle as substrates, thereby necessitating mechanisms for replenishing the intermediates. The carboxylation of pyruvate to oxaloacetate is the

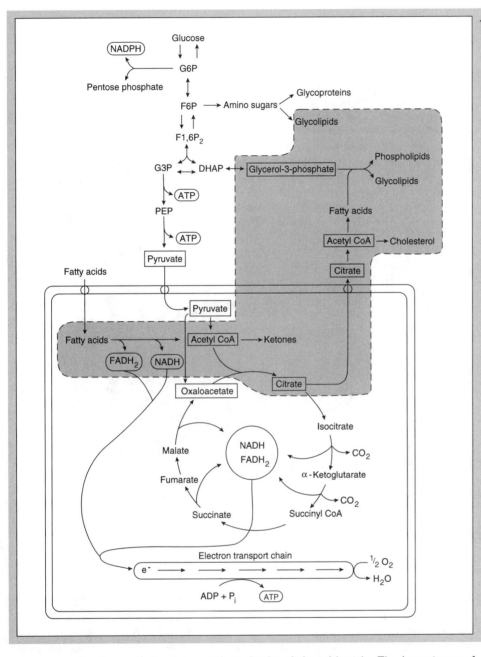

▶ FIGURE 17-2
Connections Between Pathways of Carbohydrate Metabolism and Lipid Metabolism. *The major pathways of lipid metabolism are shaded. Fatty acid oxidation occurs in the mitochondria, while both fatty acid and cholesterol synthesis occur in the cytosol. The substrate for lipogenesis is the acetyl CoA that is derived from excess carbohydrate. Glycolysis converts glucose to pyruvate, which is transported across the mitochondrial membrane and converted to acetyl CoA. Citrate acts as a shuttle for moving acetyl CoA from the mitochondrial compartment to the cytosolic compartment. Newly synthesized fatty acids are converted to triglycerides for storage or to phospholipids for membrane synthesis. G6P = glucose-6-phosphate; F6P = fructose-6-phosphate; $F1,6P_2$ = fructose-1,6-bisphosphate; DHAP = dihydroxyacetone phosphate; PEP = phosphoenolpyruvate.*

primary reaction for replacing intermediates in the citric acid cycle. The importance of this reaction is reflected in the expression "fat burns in the flame of carbohydrate," a reminder that the terminal oxidation of acetyl CoA (and fatty acids) by the citric acid cycle occurs only if there is an adequate supply of oxaloacetate, which, in turn, relies on pyruvate derived from glycolysis.

HORMONAL SIGNALS INTEGRATE CARBOHYDRATE, LIPID, AND PROTEIN METABOLISM

One of the major challenges of metabolism is to maintain a constant level of glucose in the blood, even though there may be long periods during which dietary carbohydrate is unavailable. The major consumers that are most dependent on glucose are the red blood cells (RBCs), brain, and central nervous system (CNS). The ability to maintain a constant blood glucose level depends on a multiorgan response involving the liver, muscle, and adipose tissue (Figure 17-3).

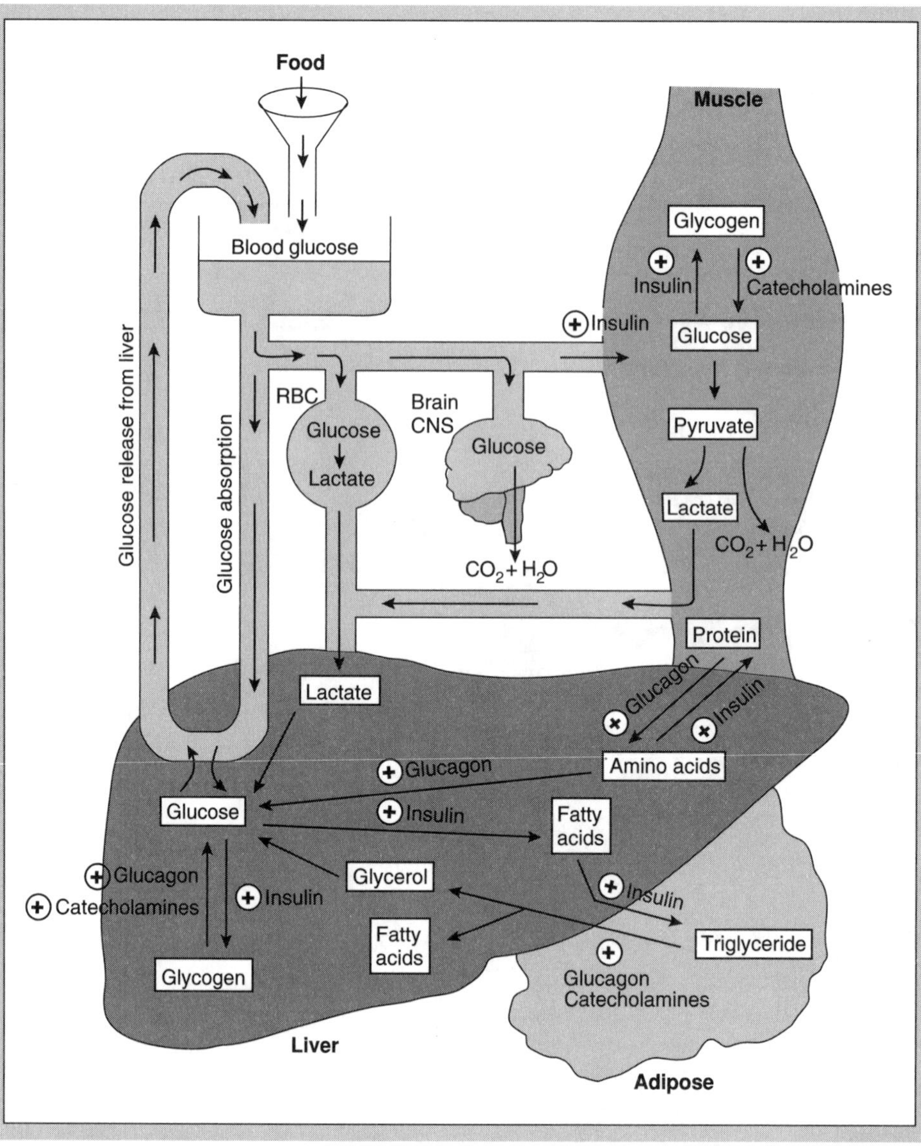

FIGURE 17-3 ▶

Role of Hormones in Fuel Storage, Mobilization, and Distribution. After a meal, insulin stimulates the pathways of fuel storage, including glycogen synthesis in liver and muscle tissue, fatty acid and triglyceride synthesis in liver and adipose tissue, and amino acid uptake and protein synthesis in muscle tissue. Between meals, fuel mobilization is stimulated by glucagon and epinephrine. Catecholamines stimulate glycogen degradation and the release of lactate from muscle tissue, and lipolysis in adipose tissue. Both glucagon and the catecholamines stimulate glycogen degradation and gluconeogenesis in the liver. The minute-to-minute regulation of fuel mobilization, distribution, and storage allows blood glucose levels to be maintained within a very narrow concentration range.

The liver is primarily responsible for the distribution of nutrients. In the well-fed state, excess glucose is converted to glycogen, and when the glycogen stores are filled, the remaining glucose is used for fatty acid synthesis. The fatty acids are subsequently stored as triglyceride in adipose tissue. In the fasting state, the primary role of the liver in carbohydrate metabolism is to supply glucose to the blood by way of glycogenolysis and gluconeogenesis. The precursors for gluconeogenesis are: (1) lactate, derived from anaerobic glycolysis in the RBC and skeletal muscle; (2) glycerol, derived from triglyceride hydrolysis in adipose tissue; and (3) amino acids, derived from protein degradation in skeletal muscle. Fatty acids, derived from lipolysis in adipose tissue, are oxidized by the liver to supply the ATP required for gluconeogenesis.

The hormones primarily responsible for coordinating the synthesis, storage, and distribution of glucose are insulin, glucagon, and the catecholamines. The effects of insulin are opposed by the effects of glucagon and the catecholamines, as shown in Figure 17-3.

Insulin

Insulin is an anabolic hormone that promotes storage of excess glucose following a meal. Insulin stimulates glycogenesis and fatty acid synthesis in the liver, triglyceride synthesis in adipose tissue, and glucose uptake and glycogenesis in muscle tissue. The uptake of amino acids, as well as protein synthesis in muscle tissue, is also stimulated by insulin.

Glucagon

Glucagon is a catabolic hormone that promotes the release of glucose into the blood by the liver between meals. Glycogenolysis and gluconeogenesis are both stimulated by glucagon. Protein degradation in muscle supplies the liver with carbon skeletons that are used as substrates for gluconeogenesis, while lipolysis in adipose tissue supplies the liver with glycerol that is converted to glucose and fatty acids that are oxidized for generating ATP.

Catecholamines

The catecholamines, like glucagon, oppose the action of insulin by promoting the release of glucose into the blood. The catecholamines directly stimulate glycogenolysis and gluconeogenesis in the liver, lipolysis in adipose tissue, and the release of amino acids and lactate by muscle tissue. Additionally, the catecholamines modulate the levels of the other two hormones by stimulating the release of glucagon by pancreatic α-cells and inhibiting the release of insulin by pancreatic β-cells.

REVIEW QUESTIONS

Directions: The groups of questions below consist of lettered choices followed by several numbered items. For each numbered item, select the appropriate lettered option with which it is most closely associated. Each lettered option may be used once, more than once, or not at all.

Questions 1–5

For each description below, select the compound with which it is most closely associated.

    (A) 6-Phosphogluconate (6-PG)

    (B) Glucose

    (C) Glucose-1-phosphate (G1P)

    (D) Glucose-6-phosphate (G6P)

    (E) Fructose-6-phosphate (F6P)

    (F) Dihydroxyacetone phosphate (DHAP)

1. The intermediate common to glycogenesis and glycogenolysis

2. The precursor of amino sugars

3. The first intermediate committed to the pentose phosphate pathway

4. The intermediate that connects galactose and glucose metabolism

5. The intermediate that connects fructose and glucose metabolism

Questions 6–10

For each description below, select the compound with which it is most closely associated.

    (A) Oxaloacetate

    (B) Pyruvate

    (C) Citrate

    (D) Dihydroxyacetone phosphate (DHAP)

    (E) Glycerol-3-phosphate

    (F) Succinyl CoA

    (G) Acetyl CoA

6. A compound that links glycolysis with the citric acid cycle

7. A compound that allows acetyl CoA to be translocated from the mitochondrial matrix to the cytosol

8. A compound that donates the glycerol backbone to both phospholipids and triglycerides

9. A common intermediate in fatty acid and cholesterol synthesis

10. An intermediate in the citric acid cycle that links amino acid metabolism with gluconeogenesis

ANSWERS AND EXPLANATIONS

1–5. The answers are: 1-C, 2-E, 3-A, 4-C, 5-F. G1P is required for glycogenesis and is the product of glycogenolysis. F6P is the precursor of *N*-acetylglucosamine and *N*-acetylgalactosamine, the two primary amino sugars. The first intermediate that is committed to the pentose phosphate pathway is 6-PG. It has no other significant function in human biochemistry. Galactose metabolism by the liver produces G1P, a compound that links the pathways of glucose and galactose metabolism. The metabolism of fructose by the liver produces DHAP and glyceraldehyde-3-phosphate, both intermediates in glycolysis. G6P is derived from glucose and is the immediate precursor of 6-GP, F6P, and G1P.

6–10. The answers are: 6-G, 7-C, 8-E, 9-G, 10-A. Acetyl CoA forms a bridge linking glycolysis with the citric acid cycle. It is derived from pyruvate, the end product of glycolysis, and it is the substrate for the citric acid cycle. Citrate acts as a carrier of acetyl CoA groups across the inner mitochondrial membrane. It is formed from acetyl CoA in the mitochondrial matrix and is cleaved, releasing acetyl CoA after being transported to the cytosol. Glycerol-3-phosphate is the donor of the glycerol backbone in both phospholipid and triglyceride synthesis. It is formed by the reduction of DHAP. Acetyl CoA is a common intermediate in the pathways of fatty acid and cholesterol synthesis. Oxaloacetate is an intermediate in both the citric acid cycle and gluconeogenesis. It is also produced by the catabolism of aspartic acid and asparagine. Several other amino acids are degraded to succinyl CoA, which can also be used as a substrate for gluconeogenesis, but succinyl CoA must first be converted to oxaloacetate, which is then translocated to the cytosol and converted to phosphoenolphosphate.

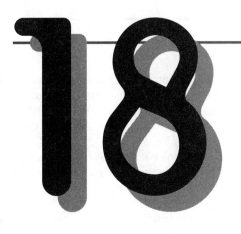

18

INTRODUCTION TO LIPID METABOLISM: DIGESTION AND ABSORPTION OF DIETARY FAT

CHAPTER OUTLINE

INTRODUCTION OF CLINICAL CASE

A 15-year-old girl was brought to the hospital by her aunt because of chronic diarrhea and a persistent cough. She had been diagnosed with cystic fibrosis 3 years earlier on the basis of a positive sweat test and no fecal tryptic activity. At that time, pancreatic extracts and multivitamins were prescribed. However, she did not keep any of her clinic appointments and was not seen again until the current admission. The patient reported that she had continued to take pancreatic extracts and vitamins until 6 months ago, when her parents were divorced, and she came to live with her aunt. Her aunt said that she did not know about the prior diagnosis, and that her niece had not been taking any medications during the last 6 months. The patient was admitted to the hospital for further examination. Sputum cultures revealed the presence of *Pseudomonas aeruginosa*, and she was started on an antibiotic immediately. Although her aunt said that she had a hearty appetite, the patient's height was 59″, and she weighed 82 lbs. She complained of dry eyes and poor night vision. Absorption studies showed a loss of 40% of fat intake. Laboratory analysis showed a serum vitamin A concentration of 0.4 µg/dL (normal: 150 µg/dL). An ophthalmologic consultation confirmed that the patient had night blindness and diminished day vision. She was treated with oral pancreatic enzymes and multi-vitamins, plus an additional 10,000 units of vitamin A per day. A diet was recommended that was high in protein, milk, and butter but low in other fats. Within 6 weeks, she had gained 5 lbs, her cough was gone, and her vision was almost normal.

LIPID METABOLISM AND HUMAN DISEASE

Lipids are essential to the structure and maintenance of living cells, where they serve as structural components of membranes, the major source of energy, and precursors to a variety of specialized regulatory molecules, such as steroid hormones, prostaglandins, and leukotrienes. Many human diseases involve disorders in lipid metabolism that can affect people either early or late in life and may be either mild or fatal. Some disorders, such as atherosclerosis and obesity, develop over many years and may have both genetic and environmental components, whereas others may involve a specific genetic mutation that can be detected in utero [1]. Some of the disorders in lipid metabolism are summarized in Table 18-1. In addition to the disorders listed, there are several commonly occurring diseases involving the metabolism of lipoproteins that are discussed in Chapter 19.

TABLE 18-1 ▶
Disorders in Lipid Metabolism

Disorders	Accumulated Lipid	Characteristic Features
Common disorders		
Obesity	Triglyceride (adipose tissue)	High risk for heart disease and diabetes
Atherosclerosis	Cholesterol (blood)	High risk for heart disease and stroke
Fatty liver	Triglyceride (liver)	Caused by chronic alcohol intake
Cholelithiasis	Gallstones (bile)	Impaired lipid absorption
Ketoacidosis	Ketones (blood)	Occurs in uncontrolled diabetes, starvation, and alcoholism
Rare disorders		
Carnitine deficiency	Triglyceride (many cells)	Impaired fatty acid oxidation
Sphingolipidoses	Partially degraded sphingolipids	Specific lysosomal hydrolase deficiency
Refsum's disease	Branched-chain fatty acids (brain)	Specific peroxisomal enzyme deficiency

CLASSIFICATION OF LIPIDS

The biologically important lipids are both structurally and functionally diverse, and they can be classified into six major groups: fatty acids, triglycerides, ketones, cholesterol, phospholipids, and sphingolipids (Table 18-2). Minor classes of lipids include bile acids, steroid hormones, fat-soluble vitamins, and the eicosanoids. Abnormalities in lipid transport, metabolism, or both are found in many human diseases including obesity, hyperlipidemias, diabetes, and sphingolipidoses. This chapter introduces generic structures and nomenclature for the major classes of lipids (Figure 18-1). The digestion and absorption of dietary lipid are also discussed.

TABLE 18-2
Lipids and Their Functions

Class	Function
Fatty acids	Metabolic fuel, precursors for eicosanoids, and building blocks for phospholipids and sphingolipids
Triglycerides	Storage form and major transport form of fatty acids
Ketones	Soluble metabolic fuel for skeletal muscle, heart, kidney, and brain
Cholesterol	Structural component of plasma membrane and precursor for steroid hormones, vitamin D, and bile acids
Phospholipids	Major building blocks of membranes, storage sites for polyunsaturated fatty acids, and components of signal transduction pathways
Sphingolipids	Structural components of membranes and surface antigens

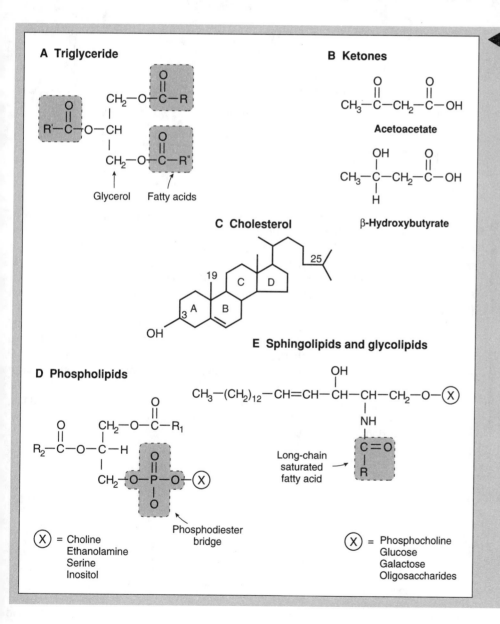

FIGURE 18-1

Structures of Major Classes of Lipids. (A) Triglycerides contain three fatty acids esterified to a glycerol backbone. (B) Ketones are small water-soluble acids. β-Hydroxybutyrate is the reduced form of acetoacetate. (C) Cholesterol has a fused four-ring nucleus that has an 8-carbon side chain attached to the D ring, and a hydroxyl group attached to the A ring. The hydroxyl group is usually esterified with a fatty acid. (D) Phospholipids are made up of two alcohols, which are linked by a phosphodiester bridge. One alcohol is always diacylglycerol, and the other, designated as X, varies. (E) Sphingolipids contain a long-chain amino alcohol. The amino group always has a long-chain saturated fatty acid attached by an amide bond, and the terminal hydroxyl group has varying substituents, designated as X.

Fatty Acids

Fatty acids serve as a major fuel for most cells, and they are precursors for all other classes of lipids. Fatty acids have a carboxyl group at one end and a hydrocarbon chain of varying length at the other end, making them amphipathic molecules. Fatty acids are rarely found free in cells, rather they are found as derivatives of coenzyme A (CoA) or as components of more complex structures, such as triglycerides, phospholipids, and sphingolipids.

Numbering Systems. Fatty acid metabolism uses two numbering systems. The *C-numbering system* starts at the carboxyl end, with the carboxyl group being C-1. Using this system, the α-carbon is always adjacent to the carboxyl group. The *ω-numbering system*, which is used widely by nutritionists, starts at the methyl end of the fatty acid and proceeds toward the carboxyl end. These numbering systems are illustrated below.

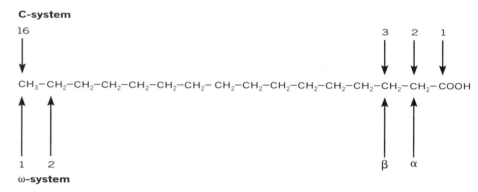

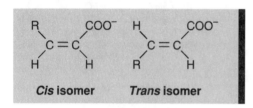

Cis isomer   Trans isomer

Unsaturated Fatty Acids. Two types of fatty acids occur in nature, saturated and unsaturated. Saturated fatty acids have no double bonds, while unsaturated fatty acids are either *monounsaturated*, having one double bond, or *polyunsaturated*, having two or more double bonds. Almost all naturally occurring fatty acids exist as the *cis isomers*, although *trans isomers* are intermediates in the oxidation of fatty acids. The polyunsaturated fatty acids (PUFAs) are further classified as either ω-3, ω-6, or ω-9, depending on the position of the double bond from the ω-end.

The nomenclature for designating the positions of double bonds in fatty acids is illustrated below with the structure of linoleic acid, a fatty acid with 18 carbons and two double bonds. Using the C-numbering system, one double bond is between carbons 9 and 10, and the other is between carbons 12 and 13. The abbreviated description of linoleic acid is C18:2(Δ9,12), where the number immediately following C is the total number of carbons, the number following the colon is the total number of double bonds, and the numbers in parenthesis indicate the position of the double bond, with the first carbon of each double bond given. Some designations include Δ to indicate double bonds, whereas in others the Δ is omitted.

Polyunsaturated Fatty Acids
Fish oils contain high concentrations of ω-3 fatty acids, whereas ω-6 and ω-9 fatty acids are present in high amounts in vegetable fat.

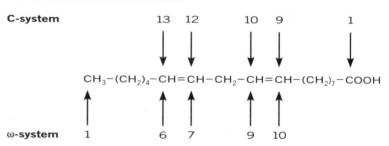

Using the ω-system, linoleic acid is described simply as having double bonds at ω-6 and ω-9 carbons.

Essential Fatty Acids. Three PUFAs are particularly important in human physiology: linoleic acid, linolenic acid, and arachidonic acid. Linoleic and linolenic acids are essential fatty acids that must be supplied by the diet. Arachidonic acid can be synthesized from linoleic acid and is essential only if there is a deficiency in linoleic acid. These

Essential Fatty Acid Deficiency
A deficiency of linoleic or linolenic acid in the diet causes skin lesions, loss of hair, weight loss, leaky red blood cells, kidney damage, sterility, and possibly death.

PUFAs are precursors for prostaglandins, thromboxanes, and leukotrienes, all classes of regulatory molecules having many diverse functions.

Triglycerides

Triglycerides, also known as triacylglycerols or as neutral fats, contain a glycerol backbone in which all three hydroxyl groups are esterified with a fatty acid. Diglycerides and monoglycerides are produced when one or two fatty acids are removed, respectively. The molecular weight of a triglyceride is usually less than 1000, but they are often considered macromolecules because they associate into large anhydrous oil drops. The major function of triglyceride is to provide a storage form for the energy-rich fatty acids. Under normal conditions triglycerides are stored almost exclusively in adipose tissue.

Ketones

Ketones are C_4 acids, which are formed when excessive fatty acid and amino acid degradation occurs during fasting and starvation. The two primary ketones are acetoacetate and β-hydroxybutyrate (see Figure 18-1). In contrast to long-chain fatty acids, which are relatively insoluble, the ketones are soluble fuels, which can be readily transported in the blood.

Cholesterol

Cholesterol is a component of membranes and a precursor for several biologically important compounds, including the bile acids, vitamin D, and the steroid hormones. All of these compounds contain the steroid nucleus, a fused four-member ring system, containing 19 carbon atoms. For example, cholesterol, a 27-carbon compound, has an 8-carbon side chain attached to the D ring and a hydroxyl group attached to C-3 of the A ring (see Figure 18-1). Most of the cholesterol in the body exists as a cholesterol ester with a fatty acid attached to the hydroxyl group at C-3. The conversion of cholesterol to bile acids and steroid hormones involves shortening the side chain attached to the D ring and adding additional hydroxyl groups to specific positions of the steroid nucleus. These pathways are considered in a later chapter.

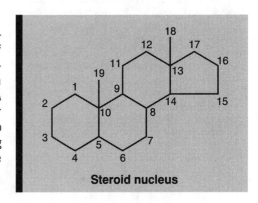

Steroid nucleus

Phospholipids

The phospholipids are a family of amphipathic molecules that serve as the primary building blocks of membranes. They contain two alcohols linked together through a phosphodiester bridge. One alcohol is diacylglycerol (DAG), and the other can be choline, ethanolamine, serine, or inositol (see Figure 18-1). This family of lipids is collectively known as the glycerol-based phospholipids.

Sphingolipids

The sphingolipids are amphipathic molecules that are important structural components of membranes. All sphingolipids contain sphingosine, a long-chain amino alcohol, which is derived from a fatty acid and has one amino group and two hydroxyl groups. The amino group is linked via an amide bond to a long-chain saturated fatty acid, and the terminal hydroxyl group can be linked to a variety of compounds, each generating a different kind of sphingolipid (see Figure 18-1).

METABOLIC INTERCONVERSIONS OF LIPIDS

Most of the major classes of lipids are interconvertible, with the primary intermediates being *acetyl CoA* and *fatty acids* (Figure 18-2). The interconversions between acetyl CoA, fatty acids, and triglycerides are regulated primarily by the relative concentration of insulin and glucagon. Following a meal, when blood glucose and insulin levels are transiently elevated, excess glucose is converted to fatty acids by the liver and stored as triglycerides in adipose tissue. Cholesterol synthesis, which uses acetyl CoA as the substrate, also increases under the influence of insulin. These processes are collectively known as *lipogenesis*. Conversely, when blood glucose begins to drop and glucagon is transiently elevated, fatty acids are mobilized from triglyceride stores and distributed to various tissues, where they are oxidized as a source of energy. In cases of prolonged fasting and starvation, when glucagon is persistently elevated, fatty acids are mobilized and degraded faster than the acetyl CoA is used. Under these conditions, the excess acetyl CoA is converted by the liver to ketones and released into the circulation as a soluble metabolic fuel that can be oxidized by various tissues.

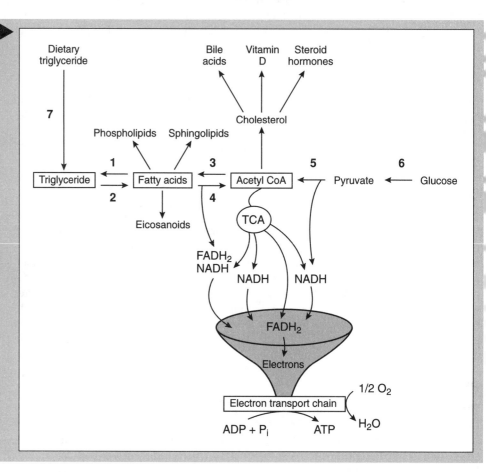

FIGURE 18-2 ▶

Metabolic Interconversion of Lipids. *Triglycerides, fatty acids, and acetyl CoA are readily interconverted. Fatty acids are used as building blocks for more complex lipids that perform specialized functions, and acetyl CoA is the building block for cholesterol. The central pathways of lipogenesis and lipolysis are identified by numbers as follows: (1) triglyceride synthesis; (2) triglyceride hydrolysis; (3) fatty acid synthesis; (4) β-oxidation of fatty acids; (5) pyruvate dehydrogenase; (6) glycolysis; (7) digestion, absorption, and distribution of dietary lipid. TCA = tricarboxylic acid cycle; NADH = the reduced form of nicotinamide adenine dinucleotide; $FADH_2$ = the reduced form of flavin adenine dinucleotide; ADP = adenosine diphosphate; ATP = adenosine triphosphate; and P_i = inorganic phosphate.*

DIGESTION AND ABSORPTION OF DIETARY FAT

Dietary fat consists mainly of triglyceride, with smaller amounts of cholesterol, cholesterol esters, and phospholipids. Digestion of triglyceride begins in the mouth and stomach, but normally most of triglyceride digestion occurs in the small intestine. The products of fat digestion diffuse into intestinal mucosal cells, where they are re-esterified and assembled into chylomicrons, large lipoproteins that act as carriers of dietary triglyceride and cholesterol esters.

Digestion in the Mouth and Stomach

Small amounts of triglyceride are hydrolyzed to fatty acids and DAG by *lingual lipase*, an enzyme secreted by the lingual glands of the mouth and swallowed with the saliva into the stomach. Lingual lipase and *gastric lipase*, an enzyme produced by the stomach, are both acid-stable lipases with a pH optimum of around 4. The hydrolysis of fat in the mouth and stomach is slow because it has not been emulsified. These acid-stable lipases normally account for about 10% of triglyceride hydrolysis in adults and as much as 40%–50% in infants, whose source of fat is milk. Homogenized milk contains triglycerides that are highly emulsified.

Intestinal Digestion

An overview of digestion of dietary lipids in the small intestine is shown in Figure 18-3. Dietary fat requires emulsification before it can be efficiently degraded by enzymes. Lipolysis in the small intestine is regulated by two hormones, cholecystokinin (CCK) and secretin. In response to secretin, the pancreas releases a solution enriched in bicarbonate, which helps neutralize the acidic contents of the stomach. In response to CCK, the exocrine pancreas releases a battery of digestive enzymes, and the gallbladder contracts, releasing bile into the small intestine. The major function of bile is to provide the emulsifying agents.

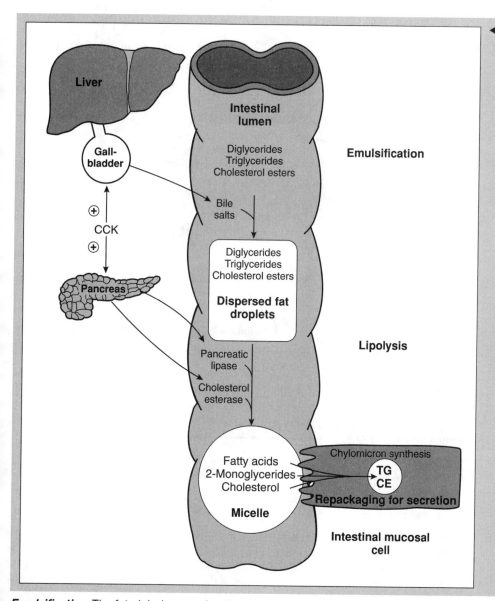

FIGURE 18-3
Digestion of Dietary Lipids. *Emulsification of dietary fat requires bile salts, which are released into the intestinal lumen from the gallbladder. The dispersed fat is hydrolyzed by pancreatic enzymes to a mixture of fatty acids, 2-monoglycerides, and cholesterol. The products of these reactions, together with bile salts, form mixed micelles, which carry the products to the brush border of the intestinal mucosal cells. Fatty acids, 2-monoglycerides, and cholesterol diffuse into the cells, where they are repackaged for secretion. CCK = cholecystokinin; TG = triglyceride; CE = cholesterol ester.*

Emulsification. The fat globules entering the small intestine are too large to be hydrolyzed efficiently by lipases. The *bile salts* are the major emulsifying agents, dispersing the large fat globules into smaller particles, which provide a larger surface area upon which the digestive enzymes can act. The smaller lipid particles have the polar groups of the bile salts on the periphery, surrounding a core of neutral lipid that consists mainly of triglyceride (Figure 18-4). The bile salts also form mixed micelles with the products of intestinal fat digestion and act as carriers of these products to the brush border of mucosal cells for absorption.

Lipolysis. Enzymes that are of particular importance to lipid digestion in the small intestine are pancreatic lipase, cholesterol esterase, and phospholipase A_2. A small protein, colipase, is also released from the pancreas and is required for the binding of

Breast Milk Lipase
Newborns who are breastfeeding obtain about half of their calories from lactose and half from triglyceride. Breast milk contains a lipase with properties very similar to those of pancreatic lipase. Until it reaches the gastrointestinal track, the enzyme has little activity because of the absence of bile salts in milk. This enzyme is also present in fresh cows' milk, but it is inactivated by pasteurization.

FIGURE 18-4 ▶

Emulsification of Fat. *(A) The structure of glycolate. This bile salt is an effective emulsifying agent. (B) A schematic structure of glycholate, emphasizing its amphipathic nature. The hydrophilic side chain and all of the hydroxyl groups are on one surface, and the hydrophobic ring system is on the other surface. (C) A schematic representation of emulsified fat, showing triglyceride surrounded by bile salts. Higher concentrations of bile salts result in smaller mixed micelles. Pancreatic lipase binds to the surface of the mixed micelle and hydrolyzes the triglyceride. Colipase is required for binding the enzyme to the micelle.*

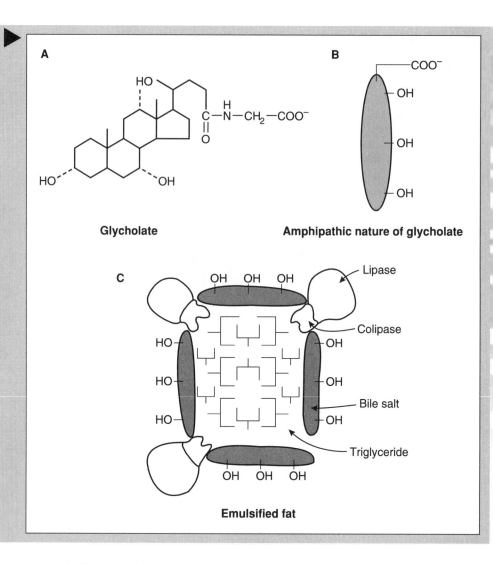

A

Glycholate

B

Amphipathic nature of glycholate

C

Lipase

Colipase

Bile salt

Triglyceride

Emulsified fat

pancreatic lipase to the small dispersed lipid particles. The reactions catalyzed by these pancreatic enzymes are shown in the following equations.

$$\text{Triglyceride} + H_2O \xrightarrow{\text{pancreatic lipase}} \text{2-monoglyceride} + \text{fatty acid}$$

$$\text{Cholesterol ester} + H_2O \xrightarrow{\text{cholesterol esterase}} \text{cholesterol} + \text{fatty acid}$$

$$\text{Phospholipid} + H_2O \xrightarrow{\text{phospholipase } A_2} \text{lysophospholipid} + \text{fatty acid}$$

Pancreatic lipase releases the fatty acids from carbons 1 and 3 of the triglyceride backbone, forming 2-monoglyceride. Phospholipase A_2 releases the fatty acid from carbon 2 of phospholipids, generating lysophospholipids, which are also good emulsifying agents. A summary of the lipases involved in the digestion of dietary fat is provided in Table 18-3.

TABLE 18-3 ▶

Lipases Involved in Digestion of Dietary Fat

Enzyme	Origin	Substrate	Products
Lingual lipase	Mouth	Triglyceride	Diglyceride and fatty acid
Gastric lipase	Stomach	Triglyceride	Diglyceride and fatty acid
Pancreatic lipase	Pancreas	Triglyceride and diglycerides	2-Monoglyceride and fatty acid
Cholesterol esterase	Pancreas	Cholesterol ester	Cholesterol and fatty acid
Phospholipase A_2	Pancreas	Phospholipid	Lysophospholipid and fatty acid

Absorption and Re-esterification of Dietary Lipid in Intestinal Mucosal Cells

The end products of lipid digestion are delivered to the luminal surface of the intestinal mucosal cells, where they diffuse across the brush-border membrane into the cell, leaving the bile salts behind. Once inside the intestinal cell, triglycerides and cholesterol esters are reformed, packaged into chylomicrons, and secreted (Figure 18-5).

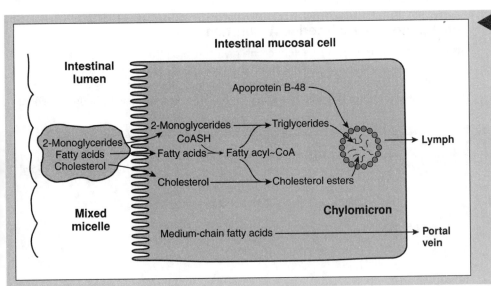

FIGURE 18-5
Repackaging of Dietary Fat by Intestinal Mucosal Cells. Long-chain fatty acids are converted to fatty acyl~CoA and re-esterified with 2-monoglyceride, forming triglyceride, and cholesterol is converted to cholesterol ester. The triglycerides and cholesterol esters are packaged into the core of chylomicrons, which are released by exocytosis into the lymphatic system. Medium-chain fatty acids are released directly into the portal blood.

Activation of Fatty Acids. Esterification of fatty acids requires that they first be converted to fatty acyl CoA, a reaction that is catalyzed by a family of *fatty acyl CoA synthetases* that recognize fatty acids of different chain lengths, designated as R in the following equation. The reaction requires adenosine triphosphate (ATP) as a source of energy for forming the energy-rich thioester bond between the fatty acid and CoA. The formation of fatty acyl CoA requires two high-energy phosphate bonds, as indicated by the formation of adenosine monophosphate (AMP) and PP_i. The high-energy bond in the PP_i is subsequently hydrolyzed to two molecules of P_i by the action of *pyrophosphatase.*

$$R\text{-COOH} + \text{CoASH} + \text{ATP} \xrightarrow{\text{fatty acyl CoA synthetase}} R\text{-}\overset{\displaystyle O}{\overset{\displaystyle \|}{C}}\text{~SCoA} + \text{AMP} + PP_i$$

Esterification Reactions. Triglycerides are reformed by the transfer of the fatty acyl group from the CoA derivatives to the glycerol backbone, a reaction catalyzed by *fatty acyl CoA transferase.* The energy driving this reaction is supplied by cleavage of the thioester bond of fatty acyl CoA. Similarly, cholesterol esters are reformed in a reaction catalyzed by *acyl CoA:cholesterol acyltransferase (ACAT).* Long-chain fatty acids, having 12 or more carbon atoms, are repackaged into triglyceride. However, medium- and short-chain fatty acids, having 10 or fewer carbons, are released into the portal blood, where they bind to serum albumin and are transported directly to the liver.

Chylomicrons and the Transport of Dietary Fat

The neutral lipids, triglycerides and cholesterol esters, are very insoluble in aqueous solutions, and their delivery to other tissues requires a special transport mechanism that prevents them from precipitating out of solution.

Chylomicron Assembly. The neutral lipids, together with protein and phospholipids, are packaged into large lipoprotein particles known as chylomicrons. The chylomicrons are a family of heterogeneous particles, having an outer hydrophilic-membrane surface layer that forms a shell around a large hydrophobic core. The hydrophilic shell consists of apoproteins, phospholipids, and free cholesterol, while the inner core is made primarily of triglyceride, with small amounts of cholesterol esters and fat-soluble vitamins. Most of

Therapeutic Use of Medium-Chain Triglycerides

Triglycerides containing medium-chain fatty acids have important therapeutic use for patients with malabsorption syndromes. In contrast to long-chain triglycerides, they can be absorbed intact and hydrolyzed completely to fatty acids and glycerol inside the intestinal mucosal cells. They are not re-esterified but are absorbed directly into the portal blood and transported by albumin to the liver. Medium-chain fatty acids have 10 carbons or less.

Lipid Composition of Chylomicrons
Lipids make up 98%–99% of the chylomicron particle, with protein comprising 1%–2%. The distribution of lipids among the major classes is as follows:

Triglyceride	*88%*
Phospholipid	*8%*
Cholesterol ester	*3%*
Cholesterol	*1%*

the protein in the nascent chylomicron particle is apoprotein B-48, which is synthesize by the intestinal cells.

Chylomicron Secretion. Chylomicrons are released by exocytosis into the lymphati capillaries and carried to the thoracic duct, where they enter the general circulatior Since chylomicrons are too large to enter the portal circulation, the peripheral tissue have access to the energy-rich triglycerides without their having been previously pro cessed by the liver. The mechanisms that allow tissues to take up fatty acids fror lipoproteins are discussed in the following chapter.

Time Course of Triglyceride Absorption

After a high-fat meal, the chylomicrons give the blood a milky appearance. The tri glyceride concentration of plasma can rise to as high as 1000 mg/dL, depending on the amount of fat consumed. It begins to increase about 2 hours after a meal, and from 6 to 8 hours are required for the concentration to return to its basal level (Figure 18-6).

FIGURE 18-6 ▶

Time Course of Dietary Triglyceride Absorption into the Blood. *An increase in serum triglyceride begins about 2 hours after ingestion of dietary fat, peaks after 3 to 4 hours, and returns to normal after 6 to 8 hours.*

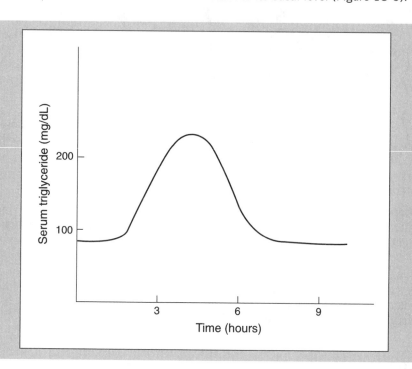

ABNORMALITIES IN LIPID DIGESTION AND ABSORPTION

Steatorrhea
Failure to digest and absorb lipids leads to the excretion of excessive amounts of fat in the feces. Quantitative determination of fecal fat is commonly used to establish the presence of steatorrhea. Normally, fecal fat excretion is less than 6% of the ingested fat.

Although many conditions can lead to impaired absorption and steatorrhea, the most common causes are related to bile salt deficiency, pancreatic enzyme deficiency, or defective chylomicron synthesis. Lipid malabsorption can also lead to a deficiency in the fat-soluble vitamins A, D, E, and K.

Bile Salt Deficiency

The bile salts are synthesized in the liver and stored in the gallbladder. A deficiency of bile salts in the small intestine can result from liver disease that impairs synthesis, an obstruction in the bile duct that impairs delivery, or an overgrowth of intestinal bacteria that converts bile salts to bile acids and diminishes their efficiency as emulsification agents. Lipid malabsorption caused by bile salt deficiency results in stools that have a characteristic chalky, clay color.

Pancreatic Enzyme Deficiency

Malabsorption that is the result of pancreatic enzyme deficiency may occur secondary to pancreatitis or cystic fibrosis, where there is a blockage in the pancreatic duct. When pancreatic lipase is less than 10% of the normal level, severe weight loss may be observed because of the loss of metabolic fuel in the feces. The steatorrhea may be reduced by supplemental pancreatic enzyme preparations that are taken orally.

Defective Chylomicron Synthesis

The inability to synthesize apoprotein B-48 leads to the accumulation of triglyceride in the intestinal mucosal cells and to low circulating levels of chylomicrons, as well as some of the other lipoproteins. This condition is known as *congenital abetalipoproteinemia*.

Congenital Abetalipoproteinemia
A deficiency in apoprotein B is characterized by the accumulation of triglyceride in the intestinal mucosal cells and liver, and by low concentrations of chylomicrons, very-low density lipoproteins, and low-density lipoproteins. The circulating levels of triglyceride and cholesterol are both very low. The inability to synthesize apoprotein B abolishes the normal mechanism for transporting both dietary lipids and lipids that are synthesized endogenously.

RESOLUTION OF CLINICAL CASE

The patient presented at the beginning of this chapter showed all the features of vitamin A deficiency secondary to cystic fibrosis. Cystic fibrosis is an inherited disorder of electrolyte transfer across cell membranes. It occurs in 1 of every 2000 live births. One of the most common clinical features is chronic respiratory problems, characterized by thick, sticky mucus and infection. There is also a failure of the exocrine pancreas to secrete digestive enzymes, resulting in malabsorption of lipid and protein. Diagnosis of cystic fibrosis is confirmed by an increased loss of chloride in sweat [2]. The loss of 40% of the dietary fat seen in this patient, when submitted to absorption tests, is consistent with malabsorption. Under normal conditions, 6% or less of the dietary fat is lost in the feces. Patients with cystic fibrosis are frequently underweight, and they may have deficiencies in the fat-soluble vitamins. This patient had a profound deficiency in vitamin A and a related visual impairment. The diet recommended for this patient included milk and butter as the major sources of fat. These sources are enriched in short- and medium-chain fatty acids that can be directly absorbed into the portal circulation. Following treatment with oral pancreatic enzymes and vitamin A supplementation, the patient's vision was almost normal within several weeks.

REVIEW QUESTIONS

Directions: For each of the following questions, choose the **one best** answer.

1. Most dietary lipids are packaged and secreted from intestinal cells in which of the following forms?

    (A) Micelles

    (B) Chylomicrons

    (C) Triglycerides

    (D) Ketones

    (E) Short-chain fatty acids

2. Which of the following statements most accurately describes digestion of triglyceride in the stomach?

    (A) The enzymes responsible have a pH optimum of around 7

    (B) Colipase is required for efficient digestion

    (C) Lingual lipase cleaves a fatty acid from triglyceride, producing diglyceride

    (D) Triglyceride droplets are dispersed by the action of bile salts

    (E) Most of the triglyceride hydrolysis is catalyzed by pancreatic lipase

3. Which of the following statements would be descriptive of a patient suspected of having cystic fibrosis?

    (A) A deficiency in vitamin A, but not vitamin E, would likely occur

    (B) Lipid digestion, but not protein digestion, would be impaired

    (C) Inclusion of butter in the diet is recommended because it is easily emulsified

    (D) Fecal fat would comprise more than 6% of the ingested fat

    (E) The content of chloride in sweat would be decreased relative to the normal value

Directions: The group of questions below consists of lettered choices followed by several numbered items. For each numbered item, select the appropriate lettered option with which it is most closely associated. Each lettered option may be used once, more than once, or not at all.

Questions 5–9

For each of the lipids listed below, select the compound that is its precursor.

    (A) Linoleic acid

    (B) Cholesterol

    (C) Ceramide

    (D) Glycerol

    (E) Acetyl CoA

    (F) Vitamin D

5. Bile acids

6. Eicosanoids

7. Triglyceride

8. Sphingolipid

9. Cholesterol

ANSWERS AND EXPLANATIONS

1. The answer is C. Most of the dietary lipid is triglyceride, which is degraded to 2-monoglyceride and fatty acids in the intestine. These products are incorporated into micelles and delivered to the brush-border membrane, where they diffuse in the cell and get converted back to triglycerides. The triglycerides, along with apoprotein B-48 and small amounts of cholesterol ester, are incorporated into chylomicrons and secreted into the lymphatic system. Ketones are neither present in dietary fat nor synthesized in the intestine. Short-chain fatty acids are absorbed directly into the portal blood.

2. The answer is C. Lingual lipase is produced in the mouth but exerts most of its action in the stomach. It is an acid-stable enzyme with a pH optimum of about 4. Pancreatic lipase is the major enzyme for hydrolyzing triglyceride in the small intestine, and it requires colipase to bind to the dispersed fat particles that result from emulsification. Emulsification does not occur in the stomach.

3. The answer is D. In a normal individual, the feces contain 6% or less of the dietary fat. In a person with cystic fibrosis, both lipid and protein digestion are impaired as the result of a deficiency in pancreatic enzymes in the gastrointestinal tract. Therefore, a greater proportion of fat is excreted in the feces. Since the fat-soluble vitamins are absorbed along with the other dietary fat, there would likely be a deficiency in all of these vitamins (A, D, E, K). Diagnosis of cystic fibrosis is made by observing an increased loss of chloride in sweat. Diets that are enriched in short- and medium-chain fatty acids (butter contains a C_4 fatty acid) are beneficial because they can be absorbed directly from the intestinal cell into the portal blood.

5–9. The answers are: 5-B, 6-A, 7-D, 8-C, 9-E. Bile acids are synthesized from cholesterol. Most eicosanoids are synthesized from arachidonic acid, which is synthesized from linoleic acid in the diet. Triglycerides contain a glycerol backbone. Sphingolipids are derived from ceramide, which consists of a long-chain saturated fatty acid linked via amide linkage to sphingosine. All of the carbons in cholesterol are derived from acetyl CoA.

REFERENCES

1. Marinetti GV: *Disorders of Lipid Metabolism*, New York, NY: Plenum Press, 1990, pp 1–30.
2. Welsh MJ, Tsui L-C, Boat TF, et al: Cystic fibrosis. In *Metabolic and Molecular Bases of Inherited Disease*, 7th ed. Edited by Scriver CR, Beaudet AL, Sly WS, et al. New York, NY: McGraw-Hill, 1995, pp 3799–3876.

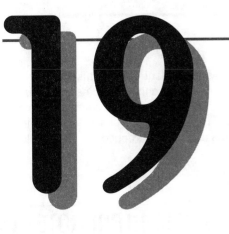

19 LIPID TRANSPORT: LIPOPROTEIN STRUCTURE, FUNCTION, AND METABOLISM

CHAPTER OUTLINE

INTRODUCTION OF CLINICAL CASE

An 8-year-old girl was admitted to the hospital for a heart and liver transplant. There was a history of coronary heart disease in her family. When the patient was 2 years old, xanthomas began to appear on her legs, and at age 4, they were also present on her elbows. At age 7, she was admitted to the hospital with symptoms of myocardial infarct. At that time, her plasma cholesterol concentration was 1240 mg/dL, and her triglyceride level was 350 mg/dL. The patient was put on a low-fat diet and started on cholestyramine and lovastatin. Her mother and father had plasma cholesterol concentrations of 355 mg/dL and 310 mg/dL, respectively. Both parents appeared to be in good health. Two weeks after the myocardial infarct, the patient had a coronary artery bypass. During the past year, she has had periodic bouts of severe angina, a second bypass operation, and was put on the waiting list for a combined heart and liver transplant. During this time, although the patient remained on a low-fat diet and continued with cholestyramine and lovastatin, her plasma cholesterol level remained around 1000 mg/dL. The transplantation appeared to be successful, with good cardiac and hepatic function observed soon after the operation. Over the next 2 months, her plasma cholesterol dropped to 260 mg/dL, and the xanthomas began to regress.

PLASMA LIPOPROTEINS

The plasma lipoproteins are large water-soluble macromolecular complexes that transport insoluble lipids in the blood. Lipoproteins consist of a core, containing triglyceride and cholesterol ester, and a surface coat or monolayer containing proteins, phospholipids, and unesterified cholesterol (Figure 19-1). The surface monolayer makes the complex soluble in aqueous solutions. The protein components are commonly referred to as apoproteins or apolipoproteins.

Classes of Lipoproteins

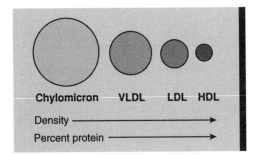

Lipoproteins are commonly divided into five major classes based on their density: (1) chylomicrons, (2) very low-density lipoproteins (VLDLs), (3) intermediate-density lipoproteins (IDLs), (4) low-density lipoproteins (LDLs), (5) and high-density lipoproteins (HDLs). The density is inversely proportional to the triglyceride content and directly proportional to the protein content. Chylomicrons, containing about 1%–2% protein and 98%–99% triglyceride, have the lowest density, while HDLs containing about 50% protein and 50% lipid have the highest density. As the density increases, both the size of the core and the diameter of the particle decrease (Table 19-1).

Separation of Lipoproteins

The lipoproteins can be separated by centrifugation on the basis of their densities. When placed in a centrifugal field, the rate at which each lipoprotein floats upward through a solution of salt depends on the relative amount of triglyceride. Chylomicrons float most rapidly, while HDLs have the slowest rate of flotation. The lipoproteins can also be

FIGURE 19-1 ▶

Generalized Lipoprotein Structure. *The proteins, phospholipids, and unesterified cholesterol are in the outer shell, where their hydrophilic groups interact with the aqueous environment. The inner core is composed of the neutral lipids, triglycerides and cholesterol esters, which aggregate into large insoluble oil droplets.*

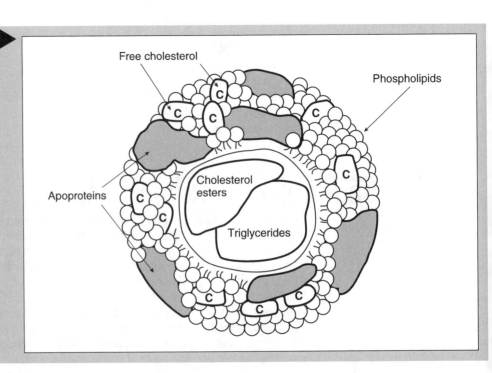

TABLE 19-1
Properties of Plasma Lipoproteins

Lipoprotein	Diameter (nm)	Density (g/ml)	Composition		Percentage of Total Lipid			
			% Protein	% Lipid	TG	CE	C	PL
Chylomicron	80–900	0.92–0.96	2	98	88	3	1	8
Very low-density lipoprotein	25–75	0.95–1.006	10	90	56	15	8	20
Low-density lipoprotein	17–26	1.006–1.063	21	79	13	48	10	28
High-density lipoprotein	4–10	1.063–1.125	52	48	13	29	6	46

Note. TG = triglyceride; CE = cholesterol ester; C = free cholesterol; PL = phospholipid.
Source: Adapted with permission from Murray RK, Granner DK, Mayes PA, et al: *Harper's Biochemistry*, 23rd ed. Norwalk, CT: Appleton and Lange, 1993, p 251.

separated on the basis of their electrophoretic mobilities. The relationship between the electrophoretic mobility and flotation rate is shown in Figure 19-2.

Both electrophoresis and centrifugation are used extensively in the clinical laboratory for diagnostic purposes. For example, the measurement of serum cholesterol and triglyceride levels in plasma is not sufficient for making a diagnosis because these lipids are present in several different interactive lipoprotein complexes. Qualitative data on the relative proportion of each lipoprotein can be obtained by electrophoresis. However, a quantitative analysis of the lipid composition and the content of each lipoprotein requires prior separation of the lipoprotein classes by centrifugation.

Apoprotein Functions

There are four major types of apoproteins: apo A, apo B, apo C, and apo E. All four classes are synthesized by the liver, while only apo A and apo B are made by intestinal cells. Although several subtypes of the apoproteins have been identified, the functions of all of the subtypes are not completely understood. The apoproteins found in each class of lipoproteins are summarized in Table 19-2. The apoproteins perform several dynamic functions, as well as serving as essential structural components of the lipoproteins [2].

Apoprotein Class	Major Function
Apo A	Reverse cholesterol transport
Apo B	LDL receptor binding and clearance
Apo C	Regulation of LpL
Apo E	Remnant receptor binding and clearance

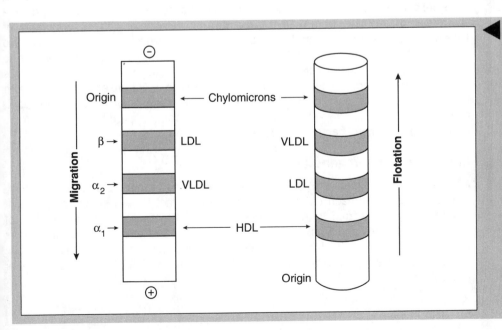

FIGURE 19-2
Separation of Plasma Lipoproteins by Electrophoresis and by Centrifugation. *The migration in an electric field at pH 8.6 is shown on the left, where the chylomicrons remain at the origin, and high-density lipoprotein (HDL) is the most rapidly migrating lipoprotein. The positions at which the serum α_1-, α_2-, and β-globulins migrate are indicated by the arrows on the left. The relative rate at which the lipoproteins float from the bottom to the top of a centrifuge tube containing a salt solution is shown on the right. LDL = low-density lipoprotein; VLDL = very low-density lipoprotein.*

TABLE 19-2

Plasma Lipoprotein Function and Apoprotein Composition

Lipoprotein	Source	Function	Apoproteins
Chylomicron	Intestine	Transport dietary triglyceride to peripheral tissues	Apo B-48, apo C-II, and apo E
Very low-density lipoprotein (VLDL)	Liver	Transport endogenous triglyceride to peripheral tissues	Apo B-100, apo C-II, and apo E
Intermediate-density lipoprotein (IDL)	Plasma VLDLs	Triglyceride transport and precursor of LDL	Apo B-100, apo C-II, and apo E
Low-density lipoprotein (LDL)	Plasma IDLs	Transport cholesterol to peripheral tissues	Apo B-100
High-density lipoprotein	Liver and intestine	Reservoir of apoproteins and reverse cholesterol transport	Apo A, apo C, and apo E

Structural Role. Apo B is an integral component of the surface monolayer of all lipoproteins except HDL. Apo B has two forms, apo B-48, which is found in chylomicrons, and apo B-100, which is found in VLDL, IDL, and LDL. Apo B-48 is a truncated form of apo B-100; both proteins are encoded by the same gene. Apo A-I is an integral structural protein of HDL.

Receptor Binding and Clearance. Apo B and apo E recognize specific receptors on the surfaces of cells. All cells have receptors, known as *LDL receptors*, which bind apo B-100, allowing IDL and LDL to be taken up by endocytosis. The liver has an additional receptor, known as the *remnant receptor*, which binds apo E and allows the remnants of partially degraded chylomicrons and VLDLs to be cleared from the plasma.

Enzyme Cofactors. Two apoproteins, apo C-II and apo A-I, are cofactors for extracellular enzymes involved in lipoprotein metabolism. Apo C-II activates *lipoprotein lipase* (LpL), an enzyme that hydrolyzes lipoprotein triglyceride to fatty acids and glycerol. Apo A-I activates *lecithin–cholesterol acyltransferase* (LCAT), an enzyme that is essential for the transfer of cholesterol from peripheral tissues to the liver, where it can be metabolized and excreted.

Source and Function of Lipoproteins

Chylomicrons are synthesized only in the intestinal mucosal cells, where they are assembled as vehicles for transporting dietary fat. VLDLs are synthesized only in the liver, and their function is to transport endogenous triglyceride to extrahepatic tissues. IDLs and LDLs are derived from the metabolism of VLDLs that occurs in the plasma. The progressive release of fatty acids from VLDL triglyceride produces a heterogeneous population of IDLs, which can be further degraded to LDLs. The progressive transformation of VLDLs to IDLs to LDLs is accompanied by a change in the neutral lipid core, with triglyceride becoming depleted and cholesterol ester becoming enriched. The major function of LDLs is to deliver cholesterol from the liver to peripheral tissues. HDLs are synthesized by both liver and intestinal mucosal cells. They act as a circulating reservoir of apo C and apo E, and they are essential for the transport of cholesterol from the peripheral tissues to the liver, where cholesterol can be metabolized.

Lipoprotein Heterogeneity

Although the lipoproteins are characterized as belonging to four major classes, heterogeneity exists within each class. The lipoproteins do not have a static composition. Heterogeneity arises from triglyceride degradation that occurs in the capillary bed of extrahepatic tissues and from the continuous exchange of apo C and E that occurs between HDL and the other lipoproteins, chylomicrons, VLDLs, and IDLs. The metabolic fate of a lipoprotein is determined by the complement of apoproteins in that particular lipoprotein.

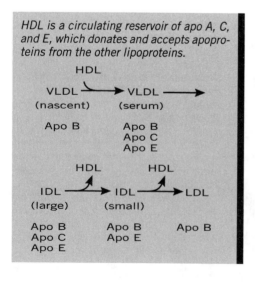

HDL is a circulating reservoir of apo A, C, and E, which donates and accepts apoproteins from the other lipoproteins.

LIPOPROTEIN METABOLISM

Chylomicron Metabolism

Chylomicrons transport dietary triglyceride from the gastrointestinal tract to various tissues. The half-life of chylomicrons in the plasma is about 15 minutes. Normally, after an overnight fast, they have disappeared from the plasma. The nascent chylomicrons, which are synthesized in the intestinal mucosal cells, contain apo B-48, which is required for secretion. Following secretion, chylomicrons acquire apo C and apo E from circulating HDL. An overview of chylomicron metabolism is shown in Figure 19-3.

Role of Lipoprotein Lipase (LpL). The triglycerides in circulating chylomicrons are hydrolyzed to free fatty acids and glycerol by LpL, an extracellular enzyme attached to the luminal walls of capillaries, particularly in adipose tissue and heart and skeletal muscle. LpL is synthesized and secreted by adipose tissue, heart, and muscle and is anchored to the capillary membrane by interaction with glycosaminoglycans (GAGs). The fatty acids released by the action of LpL move across the membrane and into the peripheral tissues, where they are either reconverted to triglyceride for storage (adipose tissue) or oxidized for energy (heart and muscle). LpL is activated by apo C-II, which is present on the surface of the chylomicron. The hydrolysis of triglyceride by LpL results in smaller lipoprotein particles, known as *chylomicron remnants.*

Fate of Chylomicron Remnants. As the chylomicron remnants are progressively depleted of triglyceride, they become more enriched with cholesterol esters, and as the remnants become smaller, apo C is eventually returned to circulating HDLs, leaving only apo B-48 and apo E in the surface monolayer. The chylomicron remnants are cleared from the

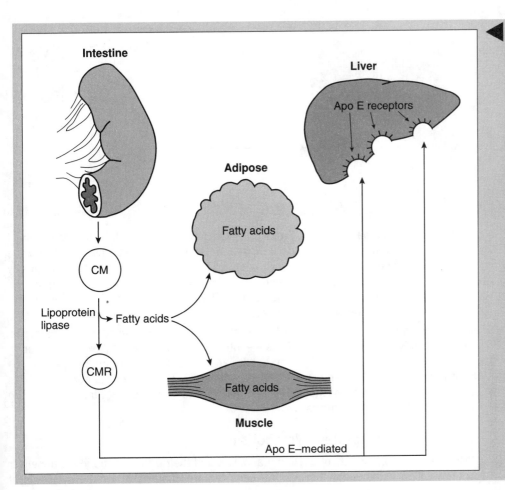

FIGURE 19-3
Metabolism of Chylomicrons. Chylomicrons transport dietary fat from the intestine to other tissues. Triglyceride is hydrolyzed to fatty acids in the capillary beds of muscle and adipose tissue, releasing fatty acids to these tissues. The chylomicron remnants bind to apo E receptors on the liver and are taken up by endocytosis. The ratio of triglyceride to cholesterol ester in the nascent chylomicron is about 10:1, whereas in the chylomicron remnant it is about 1:1. CM = chylomicrons; CMR = chylomicron remnants.

plasma by the liver, where they bind to receptors and are taken up by receptor-mediated endocytosis. Apo E binds to the remnant receptor, whereas both apo E and apo B-48 are required for the binding of chylomicron remnants to the LDL receptor. The vesicles formed by endocytosis fuse with lysosomes, where the remnants are degraded by acid hydrolases to a mixture of amino acids, fatty acids, and free cholesterol. The lipids that are delivered to the liver via chylomicron remnants are repackaged into VLDLs and returned to the plasma.

Very Low-Density Lipoprotein Metabolism

VLDLs transport triglyceride and cholesterol from the liver to extrahepatic tissues. The triglycerides and cholesterol esters that are incorporated into VLDLs are derived from de novo synthesis and from degradation of chylomicron remnants. The nascent VLDLs released by the liver contain apo B-100, which is essential for secretion. Apo C and E are acquired from HDL after the VLDLs are secreted into the plasma. An overview of VLDL metabolism is shown in Figure 19-4.

Effect of LpL on VLDLs. The triglycerides in plasma VLDLs are hydrolyzed by LpL, releasing fatty acids that are taken up primarily by adipose tissue and heart and skeletal muscle, resulting in a heterogeneous population of IDLs. The IDLs are smaller and more dense than VLDLs, and they are enriched in cholesterol esters. LpL activity is dependent on apo C-II, which is present in both VLDLs and the larger forms of IDLs. The regulation of LpL is tissue-specific. Insulin stimulates LpL synthesis in adipose tissue, where fatty acids are stored. As the IDLs become progressively smaller, apo C-II is transferred back to HDL, resulting in IDLs that have little affinity for LpL. These small IDLs are either taken up by the liver or they are further metabolized to LDLs.

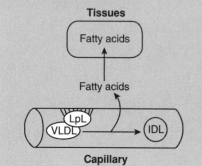

LpL is anchored to the luminal wall of capillaries by GAGs and can be released by heparin. Lipoproteins containing apo C-II bind to LpL. Hydrolysis of triglyceride releases fatty acids, which diffuse across the capillary wall into the tissues.

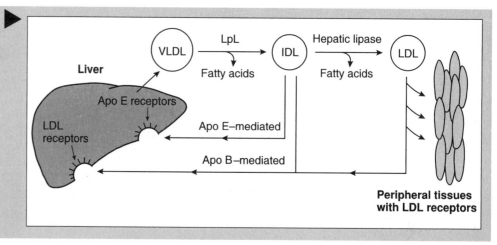

FIGURE 19-4
Metabolism of Very Low-Density Lipoproteins (VLDLs). The VLDL pathway transports endogenous lipids from the liver to the peripheral tissues. Triglyceride is hydrolyzed by lipoprotein lipase (LpL) in the capillary bed of tissues, releasing fatty acids to the tissues as the VLDL particle gets transformed into intermediate-density lipoprotein (IDL) and low-density lipoprotein (LDL). IDL binds to receptors on the liver and can be internalized, or it can be converted to LDL. LDL is taken up by all tissues that have LDL receptors.

Effect of Hepatic Lipase on IDLs. Since LpL has a low affinity for IDLs, the conversion of IDLs to LDLs is mediated by *hepatic lipase,* an extracellular enzyme located on the sinusoidal surfaces of the liver. Approximately 25% of the IDLs are converted to LDLs by the action of hepatic lipase, which hydrolyzes both triglyceride and phospholipids. All LDLs in humans are derived from IDLs. Since LDLs contain only apo B, the transformation of IDLs to LDLs also involves the return of apo E to the circulating HDLs.

Internalization of IDLs by Liver. IDLs are sometimes referred to as VLDL remnants. Approximately 75% of the plasma IDLs are internalized by the liver following interaction with surface receptors. The IDLs contain both apo E and apo B-100, and, therefore, can bind to both remnant receptors and LDL receptors [2]. The greater the number of IDLs that is internalized by these mechanisms, the lower the level of circulating LDLs and the lower the risk of atherosclerosis.

Low-Density Lipoprotein Metabolism

LDLs are the end products of VLDL metabolism, and their primary function is to deliver cholesterol to extrahepatic tissues. All cells require cholesterol for the synthesis of

And the Point Is . . .
IDLs have two fates:

IDL
- 75% internalized by liver (mediated by apo E)
- 25% converted to LDL (mediated by hepatic lipase)

plasma membranes, and some cells require additional cholesterol for the synthesis of specialized products such as steroid hormones, vitamin D, and bile acids. Cellular cholesterol can be obtained either by de novo synthesis or from receptor-mediated endocytosis of LDL. Each LDL particle has an oily core consisting of about 1500 molecules of cholesterol esters. The core is surrounded by a hydrophilic shell containing phospholipid, unesterified cholesterol, and a single molecule of apoprotein B-100. About 70% of the total cholesterol in plasma is found in LDL particles. A summary of the uptake and metabolism of LDLs is shown in Figure 19-5.

LDL Receptor-Mediated Endocytosis. All nucleated cells contain LDL receptors that recognize apo B-100 of the LDL particle. LDL receptors are located in discrete regions of the plasma membrane known as "coated pits." The intracellular side of the pit is coated with *clathrin*, a protein that polymerizes, forming a scaffold of protein that stabilizes the structure of the pit. Internalization of LDL begins within 2 to 5 minutes after binding and occurs in several steps. (1) Endocytosis of the LDL–receptor complex results in an intracellular vesicle that is coated with clathrin. (2) The clathrin coat is shed because of depolymerization, resulting in an endosome. (3) The endosome is transformed into an uncoupling vesicle known as a compartment for uncoupling of receptor and ligand (CURL). The CURL has a pH between 5.0 and 5.5, which promotes dissociation of LDL from its receptor. (4) The receptor-rich regions bud, forming recycling vesicles that return the receptors to the plasma membrane. (5) The endosome containing the LDL particle fuses with a lysosome, where the apoproteins are degraded to amino acids, and the cholesterol esters are hydrolyzed to free cholesterol and fatty acids.

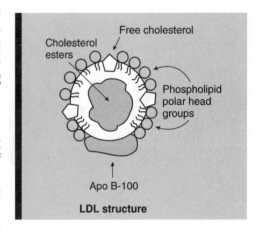

LDL structure

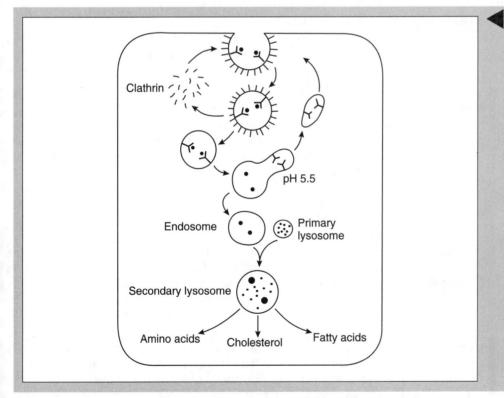

◀ *FIGURE 19-5*
Receptor-Mediated Uptake and Metabolism of Low-Density Lipoproteins (LDLs). LDL binds to receptors that cluster in clathrin-coated pits. Following endocytosis, the clathrin coat is released, the endosome becomes acidified, and LDL dissociates from the receptor. The receptors segregate and are recycled to the plasma membrane. Endosomes fuse with primary lysosomes, forming secondary lysosomes, where the LDL particles are hydrolyzed to amino acids, fatty acids, and free cholesterol.

Coordinate Control of Cholesterol Uptake and Synthesis. The intracellular concentration of free cholesterol is carefully regulated to meet the needs of the cell. Cholesterol derived from the uptake and degradation of lipoproteins affects three processes that influence the cellular concentration of cholesterol. (1) The activity of hydroxymethylglutaryl CoA (HMG CoA) reductase is inhibited. This enzyme catalyzes the rate-limiting step in the pathway of cholesterol synthesis. (2) The activity of acyl CoA:cholesterol acyltransferase (ACAT) is stimulated. ACAT converts free cholesterol to cholesterol ester, which is stored

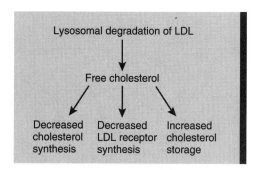

Lysosomal degradation of LDL

↓

Free cholesterol

↓ ↓ ↓

Decreased cholesterol synthesis | Decreased LDL receptor synthesis | Increased cholesterol storage

LCAT	ACAT
Extracellular	Intracellular
Fatty acid donor: lecithin	Fatty acid donor: acyl CoA
Reverse cholesterol transport	Cholesterol storage
Activated by apo A-I	Activated by cholesterol

in small intracellular oil droplets. (3) The synthesis of new *LDL receptors* is decreased, resulting in decreased LDL uptake. Cholesterol decreases the rate of transcription of the LDL-receptor gene.

Scavenger Receptors and LDL Uptake. The uptake of LDL by the pathway of receptor-mediated endocytosis described above is responsible for the clearance of about 75% of the LDL from the plasma. The remaining 25% is removed by low-affinity receptors, known as scavenger receptors, which are found on macrophages. Although these receptors have a low affinity for LDL, they have a high affinity for chemically modified forms of LDL, particularly oxidized LDL. In macrophages, unlike other cells, the synthesis of scavenger receptors is not regulated by the accumulation of intracellular cholesterol. Therefore, the uptake of oxidized LDLs occurs in an uncontrolled manner. As intracellular cholesterol accumulates, macrophages are converted to *foam cells*. The accumulation of foam cells in a particular region of the blood vessel walls results in the formation of *fatty streaks*. Fatty streaks are not necessarily harmful and can be reversed in the early stages of their formation. However, if foam cells continue to form over a long period of time, they become a part of *atherogenic plaques*.

High-Density Lipoprotein Metabolism

The major site of HDL synthesis is the liver, although small amounts can be derived from the small intestine. Excess surface components of circulating chylomicron remnants and IDLs can also pinch off, forming HDLs. HDLs contain apo A, apo C, and apo E. The nascent HDLs are disc-like particles that are rich in surface components (phospholipids, free cholesterol, apoproteins), but they contain very little cholesterol ester and triglyceride. The functions of HDL are discussed below.

HDLs AND APOPROTEIN EXCHANGE

HDLs serve as a circulating repository for apoproteins. Apo C and apo E are transferred back and forth between HDLs, and the other lipoproteins. The major apoprotein associated with HDL is apo A, which is not exchanged with the other lipoproteins and is uniquely associated with HDL function.

HDL AND REVERSE CHOLESTEROL TRANSPORT

The pathway of reverse cholesterol transport results in the net transfer of free cholesterol from peripheral tissues to the liver, where it can be processed for excretion. This pathway is mediated by HDL, although HDL does not directly carry much of the cholesterol to the liver. Instead, HDL acquires free cholesterol from peripheral tissues and transfers it to VLDL remnants (also known as IDLs) and chylomicron remnants, which can be readily taken up by the liver. Three proteins are central to the process of reverse cholesterol transport: apo A-I, LCAT, and cholesterol ester transfer protein (CETP). This process is illustrated in Figure 19-6.

Uptake of Cholesterol by HDL. The first step in reverse cholesterol transport is the transfer of free cholesterol from peripheral tissues to HDL. The HDL particle interacts with peripheral tissues, resulting in the translocation of cholesterol from intracellular sites to the plasma membrane, where it is transferred to HDL. The binding of HDL to the surface of cells in the periphery is believed to be mediated by apo A-I.

Esterification of HDL Cholesterol. The free cholesterol acquired by HDL is rapidly converted to cholesterol ester in a reaction catalyzed by LCAT, an enzyme that is associated with HDL. LCAT transfers a fatty acid from the 2 position of lecithin (phosphatidylcholine) to the hydroxyl group of cholesterol, producing a cholesterol ester and lysolecithin. The activity of LCAT is stimulated by apo A-I. The cholesterol esters formed in this reaction can be transferred either to the core of the HDL particle or to other lipoprotein remnants.

Transfer of Cholesterol Esters from HDL to Lipoprotein Remnants. The transfer of cholesterol esters from HDLs to VLDL and chylomicron remnants is mediated by CETP, a protein associated with HDL. The space in the remnant particles that becomes filled with cholesterol esters is created by the depletion of triglyceride as a result of hydrolysis by LpL. Therefore, the pathway of reverse cholesterol transport is closely linked with the pathway of LpL-catalyzed triglyceride hydrolysis.

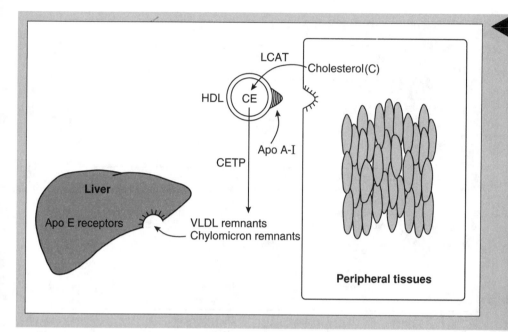

FIGURE 19-6
Reverse Cholesterol Transport. High-density lipoprotein (HDL) mediates the transport of cholesterol from peripheral tissues to the liver, where it can be processed for excretion. Apoprotein A-I (apo A-I) on the surface of HDL binds to receptors on peripheral tissues and promotes the movement of free cholesterol from the tissues to HDL, where it is converted to cholesterol ester by lecithin-cholesterol acyltransferase (LCAT). Cholesterol esters are subsequently transferred to lipoprotein remnants, which can be taken up by the liver. Transfer of cholesterol esters from HDL to remnants is catalyzed by cholesterol ester transfer protein (CETP). C = free cholesterol; CE = cholesterol ester; VLDL = very low-density lipoprotein.

Uptake of Cholesterol-Enriched Remnants by the Liver. Both VLDL remnants and chylomicron remnants contain apo E and apo B, which allow these particles to bind to receptors and be cleared by the liver. The liver converts most of the cholesterol to bile acids, which can be excreted in the feces. A small amount of free cholesterol is used in the synthesis of bile, and some cholesterol is repackaged into VLDL and secreted into the plasma.

HDL HETEROGENEITY

HDLs consist of two major forms, HDL_2 and HDL_3, which differ in size, density, and cholesterol content. HDL_2 particles are larger and have a higher cholesterol content than HDL_3. Hepatic lipase can convert the larger HDL_2 to the smaller HDL_3, which is capable of acquiring more cholesterol from peripheral cells during reverse cholesterol transport. A minor form, HDL_1, contains apo E, which can bind to remnant receptors and be taken up by the liver.

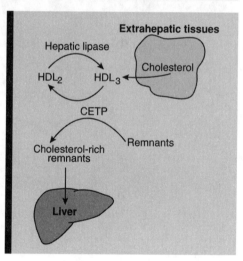

ABNORMALITIES IN LIPOPROTEIN METABOLISM

The concentration of plasma lipids and lipoproteins varies with many factors, including age, sex, physical activity, nutrition, and genetic makeup. A person within a given population is said to have hyperlipidemia if his or her plasma levels of cholesterol, triglyceride, or both are in the upper 5% of the population. Similarly, a person is said to have hypolipidemia if the lipid levels are in the lower 5% of the population. These conditions can be further classified as hyper- or hypolipoproteinemias, based on specific changes in the plasma-lipoprotein profiles. Inherited defects in lipoprotein metabolism result in primary hyperlipoproteinemia in some individuals. More commonly, however, these abnormalities are secondary to other diseases, such as hypothyroidism, diabetes, alcohol abuse, and atherosclerosis.

Primary Hyperlipidemia

The values given in Table 19-3 represent the ninety-fifth percentile of the North American population and are the cutoff values for defining hyperlipidemia. Hyperlipidemia is classified into five major phenotypes (I–V), based on the total plasma lipid levels and the type of lipoprotein that accumulates (Table 19-4). These phenotypes result from defects in either lipoprotein synthesis, metabolism, or uptake by tissues. In many cases, the defect can be traced to an abnormal form of a specific apoprotein, receptor, or enzyme.

Increased circulating levels of HDL provide protection against cardiovascular disease, whereas increased levels of chylomicrons, VLDL, and LDL have been associated with an increased risk of cardiovascular disease. Premenopausal women, vegetarians, and physically active people tend to have high levels of HDL. Inactivity, smoking, and obesity, on the other hand, have been associated with low HDL levels.

TABLE 19-3 ▶

Cutoff Values for Hyperlipidemia[a]

Age (yr)	Cholesterol (mg/dL)	Triglyceride (mg/dL)
1–9	200	120
10–19	205	140
20–29	210	140
30–39	240	150
40–49	265	160
>50	265	190

Source: Reprinted with permission from Bhagavan NV: *Medical Biochemistry.* Boston, MA: Jones and Bartlett, 1992, p 458.
[a] Measurements were made after an overnight fast and represent the 95th percentile for the North American population. Hyperlipidemia is defined by values above these cutoff levels.

TABLE 19-4 ▶

Types of Hyperlipoproteinemia

Type	Elevated Lipoprotein	Elevated Lipid	Deficiency or Defect	Appearance of Fasting Plasma
Ia	Chylomicron	Triglyceride	Lipoprotein lipase (LpL)	Milky
Ib	Chylomicron	Triglyceride	Apoprotein C-II	Milky
IIa	LDL	Cholesterol	LDL receptor	Clear
IIb	LDL and VLDL	Cholesterol	LDL receptor or apo B-100	Turbid or clear
III	β-VLDL[a]	Cholesterol and triglyceride	Abnormal apo E	Turbid
IV	VLDL	Cholesterol and triglyceride	VLDL overproduction or underutilization	Turbid or milky
V	VLDL Chylomicron	Cholesterol and triglyceride	LpL deficiency or hepatic lipase deficiency	Turbid or milky

Note. LDL = low-density lipoprotein; VLDL = very low-density lipoprotein.
Source: Adapted with permission from Marinetti GV: *Disorders of Lipid Metabolism.* New York, NY: Plenum Press, 1990, p 108.
[a] These VLDLs migrate in the region of the β-globulins during electrophoresis. The β-VLDLs are remnants of chylomicrons and VLDLs that contain an abnormal form of apo E-2.

Structure of LDL Receptor
Mutations in the gene for the LDL receptor result in familial hypercholesterolemia.

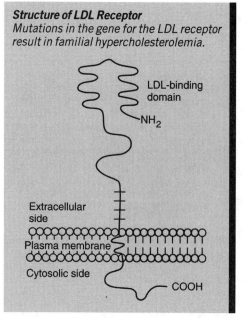

Familial Hypercholesterolemia (FH). This disorder, also known as *type II hyperlipoproteinemia*, results from an inherited defect in the LDL receptor. About 1 in 500 people are heterozygous for the FH gene. Carriers for FH have an LDL cholesterol level that is about twice that of the normal value. In the homozygous condition, the plasma cholesterol level may reach 5–8 times the normal value. A large number of mutations have been identified in the LDL-receptor gene. These mutations can impair the synthesis of LDL receptors, the transport of the receptor to the membrane, the binding of LDL to the receptor, or the clustering of LDL receptors in the coated pits. Affected individuals frequently have xanthomas and premature coronary artery disease.

Hypertriglyceridemia. A *type I hyperlipoproteinemia*, hypertriglyceridemia is generally caused by the inability to clear chylomicrons from the plasma. The molecular basis for the defect is due either to a deficiency in LpL or apo C-II, which is required for normal LpL activity.

Combined Hypercholesterolemia and Hypertriglyceridemia. Reduced uptake of chylomicron and VLDL remnants leads to an accumulation of both cholesterol and triglyceride (*type III hyperlipoproteinemia*). A deficiency in apo E is the most common cause of this type of hyperlipidemia. Electrophoresis of plasma from individuals with this condition reveals an abnormal band of lipoprotein (β-VLDL), which is a mixture of remnant particles. This type of hyperlipidemia is sometimes referred to as *dysbetalipoproteinemia* because of the accumulation of β-VLDL.

Primary Hypolipidemia

In general, hypolipidemia is less common than hyperlipidemia. Several conditions have been observed, however, where there is a decrease or an absence of one or more of the major plasma lipoproteins.

Abetalipoproteinemia. This type of hypolipidemia arises from an absence of apo B-100 and apo B-48. It is characterized by very low levels of plasma lipids and by a deficiency in all of the lipoproteins that normally contain apo B (i.e., chylomicrons, VLDL, IDL, LDL). Two striking features of this disease are retinitis pigmentosa, a condition that can lead to total blindness, and the presence of distorted red blood cells, also known as acanthocytes. These cells have a thorny appearance due to protoplasmic projections. Both the retinitis pigmentosa and acanthocytosis can be arrested with large doses of vitamin E.

Tangier Disease. Tangier disease is a rare autosomal recessive disease that is characterized by a deficiency in HDL, the intracellular accumulation of cholesterol, and elevated serum triglyceride. The serum level of apo A-I is between 1% and 3% of the normal level. The disease is usually seen in early childhood, with the appearance of enlarged, yellow–orange tonsils that are filled with foam cells. The serum lipid profile is unique, having decreased cholesterol and elevated triglycerides. The uptake of both chylomicrons and VLDL remnants is impaired as the result of a deficiency of apo E, accounting for the elevated triglyceride. Apo E is normally donated to these lipoproteins by HDL. Despite the low levels of HDL, premature atherosclerosis does not occur in Tangier disease.

Fish Eye Disease (FED). The lipoprotein profile in FED shows a marked reduction in HDL, an elevation in VLDL triglyceride, and normal LDL cholesterol levels. The activity of LCAT appears to be about 20% that of normal. In FED, the cornea becomes opaque, resulting in visual impairment. The eyes of people with FED are similar in appearance to the eyes of a boiled fish.

LOWERING PLASMA LIPIDS

Because of the strong associations among atherosclerosis, coronary heart disease, and serum cholesterol levels, much attention has been focused on methods for lowering serum cholesterol. These strategies fall into two major categories: dietary measures and drugs that lower plasma cholesterol.

Dietary Recommendations

In uncomplicated hyperlipoproteinemia, the first approach is dietary intervention and increased physical activity. The dietary focus is on reducing the intake of cholesterol, saturated fat, and total calories. Strategies include the curtailment of red meat, organ meats, whole milk, and baked goods prepared with saturated fats. Overall caloric intake is reduced to establish an ideal body weight. The guidelines from the National Cholesterol Education Program call for a trial of dietary modification for 3–6 months before considering drugs [5].

Cholesterol-Lowering Drugs

Several classes of drugs are available for treatment of hyperlipoproteinemias. They either decrease the production of cholesterol or increase the removal of cholesterol-enriched lipoproteins from the plasma.

Cholestyramine. Cholestyramine is a resin that binds bile acids in the small intestine and prevents them from being reabsorbed by the liver. The drug taken orally results in the excretion of bile acids in the feces. The impaired ability to reabsorb bile acids results in the increased use of cholesterol by the liver for bile acid synthesis.

Inhibitors of HMG CoA Reductase. Drugs such as mevinolin and lovastatin are structural analogs of HMG CoA that inhibit cholesterol synthesis. HMG CoA reductase catalyzes the rate-limiting step in cholesterol synthesis.

Nicotinic Acid. The production of VLDLs by the liver is inhibited by nicotinic acid. Decreased plasma VLDL, in turn, decreases the production of IDL and LDL.

Fibric Acid Derivatives. These drugs have multiple effects on plasma lipids. For example, the primary effect of clofibrate is to inhibit LpL, whereas the primary effect of gemfibrozil is to inhibit the secretion of VLDLs.

Probucol. Probucol is an antioxidant that significantly reduces plasma cholesterol but has no effect on triglycerides. The mechanism of probucol in humans is not clear, but in animals, it appears to stimulate clearance of LDL by the liver by a mechanism that is independent of receptors.

RESOLUTION OF CLINICAL CASE

The patient introduced at the beginning of this chapter is homozygous for familial hypercholesterolemia (FH). The diagnosis was initially suspected on the basis of her family history of coronary heart disease and by the appearance of xanthomas at such an early age. The diagnosis was subsequently confirmed at age 7 by cell culture studies of her fibroblasts, which showed she had no functional LDL receptors. The cholesterol levels in her parents were consistent with levels expected in heterozygous FH. Homozygous FH patients usually die by the age of 20 as a result of a myocardial infarct, and in some cases, they die as early as 4 or 5 years of age. Although this patient was receiving cholestyramine and lovastatin, her cholesterol levels were not reduced markedly by these drugs, a result typical for homozygous FH, although heterozygotes usually respond well to these drugs. The rationale for treating FH is always directed toward increasing the number of functional receptors on the surface of cells so that LDL can be cleared from the circulation. In heterozygotes, there is one functional LDL-receptor gene, whose expression is controlled by the intracellular level of cholesterol [6]. Therefore, drugs that lower the intracellular concentration of cholesterol induce the synthesis of new LDL receptors. In homozygous FH, both genes for the LDL receptor are defective, and the only way to increase the number of functional receptors is by organ transplantation. Liver is the organ of choice for transplantation, since about 70% of the total LDL receptors in the body are on the surface of the liver. A combined heart and liver transplant is often recommended because of advanced coronary heart disease. Indeed, in this patient, the heart that was removed showed advanced atherosclerosis.

REVIEW QUESTIONS

Directions: For each of the following questions, choose the **one best** answer.

1. A 25-year-old medical student experienced severe epigastric pain after eating a meal containing a large amount of fat. Analysis of plasma apoproteins showed a deficiency of apoprotein C-II (apo C-II). Other apoproteins were normal. Plasma electrophoresis showed an abnormal lipoprotein profile. Which of the following patterns of lipoproteins would most likely be seen in this individual?

    (A) Elevated high-density lipoproteins (HDLs) and low-density lipoproteins (LDLs)

    (B) Elevated chylomicrons and very low-density lipoproteins (VLDLs)

    (C) Elevated chylomicrons and decreased VLDLs

    (D) Decreased chylomicrons and elevated VLDLs

    (E) Decreased chylomicrons and VLDLs

2. Which of the following lipoproteins would account for most of the plasma cholesterol in a 27-year-old, healthy man who saw a physician for an annual physical examination?

    (A) High-density lipoproteins (HDLs)

    (B) Chylomicrons

    (C) Very low-density lipoproteins (VLDLs)

    (D) Low-density lipoproteins (LDLs)

    (E) Intermediate-density lipoproteins (IDLs)

3. A patient with a deficiency in lipoprotein lipase (LpL) would be expected to have which of the following plasma lipoprotein profiles?

    (A) Elevated levels of low-density lipoprotein with no other changes

    (B) Elevated levels of very low-density lipoprotein (VLDL) with no other changes

    (C) Elevated levels of chylomicrons and low levels of VLDL

    (D) Elevated levels of both chylomicrons and VLDL

    (E) Low levels of both chylomicrons and VLDL

4. Which of the following conditions would most likely result in the accumulation of cholesterol in extrahepatic tissues?

    (A) A deficiency in lipoprotein lipase (LpL)

    (B) A deficiency in acyl CoA:cholesterol acyltransferase (ACAT)

    (C) A deficiency in apoprotein A-I (apo A-I)

    (D) A high level of high-density lipoprotein (HDL)

    (E) A high level of lecithin–cholesterol acyltransferase (LCAT)

5. Which of the following characteristics describes familial hypercholesterolemia (FH)?

    (A) The plasma cholesterol in homozygous FH is about twice the normal level.

    (B) An impaired ability to internalize low-density lipoproteins (LDLs) is seen in homozygous but not heterozygous FH.

    (C) The mutation responsible for FH is in the gene that encodes apoprotein B-100.

    (D) Homozygotes for FH are unable to metabolize chylomicrons normally.

    (E) Treatment with cholestyramine and mevinolin are effective in lowering plasma cholesterol in heterozygous but not homozygous FH.

Directions: The groups of questions below consist of lettered choices followed by several numbered items. For each numbered item, select the appropriate lettered option with which it is most closely associated. Each lettered option may be used once, more than once, or not at all.

Questions 6–10

For each function described below, chose the lipoprotein, enzyme, or cell that is responsible for that function.

(A) Lecithin–cholesterol acyltransferase (LCAT)
(B) Apoprotein (apo E)
(C) High-density lipoprotein (HDL)
(D) Acyl CoA:cholesterol acyltransferase (ACAT)
(E) Beta–very low-density lipoproteins (β-VLDL)
(F) Foam cell

6. Catalyzes the extracellular esterification of cholesterol

7. Accumulates in plasma due to a deficiency in apo E

8. Accumulates in Tangier disease

9. Binds to remnant receptors

10. Mediates cholesterol transport from peripheral tissues to the liver

ANSWERS AND EXPLANATIONS

1. The answer is B. Apo C-II is required as a cofactor for lipoprotein lipase (LpL). A deficiency in apo C-II results in elevated chylomicrons and VLDL, since both are degraded by LpL. LDL and IDL levels would be decreased, since they are formed by the degradation of VLDL.

2. The answer is D. LDL is the major carrier of cholesterol in plasma. Although chylomicrons contain dietary cholesterol, and VLDL and IDL are precursors for LDL, plasma lipids are usually measured after an overnight fast. After an overnight fast, the chylomicrons have been cleared from the plasma, and most of the VLDL and IDL have been converted to LDL.

3. The answer is D. LpL hydrolyzes triglyceride in chylomicrons and VLDL. A deficiency of this enzyme results in an accumulation of both lipoproteins.

4. The answer is C. Apo A-I is found in HDL and plays an important role in reverse cholesterol transport. It binds to peripheral tissues and stimulates the uptake of cholesterol by HDL. High levels of HDL and LCAT would promote reverse cholesterol transport from extrahepatic tissues to the liver. A deficiency in ACAT would result in decreased cholesterol ester formation in tissues, whereas a deficiency in LpL would result in the accumulation of triglyceride-rich lipoproteins in the plasma.

5. The answer is E. Cholestryamine and mevinolin are drugs that promote a decrease in intracellular cholesterol, thereby inducing the synthesis of new LDL receptors. The genetic defect in FH is in the LDL receptor, and the synthesis of new receptors requires the presence of at least one functional gene for the LDL receptor. Both homozygotes and heterozygotes have an impaired ability to internalize LDL, resulting in plasma concentrations of LDL cholesterol that are about two times the normal concentrations in heterozygotes and up to eight times the normal concentrations in homozygotes. Chylomicron metabolism is not affected in FH.

6–10. The answers are: 6-A, 7-E, 8-F, 9-B, 10-C. The formation of extracellular and intracellular cholesterol ester is catalyzed by LCAT and ACAT, respectively. Apo E binds to remnant receptors on the liver and allows both chylomicron and VLDL remnants to be cleared. A deficiency in apo E results in the appearance of β-VLDL, a mixture of remnants that have an abnormal electrophoretic migration. Tangier disease is characterized by a deficiency in HDL, which results in impaired reverse cholesterol transport and the accumulation of foam cells in the tonsils, giving them a swollen yellow–orange appearance. HDL mediates the transport of cholesterol from peripheral tissues to the liver, where it can be converted to bile acids and excreted.

REFERENCES

1. Murray RK, Granner DK, Mayes PA, et al: *Harper's Biochemistry*, 23rd ed. Norwalk, CT: Appleton and Lange, 1993, p 251.
2. Havel RJ, Kane JP: Structure and metabolism of plasma lipoproteins. In *Metabolic and Molecular Bases of Inherited Disease*, 7th ed. Edited by Scriver CR, Beaudet AL, Sly WS, et al. New York, NY: McGraw-Hill, 1995, pp 1841–1851.
3. Bhagavan NV: *Medical Biochemistry*. Boston: Jones and Bartlett, 1992, p 458.
4. Marinetti GV: *Disorders of Lipid Metabolism*. New York, NY: Plenum Press, 1990, p 108.
5. Expert panel on detection, evaluation, and treatment of high blood cholesterol in adults: Report of the National Cholesterol Education Program (NCEP). *JAMA* 269:3015, 1993.
6. Goldstein JL, Hobbs HH, Brown MS: Familial hypercholesterolemia. In *Metabolic and Molecular Bases of Inherited Disease*, 7th ed. Edited by Scriver CR, Beaudet AL, Sly WS, et al. New York, NY: McGraw-Hill, 1995, p 1981.

20 FATTY ACID METABOLISM

CHAPTER OUTLINE

INTRODUCTION OF CLINICAL CASE

A 10-month-old girl was brought to the hospital in a coma. Her mother reported that she seemed to be fine when she went to sleep the previous night. She took her milk, was playful, and went to sleep about an hour after eating. However she awoke the next morning with seizures, which progressed to coma. When she arrived at the hospital, her blood glucose was 20 mg/dL. Glucose administration was started immediately, and her condition rapidly improved. The family history revealed that a sister had been hospitalized twice with hypoglycemic episodes between the ages of 8 months and 15 months and that she had died at the age of 18 months after a 15-hour fast. Analysis of the 10-month-old patient's blood showed no abnormalities in her blood cell count; her plasma levels of urea, bicarbonate, lactate, pyruvate, alanine, and ammonia were normal. No abnormal organic acids were found in either the plasma or urine. While in the hospital, the patient was submitted to a carefully monitored fast, during which her plasma glucose fell to 19 mg/dL within 16 hours and was not increased by intramuscular injection of glucagon. Her levels of plasma ketone bodies did not change during the fast. A liver biopsy showed normal mitochondria but a large accumulation of extramitochondrial fat. The carnitine concentration in the liver was normal, but carnitine acyltransferase activity was undetectable. At the end of the fast, the patient was given medium-chain triglycerides orally, and her blood glucose increased from 23 mg/dL to 140 mg/dL, acetoacetate levels increased from 3 mg/dL to 86 mg/dL, and β-hydroxybutyrate increased from 5 mg/dL to 205 mg/dL. The patient was dismissed from the hospital with instructions to be fed eight meals per day.

OVERVIEW OF FATTY ACID METABOLISM

There are three major pathways of fatty acid metabolism: (1) fatty acid synthesis, which occurs primarily in the liver; (2) fatty acid storage and mobilization, which occurs in adipose tissue; and (3) fatty acid oxidation, which occurs in most tissues. Examples of fatty acids that play important roles in human biochemistry are shown in Table 20-1. When fatty acid oxidation occurs faster than acetyl CoA is being used, ketone synthesis occurs. Ketones are synthesized in the liver and used as fuel by several extrahepatic tissues. The shift among fatty acid synthesis, storage, mobilization, and oxidation is controlled by a number of hormones, including insulin, glucagon, epinephrine, adrenocorticotropic hormone (ACTH), growth hormone, and corticosteroids.

TABLE 20-1 ▶

Fatty Acids of Importance in Human Metabolism

Name	Structure[a]	Properties
Acetic acid	2:0	Formed from glucose and amino acid degradation
Propionic acid	3:0	Formed from odd-chain fatty acids and branched-chain amino acids
Butyric acid	4:0	Found in cows' milk and butter
Decanoic acid	10:0	Major fatty acid in milk triglycerides
Palmitic acid	16:0	End product of fatty acid synthesis in most tissues
Stearic acid	18:0	Major fatty acid in gangliosides
Oleic acid	18:1 (Δ9)	Lowers plasma low-density lipoproteins when substituted for saturated fatty acids
Linoleic acid	18:2 (Δ9,12)	Essential fatty acid and precursor of arachidonic acid
Linolenic acid	18:3 (Δ9,12,15)	Essential fatty acid
Arachidonic acid	20:4 (Δ5,8,11,14)	Precursor of most eicosanoids
Lignoceric acid	24:0	Found in sphingolipids and glycolipids

[a] The nomenclature used here to describe the length and the position of double bonds is discussed in Chapter 18.

Synthesis and Storage Promoted by Insulin

The pathways of fatty acid synthesis and storage predominate in the well-fed state. The transient rise in blood glucose following a meal stimulates the release of insulin by the pancreas. The anabolic effects of insulin on fatty acid metabolism are illustrated in Figure 20-1. Insulin exerts its major effects on fatty acid metabolism by coordinating metabolic pathways in liver and adipose tissue.

Liver. In the well-fed state, excess dietary glucose and amino acids are converted to acetyl coenzyme A (CoA), the substrate for fatty acid synthesis. The conversion of glucose to fatty acids involves glycolysis, the pyruvate dehydrogenase (PDH) reaction, and the pathway of fatty acid synthesis. Insulin stimulates each of these processes. Newly synthesized fatty acids are converted to triglycerides, packaged into very low-density lipoproteins (VLDLs), and secreted by the liver into the blood.

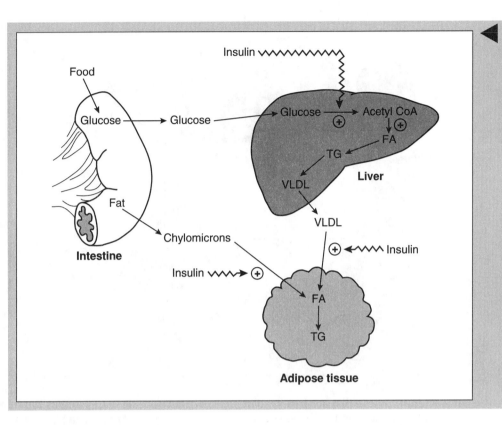

FIGURE 20-1
Effect of Insulin on Fatty Acid Synthesis and Storage. The conversion of excess dietary glucose to fatty acids in the liver is stimulated by insulin. The release of fatty acids from chylomicrons and VLDLs in the capillary bed of adipose tissue is stimulated by insulin. FA = fatty acids; TG = triglyceride; VLDL = very-low density lipoprotein.

Adipose Tissue. Most of the fatty acids in the blood are found in triglycerides, which are transported by chylomicrons and VLDLs. Fatty acids are released from chlyomicron-triglyceride and VLDL-triglyceride by the action of *lipoprotein lipase (LpL),* an extracellular enzyme whose presence in the capillary bed of adipose tissue is stimulated by insulin. The fatty acids diffuse into the adipocytes and are re-esterified to triglyceride for storage.

Mobilization and Oxidation Promoted by Glucagon and Epinephrine

The conditions that promote fatty acid mobilization from adipose tissue are fasting, physical exercise, and stress.

Adipose Tissue. The major hormones that stimulate triglyceride degradation in adipose tissue are glucagon, epinephrine, and ACTH (see Figure 20-2). Circulating glucagon levels are related to the concentration of blood glucose, whereas epinephrine and ACTH levels are increased by physical exercise and stress. Glucocorticoids and growth hormone can also promote a more chronic stimulation of triglyceride degradation.

Tissues That Oxidize Fatty Acids for Energy. The rapid release of fatty acids from adipose tissue ensures that tissues such as liver, muscle, heart, and kidney have an adequate supply of circulating fuel under a variety of physiologic conditions (see Figure 20-2). All tissues except the brain and red blood cells (RBCs) can use fatty acids as a fuel for generating energy.

Transport by Albumin

In general, fatty acids do not exist as free fatty acids in solution because of their marked affinity for proteins. The term "free fatty acid" usually means unesterified fatty acid. The major extracellular protein for binding and transporting free fatty acids is serum albumin. In the plasma, more than 99% of the free fatty acids are noncovalently bound to albumin. Albumin has at least 10 binding sites for fatty acids, with three high-affinity sites. Under most conditions, an average of 0.5 to 1.5 fatty acid molecules are bound per molecule of albumin. The small proportion of serum fatty acids that are actually free in solution (< 1% of the total) can diffuse across the membrane of tissues, where they bind to an intracellular fatty acid–binding protein (FABP). The equilibrium between albumin-bound

Contribution of Plasma Free Fatty Acids to Daily Energy Requirement
Plasma fatty acids turn over rapidly, having a half-life of about 1.5 minutes. The large reserve of albumin-bound fatty acids, coupled with the short half-life, results in a total turnover of about 200 g of fatty acids per day. The potential caloric value of these fatty acids is about 1800 kcal/day, assuming they are completely oxidized.

Transport Properties of Albumin
One of the major functions of albumin is to transport small hydrophobic molecules that have a low solubility in aqueous solutions. In addition to transporting fatty acids from adipocytes to other tissues, albumin transports bilirubin, steroid hormones, and a number of insoluble drugs that compete for the same binding sites.

FIGURE 20-2 ▶

Effect of Glucagon and Epinephrine on Fatty Acid Mobilization and Oxidation. *Glucagon, epinephrine, and other hormones that increase cAMP levels in adipose tissue stimulate the hydrolysis of triglyceride to fatty acids and glycerol. Glycerol is used by the liver for gluconeogenesis, and fatty acids are oxidized by the liver, heart, kidney, and muscle for energy. cAMP = cyclic adenosine monophosphate; ATP = adenosine triphosphate; FA = fatty acid; TG = triglyceride; ACTH = adrenocorticotropic hormone; CO_2 = carbon dioxide.*

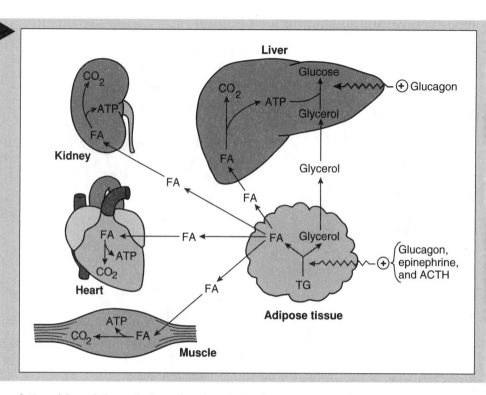

fatty acids and those that are free in solution is constantly being readjusted as the free fatty acids are taken up by tissues. Once inside the cell, the fatty acids can be translocated into the mitochondria where they are oxidized for energy, or they can be used by the smooth endoplasmic reticulum (SER) for synthesis of complex membrane lipids.

FATTY ACID SYNTHESIS

Fatty acids are synthesized by an elongation process in which two-carbon fragments, C_2 units, are added sequentially to the carboxyl end of the growing fatty acid. Acetyl CoA, derived primarily from glucose and amino acids, is the building block for fatty acids (Figure 20-3). The synthesis of palmitic acid (16:0) from acetyl CoA can be described by the following equation, in which NADPH = the reduced form of nicotinamide-adenine dinucleotide phosphate; H^+ = hydrogen ion; ADP = adenosine diphosphate; P_i = inorganic phosphate; and $NADP^+$ = the oxidized form of nicotinamide-adenine dinucleotide phosphate.

$$8 \text{ Acetyl CoA} + 7 \text{ ATP} + 14 \text{ NADPH} + 14 \text{ H}^+ + \text{H}_2\text{O} \longrightarrow$$

$$\text{palmitic acid} + 8 \text{ CoA} + 7 \text{ ADP} + 7 \text{ P}_i + 14 \text{ NADP}^+$$

Fatty acid synthesis occurs in three phases: (1) the accumulation of substrates in the appropriate cellular compartments; (2) the utilization of substrates to form palmitic acid; and (3) the elongation and desaturation of palmitate to generate a diverse family of fatty acids.

Source of Carbons for Fatty Acid Synthesis

$$CH_3-CH_2-(CH_2-CH_2)_n-CH_2-COOH$$

Acetyl CoA   **Malonyl CoA**

Substrates for Fatty Acid Synthesis

Three substrates are required for the synthesis of fatty acids: acetyl CoA, malonyl CoA, and NADPH. The initial two carbons incorporated into the fatty acids are donated by acetyl CoA and are found at the ω-end of the fatty acid. All other carbon atoms are donated by malonyl CoA. Therefore, most of the acetyl CoA in the equation above must be converted to malonyl CoA before it can be used. The pathway of fatty acid synthesis is reductive in nature, requiring 2 mols of NADPH for each C_2 unit donated by malonyl CoA.

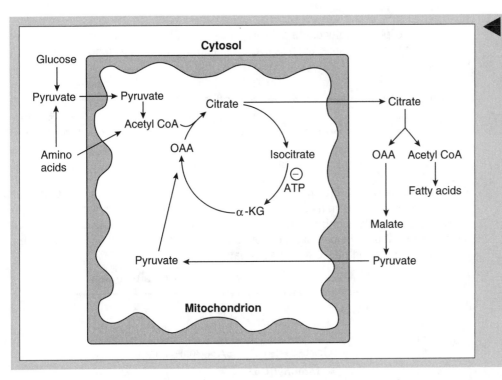

FIGURE 20-3
Synthesis of Fatty Acids from Excess Glucose and Amino Acids. Excess dietary glucose and amino acids are degraded to acetyl CoA and used by the liver for fatty acid synthesis. Acetyl CoA is transported to the cytosol as citrate, which is cleaved to oxaloacetate and acetyl CoA. Oxaloacetate is converted to pyruvate, which reenters the mitochondria and is carboxylated to oxaloacetate, completing the citrate cycle. The accumulation of ATP inhibits isocitrate dehydrogenase, resulting in the accumulation of isocitrate and citrate. OAA = oxaloacetate; α-KG = α-ketoglutarate; ATP = adenosine triphosphate.

Citrate Shuttle. Acetyl CoA is formed in the mitochondrial matrix, but fatty acid synthesis occurs in the cytosol. Since the inner mitochondrial membrane (IMM) is impermeable to acetyl CoA, it is translocated to the cytosol as citrate. Citrate is formed in the mitochondria by condensation of acetyl CoA and oxaloacetate. This reaction is catalyzed by *citrate synthase*, the first enzyme in the tricarboxylic acid (TCA) cycle. The accumulation of citrate in the mitochondria occurs only when the energy state of the cell is high. Under these conditions, ATP inhibits isocitrate dehydrogenase. The equilibrium between isocitrate and citrate favors the accumulation of citrate. After translocation to the cytosol, citrate is cleaved back to oxaloacetate and acetyl CoA by *citrate lyase*, thereby providing a source of acetyl CoA in the cytosol that can be used for fatty acid synthesis. The same two carbons that were added to oxaloacetate in the mitochondria are released as acetyl CoA in the cytosol. The reaction catalyzed by citrate lyase is shown in the following equation.

$$\text{Citrate + ATP + CoA} \xrightarrow{\text{\textbf{citrate lyase}}} \text{acetyl CoA + oxaloacetate + ADP + P}_i$$

Sources of NADPH. The NADPH required for fatty acid synthesis comes from two sources, the citrate shuttle and the pentose phosphate pathway. In addition to providing a source of cytosolic acetyl CoA, the citrate shuttle also releases oxaloacetate in the cytosol (see Figure 20-3). Since the IMM is impermeable to oxaloacetate, it is returned to the mitochondria either as malate or pyruvate. *Malate dehydrogenase* (malate DH) catalyzes the reduction of oxaloacetate to malate in a reaction that uses the reduced form of nicotinamide adenine dinucleotide (NADH). This reaction generates the oxidized form of nicotinamide adenine dinucleotide (NAD+). The next reaction, catalyzed by *malic enzyme*, converts malate to pyruvate in a reaction that generates NADPH. The sum of these two reactions effectively transfers reducing equivalents from cytosolic NADH to cytosolic NADPH, thereby providing some of the reducing power needed for fatty acid synthesis.

$$\text{Oxaloacetate} \xrightarrow[\substack{\text{NADH} \quad \text{NAD}^+}]{\textbf{malate DH}} \text{malate} \xrightarrow[\substack{\text{NADP}^+ \quad \text{NADPH}}]{\textbf{malic enzyme}} \text{pyruvate + CO}_2$$

The other source of NADPH is the pentose phosphate pathway. The NADPH-producing reactions are shown below, and are catalyzed by glucose-6-phosphate dehydrogenase

(G6PD) and 6-phosphogluconate dehydrogenase (6-PGD). Tissues that are actively engaged in fatty acid synthesis, such as liver and lactating mammary gland, are enriched in these enzymes.

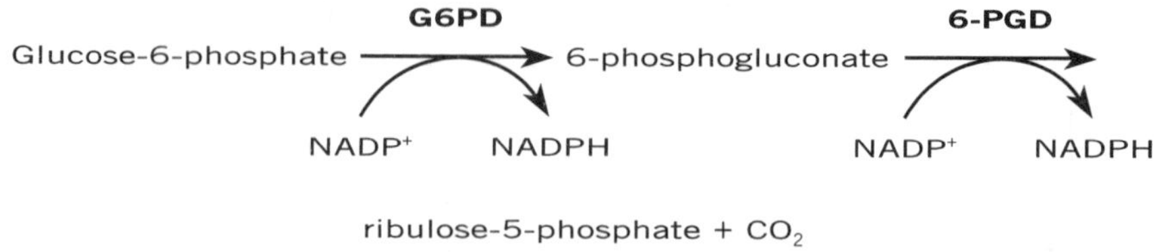

$$Glucose\text{-}6\text{-}phosphate \xrightarrow[\text{NADP}^+ \quad \text{NADPH}]{\textbf{G6PD}} 6\text{-}phosphogluconate \xrightarrow[\text{NADP}^+ \quad \text{NADPH}]{\textbf{6-PGD}}$$

$$ribulose\text{-}5\text{-}phosphate + CO_2$$

Source of Malonyl CoA. Malonyl CoA, formed by the carboxylation of acetyl CoA, has a unique role in metabolism. Its only known functions are to serve as an activated donor of acetyl groups in fatty acid biosynthesis and to help coordinate fatty acid synthesis with fatty acid oxidation. The carboxylation of acetyl CoA is catalyzed by acetyl CoA carboxylase and is described by the following equation.

$$\underset{\textbf{Acetyl CoA}}{CH_3-\overset{\overset{\displaystyle O}{\|}}{C}\sim SCoA} + HCO_3^- + ATP \xrightarrow{\hspace{1cm}\textbf{acetyl CoA carboxylase}\hspace{1cm}}$$

$$\underset{\textbf{Malonyl CoA}}{{}^-OOC\sim CH_2-\overset{\overset{\displaystyle O}{\|}}{C}\sim SCoA} + ADP + P_i$$

Acetyl CoA carboxylase requires biotin as a cofactor, and bicarbonate (HCO_3^-) and ATP are required as substrates. Some of the energy released by the hydrolysis of ATP is conserved in the newly formed carbon–carbon bond and is used to drive subsequent elongation reactions in fatty acid synthesis.

Fatty Acid Synthase Complex

The synthesis of fatty acids is catalyzed by fatty acid synthase (FAS), a multienzyme complex that catalyzes the overall reaction shown in the following equation.

$$Acetyl\sim CoA + 7\ malonyl\sim CoA + 14\ NADPH + 7\ H^+ \xrightarrow{\hspace{1cm}\textbf{FAS}\hspace{1cm}}$$

$$palmitic\ acid + 7\ CO_2 + 14\ NADP^+ + 8\ CoA + 6\ H_2O$$

In most tissues, the product of fatty acid synthesis is palmitic acid. The FAS complex consists of seven enzymes and acyl carrier protein (ACP), to which the intermediates are attached during elongation. The FAS complex catalyzes the sequential addition of C_2 units to the carboxyl end of the growing fatty acyl chain. Each new C_2 addition requires malonyl CoA and is accompanied by the release of carbon dioxide. The energy released by decarboxylation is used to drive the formation of the new C–C bond created by elongation. After a C_2 group is added, the product is fully reduced to a saturated acyl group. These reduction reactions require 2 mols of NADPH per elongation step.

Priming Reactions. The initial condensation reaction involves an acetyl group and a malonyl group. However, before this reaction can occur, the acetyl group and the malonyl group are transferred from their CoA derivatives to the condensing enzyme and ACP, respectively. Both the condensing enzyme and ACP have sulfhydryl groups that form thioesters with the substrates (Figure 20-4). These priming reactions are catalyzed by acetyl transacetylase and malonyl transacetylase.

Core Reactions of Fatty Acid Synthesis. Each elongation step consists of four core reactions, which are repeated until the fatty acid is completely synthesized. (1) The *condensation* of malonyl-ACP with the acyl-condensing enzyme produces a β-keto-acyl-ACP intermediate and releases the condensing enzyme; (2) the *reduction* of β-ketoacyl-ACP by NADPH generates a β-hydroxyacyl-ACP intermediate; (3) the *dehydration* of the β-hydroxyacyl-ACP introduces a double bond between the α- and β-carbons; and (4) *reduction* of the double bond by NADPH produces a fully saturated fatty acid. At

---

Fatty Acid Synthesis in the Mammary Gland
The major product of fatty acid synthesis in the lactating mammary gland is decanoic acid (10:0). The mammary gland contains decanoyl deacylase, an enzyme that releases the 10:0 fatty acid from the ACP before it can be further elongated. The presence of medium-chain fatty acids in milk may offer advantages to the neonate. Medium-chain fatty acids are directly absorbed from the intestinal cell into the portal blood and do not have to be packaged into chylomicrons. Additionally, they are not dependent on the carnitine shuttle for entry into the mitochondria where they are oxidized.

Sequence of Reactions in Fatty Acid Synthesis
Condensation, reduction, dehydration, and reduction.

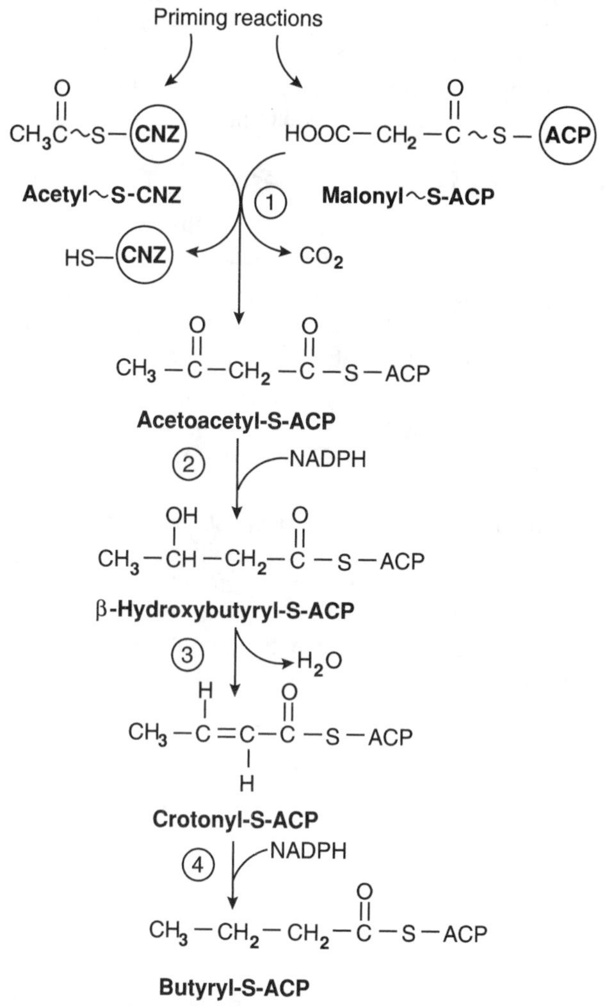

FIGURE 20-4
Core Reactions of Fatty Acid Synthesis. *The acetyl and malonyl groups are primed for condensation by becoming covalently linked to condensing enzyme (CNZ) and acyl carrier protein (ACP), respectively. Enzymes catalyzing the reactions are: 1 = condensing enzyme (also known as synthase); 2 = β-ketoacyl reductase; 3 = dehydratase; and 4 = enoyl reductase.*

the end of the first cycle, the C_4 fatty acid (butyric acid) is transferred from ACP to the condensing enzyme. The ACP is primed with another malonyl group in preparation for the next cycle of elongation. When the fatty acid has reached the length of palmitic acid (16:0), it can either be released as free palmitic acid or transferred to CoA, giving palmitoyl CoA.

Modification of Palmitic Acid

In most tissues, the elongation process stops when the chain length reaches 16 carbons. Palmitic acid (16:0) can be elongated and desaturated by auxiliary enzymes to provide a variety of fatty acids. Humans can synthesize all of the fatty acids they need except linoleic and linolenic acid, which are essential components of the diet.

Elongation Reactions. Two elongation systems exist in humans, a mitochondrial and a microsomal system. Both systems elongate palmitic acid to a variety of saturated fatty acids by the sequential addition of C_2 units to the carboxyl end. The mitochondrial system uses acetyl CoA and either NADH or NADPH as the reducing agent, whereas the microsomal system uses malonyl CoA as a C_2 donor and NADPH as the reducing agent. After an elongation reaction, the intermediates have to be fully reduced. These intermediates are similar to those generated by the FAS complex, but they are not attached to ACP, and the enzymes involved are different gene products.

Desaturation Reactions. The introduction of double bonds is catalyzed by a family of microsomal enzymes known as *desaturases*. These enzymes have slight differences in their active sites, which allow double bonds to be introduced into different, but specific, locations in the fatty acid. The insertion of a double bond requires molecular oxygen, NADPH, and three types of subunits: cytochrome b_5 reductase containing tightly bound flavin adenine dinucleotide (FAD); cytochrome b_5 containing heme; and desaturase, a protein containing iron–sulfur centers. A key intermediate in this reaction is the addition of a hydroxyl group, followed by the elimination of water, resulting in a double bond.

Regulation of Fatty Acid Synthesis

The rate-limiting step in fatty acid synthesis is the formation of malonyl CoA, catalyzed by acetyl CoA carboxylase. This enzyme is subject to multiple types of regulation.

Allosteric Regulation. Acetyl CoA carboxylase is allosterically activated by citrate and inhibited by palmitoyl CoA. In the presence of citrate, the enzyme polymerizes into long filaments that are highly active. Palmitoyl CoA prevents the polymerization.

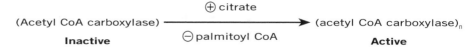

$$\text{(Acetyl CoA carboxylase)} \xrightarrow[\ominus\ \text{palmitoyl CoA}]{\oplus\ \text{citrate}} \text{(acetyl CoA carboxylase)}_n$$

Inactive   **Active**

Covalent Regulation. Acetyl CoA carboxylase is also regulated by phosphorylation and dephosphorylation (Figure 20-5). The equilibrium between the phosphorylated and dephosphorylated forms is controlled by the glucagon to insulin ratio in the plasma. Phosphorylation is catalyzed by cyclic adenosine monophosphate (cAMP)–dependent protein kinase and results in the inactivation of the enzyme. Activation is achieved by dephosphorylation, which is catalyzed by protein phosphatase.

FIGURE 20-5 ▶

Hormonal Regulation of Acetyl CoA Carboxylase. Glucagon stimulates the phosphorylation and inactivation of acetyl CoA carboxylase. Insulin antagonizes the glucagon effect. Acetyl CoA carboxylase–P = the phosphorylated form of the enzyme.

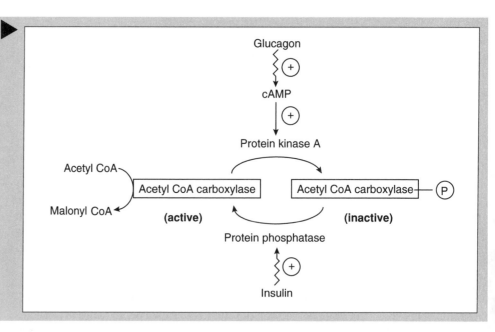

Induction of Enzyme Synthesis. Insulin induces the synthesis of several enzymes that are involved either directly or indirectly in fatty acid synthesis, including acetyl CoA carboxylase, FAS, citrate lyase, malic enzyme, G6PD, and 6-PGD.

FATTY ACID STORAGE AND MOBILIZATION

Under normal conditions, more than 95% of the triglyceride is stored in adipose tissue, with the remainder found primarily in the liver and muscle. The amount of triglyceride found in the liver increases during starvation, in uncontrolled diabetes, or in any other condition where fat is rapidly mobilized from adipose tissue and oxidized for energy.

Fat Cells

The fat cells of adipose tissue are modified fibroblasts that have between 80% and 95% of their cell volume filled with triglycerides. The triglycerides are usually in a liquid form, and they constitute about 99% of the total lipid and 80% of the weight of the adipocyte. Adipose tissue triglyceride contains at least 20 different kinds of fatty acids, the major ones being oleic, palmitic, linoleic, stearic, and myristic acids.

Turnover of Triglyceride in Fat Cells

High concentrations of lipases are found in adipose tissue. *Extracellular LpL* releases fatty acids from chylomicron-triglyceride and VLDL-triglyceride in the blood. The fatty acids are taken up by adipose tissue and converted to triglyceride for storage. *Intracellular lipases* hydrolyze fatty acids from triglyceride stores so that they can be transported to other tissues and oxidized for energy. Because of the high activity of both of these intracellular and extracellular lipases, the triglyceride content of the fat cell turns over rapidly and is renewed about once every 2–3 weeks [1]. Therefore, metabolism in adipose tissue is a dynamic process. The fat stored today is not the same fat that was stored last month. The reactions involved in the synthesis and degradation of triglyceride in adipose tissue are summarized in Figure 20-6.

Fat Stores in the Neonate
The human being is one of the few mammals born with fat stores, which begin to accumulate during the thirtieth week of gestation.

Fatty Acid Composition of Adipose Tissue

Fatty Acid	% of Total
Oleic acid (18:1)	45
Palmitic acid (16:0)	20
Linoleic acid (18:2)	10
Stearic acid (18:0)	6
Myristic acid (14:0)	4
Others	15

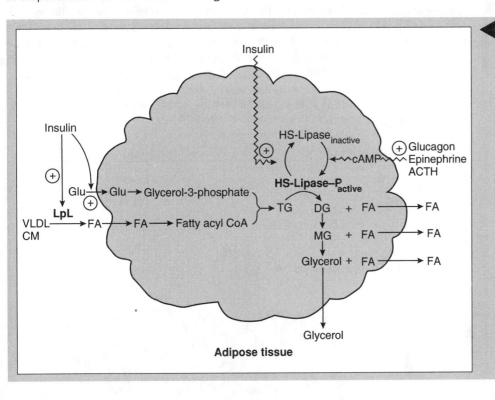

Adipose tissue

◀ **FIGURE 20-6**
Triglyceride Metabolism in Adipose Tissue. *Insulin stimulates triglyceride synthesis and inhibits degradation. Glucagon, epinephrine, and ACTH stimulate triglyceride degradation by activating hormone-sensitive lipase. HS-lipase = hormone-sensitive lipase; Glu = glucose; FA = fatty acid; VLDL = very low-density lipoprotein; CM = chylomicron; TG = triglyceride; DG = diglyceride; MG = monoglyceride; cAMP = cyclic adenosine monophosphate; ACTH = adrenocorticotropic hormone.*

Effect of Insulin on Adipose Tissue. Insulin stimulates triglyceride synthesis in adipocytes by increasing the availability of substrates. Increased fatty acid uptake results from the stimulation of LpL, while an increase in glucose uptake and glycolysis provides a source of glycerol for triglyceride synthesis. The glycerol backbone of triglycerides is derived from dihydroxyacetone phosphate, an intermediate in glycolysis.

Effect of Glucagon, Epinephrine, and ACTH on Adipose Tissue. The most important intracellular lipase in adipose tissue is *hormone-sensitive lipase*, which initiates triglyceride degradation by removing the fatty acid from either the C-1 or C-3 position of the glycerol backbone. The diglyceride is subsequently hydrolyzed to free glycerol and fatty acids, which are released into the blood and transported to other tissues. Hormone-sensitive lipase catalyzes the rate-limiting step in triglyceride degradation. It is activated by a large number of hormones, including glucagon, epinephrine, norepinephrine, and ACTH. All of these hormones increase the intracellular concentration of cAMP and pro-

Expansion of Adipose Tissue and Obesity
The rate of fat-cell formation is most rapid in early life. As the rate of fat storage increases, the number of fat cells increases. In obese children, the number of fat cells is often 2–3 times higher than in children of normal weight. However, after adolescence the number of fat cells remains relatively constant. In people who become obese in middle age, most of the obesity comes from increased fat storage in cells that are already present. When adult body weight reaches 170% of ideal, a maximum cell size is reached, after which cell number and obesity are highly correlated [2].

mote phosphorylation of hormone-sensitive lipase. Conversely, insulin inhibits the activity of hormone-sensitive lipase, both by decreasing the concentration of cAMP and by activating protein phosphatase.

FATTY ACID OXIDATION

Fatty acids are an important source of energy for the heart, skeletal muscle, kidney, and liver. Most fatty acid oxidation occurs in the mitochondria, although peroxisomes oxidize very long-chain fatty acids and branched-chain fatty acids. As soon as fatty acids enter the cell, they are converted to fatty acyl CoA (see Chapter 19).

Carnitine Shuttle

The IMM is impermeable to fatty acyl CoA, and entry into mitochondria is mediated by the carnitine shuttle. This shuttle consists of two enzymes and a carnitine transport protein (Figure 20-7). The first enzyme, *carnitine acyltransferase-1 (CAT-1)*, is located on the outer surface of the IMM, where it transfers the fatty acid from CoA to carnitine, forming acylcarnitine. The acylcarnitine is then transported across the membrane by the carnitine transporter. The second enzyme, *carnitine acyltransferase-2 (CAT-2)*, is located on the inner surface of the mitochondrial membrane, where it transfers the acyl group back to CoA as it enters the matrix. Separate pools of CoA are found inside and outside the mitochondrial matrix. Medium- and short-chain fatty acids, having chain lengths less than or equal to C_{12}, enter the mitochondrial matrix independent of carnitine. The enzymes in the carnitine shuttle are also known as "carnitine *O*-palmitoyl transferase 1 and 2" and may be seen abbreviated as PAT-1 and PAT-2.

Carnitine Deficiency
Although carnitine is not a dietary requirement, deficiencies are often seen in premature infants, who have not gained the ability to synthesize carnitine, as well as in patients with kidney disease, who are losing carnitine in the urine. Patients with organic aciduria also develop secondary carnitine deficiencies as a result of the excretion of organic acids conjugated with carnitine in the urine. Signs and symptoms of carnitine deficiency include hypoglycemia resulting from impaired gluconeogenesis, impaired fatty acid oxidation and ketogenesis, and elevated plasma fatty acid levels.

FIGURE 20-7
Carnitine Shuttle. *Carnitine is required to translocate fatty acids from the cytosol to the mitochondrial matrix. Both the entry of acylcarnitine and the exit of free carnitine are mediated by the carnitine transporter (CT). Carnitine acyltransferase-1 (CAT-1) is located on the outer surface of the inner mitochondrial membrane (IMM), and carnitine acyltransferase-2 (CAT-2) is on the inner surface. Carnitine is synthesized from trimethyllysine, which is released from the degradation of muscle protein.*

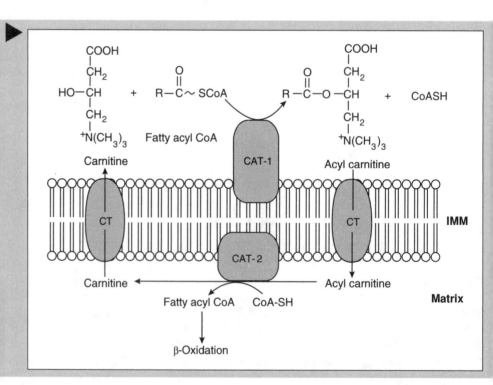

Core Reactions of β-Oxidation

The oxidation of fatty acids is a cyclic process involving four enzymes that sequentially remove acetyl CoA from the carboxyl end of the fatty acid. Each cycle of β-oxidation produces one molecule each of acetyl CoA, the reduced form of flavin adenine dinucleotide ($FADH_2$), and NADH. The reactions involved are shown in Figure 20-8. The first step in β-oxidation is a FAD-linked dehydrogenation reaction that introduces a double bond between the α- and β-carbon atoms. This reaction is catalyzed by *fatty acyl CoA dehydrogenases* that are specific for fatty acids of different chain lengths. In the second reaction, water is added across the double bond, producing β-hydroxyacyl CoA. The hydroxyl group is then oxidized in a NAD-linked dehydrogenation reaction, producing β-ketoacyl CoA. The final reaction in each cycle of β-oxidation is a thiolytic cleavage that releases acetyl CoA. The cycle is repeated until the fatty acid has been completely degraded to acetyl CoA.

Sequence of Reactions in Fatty Acid Oxidation
Dehydrogenation (FAD-dependent), hydration, dehydrogenation (NAD-dependent), and cleavage.

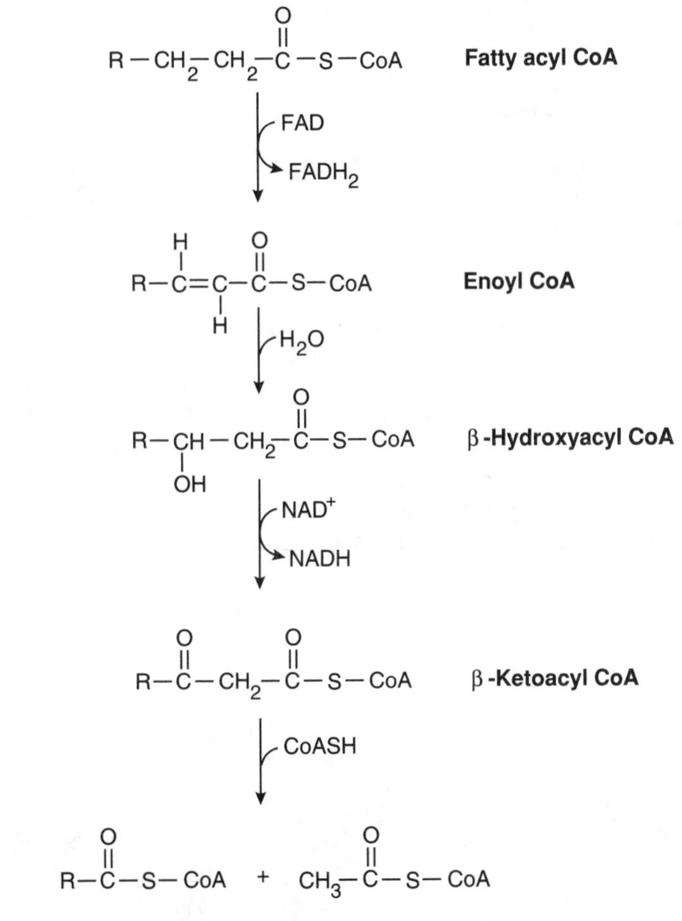

FIGURE 20-8
β-Oxidation of Fatty Acids. *Each cycle of β-oxidation includes four reactions, which start with the oxidation of fatty acyl CoA and end with the removal of acetyl CoA by thiolytic cleavage. For even-numbered fatty acids, the products are acetyl CoA, $FADH_2$, and NADH. For odd-numbered fatty acids, the final thiolytic cleavage gives acetyl CoA and propionyl CoA from the ω-end. R = alkyl group.*

There are three isozymes of fatty acyl CoA dehydrogenase: long-chain acyl CoA dehydrogenase (LCAD), medium-chain acyl CoA dehydrogenase (MCAD), and short-chain acyl CoA dehydrogenase (SCAD) that work on C_{12}–C_{18}, C_6–C_{12}, and C_4–C_6 fatty acids, respectively. The complete oxidation of a long-chain fatty acid requires all three of the isozymes, with MCAD and SCAD becoming the preferred isozymes as the fatty acid gets progressively shorter. Genetic deficiencies in each of these enzymes have been identified as discrete clinical entities.

Energetics of Fatty Acid Oxidation

Fatty acids are a dense source of energy because they are highly reduced and have little water associated with them. The complete oxidation of a fatty acid to carbon dioxide and water results in considerably more energy than that obtained from the complete

Medium-Chain Fatty Acyl CoA Deficiency
MCAD deficiency is found in about 1 in 10,000 births, and it has a wide variation in clinical presentation. Episodes of vomiting, lethargy, hypoglycemia, and hyperammonemia are common. MCAD deficiency is often mistaken for Reye's syndrome, a virally precipitated condition with many of the same symptoms. It is estimated that about 10% of the cases of sudden infant death syndrome may be the result of MCAD deficiency.

oxidation of the same amount of carbohydrate. The following equation describes the β-oxidation of palmitoyl CoA.

$$\text{Palmitoyl}{\sim}\text{CoA} + 7\ NAD^+ + 7\ FADH_2 + 7\ CoASH \longrightarrow$$

$$8\ \text{acetyl}{\sim}\text{CoA} + 7\ NADH + 7\ FADH_2$$

Although there is no ATP directly produced by β-oxidation, the products of the pathway can be further oxidized by the TCA cycle and oxidative phosphorylation. The oxidation of each mol of acetyl CoA to carbon dioxide and water can support the synthesis of 12 mols of ATP, while each mol of NADH and $FADH_2$ supports the synthesis of 3 mols and 2 mols of ATP, respectively, for a total of 131 mols of ATP per mol of palmitoyl CoA. If oxidation starts with free palmitic acid, the net ATP yield is 129 mols of ATP because two high-energy bonds are hydrolyzed in converting palmitic acid to palmitoyl CoA.

Coordinate Regulation of Fatty Acid Oxidation and Fatty Acid Synthesis

The conditions that promote fatty acid synthesis inhibit fatty acid oxidation, and vice versa, thus preventing futile cycling. The coordinate regulation of these opposing pathways is achieved by both allosteric regulation and hormonal regulation. The key enzymes involved in the coordinate regulation are CAT-1 and acetyl CoA carboxylase in the liver and hormone-sensitive lipase in adipose tissue.

Allosteric Effectors. The rate-limiting step in fatty acid oxidation is catalyzed by CAT-1, which is allosterically inhibited by *malonyl CoA*. Thus, the accumulation of malonyl CoA simultaneously provides substrate for fatty acid synthesis and blocks the entry of fatty acids into the mitochondria where β-oxidation occurs (Figure 20-9). The rate-limiting step in fatty acid synthesis is catalyzed by acetyl CoA carboxylase, the enzyme that synthesizes malonyl CoA. Acetyl CoA carboxylase is allosterically activated by *citrate*, which carries acetyl CoA from the mitochondria into the cytosol. *Palmitoyl CoA*, the end product of fatty acid synthesis, inhibits acetyl CoA carboxylase.

FIGURE 20-9 ▶

Coordinate Regulation of Fatty Acid Synthesis and Oxidation by Allosteric Effectors. The target enzyme for the regulation of fatty acid synthesis is acetyl CoA carboxylase, which is activated by citrate and inhibited by palmitoyl CoA. Fatty acid oxidation is regulated by controlling the rate at which fatty acids enter the mitochondria. Carnitine acyltransferase-1 (CAT-1) is allosterically inhibited by malonyl CoA.

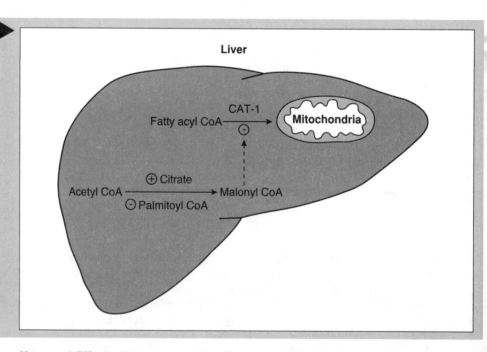

Hormonal Effects. Hormone-sensitive lipase and acetyl CoA carboxylase both exist in phosphorylated and dephosphorylated forms. The phosphorylation of these enzymes is promoted by hormones that increase intracellular cAMP levels, such as glucagon, epinephrine, and ACTH (Figure 20-10). Hormone-sensitive lipase is activated by phosphorylation, thereby increasing the supply of fatty acids that are available to various tissues for oxidation. Acetyl CoA carboxylase and fatty acid synthesis are inhibited by phosphorylation. Conversely, insulin promotes dephosphorylation of hormone-sensitive lipase and acetyl CoA carboxylase, resulting in decreased triglyceride hydrolysis in adipocytes and increased fatty acid synthesis in liver.

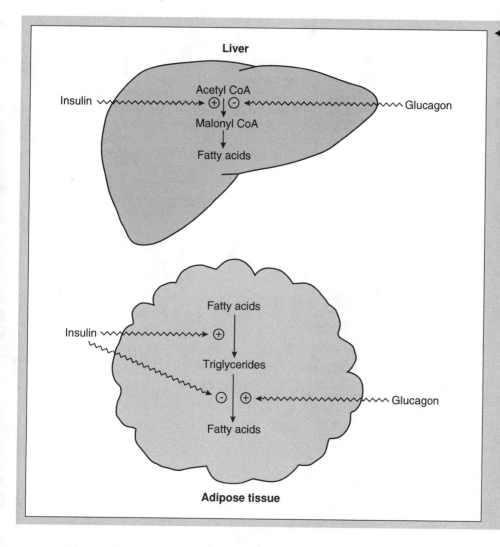

◀ **FIGURE 20-10**
Coordinate Regulation of Fatty Acid Metabolism by Insulin and Glucagon. *Insulin stimulates fatty acid synthesis in the liver and triglyceride synthesis in adipose tissue, and it inhibits lipolysis in adipose tissue. Conversely, glucagon inhibits fatty acid synthesis in the liver, and it stimulates lipolysis in adipose tissue. The enzymes affected are acetyl CoA carboxylase in the liver and hormone-sensitive lipase in adipose tissue. Insulin and glucagon control the equilibrium between the phosphorylated and dephosphorylated forms of these enzymes.*

Peroxisomal Fatty Acid Oxidation

Peroxisomes are important in the oxidation of very long-chain fatty acids and branched-chain fatty acids.

Very Long-Chain Fatty Acids. The oxidation of fatty acids having chain lengths equal to C_{26} or longer begins in peroxisomes and is completed in mitochondria. The peroxisomal pathway is analogous to the mitochondrial pathway, but different isozymes are found in the two subcellular compartments, and the $FADH_2$ formed in peroxisomes cannot lead to ATP synthesis. FAD is regenerated by oxygen, with the formation of hydrogen peroxide. When fatty acids have been reduced to a chain length of C_8, they leave the peroxisomes and are taken up by mitochondria, where oxidation is completed.

Branched-Chain Fatty Acids. Phytanic acid is a C_{20} fatty acid having methyl groups attached to carbons 3, 7, 11, and 15. It is derived from the oxidation of phytol, a major component of chlorophyll, and is present in almost all vegetables, as well as in milk and fat products derived from ruminants. Phytanic acid cannot undergo the first step of β-oxidation because of the presence of a methyl group on the β-carbon. The oxidation of phytanic acid requires hydroxylation of the α-carbon atom, followed by oxidation and decarboxylation, resulting in a C_{19} fatty acid. These reactions are catalyzed by an enzyme complex known as *α-hydroxylase*. The C_{19} fatty acid can be further degraded by β-oxidation. A genetic deficiency in α-hydroxylase results in *Refsum's disease* [3].

Refsum's Disease
This disease is caused by the accumulation of phytanic acid in nerve tissue, secondary to a genetic defect in the peroxisomal enzyme, α-hydroxylase, and the inability to oxidize phytanic acid. Clinical symptoms include retinitis pigmentosa, peripheral neuropathy, and ataxia. Treatment involves elimination of dietary sources of phytol.

Phytanic Acid

KETONE BODY METABOLISM

Ketone bodies play an important role in fuel homeostasis by providing fuel for muscle and brain tissue during periods of fasting and starvation. When the circulating concentration of ketone bodies reaches 1–3 mM, they begin to be taken up by extrahepatic tissues and oxidized. Normally, the concentration of ketone bodies in the blood is less than 0.2 mM. After fasting for 3 days, the concentration is about 3 mM, and by 3 weeks of fasting, it increases to about 7 mM [2]. Ketone bodies also play an important role in the adaptations that allow tissue protein to be conserved during starvation. The product of ketogenesis is acetoacetate, which can be reduced to β-hydroxybutyrate. Both are small water-soluble acids, having pK_a values of approximately 3.7, and both are completely dissociated within the physiologic pH range. The synthesis and utilization of ketone bodies are summarized in Figure 20-11.

Diabetic Ketoacidosis
The lack of insulin in untreated type I diabetes leads to the uncontrolled release of fatty acids from adipose tissue and the subsequent oxidation by the liver, with the overflow of acetyl CoA being used for ketone synthesis. Extremely high levels of ketone bodies (10–20 mM) can accumulate in the blood, resulting in metabolic acidosis that, if untreated, can be fatal.

FIGURE 20-11 ▶

Ketone Body Metabolism. Ketone bodies are synthesized in the liver and used by extrahepatic tissues. The liver enzymes involved in synthesis are as follows: 1 = thiolase; 2 = hydroxymethylglutaryl CoA (HMG CoA) synthase; 3 = HMG CoA lyase; 4 = β-hydroxybutyrate dehydrogenase. The enzymes in extrahepatic tissues that are involved in oxidation are: 5 = β-hydroxybutyrate dehydrogenase; 6 = succinyl CoA: acetoacetate CoA transferase; 7 = thiolase.

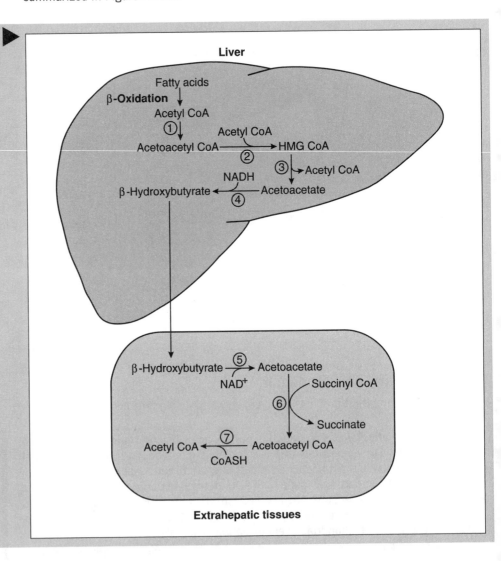

Synthesis of Ketone Bodies by the Liver

The major ketone bodies are acetoacetate and β-hydroxybutyrate. Spontaneous decarboxylation of a small fraction of the acetoacetate gives rise to acetone, which is exhaled by the lungs. Acetone is responsible for the "fruity breath" that is sometimes observed in people with uncontrolled diabetes. Ketogenesis occurs when carbohydrate availability is limited and excessive fatty acid oxidation is occurring. Synthesis occurs in the mitochondrial compartment of the liver. The two initial reactions, resulting in hydroxymethylglutaryl CoA (HMG CoA), also occur in the pathway of cholesterol synthesis (see Chapter 21). However, different isozymes are found in the mitochondria and the cytoplasm, where the synthesis of ketone bodies and cholesterol occurs, respectively.

Utilization of Ketone Bodies by Extrahepatic Tissues

The uptake and oxidation of ketone bodies by peripheral tissues is dependent on the concentration in the blood. Oxidation occurs in the mitochondria, where β-hydroxybutyrate is oxidized to acetoacetate as it crosses the inner mitochondrial membrane. Acetoacetate acquires CoA in a transfer reaction with succinyl CoA. Acetoacetyl CoA is then cleaved to two molecules of acetyl CoA. The liver is unable to use ketone bodies as fuel because the enzyme *succinyl CoA:acetoacetate CoA transferase* is not expressed in the liver. In the well-fed state, this enzyme is also absent in the brain. However, when ketone bodies accumulate in the blood to concentrations between 2 mM and 3 mM, synthesis of the enzyme in the brain is induced.

The ratio of β-hydroxybutyrate to acetoacetate is controlled by the ratio of mitochondrial NADH to NAD+. This ratio can vary from 1 to 10, but under normal circumstances is approximately 3. The ratio can be used clinically as an index of liver perfusion (oxygen availability) and liver functions.

RESOLUTION OF CLINICAL CASE

The patient introduced at the beginning of this chapter was diagnosed with hypoketonic hypoglycemia, secondary to a deficiency in hepatic carnitine acyltransferase activity. This enzyme is required to transport long-chain fatty acids into the mitochondria for oxidation. The low levels of blood glucose and ketone bodies that were seen in this patient after a few hours of fasting resulted from an impairment in β-oxidation of fatty acids. The ATP that is required for gluconeogenesis is derived from fatty acid oxidation. The analysis of plasma revealed normal levels of gluconeogenic substrates, and the analysis of liver biopsy material showed that normal levels of carnitine were present. The entry of medium-chain fatty acids into the mitochondria is not dependent on the carnitine shuttle. Thus, oral administration of medium-chain triglycerides resulted in an increase in the levels of both blood glucose and ketone bodies, indicating that the pathway of β-oxidation was functioning normally. The treatment for this condition is to rigorously avoid hypoglycemia by frequent feedings.

REVIEW QUESTIONS

Directions: For each of the following questions, choose the **one best** answer.

1. During fatty acid synthesis, acetyl CoA appears in the cytosol as a result of which of the following enzymes?

    (A) Malic enzyme

    (B) Isocitrate dehydrogenase

    (C) Citrate synthase

    (D) Citrate lyase

    (E) Thiolase

2. The removal of C_2 units from a fatty acyl CoA during β-oxidation involves which of the following sequences of reactions?

    (A) Oxidation, dehydration, reduction, and cleavage

    (B) Reduction, hydration, dehydrogenation, and cleavage

    (C) Dehydrogenation, hydration, dehydrogenation, and cleavage

    (D) Reduction, dehydration, reduction, and cleavage

    (E) Hydrogenation, dehydration, hydrogenation, and cleavage

3. Which of the following processes best describes the events occurring after 1 week of fasting?

    (A) Glucose is the major fuel for skeletal muscle

    (B) Ketones are used by the brain for energy

    (C) Protein is oxidized by the liver for ATP synthesis

    (D) Fatty acids are transported from the liver to adipose tissue

    (E) The ratio of insulin to glucagon in the blood is elevated relative to a 10-hour fast

4. Which of the following tissues cannot use ketones as a source of fuel?

    (A) Kidney

    (B) RBCs

    (C) Muscle

    (D) Adrenal cells

    (E) Brain

5. A deficiency in medium-chain fatty acyl CoA dehydrogenase (MCAD) results in which of the following conditions?

    (A) Increased synthesis of ketone bodies

    (B) High levels of blood glucose

    (C) Low levels of plasma ammonia

    (D) Elevated levels of plasma fatty acids

    (E) Low levels of carnitine

ANSWERS AND EXPLANATIONS

1. The answer is D. Citrate lyase cleaves cytoplasmic citrate to acetyl CoA and oxaloacetate. Citrate is synthesized in the mitochondrial matrix by citrate synthase, and it only accumulates in the well-fed state when the activity of isocitrate dehydrogenase is inhibited by ATP. Malic enzyme catalyzes the oxidative decarboxylation of malate, producing pyruvate and NADPH. Thiolase cleaves acetyl CoA groups from the β-ketoacyl CoA intermediates during β-oxidation.

2. The answer is C. The first and last steps of β-oxidation are dehydrogenation and cleavage, respectively, thus eliminating all possible answers except C and A (oxidation and dehydrogenation are equivalent). The second step is hydration, and the third step is dehydrogenation.

3. The answer is B. After a week of fasting, the brain has started to oxidize ketones. Thus, the amount of glucose that must be synthesized is decreased, and the protein that provides precursors for gluconeogenesis is conserved. The insulin to glucagon ratio is decreased relative to the ratio after a 10-hour fast. In the fasting state, fatty acids are transported from adipose tissue to the liver and other tissues.

4. The answer is B. RBCs have no mitochondria and cannot oxidize either fatty acids or ketone bodies. The only other tissue that is unable to oxidize ketone bodies is the liver. The liver cannot convert acetoacetate to acetoacetyl CoA because it does not express the enzyme that transfers CoA from succinyl CoA to acetoacetate.

5. The answer is D. A deficiency in MCAD decreases the ability of mitochondria to extract energy from fatty acids for ATP synthesis. The plasma levels of fatty acids are elevated, secondary to the stimulatory effect of glucagon on triglyceride hydrolysis in the adipocyte. Long-chain fatty acids are partially degraded but stop when the chain length gets to C_{12}. Decreased ATP production impairs both gluconeogenesis and urea synthesis, resulting in low levels of glucose and high levels of ammonia in the blood. The synthesis of ketone bodies is decreased, since there is no excess of acetyl CoA. The levels of carnitine are unaffected.

REFERENCES

1. Ruderman NB, Tornheim K, Goodman MN: Fuel homeostasis and intermediary metabolism of carbohydrate, fat, and protein. In *Principles and Practice of Endocrinology and Metabolism*, 2nd ed. Edited by Becker KL. Philadelphia, PA: J. P. Lippincott, 1995, pp 1174–1187.
2. Hirsh J, Salans LB, Aronne LJ: Obesity. In *Principles and Practice of Endocrinology and Metabolism*, 2nd ed. Edited by Becker KL. Philadelphia, PA: J. P. Lippincott, 1995, pp 1155–1164.
3. Murray RK, Granner DK, Mayes PA, et al: *Biochemistry*, 23rd ed. Norwalk, CT: Appleton and Lange, 1993, p 230.

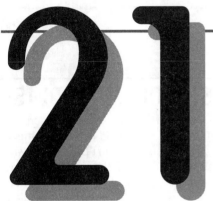

CHOLESTEROL AND STEROL METABOLISM

INTRODUCTION OF CLINICAL CASE

The patient in this case is a full-term, firstborn female child of unrelated parents. She was born with ambiguous genitalia, but karyotyping confirmed a 46,XX genotype. Despite the marked sexual ambiguity, she was discharged from the hospital 3 days after birth. At 3 weeks of age, she was readmitted to the hospital for severe salt wasting. Laboratory analysis of a blood sample gave the following results (all values are expressed relative to controls of the same age and sex): plasma 17-hydroxyprogesterone was 200 times higher than normal; testosterone was 15 times higher than normal; and renin was 10 times higher than normal. Glucocorticoid and mineralocorticoid supplements were started immediately, and within a week, the patient's plasma hormone levels were within the normal range. She was dismissed from the hospital and has continued to do well. Her parents were advised that surgery would be required at a later age to correct the masculinization of her external genitalia.

CHOLESTEROL METABOLISM

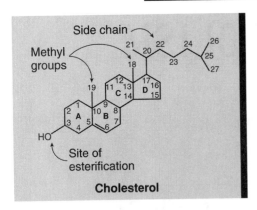

Cholesterol

Cholesterol is essential for survival in animals, where it is a structural component of membranes and the precursor for bile acids, vitamin D, and steroid hormones. It is not found in plants or prokaryotes. In plasma, cholesterol is found only in lipoproteins, which serve as transport vehicles for insoluble lipids. Cholesterol is found in the body as a mixture of free cholesterol and cholesterol esters. Most people in Western societies consume between 300 and 600 mg of cholesterol per day. About half of the dietary cholesterol is absorbed. Further reduction, however, requires severe dietary restrictions. The cholesterol content of several common foods is given in Table 21-1. Abnormalities in cholesterol metabolism are associated with many clinical conditions.

TABLE 21-1 ▶
Cholesterol Content of Common Foods

Food	Cholesterol (mg/100 g)
Milk products	
Whole milk	11
Skim milk	2
Butter	280
Cheese	100
Eggs	
Whole egg	550
Yolk	1500
Meat	
Beef, chicken, and fish	60–80
Lobster and oysters	200
Liver	300
Fruits and vegetables	0

Central Role of the Liver in Cholesterol Balance

The liver plays a key role in the distribution and balance of cholesterol in the body.

Sources of Hepatic Cholesterol. The pool of cholesterol in the liver is derived from three sources: (1) Dietary cholesterol is delivered to the liver by chylomicron remnants. (2) Cholesterol from extrahepatic tissues is delivered to the liver by reverse cholesterol transport, a process involving both high-density lipoproteins (HDLs) and remnants of very low-density lipoproteins (VLDLs) that have lost some of their triglyceride. (3) The de novo synthesis of cholesterol uses acetyl coenzyme A (acetyl CoA) that is derived primarily from dietary carbohydrate.

Fate of Hepatic Cholesterol. Cholesterol is removed from the liver by three major mechanisms: (1) Cholesterol is esterified and packaged into VLDLs; the VLDLs are secreted by the liver and catabolized to intermediate-density lipoproteins (IDLs) and low-density lipoproteins (LDLs) as they circulate in the blood. (2) A small amount of unesterified cholesterol is secreted as a component of bile. (3) Most of the cholesterol pool in the liver is converted to bile salts, which are incorporated into bile and stored in the gallbladder.

Digestion, Absorption, and Excretion of Cholesterol

Dietary cholesterol is incorporated into micelles in the intestinal lumen, where cholesterol esters are hydrolyzed by pancreatic cholesterol esterase. After absorption into the intestinal cell, cholesterol is converted back to cholesterol esters, which are incorporated into chylomicrons. Following secretion, the triglyceride content of chylomicrons is reduced by lipoprotein lipase (LpL), resulting in chylomicron remnants, which are taken up by the liver (see Chapter 19). The dietary cholesterol that is not absorbed is reduced to *coprostanol* and *cholestanol* by intestinal bacteria. These compounds are isomers that result from the reduction of the double bond in the steroid nucleus of cholesterol.

Dietary Cholesterol
Cholesterol intake should be limited to no more than 100 mg/1000 kcal, with a total cholesterol intake of no more than 300 mg/d.

De Novo Synthesis of Cholesterol

Most normal adults synthesize about 1 g of cholesterol each day. The primary site of synthesis is the liver, although other tissues, such as the adrenal cortex, ovaries, and testes synthesize cholesterol for use in steroid hormone synthesis. Cholesterol synthesis requires acetyl CoA, adenosine triphosphate (ATP), the reduced form of nicotinamide-adenine dinucleotide phosphate (NADPH), and molecular oxygen (O_2). All of the carbon atoms in cholesterol are derived from acetyl CoA. The overall synthesis of cholesterol can be described by the following equation, in which CO_2 = carbon dioxide; $NADP^+$ = the oxidized form of NADP; ADP = adenosine diphosphate; and P_i = inorganic phosphate.

$$\text{18 Acetyl CoA} + \text{18 ATP} + \text{16 NADPH} + 4\ O_2 \longrightarrow \text{cholesterol} + 9\ CO_2 + 16\ NADP^+ + \text{18 ADP} + 18\ P_i$$

An overview of cholesterol synthesis is shown in Figure 21-1. The pathway can be described in four stages: (1) the formation of hydroxymethylglutaryl CoA (HMG CoA), (2) the conversion of HMG CoA to activated isoprenoids, (3) the condensation of isoprenoids to squalene, and (4) the conversion of squalene to cholesterol.

Formation of HMG CoA. HMG CoA, a six-carbon (C_6) intermediate, is formed by the sequential condensation of three molecules of acetyl CoA. These steps are analogous to those involved in ketone synthesis (see Chapter 20), except the two pathways use different isozymes and occur in different cellular compartments. Cholesterol synthesis occurs in the cytoplasmic compartment, while ketones are synthesized in the mitochondria. The reactions and enzymes required for HMG CoA synthesis are shown in the following equation.

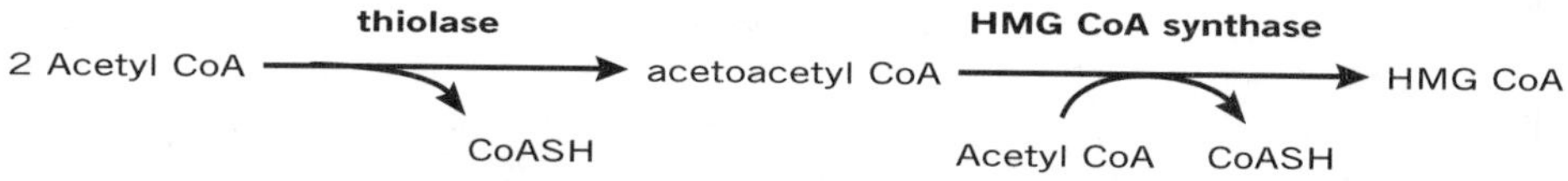
thiolase
HMG CoA synthase
2 Acetyl CoA
acetoacetyl CoA
HMG CoA
CoASH
Acetyl CoA
CoASH

Conversion of HMG CoA to Activated Isoprenoids. In the second stage of cholesterol synthesis, HMG CoA is converted to two types of C_5 intermediates, isopentenyl pyrophosphate (isopentenyl-P~P) and dimethylallyl pyrophosphate (dimethylallyl-P~P). These intermediates are known as activated isoprenoids and are used as building blocks in a number of synthetic pathways. The conversion of HMG CoA to isoprenoids is described by the following equation.

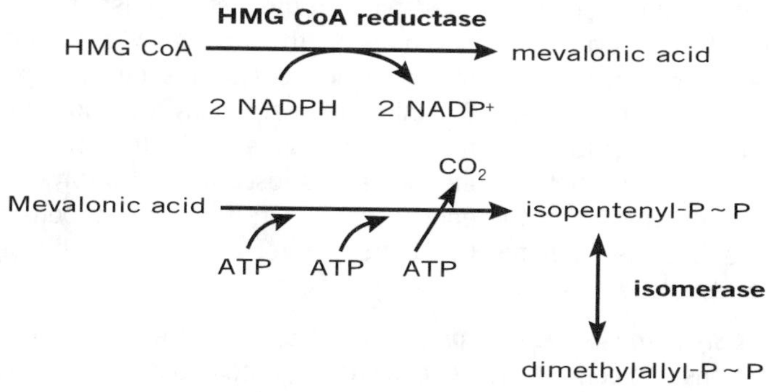
HMG CoA reductase
HMG CoA
mevalonic acid
2 NADPH
2 NADP+
CO2
Mevalonic acid
isopentenyl-P ~ P
ATP
ATP
ATP
isomerase
dimethylallyl-P ~ P

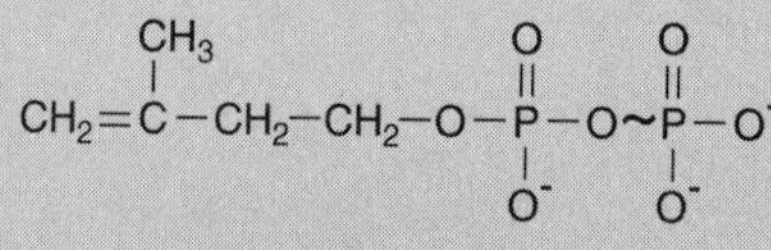

Isopentenyl-P~P

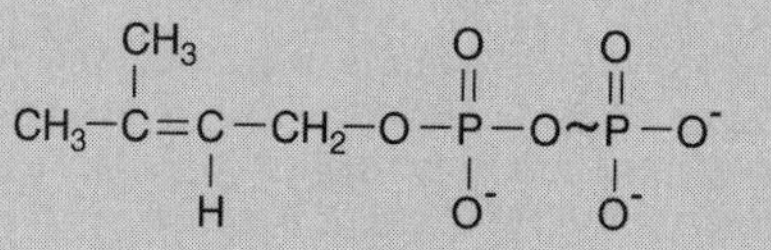

Dimethylallyl-P~P

The rate-limiting step in cholesterol synthesis is the NADPH-dependent reduction of HMG CoA to the corresponding alcohol, mevalonic acid. This reaction is catalyzed by *HMG CoA reductase*. The conversion of mevalonic acid to isopentenyl pyrophosphate requires three molecules of ATP and involves several steps. Two molecules of ATP are used to form the energy-rich pyrophosphate bonds, and the third molecule of ATP is required to decarboxylate the C_6 intermediate to isopentenyl pyrophosphate. Dimethylallyl pyrophosphate and isopentenyl pyrophosphate are interconvertible isomers. The

Cholesterol-Lowering Drugs
Inhibitors of HMG CoA reductase are used to treat hypercholesterolemia. Lovastatin and mevinolin are structural analogues of HMG CoA, which act as competitive inhibitors of HMG CoA reductase.

FIGURE 21-1 ▶

Overview of Cholesterol Synthesis. The major steps in cholesterol synthesis are shown. All of the ATP needed to synthesize cholesterol is used in the steps between mevalonate and isopentenyl pyrophosphate. The rate-limiting step in the pathway is the reduction of hydroxymethylglutaryl CoA to mevalonic acid.

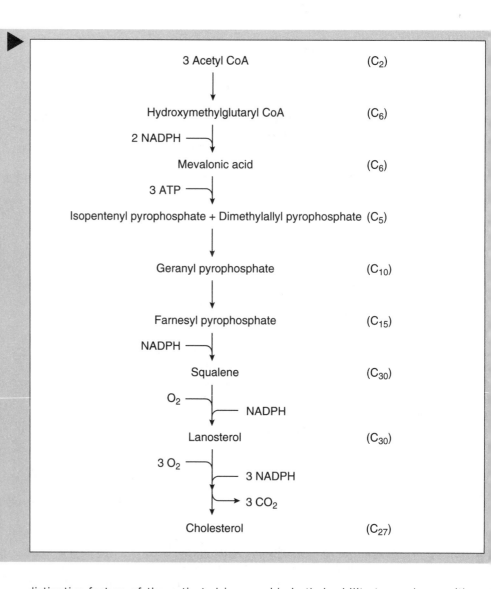

distinctive feature of the activated isoprenoids is their ability to condense with one another, forming larger molecules.

Condensation of Isoprenoids to Form Squalene. In the third stage of cholesterol synthesis, six C_5 isoprenoids condense to form squalene, a linear C_{30} precursor of cholesterol. The condensations occur in three steps. In the first step, isopentenyl pyrophosphate and dimethylallyl pyrophosphate condense to form geranyl pyrophosphate, a C_{10} intermediate. Geranyl pyrophosphate then condenses with isopentenyl pyrophosphate forming farnesyl pyrophosphate, a C_{15} intermediate. Finally, two molecules of farnesyl pyrophosphate condense to form squalene (see Figure 21-1). In each of the condensation reactions, pyrophosphate is released and subsequently hydrolyzed to inorganic phosphate, thereby providing the energy required to form the carbon–carbon bond between the various intermediates. NADPH is required in the final condensation reaction that produces squalene.

Conversion of Squalene to Cholesterol. The final stage of cholesterol synthesis involves a series of reactions that convert squalene, a linear C_{30} compound, to cholesterol, a cyclic C_{27} sterol (Figure 21-2). All of the steps in the reactions are catalyzed by enzymes that are found in the smooth endoplasmic reticulum (SER), and all of the intermediates remain bound to a *sterol carrier protein*. In the first reaction, oxygen is added to squalene forming an epoxide that undergoes cyclization to form *lanosterol*, the first intermediate in the pathway that contains the steroid nucleus. The conversion of lanosterol to cholesterol involves several steps in which three methyl groups are released from the ring as carbon dioxide, and a double bond in the side chain is reduced.

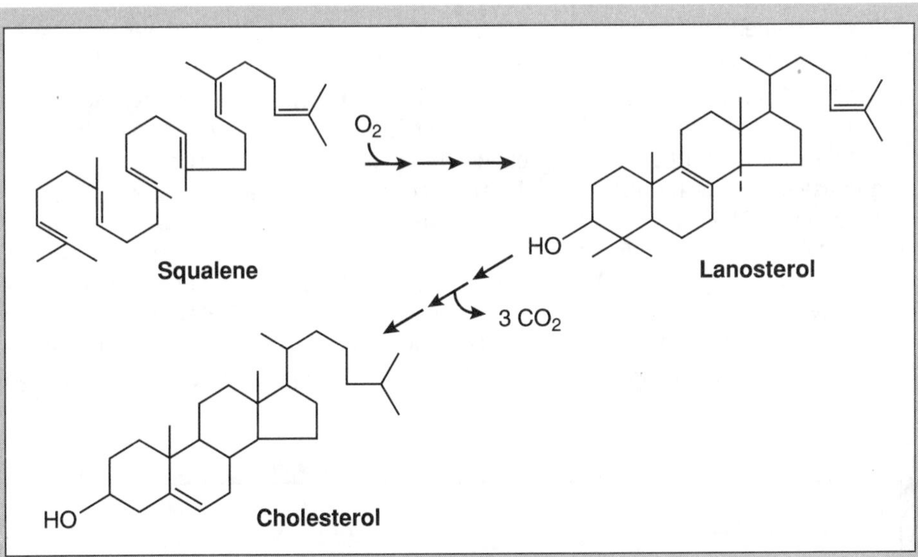

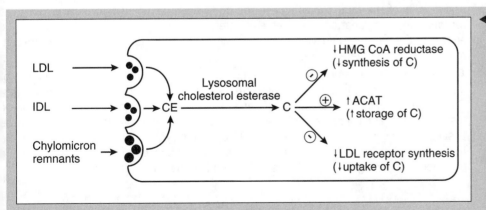

FIGURE 21-2
Conversion of Squalene to Cholesterol.
The addition of oxygen (O_2) to squalene results in an epoxide that cyclizes, forming lanosterol. In animals, the final product is cholesterol, whereas in plants and other organisms, other sterols are produced from squalene.

Regulation of Cholesterol Synthesis

The rate of cholesterol synthesis in a cell is influenced by the overall caloric intake, the uptake of cholesterol associated with chylomicrons and LDLs, and a number of hormones, including insulin, glucagon, cortisol, and triiodothyronine (T_3). These mechanisms include the transcriptional control of both HMG CoA reductase and LDL receptor synthesis, and the covalent modification of HMG CoA reductase.

Transcriptional Control of HMG CoA Reductase and LDL-Receptor Synthesis. An increase in intracellular cholesterol has a strong inhibitory effect on the activity of HMG CoA reductase (Figure 21-3). The transcription of the HMG CoA reductase gene is inhibited by cholesterol, and HMG CoA reductase also has a half-life of only 2 hours. Therefore, the decreased rate of synthesis and the rapid turnover of the enzyme result in a significant reduction in cholesterol synthesis within 3 to 4 hours after a meal. An increase in cellular cholesterol also inhibits the rate at which the LDL-receptor gene is transcribed, thereby decreasing the number of LDL receptors and the uptake of LDL from the plasma. The major source of cholesterol in cells comes from the uptake of lipoproteins. Chylomicron remnants, containing dietary cholesterol and IDLs, are taken up exclusively by the liver, whereas LDLs are taken up by almost all tissues. Following uptake of these lipoproteins

FIGURE 21-3
Effect of Chylomicron and Low-Density Lipoprotein (LDL) Uptake on Cellular Cholesterol Levels. Receptors for chylomicrons and intermediate-density lipoprotein (IDL) are found only on the liver, whereas most cells have LDL receptors. The hydrolysis of cholesterol esters occurs in lysosomes, and the resulting cholesterol decreases the rate of cholesterol synthesis and increases the rate at which free cholesterol is reesterified to cholesterol esters. These effects are mediated by cholesterol, which alters the rate of transcription for the genes encoding these enzymes and proteins. HMG CoA reductase = hydroxymethylglutaryl coenzyme A reductase; CE = cholesterol ester; C = free cholesterol; ACAT = acyl CoA:cholesterol acyltransferase.

by receptor-mediated endocytosis, free cholesterol is released from cholesterol esters by lysosomal enzymes.

Hormonal Control of Cholesterol Synthesis. Cholesterol synthesis is increased by insulin and T_3 and is decreased by glucagon and cortisol. The opposing effects of insulin and glucagon are mediated by the phosphorylation and dephosphorylation of HMG CoA reductase, whereas the effects of T_3 and cortisol are mediated by the induction and repression of HMG CoA reductase synthesis. The transient increase in insulin that occurs following a meal promotes the dephosphorylation and increased activity of HMG CoA reductase (Figure 21-4). Increased caloric intake stimulates cholesterol synthesis primarily by increasing the availability of acetyl CoA and NADPH. The pathways that supply these substrates, particularly glycolysis, the pyruvate dehydrogenase reaction, and the NADPH-producing reactions of the pentose phosphate pathway, are activated by insulin.

FIGURE 21-4 ▶
Covalent Regulation of Hydroxymethyl-glutaryl Coenzyme A Reductase (HMG CoA Reductase). The activity of HMG CoA reductase is stimulated by dephosphorylation that occurs in response to insulin binding to the surface of cells. Glucagon inactivates this enzyme by stimulating cyclic adenosine monophosphate (cAMP) formation and phosphorylation of HMG CoA reductase.

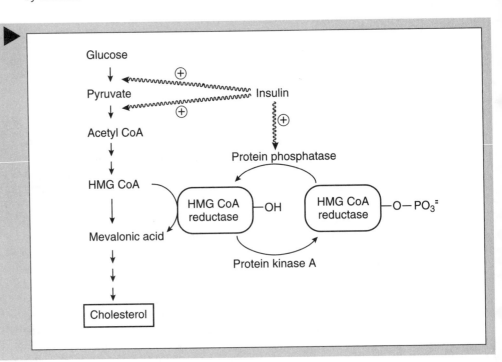

Cholesterol Ester Metabolism

About 70% of the total cholesterol in the body exists as cholesterol esters. Both the synthesis and degradation of cholesterol esters are catalyzed by a number of specific enzymes. Each of these enzymes has a characteristic localization and plays a different role in cholesterol metabolism.

Formation of Cholesterol Esters. Two major enzymes are involved in the formation of cholesterol esters. Intracellular cholesterol is converted to cholesterol esters by *acyl CoA:cholesterol acyltransferase (ACAT)*, an enzyme that is enriched in the adrenal cortex, testes, ovaries, and liver. The cholesterol esters are stored in small lipid droplets in these tissues and are used as a source of cholesterol for the synthesis of bile salts and steroid hormones. ACAT is located in the SER and catalyzes the reaction shown in the following equation. The acyl group used for esterification is donated by fatty acyl CoA.

$$\text{Cholesterol-OH + fatty acyl\sim CoA} \xrightarrow{\text{ACAT}} \text{cholesterol ester + CoA}$$

Extracellular cholesterol is converted to cholesterol esters by the action of *lecithin-cholesterol acyltransferase* (LCAT), an enzyme found associated with HDL in the plasma. LCAT transfers a fatty acid from lecithin (phosphatidylcholine) to cholesterol, forming cholesterol ester and lysolecithin. Both substrates for the LCAT-catalyzed reaction are a part of the HDL particle. This reaction plays an important role in reverse cholesterol transport. HDLs pick up cholesterol from extrahepatic tissues, and the cholesterol is esterified, so that it can be transferred into the core of the HDL particle or to other lipoprotein remnants (see Chapter 19).

$$\text{Cholesterol + lecithin} \xrightarrow{\textbf{LCAT}} \text{cholesterol ester + lysolecithin}$$

Hydrolysis of Cholesterol Esters. The hydrolysis of cholesterol esters is catalyzed by three different cholesterol esterases. *Pancreatic cholesterol esterase* is secreted into the intestinal lumen, where it hydrolyzes dietary cholesterol esters. *Lysosomal cholesterol esterase* hydrolyzes cholesterol esters that are taken up by receptor-mediated endocytosis of lipoproteins. The lysosomal enzyme has an acidic pH optimum, being most active between pH 4.5 and pH 5. A *neutral cholesterol esterase*, found in the cytosolic compartment of cells, is most active at pH 7 and hydrolyzes cholesterol esters that are stored as lipid droplets in the liver, adrenals, testes, and ovaries. The enzyme provides cholesterol to these tissues for the synthesis of bile acids or steroid hormones.

Degradation of Cholesterol

The major excretory form of cholesterol is bile acids. There are no enzymes in humans that can open the steroid ring and degrade it to smaller products. Therefore, most cholesterol is converted to bile acids and bile salts by the liver and eliminated from the body by excretion in the feces. The ring structure of cholesterol remains intact in bile acids.

BILE ACIDS AND BILE SALTS

Bile acids are synthesized by the liver and converted to bile salts by conjugation with glycine or taurine. The bile salts are secreted as a component of bile, which is concentrated and stored in the gallbladder. The major lipids in bile are the bile salts, with smaller amounts of phosphatidylcholine, free cholesterol, and bile pigments.

Primary Bile Acids

The primary bile acids, cholic acid and chenodeoxycholic acid, are synthesized by the liver. These compounds are C_{24} derivatives of cholesterol, having either two or three hydroxyl groups attached to the steroid nucleus and a side chain containing a carboxyl group (Figure 21-5). The hydroxyl groups and the side chain carboxyl group all project from the same side of the ring structure, creating amphipathic molecules that are good emulsifying agents. The negative log of the ionization constant (pK_a) of the side chain carboxyl group is about 6, and therefore, it is not totally ionized in the intestinal lumen.

Gallstones form when the components of bile precipitate out of solution. The most common gallstones consist of about 80% cholesterol. Cholesterol stones result when the bile becomes supersaturated with cholesterol. Bile that contains more than 12% cholesterol is supersaturated, and various factors, including infection or biliary stasis, can precipitate the formation of stones from a supersaturated solution of bile.

Conjugated Forms of Bile Acids

The side chain carboxyl group of the primary bile acids can form amide bonds with either glycine or taurine, resulting in bile salts. The bile salts have a lower pK_a than bile acids and are totally ionized within the pH range found in the intestine. The conjugated forms are referred to as bile salts to distinguish them from the unconjugated forms, which are only partially ionized. The bile salts are better emulsifying agents than the corresponding bile acids. The conjugated forms of cholic acid, glycholate and taurocholate, are shown in Figure 21-5.

Synthesis of Bile Salts

The reactions that convert cholesterol to bile salts can be predicted by comparing the structures of cholesterol and taurocholate (see Figure 21-5). The key types of reactions involved are hydroxylation, side-chain cleavage, and conjugation.

Bile acids

Cholic acid

Chenodeoxycholic acid

Bile salts

Glycholate

Taurocholate

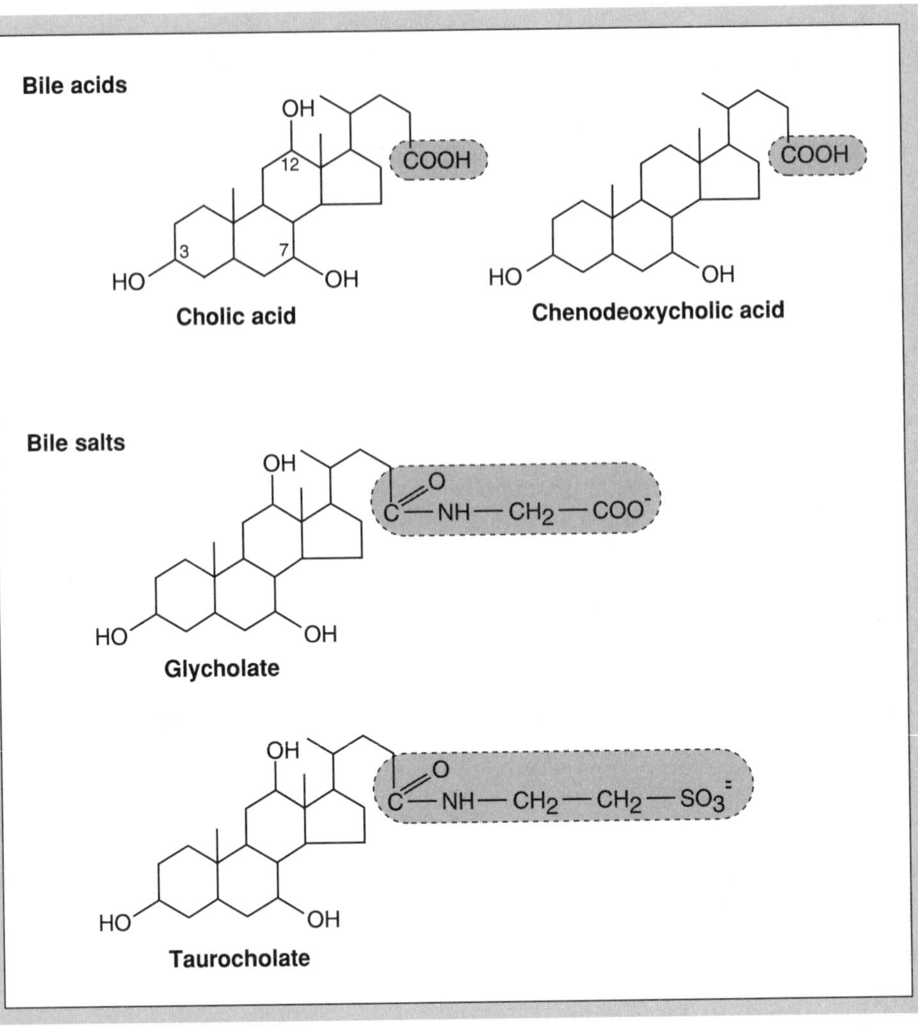

Hydroxylation. Hydroxyl groups are added to carbons 7 and 12 of the steroid nucleus by specific hydroxylases that are found in the SER. Both 7α-hydroxylase and 12α-hydroxylase require molecular oxygen, NADPH, and cytochrome P-450. These enzymes are members of a large family of enzymes known as mixed function oxygenases. The rate-limiting step in bile acid synthesis is catalyzed by *7α-hydroxylase*.

Side-Chain Cleavage. A three-carbon fragment is cleaved from the side chain of choles-terol, resulting in a C_{24} compound. The terminal carbon of the side chain is oxidized to a carboxylic acid. Both the cleavage and oxidation reactions are catalyzed by mixed function oxygenases.

Conjugation. Bile salts are formed by conjugating either glycine or taurine with the carboxyl group of a bile acid. Prior to conjugation, the side-chain carboxyl group of bile acids is activated by reaction with CoA, forming a high-energy thioester bond. The energy in the thioester bond is used to form the amide linkage between the bile acid and either glycine or taurine.

Formation of Secondary Bile Acids in the Intestine

Intestinal bacteria modify the bile salts by two types of reactions: the removal of taurine or glycine from the side chain, and the removal of the hydroxyl group from the C-7 of the steroid ring. These reactions result in the production of *deoxycholic acid*, having two hydroxyl groups, and *lithocholic acid*, having a single hydroxyl group.

Recycling of Bile Acids

Reabsorption of bile acids from the small intestine into the portal circulation is very efficient. Both primary and secondary bile acids are transported across the intestinal cells into the portal blood and returned to the liver for conjugation and use in bile

Treatment of Hypercholesterolemia with Cholestyramine
Cholestyramine is a resin that is taken orally to lower the concentration of plasma cholesterol. Cholestyramine binds bile acids in the intestine and prevents them from being reabsorbed by the enterohe-patic circulation. The decreased return of bile acids to the liver results in increased bile acid synthesis, thereby decreasing the intracellular concentration of cholesterol. The decrease in cholesterol results, in turn, in the increased synthesis of LDL receptors and uptake of LDL from the plasma.

...nthesis. The continuous recycling of bile acids between the intestine and the liver is ...own as the *enterohepatic circulation* (Figure 21-6). Although the total pool of bile ...ids is small (about 3 g), the pool is recycled about 10 times a day. Therefore, the liver ...cretes up to 30 g of bile acids per day. A small fraction, consisting of about 0.5 g/d, ...ls to be absorbed and is excreted in the feces. The bile acids lost in the feces are ...placed by the liver, which converts about 0.5 g of cholesterol to bile acids each day.

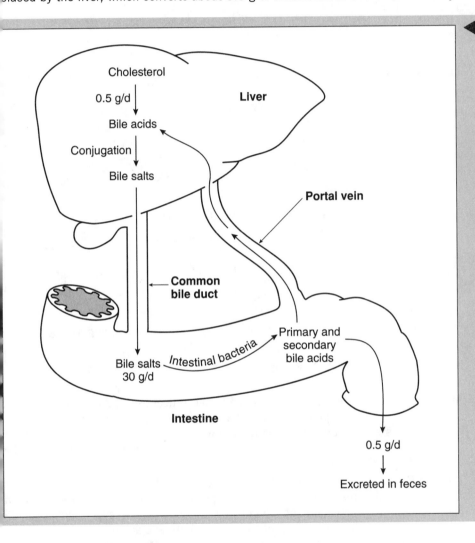

◄ FIGURE 21-6
Recycling of Bile Acids by the Enterohepatic Circulation. *Bile acids are recycled between the liver and the intestine. They are secreted into the intestine through the common bile duct and returned to the liver by the portal blood.*

STEROID HORMONE METABOLISM

...he steroid hormones are synthesized from cholesterol in the adrenal cortex, ovaries, ...estes, corpus luteum, and placenta. The structures of the most important steroid ...ormones are shown in Figure 21-7. The major hormones synthesized by the adrenal ...ortex are C_{21} derivatives of cholesterol, while the androgens and estrogens are C_{19} and ...$_{18}$ derivatives, respectively. The conversion of cholesterol to progesterone and adrenal ...teroids involves shortening the side chain to two carbons, whereas the synthesis of ...ndrogens and estrogens involves the complete removal of the side chain. Estrogen ...ynthesis also involves the removal of an additional methyl group from the steroid ...ucleus.

...drenal Steroid Hormones

...he adrenal cortex is organized into distinct layers of cells, which have different comple-
...ents of enzymes that synthesize different steroid hormones. Many different steroids are
...roduced by the adrenal cortex, but only a few are active as hormones.

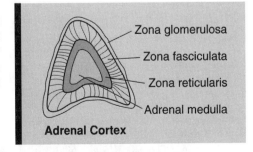

Adrenal Cortex
Zona glomerulosa
Zona fasciculata
Zona reticularis
Adrenal medulla

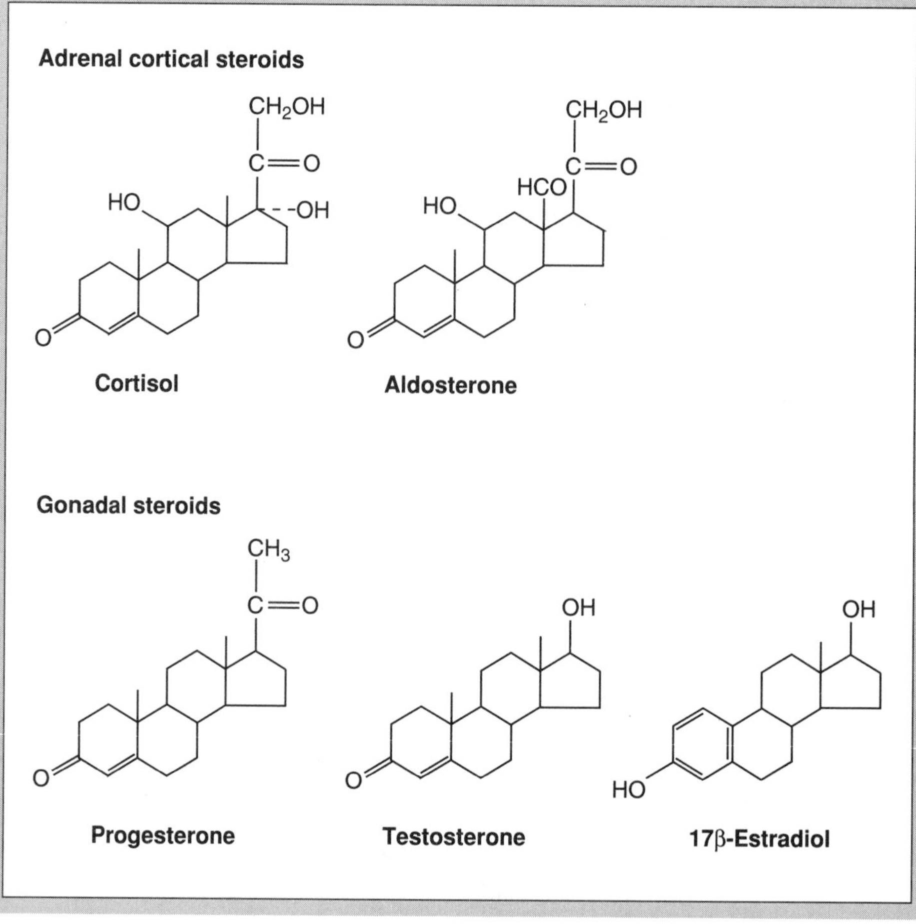

FIGURE 21-7

Major Steroid Hormones. *The major classes of steroid hormones are the adrenal corticosteroids, androgens, and estrogens. Progesterone is an intermediate in the synthetic pathway of all steroid hormones. In the corpus luteum and the placenta, progesterone is the primary end product of steroid hormone synthesis.*

Adrenal cortical steroids

Cortisol   Aldosterone

Gonadal steroids

Progesterone   Testosterone   17β-Estradiol

Mineralocorticoids. The outermost layer of adrenal cortical tissue, the *zona glomerulosa* contains the enzymes required for mineralocorticoid synthesis. The most potent mineralocorticoid is *aldosterone*, which is made exclusively in the zona glomerulosa. The primary target tissue of aldosterone is the kidney, where it promotes retention of sodium (Na^+) and excretion of potassium (K^+).

Glucocorticoids. The inner layers of the adrenal cortex, the *zona fasciculata* and *zona reticularis*, contain the enzymes required for glucocorticoid synthesis. The major glucocorticoid in humans is *cortisol*, a hormone that increases the level of blood glucose. The primary target tissues for cortisol are muscle, liver, and adipose tissue. All of these tissues contribute to glucose synthesis. Cortisol stimulates gluconeogenesis in liver, protein degradation in muscle, and mobilization of fatty acids from adipose tissue. The degradation of muscle protein supplies the liver with substrates for gluconeogenesis, while the mobilization of fatty acids from adipose tissue supplies fuel for the liver. The ATP required for gluconeogenesis is derived from the oxidation of fatty acids.

Adrenal Androgens. The *zona fasciculata* and *zona reticularis* also synthesize significant amounts of *dehydroepiandrosterone (DHEA)*, a weak androgen that can be converted to more potent androgens in extra-adrenal tissues. In postmenopausal women, DHEA is an important precursor of estrogens.

Gonadal Hormones

The testes produce androgens and spermatozoa, whereas the ovaries produce estrogen, progesterone, and ova.

Androgens. The two most potent androgens are *testosterone* and *dihydrotestosterone* (DHT). Testosterone is produced by Leydig's cells of the testes, whereas DHT is made in the seminal vesicles, prostate, external genitalia, and genital skin. DHT is formed by the NADH-dependent reduction of testosterone, a reaction that is catalyzed by *5α-reductase*. DHT exerts its androgenic effects in the cells and tissues where it is formed. The

Cushing's Syndrome
Excessive and prolonged exposure to glucocorticoids results in Cushing's syndrome. Patients with Cushing's syndrome have truncal and facial obesity but have thin arms and legs. They may also have hypertension, elevated blood glucose levels, and hirsutism. The most common cause of Cushing's syndrome is the use of glucocorticoids as anti-inflammatory drugs. Other causes include tumors of the adrenal cortex or ACTH-secreting tumors.

Testicular Feminization
A genetic defect in 5α-reductase results in a decreased ability to reduce testosterone to DHT. DHT normally exerts androgenic effects in utero that are important for sexual differentiation. Individuals with a male genotype (XY) may be born as phenotypically normal females, but they do not have ovaries and a uterus.

androgens are involved in numerous processes, including spermatogenesis, sexual differentiation, development of secondary sexual characteristics, and anabolic pathways of bone and muscle metabolism.

Estrogens and Progesterone. Estradiol is the major estrogen produced by human ovarian cells, and *progesterone* is synthesized by the corpus luteum. The ovarian hormones are responsible for the maturation and maintenance of the female reproductive system. During pregnancy, about half of the estradiol is synthesized from adrenal androgens.

Pathways of Steroid Hormone Synthesis

An overview of the pathways for steroid hormone synthesis is shown in Figure 21-8. The syntheses of all steroid hormones share two common reactions, after which the pathways diverge, leading to specific end products.

Common Reactions. In the first reaction of steroid hormone synthesis, a C_6 fragment is removed from the cholesterol side chain, producing pregnenolone. This reaction is catalyzed by *20,22-lyase*, a mitochondrial enzyme that catalyzes the rate-limiting reaction in steroid hormone synthesis. This enzyme is also known as 20,22-desmolase. The second common reaction in all pathways is catalyzed by a multienzyme complex containing two catalytic activities: *3β-hydroxysteroid dehydrogenase (3β-HSD)*, which oxidizes the hydroxyl group on the A ring to a keto group, and Δ^5, Δ^4-isomerase that shifts the double bond from the B to the A ring of the steroid nucleus, resulting in progesterone (see Figure 21-8). Both pregnenolone and progesterone are substrates for 17-hydroxylase.

Aldosterone Synthesis. The reactions that convert cholesterol to aldosterone are shown in the *left-hand column* of Figure 21-8. This particular combination of enzymes is expressed only in the zona glomerulosa of the adrenal cortex. The sequential hydroxylation of progesterone by *21-hydroxylase* and *11-hydroxylase* results in the formation of the 11-deoxycorticosterone and corticosterone, respectively. The C-18 methyl group that extends between the C and D rings of the steroid nucleus is subsequently oxidized to an aldehyde, forming aldosterone. The oxidation of C-18 occurs in two steps, which involve the addition of a hydroxyl group by *18-hydroxylase*, followed by oxidation to an aldehyde by *18-hydroxysteroid dehydrogenase (18-HSD)*. Both aldosterone and 11-deoxycorticosterone are potent mineralocorticoids. Corticosterone, however, has little mineralocorticoid activity.

Cortisol Synthesis. The sequence of reactions shown in the *second column* of Figure 21-8 are required for the synthesis of cortisol. These reactions involve three hydroxylation reactions that are catalyzed by *17-hydroxylase, 21-hydroxylase*, and *11-hydroxylase*. This particular complement of enzymes, together with 20,22-lyase, 3β-HSD, and Δ^5, Δ^4-isomerase, are present in both the zona fasciculata and zona reticularis.

Adrenal Androgen Synthesis. The major androgen produced by the adrenal cortex is DHEA. The conversion of pregnenolone to DHEA requires the sequential action of *17-hydroxylase* and *17,20-lyase*. The latter enzyme completely removes the side chain from the steroid nucleus. Under normal circumstances, most of the 17-hydroxypregnenolone is used for cortisol synthesis, with only a small fraction being converted to DHEA (see Figure 21-8). However, the amount of DHEA produced increases markedly if there is a deficiency in either 21-hydroxylase or 11-hydroxylase. Most of the DHEA produced in the adrenal gland is converted to the sulfate ester either in the adrenal cortex or in the liver. This reaction abolishes its activity as an androgen, but removal of the sulfate group restores androgen activity.

Testosterone Synthesis. Testosterone is the major androgen formed in the testes. The initial steps are identical to those in the adrenal cortex that form DHEA. In the testes, DHEA is further modified by *3β-HSD* and Δ^5, Δ^4-isomerase, producing androstenedione, which is reduced by *17β-hydroxysteroid dehydrogenase (17β-HSD)* to testosterone (see Figure 21-8).

Estradiol Synthesis. Testosterone is the precursor for estrogen synthesis. Therefore, the same reactions that occur in the testes also occur in the ovaries. The conversion of testosterone to estradiol involves the aromatization of the A ring and removal of carbon 19 from the steroid nucleus. These reactions are specific for estrogen synthesis and are catalyzed by the *19-hydroxylase–aromatase* complex (see Figure 21-8).

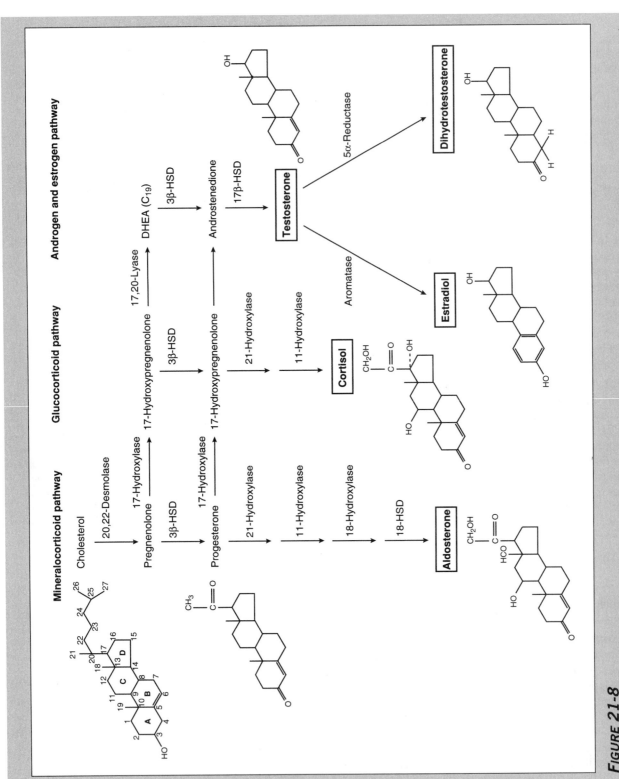

FIGURE 21-8
Pathway of Steroid Hormone Synthesis. The reactions in the left column occur in the zona glomerulosa. The reactions that convert progesterone and pregnenolone to cortisol are shown in the center column. The end product of androgen synthesis in the adrenal cortex is dihydroepiandrosterone (DHEA). In the testes, the additional enzymes are present that convert DHEA to testosterone. In the ovaries, testosterone is further converted to estrogens. The end product of steroid hormone synthesis in a particular tissue is determined by the complement of enzymes in that tissue, and the regulation of hormone synthesis by different tissues is determined by the type of receptors found on the surface of cells. 3β-HSD = 3β-hydroxy-steroid dehydrogenase; 18-HSD = 18-hydroxysteroid dehydrogenase.

Central Role of Hydroxylation Reactions in Steroid Hormone Synthesis

The major reactions in steroid hormone synthesis involve the hydroxylation of carbon atoms. In addition to the specific hydroxylases, the 20,22-lyase and the 17,20-lyase reactions are initiated by hydroxylation reactions. All of these enzymes are mixed function oxygenases (MFOs) that have similar mechanisms. Most MFOs are located in the SER, although 20,22-lyase, 11-hydroxylase, and 18-hydroxylase are mitochondrial enzymes. All MFOs are multienzyme complexes that require molecular oxygen and NADPH and consist of three types of proteins, a flavoprotein with tightly bound flavin adenine dinucleotide (FAD), a nonheme iron protein with iron–sulfur centers, and a cytochrome P-450, which contains heme. These proteins form a miniature electron transport chain that uses NADPH to reduce molecular oxygen to two hydroxyl groups (Figure 21-9). One hydroxyl group is inserted into the steroid nucleus, and the other is incorporated into water. In addition to their role in bile acid and steroid hormone synthesis, MFOs hydroxylate many other compounds, including xenobiotics, environmental carcinogens, and drugs such as phenobarbital.

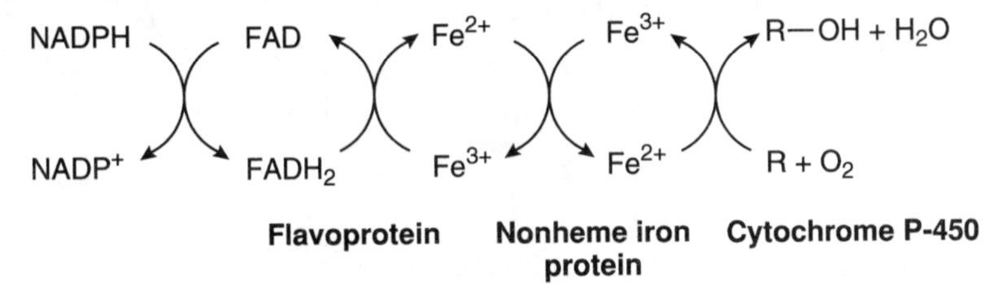

FIGURE 21-9
Mechanism of Mixed Function Oxygenases (MFOs). MFOs incorporate one atom of molecular oxygen into the substrate and the other into water. Most hydroxylation reactions are catalyzed by these enzymes. All MFOs contain cytochrome P-450.

Regulation of Steroid Hormone Synthesis

Steroid hormones are released into the plasma as they are formed. The rate of synthesis of each of the major steroid hormones is regulated by a different mechanism. In each case, however, the primary regulatory enzyme is 20,22-lyase, which is activated by phosphorylation.

Regulation of Cortisol Synthesis. The synthesis of cortisol is stimulated by adrenocorticotropic hormone (ACTH), a hormone produced by the pituitary gland. ACTH binds to receptors that are concentrated on the surface of cells in the zona fasciculata and zona reticularis of the adrenal cortex. ACTH binding results in increased intracellular cAMP, leading to the phosphorylation and activation of 20,22-lyase. The secretion of ACTH by the pituitary gland is regulated by corticotropin-releasing factor (CRF), a hormone produced by the hypothalamus in response to stress (Figure 21-10). A rise in plasma cortisol inhibits the release of CRF by the hypothalamus, resulting in decreased release of ACTH and cortisol.

Regulation of Aldosterone Synthesis. The synthesis of aldosterone is stimulated by angiotensin II, a small peptide hormone derived from angiotensinogen, a plasma protein that is made in the liver. The release of angiotensin II requires two proteolytic reactions, which are shown in the following equation.

$$\text{Angiotensinogen} \xrightarrow{\text{renin}} \text{angiotensin I} \xrightarrow{\text{ACE}} \text{angiotensin II}$$

Renin is released by the kidney in response to a decrease in blood volume. It releases a small peptide, angiotensin I, from angiotensinogen. Angiotensin I is converted to angiotensin II by the removal of two amino acids, a reaction that is catalyzed by angiotensin-converting enzyme (ACE). ACE is a protease found in the lung and plasma. Angiotensin II binds to receptors on the glomerulosa cells of the adrenal cortex and stimulates the phosphatidylinositol signaling pathway, resulting in an increase in

Congenital Adrenal Hyperplasia (CAH)
A genetic defect in any of the enzymes leading to cortisol synthesis results in a compensatory increase in circulating levels of ACTH, resulting in hyperplasia of the adrenal gland. In addition to insufficient cortisol, intermediates behind the block accumulate, leading to various clinical symptoms. The most common enzyme defect in CAH is in 21-hydroxylase activity, although defects in all of the enzymes required for cortisol synthesis have been reported. The clinical symptoms resulting from a defect are usually related to both the hormone that is deficient and the intermediates that accumulate.

Drugs for Treating Hypertension
ACE is the target for a number of drugs used to treat hypertension and congestive heart failure. These include captopril, lisinopril, and enalapril, which are small peptides that are competitive inhibitors of ACE.

FIGURE 21-10 ▶
Regulation of Cortisol Synthesis. *The regulation of cortisol secretion is controlled by hormones that are synthesized and secreted by the pituitary and the hypothalamus. Stress initiates the release of corticotropin-releasing factor (CRF) by the hypothalamus. When cortisol levels rise in the plasma, receptors in the hypothalamus bind cortisol, resulting in decreased release of CRF, followed by decreased release of adrenocorticotropic hormone (ACTH) by the pituitary, and decreased release of cortisol by the adrenal cortex. Cortisol also acts directly on the pituitary to inhibit ACTH secretion. When the plasma level of cortisol decreases, these processes are reversed.*

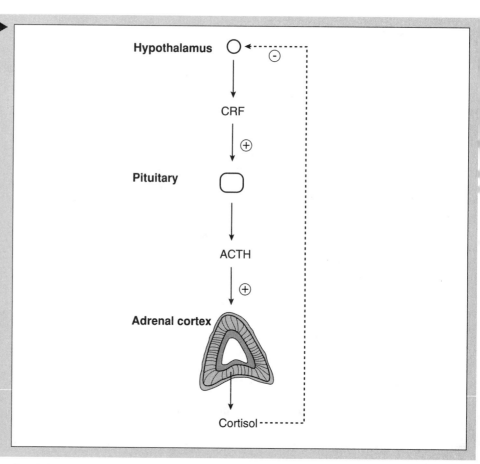

diacylglycerol and intracellular calcium. These second messengers activate protein kinases that lead to the phosphorylation and activation of both *20,22-lyase* and *18-hydroxylase.*

Regulation of Androgen and Estrogen Synthesis. Androgen and estrogen synthesis in the testes and ovaries, respectively, are regulated by luteinizing hormone (LH). The secretion of LH by the pituitary gland is regulated, in turn, by the hypothalamic hormone, gonadotropin-releasing factor (GnRF). The binding of LH to receptors on the surface of cells in the testes and ovaries results in the phosphorylation and activation of *20,22-lyase* and *17,20-lyase.*

Mechanism of Steroid Hormone Action

All steroid hormones exert their action in the nucleus of cells. The hormone-receptor complex binds to specific sequences in DNA and alters the rate of transcription of specific genes, resulting in either the induction or repression of the synthesis of one or more proteins (see Chapter 8).

Transport of Steroid Hormones

Steroid hormones are insoluble, lipophilic molecules requiring transport proteins that are synthesized by the liver. Cortisol is transported by transcortin, also known as corticosteroid-binding protein (CBG). Androgens and estrogens are transported by testosterone-estrogen–binding protein (TEBP). Aldosterone does not have a specific transport protein but binds to albumin, which serves as a nonspecific transporter for all of the steroid hormones.

Catabolism of Steroid Hormones

The steroid nucleus cannot be degraded to smaller soluble compounds for excretion. Therefore, several mechanisms are used for increasing the solubility of steroid hormones so that they can be efficiently excreted. These reactions occur in the liver and involve: (1)

he reduction of the double bond in the ring system, and (2) the conjugation of hydroxyl
roups with either sulfate or glucuronic acid, resulting in compounds that are water
oluble and readily excreted by the kidney.

RESOLUTION OF CLINICAL CASE

he patient presented at the beginning of the chapter has congenital adrenal hyperplasia
CAH) due to a deficiency in 21-hydroxylase activity. CAH is a family of inherited
isorders resulting from a genetic deficiency in any one of the enzymes required for
ortisol synthesis. The inability to synthesize adequate amounts of cortisol results in an
levation in plasma ACTH, which leads to overstimulation and hyperplasia of the adrenal
ortex. The conversion of cholesterol to cortisol requires the successive action of six
nzymes: 20,22-desmolase, 3β-hydroxysteroid dehydrogenase, Δ^5, Δ^4-isomerase, 17-
ydroxylase, 21-hydroxylase, and 11-hydroxylase. Although a defect in any of these
nzymes can cause CAH, a deficiency in 21-hydroxylase accounts for more than 90% of
ll cases of CAH [1]. Most of the clinical consequences of a 21-hydroxylase deficiency
an be attributed to either an accumulation of intermediates behind the block or a deficit
f products ahead of the block. In the case of 21-hydroxylase deficiency, the synthesis of
oth cortisol and aldosterone is decreased. The salt wasting seen in this patient is due to
educed levels of aldosterone. About 75% of patients with 21-hydroxylase deficiency are
nable to conserve sodium, and exhibit salt wasting. The decreased aldosterone also
eads to a compensatory increase in renin secretion by the kidney. The accumulation of
7-hydroxyprogesterone and 17-hydroxypregnenolone is always seen in individuals with
 deficiency in 21-hydroxylase (see Figure 21-8). These intermediates get shunted into
he pathway of adrenal androgen synthesis, resulting in virilization. Most females with
?1-hydroxylase deficiency are born with ambiguous genitalia as a result of prenatal
xposure to elevated levels of androgens, whereas males with the same deficiency show
recocious sexual development at a young age. Treatment of 21-hydroxylase deficiency
onsists of glucocorticoid supplementation and, if salt wasting occurs, mineralocorticoid
upplementation. If a family history of 21-hydroxylase deficiency has been established,
t is possible to prevent prenatal virilization of potentially affected individuals by treating
he mother with dexamethasone, a steroid that crosses the placenta and suppresses the
roduction of androgens by the fetal adrenal gland.

REVIEW QUESTIONS

Directions: For each of the following questions, choose the **one best** answer.

1. Which of the following reactions will be most directly affected by a diet high in cholesterol?

    (A) Lanosterol to cholesterol

    (B) Hydroxymethylglutaryl CoA (HMG CoA) to mevalonic acid

    (C) Acetoacetyl CoA to HMG CoA

    (D) Geranyl pyrophosphate to farnesyl pyrophosphate

    (E) Acetyl CoA to acetoacetyl CoA

2. Which of the following bile acids or bile salts is the most effective emulsifying agent?

    (A) Cholic acid

    (B) Glycodeoxycholate

    (C) Taurocholate

    (D) Lithocholic acid

    (E) Chenodeoxycholate

Questions 3 and 4

A young girl was suspected of having a partial deficiency in 11-hydroxylase activity. The diagnosis was confirmed by the measurement of several hormones and enzymes.

3. Which of the following compounds is most likely to be elevated in the plasma of this patient?

    (A) Cortisol

    (B) Aldosterone

    (C) Estradiol

    (D) 11-Deoxycorticosterone

    (E) Cholesterol

4. Which of the following symptoms is most likely to be observed in this patient?

    (A) Hypertension with virilization

    (B) Hypotension with virilization

    (C) Hypertension without virilization

    (D) Virilization without hypertension

    (E) Hypotension without virilization

5. Which steroid hormone is incorrectly paired with its regulatory hormone?

    (A) Cortisol and adrenocorticotropin (ACTH)

    (B) Aldosterone and corticotropin-releasing factor (CRF)

    (C) Estradiol and luteinizing hormone (LH)

    (D) Testosterone and LH

6. Which of the following compounds would most likely be elevated in the plasma of a patient with a renin-secreting tumor?

    (A) Cholesterol

    (B) Cortisol

    (C) Angiotensin II

    (D) Angiotensinogen

    (E) Pregnenolone

7. Which of the following sets of enzymes is required for the synthesis of estrogens?

    (A) 20,22-Lyase, 11-hydroxylase, and 17-hydroxylase

    (B) 20,22-Lyase, 21-hydroxylase, and 17,20-lyase

    (C) 3β-Hydroxysteroid dehydrogenase (3β-HSD), 17,20-lyase, and aromatase

    (D) 3β-HSD, 18-hydroxylase, and aromatase

    (E) 21-Hydroxylase, 17-hydroxylase, and aromatase

ANSWERS AND EXPLANATIONS

1. The answer is B. Dietary cholesterol inhibits the conversion of HMG CoA to mevalonic acid, the rate-limiting step in cholesterol synthesis. The major mechanism of regulation involves decreased transcription of the gene encoding HMG CoA reductase. All of the other reactions listed are involved in cholesterol synthesis but are not directly inhibited by cholesterol.

2. The answer is C. Bile salts are more effective emulsifying agents than bile acids, and the most effective emulsifying agent is the bile salt that has the largest number of hydroxyl groups attached to the steroid nucleus. Of the compounds listed, only glycodeoxycholate and taurocholate are bile salts. Taurocholate has three hydroxyl groups attached to the steroid nucleus, whereas glycodeoxycholate has only two.

3. The answer is D. The precursor immediately behind the block is 11-deoxycorticosterone. Cortisol and aldosterone would be decreased because 11-hydroxylase is required for the synthesis of both of these compounds. Estradiol and cholesterol levels would not be expected to fall outside the normal range.

4. The answer is A. Although this patient cannot make aldosterone, 11-deoxycorticosterone has potent mineralocorticoid activity and stimulates the reabsorption of sodium and the expansion of plasma volume. Since the pathways of both aldosterone and cortisol are partially blocked, both progesterone and 17-hydroxyprogesterone accumulate behind the block and are shunted into the pathways of androgen synthesis, resulting in virilization.

5. The answer is B. Aldosterone synthesis is regulated by angiotensin II. CRF is the hypothalamic hormone that stimulates the secretion of ACTH. All of the other steroid hormones are correctly paired with the regulatory pituitary hormone.

6. The answer is C. Renin cleaves angiotensin I from angiotensinogen, and angiotensin I is hydrolyzed to angiotensin II by angiotensin-converting enzyme. Therefore, the concentration of angiotensinogen is decreased, and the concentration of angiotensin II is increased in this patient. The concentration of aldosterone is elevated, whereas the concentrations of cholesterol, cortisol, and pregnenolone would not be affected.

7. The answer is C. 20,22-Lyase and 3β-HSD are required for the synthesis of all steroid hormones. The synthesis of both androgens and estrogens requires 17,20-lyase, but aromatase is required only for the synthesis of estrogens.

REFERENCES

1. Donohoue PA, Parker K, Migeon CJ: Congenital adrenal hyperplasis. In *Metabolic and Molecular Bases of Inherited Disease*, 7th ed. Edited by Scriver CR, Beaudet AL, Sly WS, et al. New York, NY: McGraw-Hill, 1995, pp 2929–2966.

22

COMPLEX LIPIDS: PHOSPHOLIPIDS, SPHINGOLIPIDS, AND EICOSANOIDS

INTRODUCTION OF CLINICAL CASE

A 1-year-old girl was referred to the hospital by her pediatrician because of slow motor development. She was born at full term and developed normally for the first 6 months. At 6–8 months of age, her mother noticed that she had difficulty holding objects, and by 1 year, she could not sit up or crawl. Upon physical examination, her motor strength was found to be about one-third of that expected for a normal child of the same age. Examination of her eyes showed red spots in the macular region of each eye. Marked hypotonia was observed in both upper and lower extremities. Her visceral organs were of normal size, and there was no evidence of skeletal abnormalities. A routine laboratory workup showed no abnormalities, and examination of bone marrow showed no evidence of foam cells. Radiologic examination showed no bone abnormalities. The patient's condition rapidly deteriorated after 1 year of age. By 13 months, she could not suck and gavage feedings were started. She began to have frequent convulsions, and by 16 months, the circumference of her head was enlarged. By 19 months, she was blind, had difficulty swallowing, and experienced frequent seizures. At 22 months, she was admitted to the hospital with pneumonia and died within 2 days. When autopsied, the visceral organs were normal in size but contained histocytes with vacuolated cytoplasm. A marked loss of neurons in the cerebral cortex was found. The neurons that remained were filled with granular deposits that stained positive with periodic acid–Schiff (PAS) reagent. The PAS-positive material was identified as a mixture of ganglioside GM_2 and globoside by chemical analysis. Analysis of lysosomal enzymes in autopsy tissue showed the levels of both hexosaminidases A and B to be less than 1% of normal control levels. Enzyme analysis of fibroblasts from both parents showed levels of both hexosaminidase A and B between 30%–50% of normal levels. Neither parent had any sign of the disease.

PHOSPHOLIPID METABOLISM

Phospholipids have both structural and dynamic roles in cells. In addition to being the major building block of membranes, they are important components of signal transduction pathways, the blood clotting system, lipoprotein particles, bile, and lung surfactant. Most phospholipids are phosphoglycerides, having a glycerol backbone. The single exception is sphingomyelin, a phospholipid having a sphingosine backbone.

Structure, Nomenclature, and Function of Phospholipids

The phosphoglycerides are a diverse family of lipids whose structures are similar to one another. More than 90% of the phospholipids in membranes can be described by the generic structure shown in Figure 22-1.

FIGURE 22-1 ▶

Major Phospholipids. The phosphate group attached to the glycerol backbone is esterified to another alcohol, represented as X. With the exception of inositol, all are amino alcohols whose structures are closely related. Inositol is a polyol. R_1 and R_2 are fatty acids.

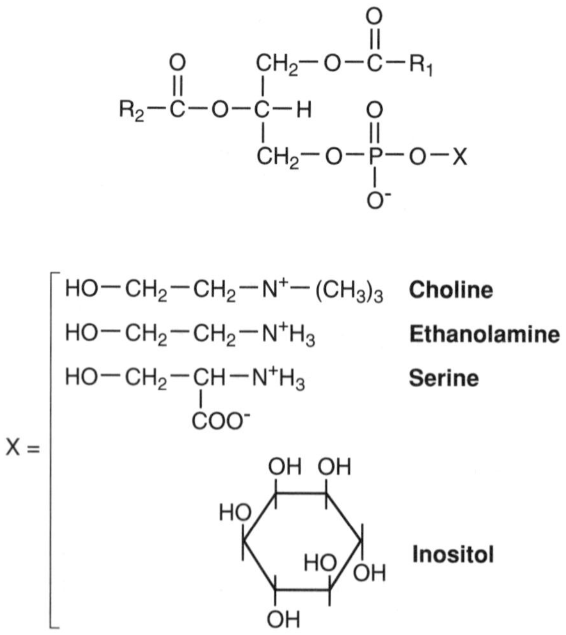

MAJOR PHOSPHOLIPIDS

The phosphoglycerides contain fatty acids esterified to both carbon positions C-1 and C-2 of the glycerol backbone, and a phosphate ester is found at C-3. The fatty acid esterified to C-1 is usually a saturated fatty acid, while the one at C-2 is unsaturated. The simplest phospholipid is phosphatidic acid, with X in Figure 22-1 being a hydrogen tom. Although phosphatidic acid is not a component of membranes, it is an intermedi-te in both the synthesis and degradation of membrane phospholipids. The major phospholipids contain phosphate that is linked to two different alcohols, one being diacylglycerol and the other either choline, ethanolamine, serine, or inositol.

Phosphatidylcholine and Phosphatidylethanolamine. Phosphatidylcholine (also known as lecithin) and phosphatidylethanolamine (also known as cephalin) are the most abundant phospholipids in the body. They are *neutral phospholipids*, having no net charge within the physiologic pH range. Phosphatidylcholine serves as a reservoir of membrane-bound arachidonic acid that can be mobilized and used for eicosanoid synthesis. A specific form of phosphatidylcholine having palmitate esterified to both C-1 and C-2, dipalmitoyl lecithin, is a surface-active agent that plays an important role in normal lung function.

Phosphatidylserine and Phosphatidylinositol. Phosphatidylserine and phosphatidylino-sitol are *acidic phospholipids*, having a net negative charge within the physiologic pH range. Phosphatidylserine is enriched in the brain, where it constitutes about 15% of the total phospholipids and serves as a precursor of phosphatidylethanolamine. Although phosphatidylinositol constitutes less than 5% of the total lipid in plasma membranes, it plays an important role in signal transduction. A number of hormones stimulate the degradation of phosphatidylinositol, resulting in the release of diacylglycerol and ino-sitol triphosphate, compounds having key regulatory functions in cells (see Chapter 8). Phosphatidylinositol is also found covalently linked to some extracellular proteins, where it acts as an anchor that tethers the protein to the surface of the plasma membrane.

MINOR PHOSPHOLIPIDS

Several phospholipids are present in small amounts in the body but have important biologic properties. These include plasmalogens, lysophospholipids, and cardiolipin (Figure 22-2).

Surfactant and Respiratory Distress Syndrome
Normal lung function depends on the presence of surfactant, which lines the walls of alveoli and prevents their collapse at the end of each respiratory cycle. The major lipid component of surfactant is di-palmitoylphosphatidylcholine. The inability to synthesize surfactant is the cause of acute respiratory distress syndrome (also known as hyaline membrane disease), which accounts for about 20% of infant mortality in the United States.

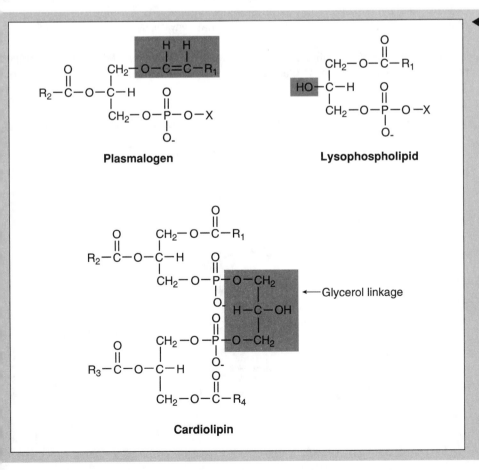

FIGURE 22-2
Minor Phospholipids. Structures for plasmalogens, lysophospholipids, and cardiolipin are shown. The shaded areas indicate the unique features of these phospholipids. Plasmalogens have alkyl ethers at C-1, and the ether is usually unsaturated. Lysophospholipids have a free hydroxyl group either at C-1 or C-2. Cardiolipin is made up of two molecules of phosphatidic acid that are linked together by a glycerol molecule. R_1, R_2, R_3, and R_4 represent fatty acids.

Plasmalogens. Plasmalogens have long-chain alkyl groups attached to C-1 of the glycerol backbone by an ether linkage. The alkyl group is usually unsaturated, containing a *cis* double bond. The most common plasmalogens are phosphatid**al**choline and phosphatid**al**ethanolamine. The ether linkage at C-1 of plasmalogens is distinguished from the ester linkage at the same position in phosphoglycerides by the use of **al** rather than **yl** in the name. Plasmalogens are found in myelin and in cardiac muscle. Platelet-activating factor (PAF) is a plasmalogen that is a potent mediator of inflammatory responses. It is synthesized and released by polymorphonuclear leukocytes.

Lysophospholipids. Lysophospholipids are produced when the fatty acid attached to either C-1 or C-2 is removed by the action of phospholipase A_1 or phospholipase A_2, respectively. The lysophospholipids are good detergents. Pancreatic phospholipase A_2 hydrolyzes dietary phosphatidylcholine to lysophosphatidylcholine, which helps emulsify dietary triglyceride.

Cardiolipin. Cardiolipin is found in the inner mitochondrial membrane and in bacterial membranes and is the only phospholipid found in humans that is known to be antigenic. It consists of two molecules of phosphatidic acid that are connected through their phosphate groups by glycerol.

Synthesis of Phospholipids

The major pathways of phosphatidylcholine and phosphatidylethanolamine synthesis use dietary choline and ethanolamine, and they are considered salvage pathways. Phospholipid synthesis occurs in the endoplasmic reticulum, and the enzymes are intrinsic membrane proteins. The salvage pathway for phosphatidylcholine synthesis involves three steps: (1) Choline is trapped in the cells by adenosine triphosphate (ATP)–dependent phosphorylation, resulting in phosphocholine. (2) Phosphocholine is activated by reaction with cytidine triphosphate (CTP), resulting in the cytidine diphosphate (CDP) derivative, CDP-choline. (3) Phosphocholine is transferred from CDP-choline to C-3 of diacylglycerol, resulting in phosphatidylcholine and cytidine monophosphate (CMP) [Figure 22-3]. An analogous salvage pathway exists for phosphatidylethanolamine.

The synthesis of phosphatidylinositol involves the activation of diacylglycerol rather than inositol. The reaction of diacylglycerol with CTP results in CDP-diacylglycerol.

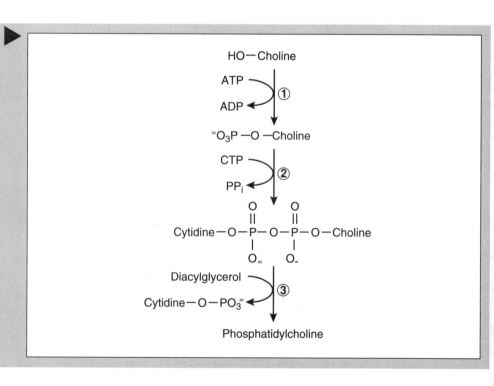

Phosphodiacylglycerol is subsequently transferred from CDP-diacylglycerol to inositol, forming phosphatidylinositol as shown in the following equation.

Cytidine-P-P-diacylglycerol + inositol $\longrightarrow$ phosphatidylinositol + cytidine-P

Interconversion of Phospholipids

Phosphatidylserine can serve as a precursor for both phosphatidylethanolamine and phosphatidylcholine (Figure 22-4). Decarboxylation of phosphatidylserine results in phosphatidylethanolamine. Phosphatidylethanolamine can be converted to phosphatidylcholine by three successive methylation reactions, each requiring *S*-adenosylmethionine (SAM) as an activated donor of methyl groups. Most of the phosphatidylcholine in the liver is derived by the methylation of phosphatidylethanolamine. The structures of choline, ethanolamine, and serine are shown in Figure 22-1. Phosphatidylserine and phosphatidylethanolamine are readily interconverted in an exchange reaction that occurs between the serine and ethanolamine polar head groups.

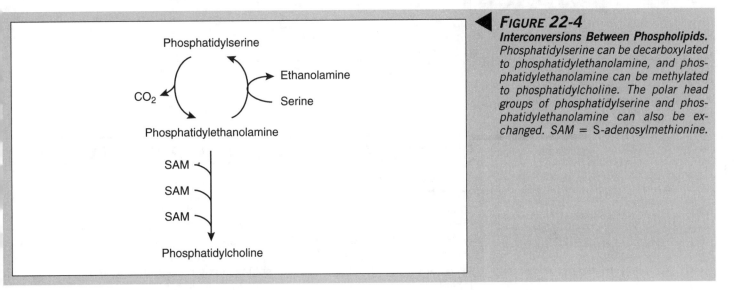

FIGURE 22-4
Interconversions Between Phospholipids. *Phosphatidylserine can be decarboxylated to phosphatidylethanolamine, and phosphatidylethanolamine can be methylated to phosphatidylcholine. The polar head groups of phosphatidylserine and phosphatidylethanolamine can also be exchanged. SAM = S-adenosylmethionine.*

Source of Glycerol Backbone in Phospholipids

The glycerol backbone found in both phospholipids and triglycerides is derived from dihydroxyacetone phosphate (DHAP), an intermediate in glycolysis. As shown in the following equation, the reduction of DHAP to glycerol-3-phosphate is catalyzed by *glycerol-3-phosphate dehydrogenase* and requires the reduced form of nicotinamide adenine dinucleotide (NADH). Glycerol-3-phosphate is converted to phosphatidic acid by the sequential transfer of fatty acids to C-1 and C-2 of the glycerol backbone. The release of inorganic phosphate (P_i) from C-3 by *phosphatide phosphatase* results in diacylglcyerol, a common precursor in the synthesis of phospholipids and triglycerides.

Phospholipid Degradation

The degradation of phospholipids requires four phospholipases: phospholipase A_1, A_2, C, and D. All of these enzymes hydrolyze ester bonds, but each is specific for a particular bond in the phospholipid molecule (Figure 22-5). Phospholipase A_2 plays an important role in the synthesis of eicosanoids, whereas phospholipase C is a key enzyme in the phosphatidylinositol signal transduction pathway (see Chapter 8).

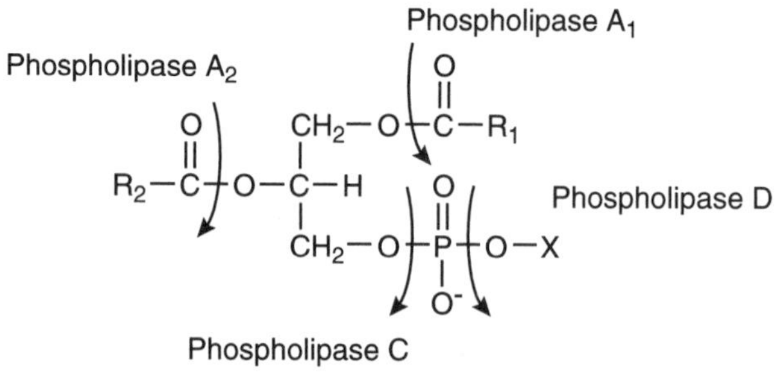

FIGURE 22-5 ▶
Specificity of Phospholipases. Phospholipases A_1, A_2, C, and D cleave the ester bonds in phospholipids at the indicated positions. X = choline, ethanolamine, serine, or inositol.

SPHINGOLIPID AND GLYCOLIPID METABOLISM

Sphingolipids and glycolipids are complex lipids that are found in plasma membranes and in the myelin sheath of neurons. There are five major classes of sphingolipids: (1) sphingomyelins, (2) cerebrosides, (3) sulfatides, (4) globosides, and (5) gangliosides. All classes, except sphingomyelin, contain one or more monosaccharides and are also classified as glycolipids. The carbohydrate portion of glycolipids has been associated with several functions, including blood group antigens, tumor antigens, and receptors for bacterial toxins. The degradation of sphingolipids occurs in lysosomes. A number of inherited diseases result from the inability to degrade sphingolipids.

Common Structural Features of Sphingolipids and Glycolipids

Ceramide is the basic structural unit of all sphingolipids and glycolipids. The structures of both sphingosine and ceramide and the precursors required for their synthesis are shown in Figure 22-6.

Sphingosine. Sphingosine is a long-chain amino alcohol that is formed from palmitoyl CoA and serine. The synthesis of sphingosine involves several reactions and requires three cofactors: the reduced form of nicotinamide-dinucleotide phosphate (NADPH), flavin adenine dinucleotide (FAD), and pyridoxal phosphate.

Ceramide. Ceramide, also known as N-acylsphingosine, is formed by the attachment of a long-chain fatty acid to the amino group of sphingosine. Ceramide has two hydroxyl groups, one attached to C-3 that is never substituted and another attached to C-1 that is always substituted in the sphingolipids and glycolipids.

Classes of Sphingolipids

The different classes of sphingolipids are generated by the addition of different chemical groups to the terminal hydroxyl group of ceramide (Figure 22-7).

Sphingomyelin. The addition of phosphocholine to ceramide results in sphingomyelin. Phosphocholine can be added directly to ceramide, or it can be transferred from either CDP-choline or phosphatidylcholine. Sphingomyelin is found in high concentrations in the RBC membrane and in the myelin sheath that surrounds neurons in the central

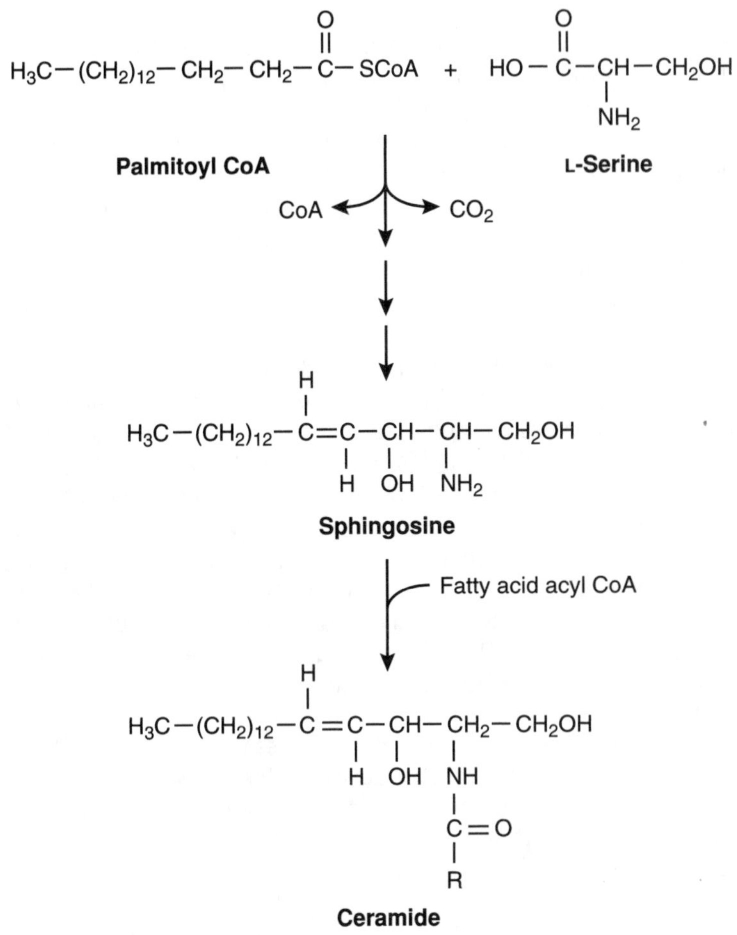

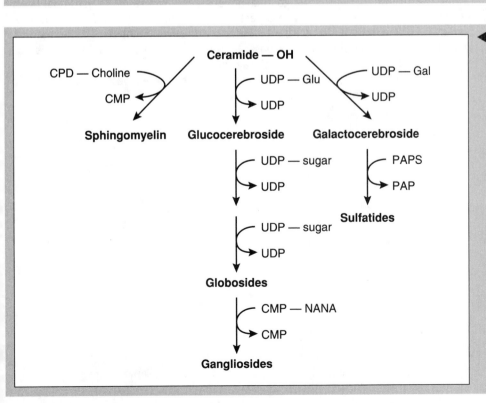

◀ **FIGURE 22-6**
Structure and Precursors of Ceramide.
Sphingosine is derived from palmitoyl CoA and serine. The addition of a fatty acid to the amino group of sphingosine results in ceramide. The fatty acids are usually C_{24} fatty acids, which may be either saturated (lignoceric acid), unsaturated (nervonic acid), or hydroxylated (cerebronic acid).

◀ **FIGURE 22-7**
Synthesis of Major Classes of Sphingolipids. *Different classes are generated by the addition of different substituents to the terminal hydroxyl group of ceramide. The precursors required for generating each of the major classes of sphingolipids are shown. Sphingomyelin is formed by the addition of phosphocholine to the hydroxyl group of ceramide. Cerebrosides are formed by addition of either glucose or galactose. Sulfatides are formed by the addition of sulfate to galactocerebroside. Globosides and gangliosides contain oligosaccharides. The defining component of a globoside is N-acetylgalactosamine (GalNAc), while that for a ganglioside is N-acetylneuraminic acid (NANA). UDP = uridine dinucleotide; CMP = cytidine monophosphate; Glu = glucose; Gal = galactose; PAPS = 3'-phosphoadenosine-5'-phosphosulfate.*

nervous system (CNS). It is the only phospholipid that is not attached to a glycerol backbone.

Cerebrosides. Cerebrosides have either glucose or galactose linked to ceramide. Galactocerebroside is found in high concentration in nerve tissue, whereas glucocerebroside is formed primarily in extraneural tissues, where its major function is as an intermediate in the synthesis of more complex glycolipids. Synthesis of the cerebrosides requires uridine diphosphate (UDP) derivatives of galactose and glucose.

Sulfatides. Sulfatides are cerebrosides in which the monosaccharide contains a sulfate ester. The most common sulfatide is sulfogalactocerebroside, which is found in nerve tissue. The addition of sulfate requires 3'-phosphoadenosine-5'-phosphosulfate (PAPS) as the activated sulfate donor. The sulfatides are acidic lipids, having a negative charge within the physiologic pH range.

Globosides. Additional monosaccharides can be added to glucocerebrosides, resulting in a family of more complex glycolipids. The addition of each monosaccharide is catalyzed by a specific glycosyltransferase. Globosides contain glucose, galactose, and N-acetylgalactosamine (GalNAc). These glycolipids are important constituents of the RBC membranes, and they contain the determinants of the ABO blood group system.

Gangliosides. Gangliosides are synthesized from glucocerebroside by the sequential addition of monosaccharides from their activated donors. Gangliosides contain a variety of oligosaccharides that consist of glucose, galactose, GalNAc, and a sialic acid, which is usually N-acetylneuraminic acid (NANA). The gangliosides, like the sulfatides, are acidic lipids due to the presence of NANA, which has a carboxylate group that is negatively charged within the physiologic pH range. Gangliosides function as receptors for cholera toxin and diphtheria toxin.

The nomenclature and classification of gangliosides (G) are based on the number of NANA residues present in the oligosaccharide. The subscript M (mono-), D (di-), and T (tri-) indicate the presence of either one, two, or three residues of NANA. Different members of each class are further identified by a subscript number (GM_1, GM_2) that indicates the specific sequence of oligosaccharides attached to ceramide.

Sphingolipidoses

During the turnover of cells, sphingolipids are degraded by a series of lysosomal hydrolases (Figure 22-8). A deficiency in several of the lysosomal hydrolases has been reported. Failure to remove a substituent interferes with subsequent steps in the pathway, resulting in a group of lipid storage diseases known as sphingolipidoses. In each disease, a characteristic intermediate in the pathway accumulates.

Some of the lipid storage diseases, together with the defective enzyme and characteristic clinical symptoms of each, are summarized in Table 22-1.

Treatment of Gaucher's Disease by Enzyme Replacement
Gaucher's disease, resulting from the inability to degrade glucocerebrosides, is the most common of the sphingolipidoses. The glucocerebroside accumulates in macrophages, resulting in enlargement of the liver and spleen. Other symptoms include anemia, thrombocytopenia, and necrosis of bone tissue. Gaucher's disease is the first lysosomal storage disease to be treated effectively by enzyme replacement therapy.

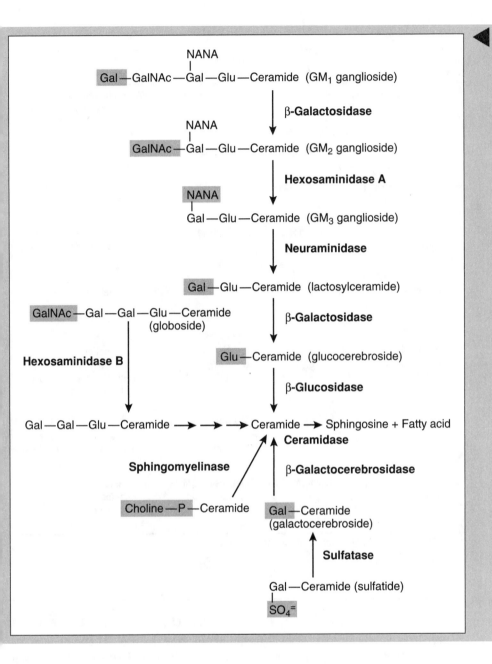

FIGURE 22-8
Sphingolipid and Glycolipid Degradation.
The group removed at each step is shaded. The name of each intermediate is given in parentheses by the structure, and the enzymes that catalyze each step are given in bold print. Gal = galactose; GalNAc = N-acetylgalactosamine; Glu = glucose; NANA = N-acetylneuraminic acid; $SO_4^=$ = sulfate.

TABLE 22-1 ▶

The Sphingolipidoses

Disease	Enzyme Deficiency	Substance Accumulated[a]	Clinical Symptoms
Tay-Sachs disease	Hexosaminidase A	Ganglioside GM_2	Mental retardation, blindness, cherry-red spot on retina, and death by age 3
Sandhoff's disease	Hexosaminidases A and B	Ganglioside GM_2	Same as Tay-Sachs but progresses more rapidly
Gaucher's disease	β-Glucocerebrosidase	Glucocerebroside	Enlargement of liver and spleen and erosion of long bones and pelvis
Niemann-Pick disease	Sphingomyelinase	Sphingomyelin	Enlarged liver and spleen, mental retardation, and foam cells in bone marrow
Krabbe's disease	Galactocerebrosidase	Galactocerebroside	Mental retardation, demyelination, psychomotor retardation, and death
Metachromatic leukodystrophy	Arylsulfatase	Sulfatide	Demyelination, mental retardation, nerves stain yellow-brown with cresyl-violet dye, and progressive paralysis
Fabry's disease	α-Galactosidase A	Ceramide trihexoside	Skin lesions, kidney disease, pain in lower extremities, and X-linked recessive inheritance
Generalized gangliosidosis	β-Galactosidase	Ganglioside GM_1 and proteoglycans	Mental retardation, hepatomegaly, skeletal involvement, and a startle response to sound

[a] See Figure 22-8 for the structure of the lipid accumulated.

EICOSANOID METABOLISM

The eicosanoids are a group of biologically active 20-carbon (C_{20}) compounds that include the prostaglandins, thromboxanes, and leukotrienes. These compounds were first discovered in semen and were assumed to be produced by the prostate gland, accounting for the name "prostaglandin." One or more eicosanoids, however, are now known to be made by all mammalian cells except RBCs. The eicosanoids are synthesized from polyunsaturated fatty acids that are stored in the phospholipids of cell membranes. The most important polyunsaturated fatty acid precursor in humans is arachidonic acid.

Essential Fatty Acids

Essential Fatty Acid Deficiency
The symptoms of a deficiency in linoleic and linolenic acids include dermatitis and poor wound healing. Deficiencies are often seen in infants receiving low-fat formulas and in patients who are fed intravenously for long periods of time. Deficiency symptoms can be reversed or prevented by including essential fatty acids in amounts equivalent to 1%–2% of the daily caloric intake in the diet.

Eicosanoids are synthesized from three polyunsaturated fatty acids: arachidonic acid (20:4, Δ5, 8, 11, 14) and eicosatrienoic acid (20:3, Δ8, 11, 14), both ω-6 fatty acids, and eicosapentaenoic acid (20:5, Δ5, 8, 11, 14, 17), an ω-3 fatty acid. The dietary precursor of the ω-6 fatty acids is linoleic acid (18:2, Δ9, 12), whereas the precursor of the ω-3 fatty acids is linolenic acid (18:3, Δ9, 12, 15). Humans are unable to insert double bonds in fatty acids at either the ω-6 or the ω-3 position. Therefore, both linoleic and linolenic acids are essential components of the diet. Dietary linoleic acid is converted to arachidonic acid and eicosatrienoic acid, whereas linolenic acid is converted to eicosapentaenoic acid. The polyunsaturated fatty acids are stored in membrane phospholipids. In humans, the most important precursor of the eicosanoids is arachidonic acid.

Cyclic Eicosanoids: Prostaglandins and Thromboxanes

The cyclic eicosanoids are related structurally to prostanoic acid, which contains a cyclopentane ring with two alkyl side chains (R), one with seven carbons (R_7) and the other with eight carbons (R_8) [Figure 22-9]. The prostaglandins can be distinguished from the thromboxanes on the basis of their ring systems. Prostaglandins have a cyclopentane ring, whereas thromboxanes have a six-member ring containing oxygen.

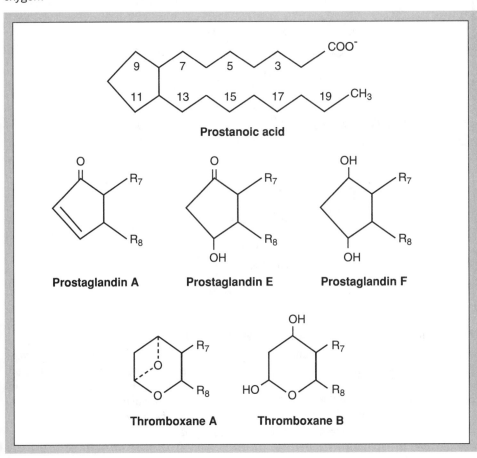

◀ **FIGURE 22-9**
Generic Structures of the Cyclic Eicosanoids. *The cyclic eicosanoids can be considered derivatives of prostanoic acid, since they have a ring structure and two side chains that have seven and eight carbons (R_7, R_8). The different classes of prostaglandins (PG) differ in ring structure and in groups attached to the ring, and they are designated by capital letters. PGA is the most oxidized class of prostaglandins, and PGF is the most reduced class. Thromboxanes have a six-member ring containing oxygen.*

NOMENCLATURE

The cyclic eicosanoids are grouped into different classes, which are identified by a capital letter (A, B, C, and so on). Each class is further defined by having three different series that are identified by numerical subscripts (Figure 22-10).

Classes. Three major classes of prostaglandins (PG) are found in humans: PGA, PGE, and PGF. These classes can be distinguished from one another by their ring systems. PGA has the most oxidized ring, containing a double bond and an attached carbonyl oxygen. PGF has the most reduced ring, having no double bonds and two attached hydroxyl groups. The oxidation state of the PGE ring is intermediate between that of PGA and PGF. A fourth class, PGI, is a special class of prostaglandins, sometimes referred to as prostacyclins, that has a two-member ring system.

Series. Each class of prostaglandins has three different series, designated as 1, 2, and 3. The 2 series is the most important series in humans. The numbers in each series indicate the total number of double bonds in the side chains attached to the ring. For example, the side chains of PGA_1, PGA_2, and PGA_3 contain one, two, and three double bonds, respectively. The series also identifies the parent polysaturated fatty acid. The 1 series is derived from eicosatrienoic acid (20:3), the 2 series from arachidonic acid (20:4), and the 3 series from eicosapentaenoic acid (20:5).

Fish Oils and Decreased Heart Disease
The antithrombogenic activity of fish oils is due to their high content of ω-3 fatty acids. Platelets synthesize thromboxanes (TX) from polyunsaturated fatty acids. The ω-3 fatty acids are precursors for TXA_3, whereas the ω-6 fatty acids are precursors for TXA_2. TXA_2 is thrombogenic, promoting the aggregation of platelets, whereas TXA_3 decreases platelet aggregation in humans. High concentrations of ω-3 fatty acids are found in herring, salmon, bluefish, and tuna.

FIGURE 22-10 ▶

Selected Prostaglandins (PG) and Thromboxanes (TX). *The three most important prostaglandins in humans are PGA₂, PGE₂, and PGF₂. A comparison of PGA₁ and PGA₂ illustrates the significance of the numerical subscript in the names of the prostaglandins. PGA₁ has only one double bond in its side chains, whereas PGA₂ has two. TXA₂ is the most important thromboxane.*

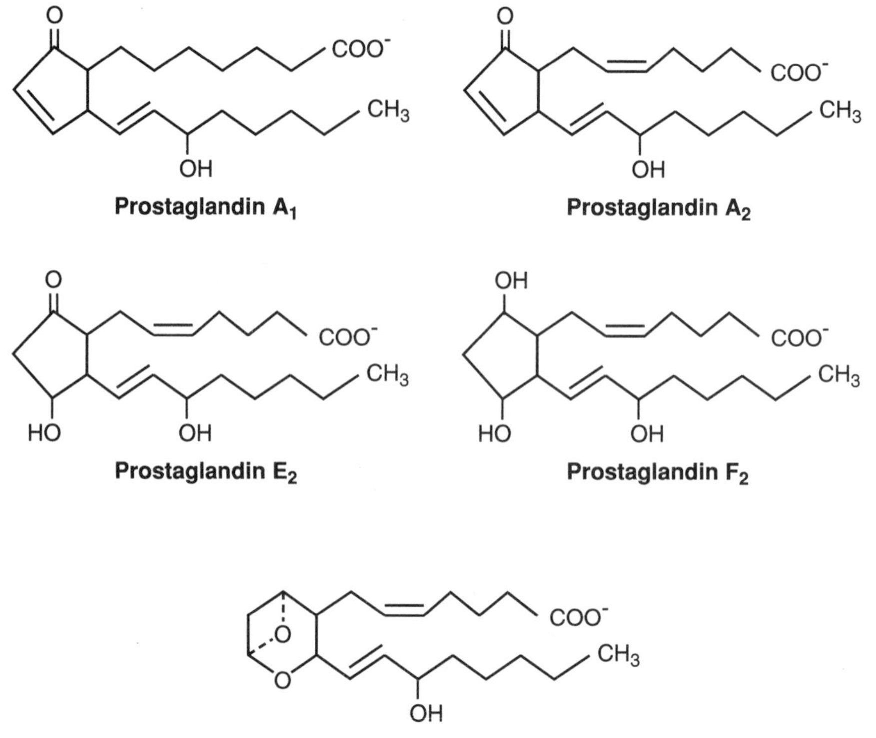

Prostaglandin A₁   Prostaglandin A₂

Prostaglandin E₂   Prostaglandin F₂

Thromboxane A₂

FUNCTIONS OF PROSTAGLANDINS AND THROMBOXANES

The eicosanoids are local hormones that exert their action either on the cell where they are produced or on neighboring cells. They are not stored but are synthesized upon demand. They are present in trace amounts and have a very short half-life, ranging from seconds to a few minutes. Many of these compounds have opposing effects on different tissues. They initiate their actions by binding to cell-surface receptors and activating signal transduction pathways. Some of the biologic effects of the cyclic eicosanoids are summarized in Table 22-2.

TABLE 22-2 ▶

Site of Synthesis and Biologic Functions of Selected Cyclic Eicosanoids

Tissue	Eicosanoid	Biologic Effect
Heart	PGE_2 and PGF_2 PGI_2	Contraction Relaxation
Peripheral vasculature	PGE_2 and PGI_2	Vasodilation and decreased blood pressure in heart, kidney, and skeletal muscle
Gastrointestinal system	PGE_2	Suppression of gastric secretion
Lungs	PGE_2 PGF_2 and TXA_2	Relaxation of bronchial smooth muscle Contraction of bronchial smooth muscle
Platelets	PGI_2 TXA_2	Inhibition of aggregation Stimulation of aggregation

Note. PGE_2 = prostaglandin E_2; PGF_2 = prostaglandin F_2; PGI_2 = prostaglandin I_2; and TXA_2 = thromboxane A_2.

Linear Eicosanoids: Leukotrienes

The leukotrienes are linear C_{20} carboxylic acids that contain three conjugated double bonds. These compounds are formed primarily in leukocytes and macrophages.

NOMENCLATURE

The leukotrienes (LT) are grouped into five classes (LTA, LTB, LTC, LTD, LTE), based on the type of substituents attached to the linear carboxylic acid (Figure 22-11). Each class has a subscript indicating the number of double bonds. The leukotrienes found in humans are derived from arachidonic acid, and all contain four double bonds (LTA_4, LTB_4, LTC_4, LTD_4, LTE_4). The addition of glutathione to LTB_4 results in LTC_4. The sequential removal of glutamate and glycine from the glutathione peptide produces LTD_4 and LTE_4, respectively.

FUNCTIONS OF LEUKOTRIENES

The leukotrienes are potent mediators of inflammatory responses. They cause degranulation of polymorphonuclear lymphocytes, stimulate smooth muscle contraction, constrict pulmonary airways, increase fluid leakage from small blood vessels, and mediate chemotaxis. The slow-reacting mediator of anaphylaxis (SRS-A) is a mixture of LTC_4, LTD_4, and LTE_4.

Leukotrienes and Inflammatory Diseases
Leukotrienes have been implicated in the pathogenesis of several inflammatory diseases, including asthma, psoriasis, rheumatoid arthritis, and inflammatory bowel disease. LTB_4 is a potent chemoattractant for leukocytes, and LTC_4, LTD_4, and LTE_4 increase vascular permeability and stimulate the constriction of smooth muscle.

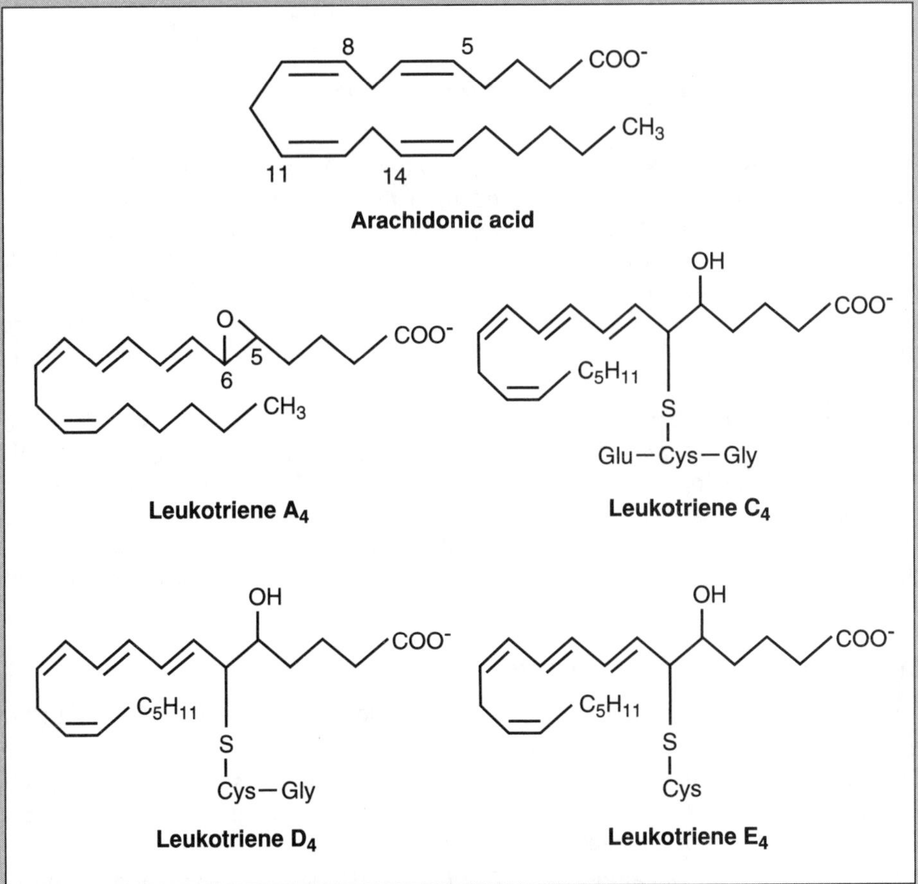

FIGURE 22-11
Selected Leukotrienes (LT). *The leukotrienes are linear derivatives of arachidonic acid, which contain three conjugated double bonds. LTA_4 is an epoxide, containing oxygen between C-5 and C-6. The tripeptide, glutathione, can combine with C-6, producing LTC_4. The sequential removal of glutamate and glycine from glutathione results in LTD_4 and LTE_4. Glu = glucose; Cys = cysteine; Gly = glycine.*

Synthesis of Eicosanoids

The synthesis of eicosanoids can be considered as occurring in two stages: (1) the mobilization of arachidonic acid from membrane stores and (2) the conversion of arachidonic acid to either prostaglandins, thromboxanes, or leukotrienes (Figure 22-12).

Release of Arachidonic Acid from Cell Membranes. Arachidonic acid is released from cell membranes by the action of phospholipase A_2. Cell stimuli such as epinephrine, angiotensin II, and thrombin increase the intracellular concentration of calcium (Ca^{2+}), which translocates cytosolic phospholipase A_2 to the membrane.

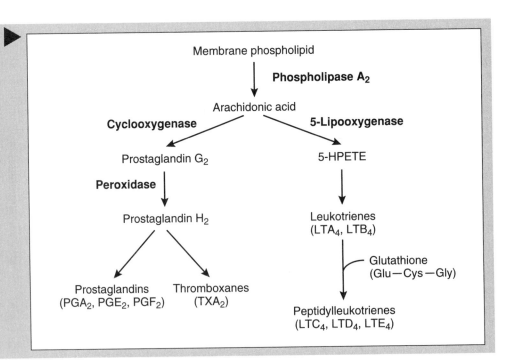

FIGURE 22-12
Synthesis of Eicosanoids. *The release of arachidonic acid from membrane phospholipid is catalyzed by phospholipase A₂, which is activated by hormones that increase intracellular Ca²⁺. The prostaglandin (PG) complex, consisting of cyclooxygenase and peroxidase, is present in most cells. Additional enzymes that convert PGH₂ to other prostaglandins vary with different types of cells. The thromboxanes are synthesized in platelets. Neutrophils are enriched in 5-lipooxygenase, the primary site of leukotriene synthesis. 5-HPETE = 5-hydroperoxyeicosatetraenoic acid.*

Prostaglandin Synthase Reaction. The step that commits arachidonic acid to the synthesis of cyclic eicosanoids is catalyzed by a multienzyme complex, prostaglandin synthase. This enzyme complex consists of two catalytic activities, cyclooxygenase, which converts arachidonic acid to PGG_2, and peroxidase, which converts PGG_2 to PGH_2. Virtually all cells contain these enzymes and can synthesize PGH_2. Other prostaglandins, as well as thromboxane A_2 (TXA_2), are derived by modification of PGH_2. Different types of cells synthesize different eicosanoids, depending on the complement of enzymes found in a particular cell.

5-Lipooxygenase Reaction. The pathway resulting in leukotriene synthesis is initiated by 5-lipooxygenase, an enzyme that catalyzes the addition of molecular oxygen to the double bond between C-5 and C-6 of arachidonic acid. The product of this reaction, 5-hydroperoxyeicosatetraenoic acid (5-HPETE), is the precursor for all of the leukotrienes. LTC_4, LTD_4, and LTE_4 have peptides or amino acids attached. The tripeptide glutathione is attached to LTC_4, and the sequential removal of one of the amino acids results in LTD_4 and LTE_4.

Inhibition of Eicosanoid Synthesis

The synthesis of eicosanoids is inhibited by two major classes of drugs: glucocorticoids and nonsteroidal anti-inflammatory drugs (NSAIDs).

Glucocorticoids. Cortisol and other corticosteroids inhibit phospholipase A_2, thereby decreasing the availability of arachidonic acid. This class of drugs inhibits the synthesis of prostaglandins, thromboxanes, and leukotrienes.

Nonsteroidal Anti-inflammatory Drugs (NSAIDs). NSAIDs such as aspirin, indomethacin, and phenylbutazone inhibit cyclooxygenase. These drugs decrease the synthesis of prostaglandins and thromboxanes but have no effect on leukotriene synthesis. Aspirin is an irreversible inhibitor of cyclooxygenase, whereas indomethacin and phenylbutazone are reversible inhibitors.

RESOLUTION OF CLINICAL CASE

The patient presented at the beginning of this chapter had Sandoff's disease, a genetic disease resulting from a deficiency in both hexosaminidase A and B. The clinical picture of Sandoff's disease is almost identical to that of Tay-Sachs, but in Tay-Sachs disease, only hexosaminidase A is deficient [1]. Patients with either one of these diseases frequently have a doll-like facial appearance, and cherry-red spots are always seen in the macular region of the eyes. Vision deteriorates rapidly, but the ability to distinguish between light and dark may be preserved. Seizures are common by the end of the first year. Difficulty in swallowing is usually seen by the second year of life, and death usually occurs by age 2 or 3 as the result of bronchopneumonia. Because of the similarities between Tay-Sachs and Sandhoff's disease, it is difficult to distinguish between them on the basis of their clinical presentations. Additional evidence that may suggest Sandoff's disease rather than Tay-Sachs is organomegaly and skeletal abnormalities, but it is not always observed [2]. A definitive diagnosis requires either the analysis of the lipids that accumulate, or direct enzyme assays, or both. In Tay-Sachs disease there is an accumulation of ganglioside GM_2, whereas in Sandoff's disease there is an accumulation of both ganglioside GM_2 and globoside. In the present case, organomegaly and bone involvement were not observed, but direct enzyme analysis showed a deficiency in both hexosaminidase A and B. The positive PAS stain observed with autopsy tissue indicated the accumulation of carbohydrate-containing material. Chemical analysis of the accumulated material showed both ganglioside GM_2 and globoside. Ganglioside GM_2 accumulates from a deficiency in hexosaminidase A, whereas globoside accumulates when there is a deficiency in hexosaminidase B.

REVIEW QUESTIONS

Directions: For each of the following questions, choose the **one best** answer.

1. Which of the following lipids is deficient in infants with respiratory distress syndrome?
    (A) Sphingomyelin
    (B) Platelet activation factor
    (C) Dipalmitoyl phosphatidylcholine
    (D) Cardiolipin
    (E) Thromboxane A_2

2. Which of the following lipids can be formed by the methylation of phosphatidyl-ethanolamine?
    (A) Phosphatidylinositol
    (B) Phosphatidylcholine
    (C) Phosphatidylserine
    (D) Sphingomyelin
    (E) Lysophosphatidylcholine

3. Which of the following monosaccharides distinguishes a ganglioside from a globoside?
    (A) Glucose
    (B) N-Acetylgalactosamine (GalNAc)
    (C) Galactose
    (D) N-Acetylneuraminic acid (NANA)
    (E) Galactose sulfate

4. Aspirin inhibits the synthesis of which of the following sets of eicosanoids?
    (A) Prostaglandin E_2 and leukotriene A_4
    (B) Thromboxane A_2 and leukotriene C_4
    (C) Prostaglandin F_2 and thromboxane A_2
    (D) Prostaglandin A_2 and 5-hydroperoxyeicosatetraenoic acid (5-HPETE)
    (E) Peptidylleukotrienes and prostaglandin E_2

5. Which of the following enzymes and pathways are correctly matched?
    (A) Phospholipase C and prostaglandin synthesis
    (B) β-Glucocerebrosidase and sphingolipid degradation
    (C) 5-Lipooxygenase and prostaglandin synthesis
    (D) Choline kinase and phosphatidylethanolamine synthesis
    (E) Phospholipase A_2 and sphingomyelin synthesis

ANSWERS AND EXPLANATIONS

1. The answer is C. Dipalmitoyl phosphatidylcholine is the major lipid component of surfactant, a complex of proteins and lipids that is synthesized by pneumocytes shortly before birth. A deficiency in surfactant in newborns results in respiratory distress syndrome.

2. The answer is B. The addition of three methyl groups to the nitrogen atom in the polar head group of phosphatidylethanolamine results in phosphatidylcholine. The methyl donor in these reactions is *S*-adenosylmethionine. The decarboxylation of phosphatidylserine results in phosphatidylethanolamine, and the deacylation of phosphatidylcholine results in lysophosphatidylcholine. The other phospholipids are not interconvertible.

3. The answer is D. The addition of NANA to a globoside results in a ganglioside. Both compounds contain glucose, galactose, and GalNAc. Neither compound contains galactose sulfate.

4. The answer is C. Aspirin inhibits cyclooxygenase, one of the enzymes in the prostaglandin synthase complex, resulting in decreased synthesis of all the prostaglandins and thromboxanes. Aspirin has no effect on the synthesis of leukotrienes or of 5-HPETE, a precursor to all of the leukotrienes.

5. The answer is B. β-Glucocerebrosidase is a lysosomal enzyme that degrades glucocerebroside to glucose and ceramide. Phospholipase C is involved in the degradation of phospholipids, hydrolyzing the phosphate ester bond between the glycerol backbone and the polar head group. 5-Lipooxygenase initiates leukotriene synthesis but has no effect on prostaglandin synthesis. Choline kinase traps dietary choline in the cell and participates in the salvage pathway of phosphatidylcholine synthesis. Phospholipase A_2 removes the fatty acid from the C-2 position of phosphoglycerides, resulting in the lysophosphoglycerides.

REFERENCES

1. Okada S, McCrea M, O'Brien JS: Sandoff's disease (GM_2 gangliosidosis type 2): clinical, chemical, and enzyme studies in five patients. *Pediat Res* 6:606–615, 1972.
2. Gravel RA, Clarke JTR, Kaback MM, et al: The GM_2 gangliosidoses. In *The Metabolic and Molecular Bases of Inherited Disease*, 7th ed. Edited by Scriver CR, Beaudet AL, Sly WS, et al. New York, NY: McGraw-Hill, 1995, pp 2839–2879.

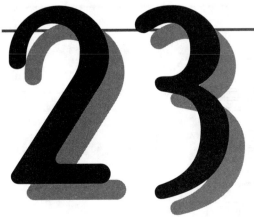

23 PATHWAYS OF LIPID METABOLISM: SUMMARY, REGULATION, AND COORDINATION

CHAPTER OUTLINE

Summary of Pathways of Lipid Metabolism
- Synthetic Pathways
- Pathways of Lipid Oxidation

Hormonal Regulation and Coordination of Lipid Metabolism
- Release of Fatty Acids from Triglyceride Stores
- Entry of Fatty Acids into Tissues
- Fatty Acid Synthesis
- Fatty Acid Oxidation
- Cholesterol Synthesis
- Ketone Body Synthesis and Oxidation

Review Questions

SUMMARY OF PATHWAYS OF LIPID METABOLISM

A summary of the major pathways of lipid metabolism and how they are related to one another is shown in Figure 23-1. The synthetic pathways of lipid metabolism are localized in the extramitochondrial compartment of the cell, whereas the oxidative pathways are located in the mitochondria.

Synthetic Pathways

The pathways of lipid synthesis are shown on the *left side* of Figure 23-1. The pathways are found in the extramitochondrial compartments of the cell, and they include the synthesis of fatty acids, triglycerides, cholesterol, phospholipids, sphingolipids, and eicosanoids.

Fatty Acid Synthesis. The key features of de novo fatty acid synthesis are shown in the *lower half* of Figure 23-1. Most fatty acid synthesis occurs in the liver, where the major substrate is excess dietary glucose, although surplus glucogenic amino acids can also be converted to fatty acids. Glucose is converted to pyruvate by glycolysis, and following transport into mitochondria, pyruvate is oxidized to acetyl coenzyme A (CoA) by pyruvate dehydrogenase (PDH), providing the substrate for fatty acid synthesis. The synthesis of fatty acids occurs in the cytosol, and since the inner mitochondrial membrane (IMM) is impermeable to acetyl CoA, citrate acts as a carrier for translocating acetyl CoA from the mitochondria to the cytosol. The end product of de novo fatty acid synthesis is palmitoyl CoA, a C_{16} fatty acyl CoA. Elongation and desaturation of palmitoyl CoA occur in the smooth endoplasmic reticulum (SER).

The condensation of acetyl CoA with oxaloacetate, forming citrate, is catalyzed by *citrate synthase*, an enzyme in the tricarboxylic acid (TCA) cycle. When the adenosine triphosphate (ATP) level in the cell is high, the TCA cycle is inhibited and citrate accumu-

FIGURE 23-1

Summary of Lipid Metabolism. *The inner mitochondrial membrane (IMM), shown in the center of the figure, separates the mitochondrial and extramitochondrial compartments of the cell. The pathways of lipid metabolism in each of these cellular compartments are listed at the bottom of the figure. FA = fatty acid; FA~CoA = fatty acyl CoA; Glu = glucose; DHAP = dihydroxyacetone phosphate; OAA = oxaloacetate; NADH = reduced nicotinamide adenine dinucleotide; NADPH = reduced nicotinamide-adenine dinucleotide phosphate; CAT-1 = carnitine acyltransferase-1; CAT-2 = carnitine acyltransferase-2; TCA = tricarboxylic acid cycle; $FADH_2$ = reduced flavin adenine dinucleotide; ATP = adenosine triphosphate; CO_2 = carbon dioxide; HMG CoA = hydroxymethylglutaryl CoA; SER = smooth endoplasmic reticulum.*

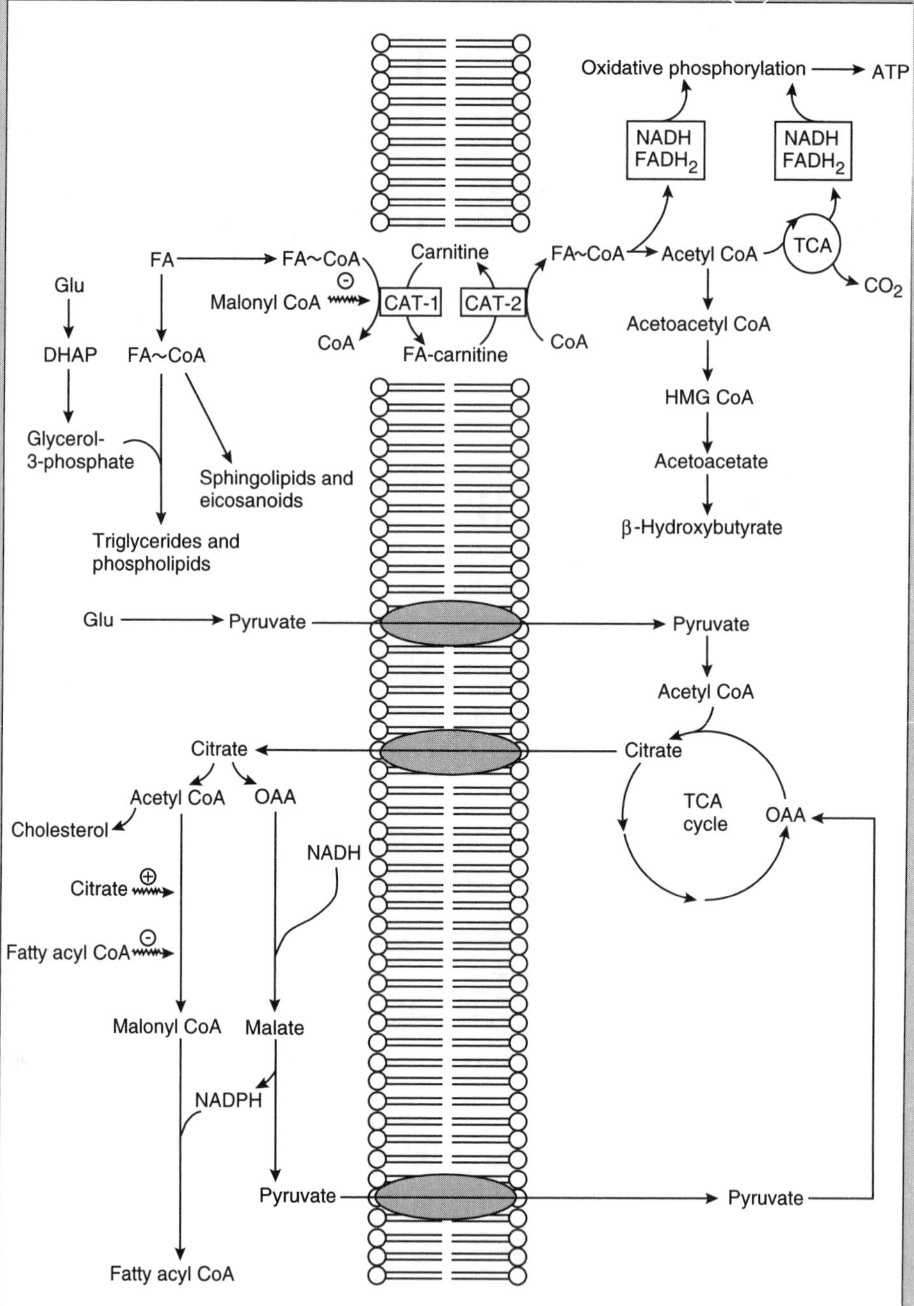

Extramitochondrial	IMM	Mitochondria
Fatty acid synthesis (cytosol)		β-Oxidation
Triglyceride synthesis (SER)		Ketogenesis (liver)
Cholesterol synthesis (SER)		Ketone oxidation (extrahepatic)
Phospholipid synthesis (SER)		Tricarboxylic acid (TCA) cycle
Sphingolipid synthesis (SER)		Oxidative phosphorylation
Eicosanoid synthesis (SER)		

lates. Following translocation to the cytosol, citrate is converted back to acetyl CoA and oxaloacetate by *citrate lyase*. Acetyl CoA is used for the synthesis of malonyl CoA, a key intermediate in the pathway of fatty acid synthesis. Cytosolic oxaloacetate is converted to pyruvate and returned to the mitochondria, where it is carboxylated to oxaloacetate, completing the citrate shuttle. The reactions that convert oxaloacetate to pyruvate also produce the reduced form of nicotinamide-adenine dinucleotide phosphate (NADPH), a substrate required for fatty acid synthesis. NADPH is produced in the reaction catalyzed by *malic enzyme*.

The rate-limiting step in fatty acid synthesis is the formation of malonyl CoA, a reaction catalyzed by *acetyl CoA carboxylase*. Acetyl CoA carboxylase is regulated by a variety of mechanisms. It is allosterically activated by citrate and inhibited by fatty acyl CoA. Hormonal regulation is mediated by insulin, which stimulates the synthesis of acetyl CoA carboxylase, and also promotes the dephosphorylation and activation of the enzyme. Additionally, insulin makes substrates available for fatty acid synthesis in the liver by stimulating both glycolysis, the PDH reaction, and the reactions of the pentose phosphate pathway that produce NADPH.

Triglyceride Synthesis. In the well-fed state, fatty acids arising from both dietary sources and de novo synthesis are converted to triglycerides for storage (see *upper left portion* of Figure 23-1). The glycerol-3-phosphate backbone of triglycerides is derived from glycolysis. The enzymes responsible for triglyceride synthesis are found in the SER.

Triglyceride formation in adipose tissue is increased by insulin. Insulin stimulates extracellular lipoprotein lipase (LpL), resulting in increased uptake of fatty acids from chylomicrons and very low-density lipoproteins (VLDLs). The uptake of glucose by adipocytes is also increased by insulin. The glucose is used primarily for synthesis of glycerol-3-phosphate.

Triglyceride formation in the liver uses fatty acids derived primarily from de novo synthesis. The triglycerides are incorporated into VLDLs and secreted into the blood. LpL releases fatty acids from lipoprotein triglyceride, and they are taken up by extrahepatic tissues.

Cholesterol Synthesis. Most cholesterol synthesis occurs in the liver. The same conditions that stimulate fatty acid synthesis also stimulate cholesterol synthesis. The cytosolic pool of acetyl CoA resulting from the cleavage of citrate can be used for both fatty acid and cholesterol synthesis. The early stages of cholesterol synthesis occur in the cytosol, whereas the later steps are catalyzed by enzymes that are found in the SER. The rate-limiting step in cholesterol synthesis is catalyzed by hydroxymethylglutaryl CoA (HMG CoA) reductase. Insulin stimulates the synthesis of cholesterol by two major mechanisms. First, insulin promotes dephosphorylation and activation of HMG CoA reductase, and second, it increases the availability of both acetyl CoA and NADPH.

Phospholipid, Sphingolipid, and Eicosanoid Synthesis. The synthesis of phospholipids, sphingolipids, and eicosanoids occurs in virtually all cells. The enzymes are found in the SER. The phospholipids and sphingolipids are necessary components of membranes, and the eicosanoids are lipid hormones that are derived from essential fatty acids. Arachidonic acid, the major precursor of eicosanoids in humans, is stored in membrane phospholipid and released by hormones and growth factors that increase cellular calcium levels.

Pathways of Lipid Oxidation

The pathways for oxidizing lipids consist of fatty acid oxidation, ketogenesis, and ketone oxidation (see *upper right portion* of Figure 23-1). The products of fatty acid and ketone oxidation are acetyl CoA, the reduced form of nicotinamide adenine dinucleotide (NADH), and the reduced form of flavin adenine dinucleotide ($FADH_2$). These products are further oxidized to carbon dioxide and water by the TCA cycle and oxidative phosphorylation, providing the energy needed for the synthesis of most of the cellular ATP.

Fatty Acid Oxidation. The fatty acids oxidized by mitochondria are derived either from triglyceride found in circulating lipoproteins or from triglyceride stored in adipose tissue. Fatty acids are released from lipoprotein triglyceride by LpL, an extracellular enzyme found in the capillary bed of tissues, and they are taken up by tissues for oxidation. Fatty acids that originate in adipose tissue are transported to other tissues by serum albumin.

The entry of fatty acids into a cell is followed by the conversion to fatty acyl CoA. The IMM is impermeable to fatty acyl CoA, and the carnitine shuttle is required for transport into the mitochondria where oxidation occurs. The products of fatty acid oxidation are acetyl CoA, NADH, and $FADH_2$.

Fatty acid oxidation is promoted by glucagon, epinephrine, adrenocorticotropic hormone (ACTH), and other hormones that mobilize fatty acids from triglyceride stores in adipose tissue. These hormones increase cyclic adenosine monophosphate (cAMP) levels in adipocytes, leading to the phosphorylation and activation of *hormone-sensitive lipase*. The synthesis of hormone-sensitive lipase is also induced by cortisol and thyroid hormones. Insulin antagonizes the effect of glucagon, epinephrine, and ACTH by promoting dephosphorylation (and inactivation) of hormone-sensitive lipase.

The coordination of fatty acid oxidation with fatty acid synthesis prevents futile cycling of fatty acids. The rate-limiting step in fatty acid oxidation is catalyzed by carnitine acyltransferase-1 (CAT-1), the enzyme that controls the entry of fatty acids into the mitochondria. The accumulation of malonyl CoA during fatty acid synthesis inhibits CAT-1 and blocks the entry of fatty acids into the mitochondria. Insulin stimulates the synthesis of malonyl CoA by the activation of acetyl CoA carboxylase.

Ketone Body Synthesis and Oxidation. Ketogenesis is a pathway for conserving excess acetyl CoA and occurs concurrently with fatty acid oxidation. If acetyl CoA is produced faster than it is oxidized by the TCA cycle, the excess is used for ketone body synthesis (see Figure 23-1, *upper right hand panel*). Ketogenesis occurs only in the liver. The liver, however, is unable to oxidize ketones. Therefore, β-hydroxybutyrate and acetoacetate are released into the blood and transported to extrahepatic tissues. The heart, muscle, and kidney readily oxidize ketone bodies. During prolonged fasting or starvation, the brain acquires the ability to oxidize ketones, an adaptative process that spares glucose and protein. Ketones, however, cannot completely replace the glucose requirement of the brain. The interorgan metabolism of ketone bodies is summarized in Figure 23-2.

FIGURE 23-2 ▶

Synthesis and Oxidation of Ketone Bodies. Ketone bodies are synthesized by the liver, but they cannot be oxidized by the liver. Following release into the blood, they are taken up by extrahepatic tissues, where they are oxidized to carbon dioxide and water. The ability of the brain to oxidize ketones is an adaptative process that occurs only in prolonged fasting or starvation. The brain cannot oxidize fatty acids. CO_2 = carbon dioxide.

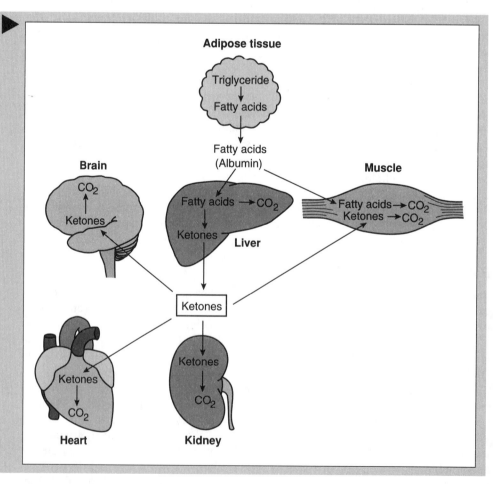

HORMONAL REGULATION AND COORDINATION OF LIPID METABOLISM

Release of Fatty Acids from Triglyceride Stores

The major storage site for triglyceride is adipose tissue. The rate of fatty acid release is determined by the activity of *hormone-sensitive lipase*. This enzyme is active only in the phosphorylated state. Glucagon, epinephrine, and ACTH are the major hormones that promote phosphorylation, while insulin promotes dephosphorylation.

Entry of Fatty Acids into Tissues

Fatty acids are transported either as free fatty acids that are bound to albumin or as triglycerides that are associated with chylomicrons and VLDLs. The uptake of free fatty acids from albumin is dependent on the concentration gradient between extracellular and intracellular fatty acids. The circulating level of free fatty acids is increased by hormones that stimulate the release of fatty acids from adipose tissue. The uptake of fatty acids from triglycerides in lipoproteins is determined by the activity of LpL, which is found in the capillary beds of most tissues, but is particularly concentrated in the capillary beds of skeletal muscle and adipose tissue. LpL synthesis is stimulated by insulin in adipose tissue but not in muscle tissue.

Fatty Acid Synthesis

The rate-limiting step in fatty acid synthesis is catalyzed by *acetyl CoA carboxylase*. This enzyme is allosterically activated by citrate and inhibited by fatty acyl CoA. The covalently active form of acetyl CoA carboxylase is the dephosphorylated form, which predominates in the well-fed state when the insulin to glucagon ratio is high. Additionally, insulin stimulates the synthesis of virtually all the enzymes that are required either directly or indirectly for fatty acid synthesis. These enzymes include citrate lyase, acetyl CoA carboxylase, the fatty acid synthase complex, malic enzyme, glucose-6-phosphate dehydrogenase, and 6-phosphogluconate dehydrogenase.

Fatty Acid Oxidation

The rate-limiting step in fatty acid oxidation is catalyzed by CAT-1. The activity of this enzyme is inhibited by insulin. The effect of insulin is mediated by malonyl CoA, an intermediate in fatty acid synthesis. The dual role of malonyl CoA as a substrate in fatty acid synthesis and an inhibitor of fatty acid oxidation ensures that these opposing pathways do not occur simultaneously.

Cholesterol Synthesis

The rate-limiting step in cholesterol synthesis is catalyzed by HMG CoA reductase. This enzyme is regulated by phosphorylation and dephosphorylation, which are controlled by the insulin to glucagon ratio. The dephosphorylated form is the active form. Therefore, in the well-fed state when insulin is high and substrates are available, the synthesis of cholesterol is increased. The activity of HMG CoA reductase is inhibited by the accumulation of cholesterol.

Ketone Body Synthesis and Oxidation

Ketone bodies are formed when fatty acids are oxidized more rapidly than acetyl CoA is used. A low level of insulin and an elevated level of glucagon are the major hormonal stimuli for fatty acid oxidation and ketone body formation. Ketone bodies are formed in the liver and released into the blood, where they are taken up and oxidized by extrahepatic tissues. The rate of uptake and oxidation is dependent on the circulating concentration of the ketone bodies.

REVIEW QUESTIONS

Directions: For each of the following questions, choose the **one best** answer.

1. Which of the following enzymes is activated by cAMP-dependent phosphorylation?

    (A) Acetyl CoA carboxylase

    (B) Lipoprotein lipase (LpL)

    (C) Hormone-sensitive lipase

    (D) Hydroxymethylglutaryl CoA (HMG CoA) reductase

    (E) Fatty acid synthase

2. Which of the following enzymes is inhibited by malonyl CoA?

    (A) Fatty acid synthase

    (B) Acetyl CoA carboxylase

    (C) Hormone-sensitive lipase

    (D) Carnitine acyltransferase-1 (CAT-1)

    (E) Hydroxymethylglutaryl CoA reductase

3. Which of the following enzymes is inhibited by insulin?

    (A) Lipoprotein lipase

    (B) Acetyl CoA carboxylase

    (C) Hydroxymethylglutaryl CoA reductase

    (D) Carnitine acyltransferase-1 (CAT-1)

    (E) Fatty acid synthase

4. Which of the following statements about the citrate shuttle is correct?

    (A) Citrate accumulates in the mitochondria when adenosine diphosphate is high

    (B) Citrate freely diffuses across the inner mitochondrial membrane (IMM)

    (C) Citrate lyase is located in the mitochondrial matrix

    (D) Cytosolic oxaloacetate is formed by the carboxylation of pyruvate

    (E) NADPH is formed by a two-step conversion of oxaloacetate to pyruvate

5. Which of the following pathways is operating during prolonged fasting and starvation but is not operating in the well-fed state or during an overnight fast?

    (A) Fatty acid oxidation in muscle

    (B) Fatty acid synthesis in the liver

    (C) Triglyceride hydrolysis in adipose tissue

    (D) Ketone oxidation in the brain

    (E) Triglyceride synthesis in adipose tissue

ANSWERS AND EXPLANATIONS

1. The answer is C. Hormone-sensitive lipase is found primarily in adipose tissue, where it catalyzes the release of fatty acids from the carbon positions C-1 and C-3 of the glycerol backbone of triglyceride. Hormones that increase the concentration of cAMP in adipose tissue result in phosphorylation and activation of this enzyme. Acetyl CoA carboxylase and HMG CoA reductase are both inhibited by cAMP-dependent phosphorylation. Neither LpL nor fatty acid synthase are covalently regulated.

2. The answer is D. CAT-1 controls the entry of fatty acids into the mitochondria and is inhibited by malonyl CoA, an intermediate in fatty acid synthesis. This mechanism is important in preventing futile cycling of fatty acids. The other enzymes listed are not affected by malonyl CoA.

3. The answer is D. The activity of CAT-1 is inhibited by insulin, although the effect is mediated by malonyl CoA. Insulin stimulates the synthesis of malonyl CoA. The activity of the other enzymes listed is stimulated by insulin.

4. The answer is E. In the conversion of oxaloacetate to pyruvate, oxaloacetate is first reduced to malate by malate dehydrogenase. Malate is subsequently oxidized and decarboxylated to pyruvate, producing NADPH. The pyruvate is transported back into the mitochondria where it is carboxylated to oxaloacetate. The accumulation of citrate occurs when ATP is high, and it is transported across the IMM by facilitated diffusion. Citrate lyase, located in the cytosol, cleaves citrate to oxaloacetate and acetyl CoA.

5. The answer is D. During a prolonged fast, the brain can adapt to using ketones as a source of fuel. During a well-fed state, fatty acid synthesis in the liver and triglyceride synthesis in adipose tissue are occurring. In an overnight fast, triglyceride hydrolysis occurs in adipose tissue, and fatty acid oxidation occurs in muscle.

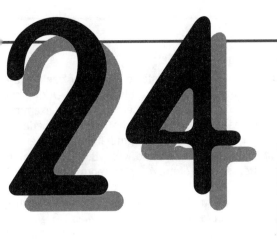

INTRODUCTION TO AMINO ACID METABOLISM: DIGESTION AND ABSORPTION OF DIETARY PROTEIN

CHAPTER OUTLINE

INTRODUCTION OF CLINICAL CASE

A 59-year-old woman was admitted to the hospital for an emergency appendectomy. She weighed 42 kg, and her height was 153 cm. A review of her medical history showed that she had lost 14 kg over the past 6 months. The patient's appetite was poor, and she reported frequent nausea and vomiting. The surgery was uncomplicated, and she was released 2 days later. Two weeks after the surgery, her sister brought her back to the hospital because the surgical incision was oozing a watery, bloody fluid. During the previous 2 weeks, her diet consisted mainly of soup and warm cereal. Physical examination indicated that the patient's weight was now 51 kg, and she had pitting edema. Pinpoint hemorrhages were noted on her legs, her skin showed light patches, and her hair could be plucked out with no sign of pain. Her temperature was 38.6°C. Laboratory analysis of blood gave the following results: serum protein, 4.3 g/dL (normal: 6–8 g/dL); albumin, 2 g/dL (normal: 3.5–5.5 g/dL); transferrin, 120 mg/dL (normal: 200–400 mg/dL); blood urea nitrogen (BUN), 5.5 mg/dL (normal: 8–23 mg/dL); and lymphocytes, 200/μL (normal: 1,500–4,000/μL). Urinary urea nitrogen excretion was 20 g/24 hr. Following a consultation with the nutritional service, central venous alimentation was started immediately. Orders were written for 500 g dextrose, 150 g protein, 5 mg zinc, and standard amounts of vitamins and electrolytes daily for a period of 2 weeks. She was also started on an antibiotic.

OVERVIEW OF NITROGEN METABOLISM

The amino acid pool in cells is derived primarily from the turnover of tissue protein. Between 125 and 220 g of protein are turned over a day. About 75% of the amino acids are used for the resynthesis of tissue protein. The remainder is used for gluconeogenesis, ketogenesis, and the synthesis of a variety of specialized products. The amino acids that are removed from the pool are replaced by de novo synthesis and by dietary protein. Unlike dietary glucose and fatty acids, there is no storage form for excess amino acids. They are degraded, primarily by the liver. Most of the nitrogen in amino acids is converted to urea and excreted, while the carbon skeletons are either oxidized to carbon dioxide and water or used for gluconeogenesis and ketogenesis (Figure 24-1).

FIGURE 24-1 ▶
Overview of Amino Acid Metabolism. The source and fate of the amino acid pool is shown. Amino acids are used for resynthesizing protein, the synthesis of several specialized products, gluconeogenesis, and ketogenesis. Excess amino acids are also oxidized by the liver to carbon dioxide (CO_2) and water (H_2O). Nonessential amino acids can be resynthesized from various intermediates in metabolism. The essential amino acids are provided by dietary protein.

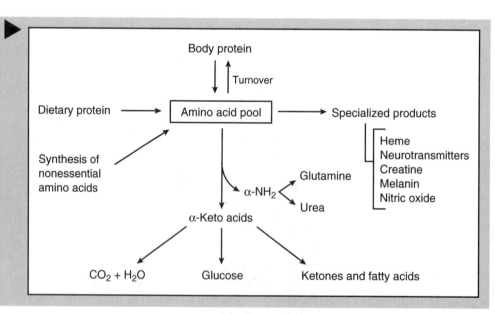

Protein Turnover

The turnover of proteins occurs at different rates. Some proteins, like immunoglobulins and collagen, have a very long half-life that is measured in years. Other proteins, particularly liver proteins and regulatory enzymes, have a short half-life that is measured in hours or days. Protein turnover occurs in all tissues but is much more active in some tissues than in others. For example, proteins of the visceral organs generally turn over at a much faster rate than those in skeletal muscle and connective tissue.

Essential Amino Acids

Of the 20 amino acids found in proteins, adults are unable to synthesize 8 of the amino acids at rates sufficient to meet the needs of the body. Infants are unable to synthesize 10 of the 20 amino acids. These essential amino acids must be supplied by the diet.

Essential Amino Acids	
Arginine[a]	Methionine
Histidine[a]	Phenylalanine
Isoleucine	Lysine
Leucine	Tryptophan
Threonine	Valine

[a] Essential only in infancy.

NITROGEN BALANCE AND DIETARY PROTEIN REQUIREMENT

Nitrogen balance is defined as the condition that exists when the nitrogen consumed in the diet is equal to the nitrogen excreted from the body. Most nitrogen is excreted in the urine as urea, with a small amount of undigested protein excreted in the feces. Positive nitrogen balance occurs when the intake of nitrogen exceeds the amount of nitrogen excreted. Conversely, negative nitrogen balance occurs when the amount of nitrogen excreted exceeds the intake. Nitrogen balance is affected by a number of normal and pathologic conditions.

Positive Nitrogen Balance

A positive nitrogen balance is associated with periods of growth, pregnancy, lactation, and recovery from metabolic stress. In all of these conditions, net protein synthesis is occurring, and the amount of nitrogen taken in exceeds the total nitrogen excreted.

Negative Nitrogen Balance

A negative nitrogen balance occurs when there is an inadequate amount of protein in the diet or in several clinical situations such as uncontrolled diabetes, infection, injury, or other trauma. In these situations, increased degradation of tissue protein provides substrate for gluconeogenesis. A diet deficient in any one of the essential amino acids results in a negative nitrogen balance, even if a large amount of protein is consumed.

Dietary Protein Requirement

The amount of dietary protein required by adults is equal to the amount needed to maintain nitrogen balance. An additional protein allowance is required by women who are pregnant or breast-feeding. During pregnancy, approximately 950 g of new protein are synthesized for the fetus and for maternal reproductive tissues. An additional 30 g of protein a day throughout the pregnancy are recommended. During lactation, an additional 20 g of protein a day are recommended for the synthesis of milk protein. Approximately 850 mL of milk are synthesized daily during lactation.

The amount of protein required by children is based on the amount needed for optimal growth, rather than on the amount needed to maintain nitrogen balance. In all age groups, the protein requirement of a particular individual is increased during periods of catabolic states, such as surgery, sepsis, and trauma.

Recommended Daily Allowance of Protein	
Infants (0–1 yr)	2.0 g/kg body weight/d
Children (1–10 yrs)	1.2 g/kg body weight/d
Adolescents	1.0 g/kg body weight/d
Adults	0.8 g/kg body weight/d

Biologic Value of Protein

The biologic value of a protein is an index of its content of essential amino acids. The biologic value of egg white is used as a reference and is arbitrarily assigned a value of 100%. Proteins from animal sources have a higher biologic value than those from plant sources. Any protein that is deficient in a single essential amino acid has little or no biologic value. However, a proper combination of different proteins of low biologic value can provide a diet of adequate biologic value. The mixed protein found in the average American diet has a composite biologic value of about 70%.

Effect of Caloric Intake on Dietary Protein Requirement

Dietary protein is used efficiently only when adequate calories are included in the diet. When the caloric intake is low, much of the protein is oxidized as a source of energy, thereby increasing the amount of protein needed to maintain nitrogen balance.

CONSEQUENCES OF DIETARY PROTEIN DEFICIENCY

Calculating the Protein Requirement for Hospitalized Patients
The recommended daily allowances are based on the assumption that individuals in a particular age category are healthy. For hospitalized patients, the amount of protein required can be calculated from the following formula [2], which is based on the amount of nitrogen that is excreted as urea within a 24-hour period.

Protein intake (g/24 hr) =
(g urinary urea nitrogen + 4) × 6.25

A small amount of nitrogen (estimated as 4 g) is lost in the stool, sweat, hair, skin, and nonurea nitrogen in the urine. Since the nitrogen content of protein is 16%, the total nitrogen losses are multiplied by 6.25 (or divided by 0.16) to calculate the amount of protein required to maintain nitrogen balance.

Consequences of Prolonged Intake of Excess Protein
Consumption of excess dietary protein for long periods of time has potentially adverse effects. Increased loss of calcium in the urine occurs and may result in osteoporosis. Because of the need to excrete excess nitrogen, sulfur, and phosphate, the work load on the kidney is also increased and has been implicated in the gradual deterioration of renal function that occurs with age.

The most common form of malnutrition is protein-calorie malnutrition. Not only is malnutrition widespread in developing countries, but it is also common in hospitalized patients, where it may be caused by an underlying disease. The development of malnutrition in the hospitalized patient usually results from a failure to recognize and meet the patient's nutritional needs [1]. Although the symptoms of protein-calorie malnutrition vary widely among individuals, most cases are usually classified as either marasmus or kwashiorkor. The distinguishing features of these two types of protein-calorie malnutrition are summarized in Table 24-1.

Marasmus

Marasmus is a chronic condition, resulting from a deficiency of both protein and energy. Severe wasting, from a loss of body fat and muscle, results in an emaciated appearance. Serum albumin levels are usually within the normal range. The patient's appetite is usually good, and the response to a diet containing skim milk and vegetable oil is rapid. Nutritional intervention in hospitalized patients should be started slowly. Overly aggressive parenteral nutrition can result in a variety of electrolyte and hemodynamic derangements that can be life-threatening. When possible, enteral nutritional support is preferable to parenteral support.

Kwashiorkor

Kwashiorkor results from a deficiency of protein, although the overall intake of calories is adequate. The onset of kwashiorkor is often precipitated by an increased demand for protein, which may result from infection or some other form of metabolic stress. In growing children who are eating a diet high in carbohydrate and low in protein, kwashiorkor is often precipitated by infection. In adults, it is often precipitated in hospitalized patients who are under acute stress. Since there is little muscle wasting or depletion of fat, kwashiorkor may not be readily noticed. Symptoms of kwashiorkor include edema, depigmentation of skin and hair, and easily pluckable hair. The blood volume is decreased, and levels of serum albumin and transferrin are severely reduced. The immune system is compromised, and slow wound healing is observed.

TABLE 24-1 ▶
Symptoms of Kwashiorkor and Marasmus

Symptom	Marasmus	Kwashiorkor
Growth failure	Present	Present
Anemia	Present	Present
Edema	Absent	Present
Hepatomegaly	Absent	Present
Depigmentation	Absent	Present
Hypoalbuminemia	Normal to mild	Severe
Muscle wasting	Severe	Absent to mild
Fat reserves	Absent	Normal to mildly diminished

DIGESTION OF DIETARY PROTEIN

The source of protein to be digested comes from both exogenous and endogenous sources. As much as 50 g of protein a day may be derived from secretions of the gastrointestinal (GI) tract and cells that have been sloughed off. Most protein is digested to a mixture of amino acids, dipeptides, and tripeptides. Under normal conditions, very little protein is excreted in the feces. Digestion is facilitated by three types of secretions elaborated by the stomach, intestine, and pancreas. These include: (1) aqueous solutions having varying pH and electrolyte compositions, which provide the environment required for optimal activity of the digestive enzymes; (2) the inactive precursors of the digestive enzymes; and (3) mucoproteins, which form highly viscous solutions and act as lubricants to facilitate passage of food through the GI tract. The digestion of protein starts in the stomach and is completed in the small intestine.

Digestion of Protein in the Stomach

The entry of food into the stomach results in the release of gastrin by the enteroendocrine cells of the mucosa. Gastrin is a peptide hormone, having receptors on the surface of both parietal cells and chief cells. Binding of gastrin to its receptors results in the release of hydrochloric acid (HCl) from parietal cells and pepsinogen from chief cells (Figure 24-2).

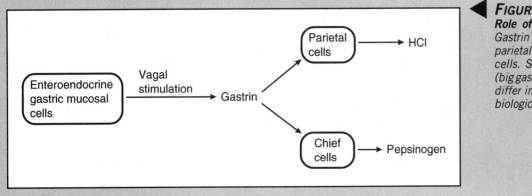

FIGURE 24-2
Role of Gastrin in Protein Degradation.
Gastrin stimulates the release of HCl from parietal cells and pepsinogen from chief cells. Several forms of gastrin are found (big gastrin, little gastrin, minigastrin) that differ in the length of the peptide. All are biologically active.

Liver Failure and Nitrogen Metabolism
Diseases of the liver impair its ability to metabolize protein. The synthesis of urea is impaired in patients with advanced liver disease. The accumulation of ammonia is toxic. Protein with high biologic value should be consumed to minimize the nitrogen load but still ensure an adequate supply of essential amino acids.

Secretion and Function of HCl. Parietal cells secrete a solution containing 0.16 mol/L HCl, along with a few other electrolytes. Intrinsic factor, a protein required for the absorption of vitamin B_{12}, is also synthesized and secreted by the parietal cells. Gastric juice has a pH of about 1 and is effective in denaturing dietary protein, making it highly susceptible to proteolysis.

Secretion and Activation of Pepsinogen. The chief cells of the stomach secrete pepsinogen, an inactive precursor of pepsin, the enzyme that hydrolyzes protein in the stomach. The activation of pepsinogen is stimulated by hydrogen ion (H^+), which cleaves a peptide bond, resulting in the formation of catalytically active pepsin. Autocatalytic activation follows, with pepsin rapidly activating other pepsinogen molecules (Figure 24-3).

Action of Pepsin. Pepsin is an endopeptidase with broad specificity, cleaving peptide bonds that are formed from carboxyl groups of aromatic amino acids, acidic amino acids, leucine, and methionine. Proteins are degraded by pepsin to a mixture of oligopeptides.

Zollinger-Ellison Syndrome
Zollinger-Ellison syndrome results from ectopic production of gastrin by pancreatic islet cell tumors. The patients spontaneously secrete HCl at a high rate, eroding the gastric mucosa and resulting in ulcers.

Digestion of Protein in the Intestinal Lumen

The movement of partially digested chyme through the duodenum stimulates the release of two hormones, secretin and cholecystokinin (CCK), as well as an enzyme, enteropeptidase.

FIGURE 24-3 ▶

Activation of Pepsinogen. *The acidic pH of the stomach initiates the conversion of pepsinogen to pepsin. At pH values greater than 2, the peptide remains associated with pepsin in a complex that is catalytically inactive. In cases of pernicious anemia where HCl production fails, the complex does not dissociate, and protein digestion in the stomach does not occur. N = N-terminus; C = C-terminus.*

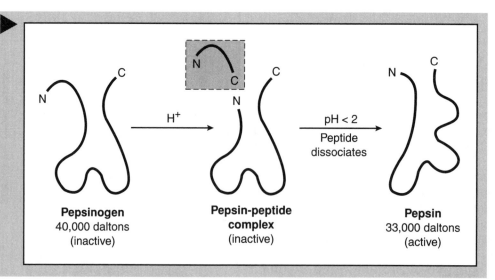

Pepsinogen
40,000 daltons
(inactive)

Pepsin-peptide complex
33,000 daltons
(inactive)

Pepsin
33,000 daltons
(active)

Effect of Secretin. Secretin stimulates the release of pancreatic juice, an alkaline secretion that is enriched in bicarbonate (HCO_3^-). The HCO_3^- neutralizes the HCl in the chyme as it enters the small intestine.

Effect of CCK. CCK stimulates the release of several inactive zymogens from the exocrine pancreas. Some of the zymogens are precursors of endopeptidases (trypsinogen, chymotrypsinogen, proelastase), and others are precursors of exopeptidases (procarboxypeptidase A, procarboxypeptidase B).

Effect of Enteropeptidase. Enteropeptidase, also known as enterokinase, initiates a cascade of proteolytic events that leads to the activation of the pancreatic zymogens. Enteropeptidase hydrolyzes a single peptide bond in trypsinogen, resulting in the release of a small peptide from the amino terminus. The removal of the peptide from trypsinogen is accompanied by a conformational change, resulting in catalytically active trypsin (Figure 24-4). Once a small amount of trypsin is formed, it catalyzes the conversion of all the remaining zymogens to their active forms.

FIGURE 24-4 ▶

Activation of Pancreatic Zymogens. *Enteropeptidase catalyzes the initial reaction that results in the activation of all the pancreatic zymogens. A peptide containing six amino acids is removed from the N-terminus of trypsinogen, forming active trypsin. N = N-terminus; C = C-terminus.*

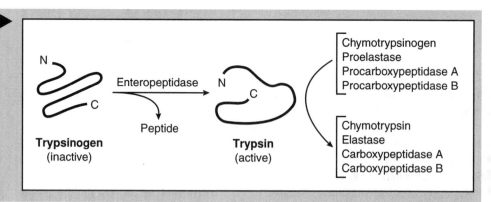

Trypsinogen
(inactive)

Peptide

Trypsin
(active)

Chymotrypsinogen
Proelastase
Procarboxypeptidase A
Procarboxypeptidase B

Chymotrypsin
Elastase
Carboxypeptidase A
Carboxypeptidase B

Specificity of Pancreatic Proteases. Each of the pancreatic proteases has a different specificity, and the products of some enzymes are substrates for others. For example, all of the peptides produced by the action of trypsin have lysine or arginine at their C-terminus. These peptides are then substrates for carboxypeptidase B, an exopeptidase that removes basic amino acids from the carboxyl end. The battery of proteases efficiently hydrolyzes the protein and peptides to a mixture of free amino acids (about 35%) and small peptides having 2–5 amino acids (about 65%). The specificity of the different enzymes involved in protein digestion is summarized in Table 24-2.

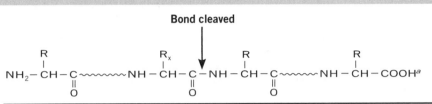

Bond cleaved

Site of Action	Enzyme	Specificity
Stomach	Pepsin	R_x = Phenylalanine, tyrosine, tryptophan, methionine, glutamic acid, and aspartic acid
Intestinal lumen	Trypsin	R_x = lysine, arginine, and histidine
	Chymotrypsin	R_x = phenylalanine, tyrosine, and tryptophan
	Elastase	R_x = alanine, serine, and glycine
	Carboxypeptidase A	Any C-terminal amino acid except lysine, arginine, and proline
	Carboxypeptidase B	C-terminal lysine and arginine
Intestinal membrane	Aminopeptidases	Most N-terminal residues of oligopeptides
Intestinal cell cytosol	Aminopeptidases	Most N-terminal residues of oligopeptides
	Dipeptidases	Most dipeptides except those X-proline[b]
	Prolidase	Dipeptides containing proline

[a] The wavy lines indicate regions of protein that are between cleavage sites.
[b] X-proline is any dipeptide with proline at the C-terminus.

Intestinal Aminopeptidases and Dipeptidases

Intestinal mucosal cells contain enzymes that catalyze the terminal steps in protein digestion. There are several aminopeptidases, having different specificities, that sequentially release amino acids from the N-terminus of peptides. There are also several peptidases that are specific for dipeptides. Most of the intestinal enzymes require metal ions (e.g., zinc, cobalt, or magnesium) for activity. The intestinal enzymes are found both in the brush-border membrane and in the cytosol of intestinal cells.

ABSORPTION OF AMINO ACIDS FROM THE INTESTINE

Amino acids arising from protein digestion in the GI tract are transported into the intestinal mucosal cells by mechanisms that are analogous to the sodium (Na^+)-dependent glucose transporters (see Chapter 10). Several transport proteins are found in the brush-border membrane that are specific for groups of structurally similar amino acids. Di- and tripeptides that escape hydrolysis also are transported into the intestinal cells by Na^+-dependent mechanisms, where they are hydrolyzed to free amino acids.

Major Amino Acid Transport Systems

Four Na^+-dependent amino acid transport systems have been well characterized. These systems transport basic amino acids, acidic amino acids, neutral amino acids, and imino acids and glycine. All are specific for L-amino acids. D-Amino acids are transported by passive diffusion. The Na^+-dependent transport systems are also found in the brush-border membrane of the kidney, where they reabsorb amino acids from the glomerular filtrate before the urine is excreted. The sustained transport of amino acids requires that Na^+ be pumped back out of the cell in exchange for potassium (K^+), a reaction that is catalyzed by Na^+,K^+-ATPase. These amino acid transporters are classified as carrier-mediated active transport systems.

Hartnup Disease and Blue Diaper Syndrome

Hartnup disease is an autosomal recessive trait that is characterized by neutral aminoaciduria. The serum levels of the neutral amino acids are lower than normal. One of the amino acids that is neither absorbed from the intestine nor reabsorbed by the kidney is tryptophan, a precursor for niacin synthesis. The decreased synthesis of niacin results in pellagra-like symptoms. In addition to excreting tryptophan, intestinal bacteria degrade unabsorbed tryptophan to several indole derivatives, including indigo blue. The inability to absorb tryptophan may be initially recognized by blue urine and is sometime called "blue diaper syndrome."

TABLE 24-3 ▶
Amino Acid Transport Systems

Transport System	Amino Acids Transported	Genetic Disease
Neutral amino acids	Alanine, glycine, serine, threonine, valine, leucine, isoleucine, phenylalanine, tyrosine, tryptophan, histidine, cysteine, methionine, and citrulline	Hartnup disease
Acidic amino acids	Glutamic acid and aspartic acid	Dicarboxylic aminoaciduria
Dibasic amino acids	Lysine, arginine, cystine and ornithine	Cystinuria
Imino acids and glycine	Proline, hydroxyproline and glycine	Joseph's syndrome

Cystinuria

Cystinuria, also known as basic amino-aciduria, is the most common genetic defect in amino acid metabolism, occurring at a frequency of 1 in 7000 individuals [3]. The levels of cystine, lysine, arginine, and ornithine in the urine are 20–30 times the normal levels. Cystine is significantly less soluble than the other basic amino acids, and at the acidic pH of urine, it precipitates out of solution, forming stones in the kidney. Cystinuria is inherited as an autosomal recessive trait.

Genetic Defects in Amino Acid Transport

Genetic diseases arising from defects in each of the amino acid transport systems have been reported (Table 24-3). Most of these conditions were initially described as defects in the renal tubular transport systems in which specific groups of amino acids were excreted in large amounts in the urine. Both the absorption of amino acids from the intestine and reabsorption from the glomerular filtrate are impaired. In most cases, these deficiencies have minimal nutritional consequences because the amino acids can be absorbed by independent di- and tripeptide transport systems.

RESOLUTION OF CLINICAL CASE

Both the history of the patient introduced at the beginning of the chapter and the laboratory findings support the diagnosis of kwashiorkor. The 25% loss in weight that she experienced during the 6 months prior to surgery, accompanied by the stress associated with surgery, were strong indicators of protein malnutrition. In general, a weight loss that is greater than 10% over a 6-month period is significant in the assessment of malnutrition [4]. Malnutrition, however, was not diagnosed in this patient until she returned to the hospital 2 weeks later. At this time, physical examination revealed pitting edema and a weight of 51 kg, which was about 20% higher than her weight just prior to surgery, although she reported eating only soup and cereal since being released from the hospital. The spuriously high weight was the result of edema. Other physical findings indicative of protein malnutrition were poor wound healing and painless pluckability of hair. The patient also had a fever, suggesting that infection may be contributing to metabolic stress. Deficiencies in vitamins and minerals are often found in patients with kwashiorkor. The pinpoint hemorrhages in this patient are consistent with vitamin C deficiency. Laboratory values confirmed severe malnutrition. Her lymphocyte count was severely reduced, indicating an impairment in her immune system and increasing her susceptibility to infections. Her total serum protein was markedly reduced, as were her levels of albumin and transferrin. The half-life of albumin is about 21 days, while that of transferrin is 8 days. Measurement of these two serum proteins are frequently used as indicators of the visceral protein compartment. The short half-life of transferrin provides a more sensitive indicator of acute changes, while the longer half-life of albumin is reflective of more chronic changes. Glucose is the primary fuel for hypoxic tissues and phagocytic white blood cells, and protein is being catabolized in this patient to provide substrate for gluconeogenesis. The low concentration of BUN is consistent with a low intake of protein.

Nutritional support was started immediately. Because of her history of poor eating, nausea, and vomiting, the route for delivery of nutrients was via central venous alimentation. The amount of urinary urea nitrogen in a 24-hour urine specimen (20 g/d) was used as the basis for calculating the amount of protein the patient needed to maintain nitrogen balance. Her estimated protein needs were 150 g/d (20 g + 4 g for stool and other nonurea nitrogen losses, multiplied by 6.25 to convert nitrogen loss to protein loss). The 500 g of dextrose per day provided 1700 kcal (intravenous dextrose solutions contain 3.4 kcal/g). Zinc was increased to about twice the recommended daily allowance because of the increased need during times of infection and wound healing.

REVIEW QUESTIONS

Directions: For each of the following questions, choose the **one best** answer.

1. A deficiency in which of the following amino acids results in negative nitrogen balance in an adult?
    - **(A)** Serine
    - **(B)** Proline
    - **(C)** Alanine
    - **(D)** Lysine
    - **(E)** Histidine

2. Which of the following symptoms is found in kwashiorkor but is absent in marasmus?
    - **(A)** Muscle wasting
    - **(B)** Growth failure
    - **(C)** Edema
    - **(D)** Anemia
    - **(E)** Normal appetite

3. Which of the following enzymes initiates the activation of pancreatic zymogens in the small intestine?
    - **(A)** Chymotrypsin
    - **(B)** Elastase
    - **(C)** Carboxypeptidase A
    - **(D)** Enteropeptidase
    - **(E)** Trypsin

4. A cab driver was hospitalized following an accident that resulted in multiple broken bones. Analysis of a 24-hour urine specimen showed a total of 16 g of urea nitrogen. How much protein should be included in his diet to maintain nitrogen balance?
    - **(A)** 200 g/d
    - **(B)** 125 g/d
    - **(C)** 150 g/d
    - **(D)** 175 g/d
    - **(E)** 100 g/d

5. Which of the following characteristics would apply to a person with cystinuria?
    - **(A)** The neutral amino acid transporter is defective
    - **(B)** Urinary cysteine excretion is elevated
    - **(C)** Gallstone formation is common
    - **(D)** The dibasic amino acid transporter is defective
    - **(E)** Urinary excretion of histidine, leucine, and arginine is increased

ANSWERS AND EXPLANATIONS

1. The answer is D. A deficiency in any one of the essential amino acids leads to net degradation of body protein and a negative nitrogen balance. Lysine is the only amino acid listed that is essential in adults. Histidine is essential only in infancy and early childhood, and serine, proline, and alanine are nonessential throughout life.

2. The answer is C. Plasma proteins are degraded and used as substrates for gluconeogenesis. In kwashiorkor, the decrease in plasma protein concentration leads to the accumulation of fluid in the extracellular space. Growth failure and anemia are seen in both kwashiorkor and marasmus. Muscle wasting is severe in marasmus and is either absent or mild in kwashiorkor. A normal appetite is found in marasmus, whereas kwashiorkor is characterized by lack of appetite.

3. The answer is D. Enteropeptidase initiates a cascade of activation reactions by converting a small portion of trypsinogen to trypsin. Once a small amount of trypsin is formed, its activation becomes autocatalytic, and it also activates chymotrypsinogen, proelastase, and carboxypeptidase A.

4. The answer is B. The total nitrogen losses are assumed to be 20 g/d (16 g of urinary urea nitrogen + 4 g for of nitrogen in the stool, skin, and sweat). Multiplication of total nitrogen losses by 6.25 converts nitrogen losses to protein losses. Therefore, to counteract the losses, 125 g of protein are required a day.

5. The answer is D. Cystine is a dimer of two molecules of cysteine that are linked by a disulfide bridge. Cystinuria results from a genetic defect in the dibasic amino acid transporter found in the brush-border membrane of both intestinal and kidney cells. Dibasic amino acids are lysine, arginine, ornithine, and cystine. Elevated levels of all of these amino acids are excreted in the urine. Both leucine and cysteine are neutral amino acids that are unaffected in cystinuria. Because of the insolubility of cystine, kidney stones are often formed in cystinuria.

REFERENCES

1. Weinsier RL, Morgan SL: *Fundamentals of Clinical Nutrition*, St. Louis, MO: C. V. Mosby, 1993, pp 129–132.
2. Blackburn GL, Bell SJ, Mullen JL: *Nutritional Medicine: A Case Management Approach.* Philadelphia, PA: W. B. Saunders, 1989, pp 116–117.
3. Levy HL: Genetic screening. In *Advances in Human Genetics*, vol 4. New York, NY: Plenum Press, 1973, p 1.
4. Detsky AS, Smalley PS, Chang J: Is this patient malnourished? *JAMA* 241:54–58, 1994.

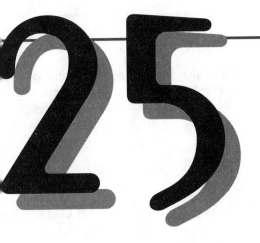

AMINO ACID CATABOLISM: DISPOSAL OF NITROGEN AND CARBON SKELETONS

CHAPTER OUTLINE

INTRODUCTION OF CLINICAL CASE

A male child was born into a family with no history of neonatal deaths. He weighed 2.9 kg at birth and appeared to be healthy until 3 days of age when he developed seizures. The mother had a history of aversion to meat, the eating of which was accompanied by episodes of vomiting and lethargy. The patient had mild alkalosis with a blood pH of 7.5 (normal: 7.35–7.45). His plasma ammonium ion (NH_4^+) level was 240 μM (normal: 25–40 μM). Plasma amino acid levels included: glutamine, 2.4 mM (normal: 350–650 μM); alanine, 750 μM (normal: 8–25 μM); arginine, 5 μM (normal: 30–125 μM); and undetectable citrulline. Urinary orotic acid excretion was 285 µg/mg creatinine (norm 0.3–10 µg/mg creatinine). Oral therapy was started by administering a combination essential amino acids (including arginine) at a dose of 1.1 g/kg/d and sodium benzoate a dose of 2 mmol/kg/d. By the seventh day, his plasma NH_4^+ level was 40 µM, and appeared clinically well.

OVERVIEW OF AMINO ACID CATABOLISM

Various organs and tissues have different functions in amino acid metabolism. Durir fasting, the plasma amino acid levels are maintained by the degradation of muscle tiss protein. In the fed state, dietary amino acids are used to replenish tissue protei Therefore, interorgan amino acid exchange is essential for maintaining homeostas

Interorgan Relationships

The major organs involved in amino acid exchange are the small intestine, liver, skelet muscle, and kidney (Figure 25-1).

FIGURE 25-1 ▶

Interorgan Amino Acid Exchange. The interchange of amino acids among the intestine, liver, muscle, and kidney occurs following a meal. The catabolism of most amino acids, except the branched-chain amino acids (BCAAs), starts in the liver. BCAA catabolism starts in the skeletal muscle. Urea synthesis can only occur in liver. Alanine (Ala) and glutamine (Gln) are carriers of amino groups from muscle to the liver and kidney, respectively. Arg = arginine.

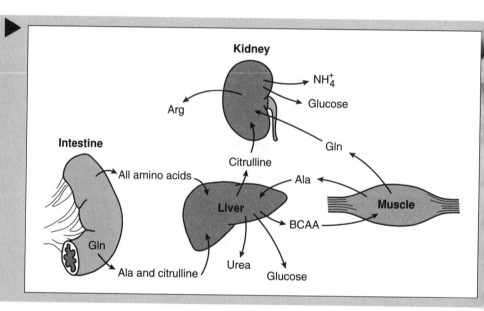

Intestine. Amino acids are absorbed from the small intestine into the portal circulatio following a meal. The amino acid composition of dietary protein is altered by th intestinal mucosal cell. These cells use glutamine and asparagine as their major sourc of energy, producing a mixture of products including carbon dioxide, NH_4^+, alanine, and citrulline. These products are released into the portal circulation, along with the dietar amino acids that are not catabolized. In the fasting state, the intestine oxidizes glu tamine that is released from skeletal muscle.

Liver. The catabolism of most amino acids starts in the liver, where the amino groups ar removed and incorporated into urea. The carbon skeletons that remain can either be oxidized to carbon dioxide and water or used as substrates for gluconeogenesis and ketogenesis. The catabolism of branched-chain amino acids (BCAAs) [valine, isoleucine leucine] cannot be initiated in the liver. The concentration of the amino acid pool leaving the liver in the fed state is 2–3 times higher than in the fasting state, and more than hal are BCAAs.

Skeletal Muscle. The catabolism of BCAAs starts in skeletal muscle, where the amino groups are transferred through a series of reactions to pyruvate, forming alanine. More than 50% of the amino acids released from skeletal muscle are alanine and glutamine Both of these amino acids act as carriers of amino groups from muscle to other tissues

anine is taken up by the liver, where the amino group is removed and incorporated into
ea. Pyruvate, the carbon skeleton derived from alanine, is used as a substrate for
uconeogenesis. Glutamine that is released by skeletal muscle is taken up by the kidney
d liver, where the amino groups can be excreted as NH_4^+ or converted to urea,
spectively. In the fasting state, some of the glutamine is taken up by intestinal cells,
here it is oxidized as a source of energy.

idney. The kidney is an ammoniagenic organ. Most of the NH_4^+ excreted in the urine
as its origin in glutamine, which is released by skeletal muscle. The release of ammonia
om glutamine occurs in two consecutive reactions that are catalyzed by *glutaminase*
nd *glutamate dehydrogenase*, respectively. Both enzymes are located in the mito-
hondria.

$$Glutamine \xrightarrow{\quad NH_4^+ \quad} glutamate \xrightarrow{\quad NH_4^+ \quad} \alpha\text{-ketoglutarate}$$

he reaction catalyzed by glutaminase is particularly important during metabolic ac-
dosis. Ammonia (NH_3) readily picks up a proton (H^+) from the medium, forming NH_4^+,
hus providing a mechanism for excreting H^+ in the urine. Essentially all of the ammonia
eleased in the kidney is excreted as NH_4^+. The α-ketoglutarate is the major substrate for
enal gluconeogenesis. The kidney also converts citrulline, a metabolite released by
ntestinal cells, to arginine.

Major Coenzymes Required for Amino Acid Metabolism

here are three coenzymes that are critical for amino acid metabolism: pyridoxal phos-
hate, tetrahydrofolate, and vitamin B_{12}.

Pyridoxal Phosphate. Pyridoxal phosphate is derived from two forms of vitamin B_6,
yridoxine and pyridoxal. Most reactions that involve the α-carbon atom of an amino acid
equire pyridoxal phosphate as a coenzyme. The aldehyde group of pyridoxal phosphate
orms a Schiff's base with the amino group of an amino acid, resulting in a labile
ntermediate that is common to many reactions in amino acid metabolism (Figure 25-2).
nzymes that catalyze these reactions are *transaminases*, amino acid *decarboxylases*,
nd some amino acid *deaminases*.

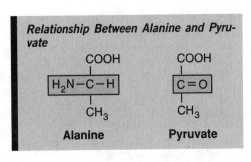

Equilibrium Between NH_3 and NH_4^+
NH_3 is readily converted to NH_4^+ by the addition of a H^+, and the terms ammonia and ammonium ion are often used interchangeably.

$$NH_3 + H^+ \rightleftharpoons NH_4^+$$

The negative log of the ionization constant of an acid (pK_a) for NH_4^+ is 9.3. Therefore, at physiologic pH, the ratio of NH_4^+ : NH_3 is about 100:1.

◀ **FIGURE 25-2**
Pyridoxal Phosphate Forms a Labile Intermediate with Amino Acids. The binding of an amino acid to pyridoxal phosphate results in labilization of the bonds attached to the α-carbon atom. Pyridoxal phosphate is bound to transaminases, racemases, decarboxylases, and dehydratases, which catalyze the cleavage of these bonds.

Tetrahydrofolate (THF). THF provides a link between two major areas of metabolism,
amino acid catabolism and nucleotide synthesis. The function of THF is to act as a carrier
of one-carbon (C_1) fragments in metabolism (Figure 25-3). The C_1 fragments are donated
to THF by intermediates in the degradation of amino acids, and the acceptors of the C_1
fragments are intermediates in the synthesis of purine and pyrimidine nucleotides.

Vitamin B_{12}. Vitamin B_{12} is required by two enzymes that catalyze key reactions in amino
acid metabolism. One reaction, involved in the catabolism of BCAAs, converts methylmalonyl coenzyme A (CoA) to succinyl CoA, and the other reaction converts homocysteine
to methionine.

FIGURE 25-3 ▶
Role of Tetrahydrofolate (THF) in Amino Acid and Nucleotide Metabolism. *The amino acids that serve as donors of C_1 fragments to THF are serine, glycine, histidine, and tryptophan. Most of the C_1 acceptors are intermediates in purine and pyrimidine synthesis. In some of the transfer reactions, THF is oxidized to dihydrofolate (DHF) and must be reduced back to THF before the coenzyme can be charged with another C_1 fragment. NADPH = the reduced form of nicotinamide-adenine dinucleotide phosphate.*

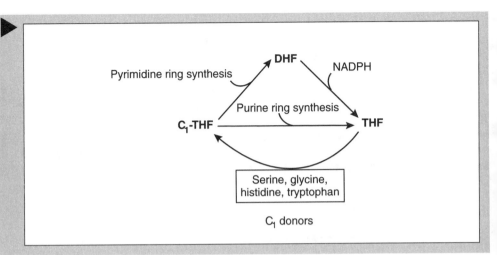

DISPOSAL OF AMINO GROUPS

The first step in the catabolism of amino acids is the removal of the amino groups. Two types of reactions exist in cells for removing amino groups, *transamination* and *deamination*. Transamination reactions channel amino groups into glutamate, which is subsequently deaminated, releasing ammonia. However, deamination reactions release ammonia directly from amino acids. Ammonia is extremely toxic to the central nervous system, and the body has evolved mechanisms for converting ammonia into two nontoxic nitrogenous compounds, urea and glutamine. Urea, the major nontoxic product, is synthesized only in the liver. Therefore, mechanisms for transferring amino groups from extrahepatic tissues to the liver are important for the safe disposal of amino nitrogen (Table 25-1).

TABLE 25-1 ▶
Major Forms of Urinary Nitrogen

Compound Excreted	Percent of Total Nitrogen Excreted
Urea	80%–90%
Creatinine	3%–4%
NH_4^+	2.5%–4.5%
Uric acid	1%–2%
Amino acids	1%–2%

Transamination Reactions

The degradation of most amino acids begins with the transfer of the amino group to an α-keto acid acceptor, as shown in the following equation. These reactions are catalyzed by transaminases, also known as aminotransferases.

$$\underset{\textbf{Amino acid}_1}{\overset{NH_2}{\underset{R_1}{H-C-COOH}}} + \underset{\textbf{α-Keto acid}_2}{\overset{O}{\underset{R_2}{H-C-COOH}}} \rightleftharpoons \underset{\textbf{α-Keto acid}_1}{\overset{O}{\underset{R_1}{H-C-COOH}}} + \underset{\textbf{Amino acid}_2}{\overset{NH_2}{\underset{R_2}{H-C-COOH}}}$$

STRATEGY AND SPECIFICITY

The strategy of transamination reactions is to transfer the amino group from a diverse group of amino acid donors to a small group of keto acid acceptors. Each transaminase is specific for one or a few amino acid donors, whereas most transaminases use α-ketoglu-

tarate as a common acceptor of amino groups. This provides a mechanism for channeling the amino groups from many different amino acids into a common product, *glutamate*. Transaminases are usually named by the amino acid that donates the amino group.

$$\text{Alanine} + \alpha\text{-ketoglutarate} \xrightleftharpoons{\text{alanine transaminase}} \text{pyruvate} + \text{glutamate}$$

$$\text{Aspartate} + \alpha\text{-ketoglutarate} \xrightleftharpoons{\text{aspartate transaminase}} \text{oxaloacetate} + \text{glutamate}$$

$$\text{Tyrosine} + \alpha\text{-ketoglutarate} \xrightleftharpoons{\substack{\text{tyrosine} \\ \text{transaminase}}} p\text{-hydroxyphenylpyruvate} + \text{glutamate}$$

REVERSIBILITY

Transamination reactions are readily reversible. This property is particularly important in the reactions catalyzed by alanine transaminase and aspartate transaminase, which have special roles in the transfer of amino nitrogen.

Alanine Transaminase. Alanine is important in transferring amino groups from skeletal muscle to the liver where they can be incorporated into urea and excreted. The amino groups that have been channeled into glutamate by various transaminase reactions in skeletal muscle are transferred to pyruvate, forming a large pool of alanine, which is transferred to the liver. In the liver, the amino groups are transferred from alanine back to α-ketoglutarate, forming glutamate.

Aspartate Transaminase. The reaction catalyzed by aspartate transaminase is especially important in the liver, where oxaloacetate acts as an acceptor of some of the amino groups that have been channeled into glutamate. Aspartate, the product of this reaction, is a direct donor of amino groups in the synthesis of urea.

> **Nomenclature of Transaminases**
> In the clinical literature, alanine transaminase is often referred to as serum glutamate:pyruvate transaminase (SGPT), and aspartate transaminase is frequently referred to as serum glutamate:oxaloacetate transaminase (SGOT).

Deamination Reactions

The catabolism of a few amino acids starts with the direct release of ammonia. These reactions are grouped into three classes of deaminations: oxidative, hydrolytic, and nonoxidative.

Oxidative Deamination of Glutamate. The oxidative deamination of glutamate is catalyzed by *glutamate dehydrogenase*, an enzyme found in high concentration in the mitochondria of the liver. This reaction uses either nicotinamide adenine dinucleotide (NAD+) or nicotinamide-adenine dinucleotide phosphate (NADP+) as an oxidizing agent and produces the reduced forms of these cofactors, NADH or NADPH. The NH_4^+ produced in this reaction is used as a substrate for urea synthesis.

$$\text{Glutamate} + \text{NAD}^+ (\text{NADP}^+) \rightleftharpoons \alpha\text{-ketoglutarate} + NH_4^+ + \text{NADH (NADPH)}$$

Hydrolytic Deamination. The side chain amide groups of asparagine and glutamine are released by hydrolysis, resulting in ammonia. These reactions are catalyzed by *glutaminase* and *asparaginase*, respectively.

$$\text{Glutamine} + H_2O \longrightarrow \text{glutamate} + NH_4^+$$

$$\text{Asparagine} + H_2O \longrightarrow \text{aspartate} + NH_4^+$$

Nonoxidative Deamination. In addition to the reactions above, several other amino acids can also be deaminated by various mechanisms. These include serine, threonine, histidine, and glycine. Most of these amino acids also can be transaminated.

Detoxification of Ammonia by the Liver

The liver is very effective in detoxifying ammonia. Following a meal, the concentration of NH_4^+ in the portal blood is approximately 0.3 mM. As the blood moves through the liver, the concentration is transiently increased to a level as high as 1.0 mM by the release of NH_4^+ from glutamine. However, by the time the blood enters the systemic circulation, the concentration has been reduced to approximately 20 µM, a reduction of about 50-

fold. The normal concentration range for NH_4^+ in the plasma is between 25 and 40 µM. Different hepatocytes have different complements of enzymes, and the arrangement of these hepatocytes, relative to the blood flow, contributes significantly to the ability of the liver to remove ammonia from the blood (Figure 25-4).

FIGURE 25-4 ▶

Ammonia Detoxification by the Liver. The periportal hepatocytes synthesize urea whereas the perivenous hepatocytes synthesize glutamine. The enzymes in the periportal hepatocytes have a high capacity for converting NH_4^+ to urea. Glutamine synthetase in the perivenous hepatocytes has a lower K_m for NH_4^+ and is effective at removing the NH_4^+ that was not converted to urea in the periportal hepatocytes. CPS-1 = carbamoyl phosphate synthetase-1; Orn = ornithine; Cit = citrulline; Arg = arginine.

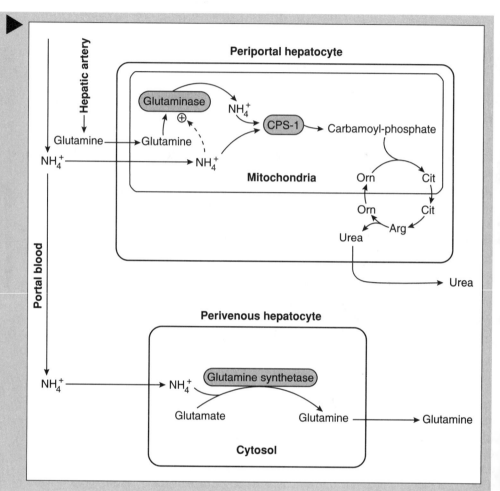

Symptoms of Hyperammonemia
Ammonia is toxic, particularly to the brain and the CNS. Hyperammonemia is characterized by vomiting, lethargy, lack of appetite, seizures, and coma. A deficiency in any of the urea cycle enzymes, except arginase, can result in hyperammonemia. The specific enzyme that is defective can be identified by the compounds that accumulate in the blood, urine, or both.

Urea Synthesis in Periportal Hepatocytes. The periportal hepatocytes are located near the portal vein and receive blood from the intestine that is enriched in nutrients. The periportal hepatocytes have high concentrations of *glutaminase, glutamate dehydrogenase,* and the *urea cycle enzymes.* NH_4^+ released from glutamine by the action of glutaminase and glutamate dehydrogenase in the mitochondrial matrix is used by carbamoyl phosphate synthetase-1 (CPS-1), the enzyme that catalyzes the first reaction in urea synthesis. The major site of ammonia detoxification occurs in the periportal hepatocytes, where urea synthesis occurs. The Michaelis constant (K_m) of CPS-1 for NH_4^+ is approximately 1.0 mM, and this enzyme is not saturated under normal conditions. NH_4^+ entering the hepatocytes allosterically activates glutaminase, resulting in the release of additional NH_4^+ that is used for urea synthesis.

Glutamine Synthesis in Perivenous Hepatocytes and Extrahepatic Tissues. The perivenous hepatocytes consist of one to three layers of cells that surround the central vein. These cells are enriched in *glutamine synthetase,* which has a low K_m for NH_4^+. Therefore, the NH_4^+ that is not converted to urea in the periportal hepatocytes is incorporated into the side chain of glutamate, forming glutamine.

All extrahepatic tissues synthesize glutamine as a means of detoxifying ammonia. Glutamine synthesis is especially important in skeletal muscle and the brain. The reaction is catalyzed by glutamine synthetase and is described by the following equation. The energy for forming the amide bond is supplied by the hydrolysis of adenosine triphosphate (ATP) to adenosine diphosphate (ADP) and inorganic phosphate (P_i).

$$\text{Glutamate} + NH_4^+ + ATP \longrightarrow \text{glutamine} + ADP + P_i$$

Glutamine can be used as a source of biosynthetic nitrogen, which is particularly important in the synthesis of purine and pyrimidine nucleotides. Alternatively, it can be released into the blood and used by the kidney as a source of NH_4^+ by the intestine as a source of energy, or it can be deaminated by the liver, where NH_4^+ can be incorporated into urea.

Pathway for Urea Synthesis

The liver is the only organ that contains all of the enzymes required for urea synthesis. Urea synthesis starts in the mitochondrial matrix and is completed in the cytosol.

STOICHIOMETRY

The overall reaction catalyzed by the urea cycle is described by the following equation (AMP = adenine monophosphate.)

$$NH_4^+ + HCO_3^- + \text{aspartate} + 3\ ATP \longrightarrow \text{urea} + \text{fumarate} + 2\ ADP + AMP + 4P_i$$

The synthesis of urea requires three molecules of ATP and the hydrolysis of four high-energy bonds. One of the nitrogen atoms in urea is supplied by NH_4^+, which is released in the mitochondria by either glutaminase or glutamate dehydrogenase. The other nitrogen atom is donated by aspartate. The remainder of the aspartate molecule is released as fumarate. The carbonyl group in urea arises from bicarbonate (HCO_3^-).

REACTIONS OF THE UREA CYCLE

The five reactions required for urea synthesis are shown in Figure 25-5. The first two reactions occur in the mitochondria, while the last three occur in the cytosol. A citrulline–ornithine antiporter, which transports ornithine into the mitochondria in exchange for citrulline, is located in the inner mitochondrial membrane (IMM).

Formation of Carbamoyl Phosphate. Carbamoyl phosphate is the first intermediate in the urea cycle, and its synthesis is catalyzed by *CPS-1*, the rate-limiting enzyme in the urea cycle. CPS-1 is a mitochondrial enzyme that requires *N*-acetylglutamate (NAG) as an allosteric activator. Two distinct isozymes that synthesize carbamoyl phosphate, CPS-1 and CPS-2, are found in cells. However, they are found in different cellular compartments, where they use different sources of nitrogen and perform different cellular functions. CPS-2 is located in the cytosol, where it participates in the synthesis of pyrimidine nucleotides, and CPS-1 is in the mitochondria, where it participates in urea synthesis.

Formation of Citrulline. The condensation of carbamoyl phosphate with ornithine is catalyzed by *ornithine transcarbamoylase (OTC)*, also a mitochondrial enzyme. In this reaction, the carbamoyl group is transferred from phosphate to the side chain amino group of ornithine, resulting in the production of citrulline and P_i. Citrulline is transported out of the mitochondria into the cytosol where the remaining reactions occur. Both ornithine and citrulline are basic amino acids and are transported in opposite directions across the IMM.

Formation of Argininosuccinate. The condensation of citrulline with aspartic acid results in the formation of argininosuccinate. This reaction occurs in the cytosol where it is catalyzed by *argininosuccinate synthetase*. The energy required for argininosuccinate synthesis is provided by the hydrolysis of ATP to one molecule of AMP and two molecules of P_i.

Formation of Arginine. The cleavage of argininosuccinate to arginine and fumarate is catalyzed by *argininosuccinate lyase*, a cytosolic enzyme that cleaves the bond between the amino group and the α-carbon of the aspartic acid moiety in argininosuccinate. The carbon skeleton of aspartic acid is released as fumarate, and the amino group becomes a part of the arginine side chain. The fumarate produced in this reaction provides a link with other pathways, including the tricarboxylic acid (TCA) cycle, gluconeogenesis, and the synthesis of aspartic acid.

Formation of Urea. The cycle is completed by removal of urea from the side chain of arginine, resulting in the regeneration of ornithine. This reaction is catalyzed by *arginase*. The high concentration of arginase in the liver prohibits the accumulation of arginine. Urea diffuses out of the liver and is transported to the kidneys, where it is

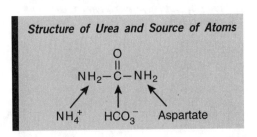

Structure of Urea and Source of Atoms

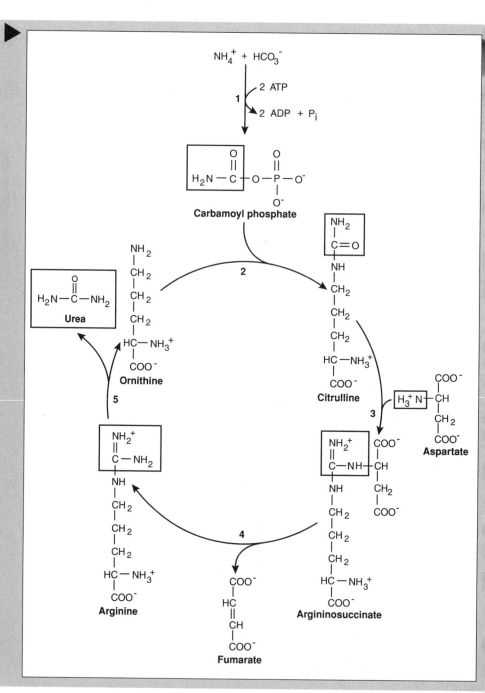

FIGURE 25-5 ▶

The Urea Cycle. The enzymes that catalyze the steps shown are identified by numbers as follows: (1) carbamoyl phosphate synthetase-1, (2) ornithine transcarbamoylase, (3) argininosuccinate synthetase, (4) argininosuccinate lyase, and (5) arginase. Enzymes 1 and 2 are located in the mitochondrial matrix, while enzymes 3, 4, and 5 are located in the cytosol.

filtered and excreted. About 25% of the urea diffuses from the blood into the colon where it is hydrolyzed by bacterial urease, resulting in most of the ammonia found in the portal blood. Ornithine is transported back into the mitochondria where it can participate in another cycle of urea synthesis.

FLOW OF NITROGEN FROM AMINO ACIDS TO UREA

The two most important reactions in the transfer of amino nitrogen from various amino acids to urea are catalyzed by the transaminases and glutamate dehydrogenase (Figure 25-6). The transaminases channel amino groups from several amino acids into glutamate. Some of the amino groups in glutamate are transferred to oxaloacetate, resulting in aspartate, while others are released as NH_4^+ by the action of glutamate dehydrogenase. Both NH_4^+ and aspartate are substrates for urea synthesis.

REGULATION OF THE UREA CYCLE

The rate at which the urea cycle operates is controlled by both short- and long-term regulatory mechanisms.

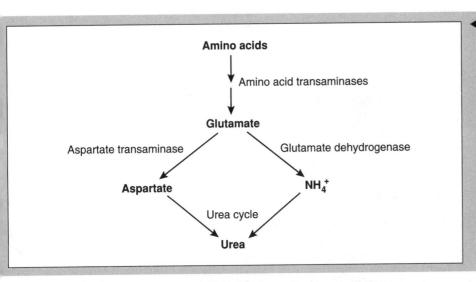

FIGURE 25-6
Pathway of Nitrogen from Amino Acids to Urea. *Transaminases and glutamate dehydrogenase are crucial in transferring amino nitrogen from the various amino acids to urea. Many transaminases act on specific amino acids to channel amino groups into glutamate, which acts as a common precursor for aspartate and NH_4^+.*

Short-Term Regulation. The minute-to-minute rate of the urea cycle is determined by the activity of CPS-1, which is allosterically activated by NAG. The synthesis of NAG, as described in the following equation, increases as the concentration of glutamate increases. Therefore, NAG synthesis and the rate of the urea cycle increase as protein degradation and amino acid transamination increase. The K_m of *NAG synthase* for glutamate is high, and it is not saturated under physiologic conditions. NAG synthase is also activated allosterically by arginine.

$$\text{Glutamate + acetyl}\sim\text{CoA} \xrightarrow{\oplus \text{ arginine}} \textit{N}\text{-acetylglutamate + CoA}$$

Long-Term Regulation. The rate at which the enzymes of the urea cycle are synthesized depends on the amount of protein in the diet. An increase in protein content over several days results in increased synthesis of all enzymes in the cycle, resulting in increased excretion of urea. The process is reversed by a shift to a low-protein diet. During starvation, when protein degradation in tissues is accelerated, the synthesis of urea cycle enzymes is also induced.

GENETIC DEFICIENCIES IN THE UREA CYCLE

Collectively, deficiencies in the urea cycle enzymes occur at a frequency of about 1 in 25,000 live births, and they usually become apparent during the neonatal period [1]. Inherited defects in each of the enzymes of the urea cycle have been described (Table 25-2). Because of the high toxicity of ammonia, neonatal hyperammonemia must be treated immediately to avoid brain damage. These disorders are associated with mental retardation, convulsions, coma, and death.

Antenatal Diagnosis of Urea Cycle Defects
The identification of fetuses at risk for a urea cycle disorder can be made by either enzyme assays or DNA analysis of cultured amniocytes.

TABLE 25-2
Inherited Defects in the Urea Cycle

Disease	Defective Enzyme	Products Accumulated
Hyperammonemia type I	Carbamoyl phosphate synthetase I	Ammonia, glutamine, and alanine
Hyperammonemia type II	Ornithine transcarbamoylase	Ammonia, glutamine, and orotic acid
Citrullinemia	Argininosuccinate synthetase	Citrulline
Argininosuccinic aciduria	Argininosuccinate lyase	Argininosuccinate
Argininemia	Arginase	Arginine

TREATMENT AND MANAGEMENT OF HYPERAMMONEMIA

Treatment of acute hyperammonemia may involve hemodialysis or exchange transfusions to lower the ammonia level rapidly (Figure 25-7). Management usually involves decreased protein intake, avoiding infections, and stimulating alternative pathways for

FIGURE 25-7 ▶

Alternative Pathways of Nitrogen Excretion. Blood ammonia levels can be lowered by feeding benzoic acid or phenylacetate, which are activated by conversion to their coenzyme A derivatives and then conjugated with glycine and glutamine, respectively. The conjugates, hippuric acid and phenylacetylglutamine, are excreted in the urine. Both of these amino acids are in equilibrium with the free NH_4^+ pool in the body.

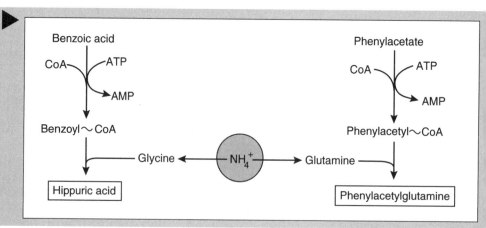

Inheritance Patterns for Urea Cycle Enzyme Deficiencies

The inheritance pattern for enzyme deficiencies in the urea cycle is autosomal recessive except for ornithine transcarbamoylase (OTC), which is an X-linked chromosomal trait. A deficiency in OTC is the most common deficiency in the urea cycle. Women who are carriers for OTC deficiency can be identified by giving a single dose of allopurinol, followed by the measurement of orotidine excretion in the urine [1]. Orotidine is an intermediate in the synthesis of pyrimidine nucleotides.

nitrogen excretion. Benzoic acid and phenylacetate activate latent pathways in the liver that conjugate glycine and glutamine with benzoic acid and phenylacetate, respectively. The products, hippuric acid and phenylacetylglutamine, are excreted in the urine. This treatment is based on the underlying principle that both glycine and glutamine are in equilibrium with the free ammonia pools in the body.

DISPOSAL OF CARBON SKELETONS

In amino acid catabolism, the carbon skeletons of all 20 common amino acids are degraded to seven products, which are intermediates in central pathways of metabolism (Table 25-3). Some of the amino acids are fragmented in such a way that they produce more than one of the seven products. The amino acids can be classified into two major classes, ketogenic and glucogenic, with a few being both ketogenic and glucogenic. The metabolic intermediates arising from the degradation of each of the common amino acids is shown in Figure 25-8.

TABLE 25-3 ▶
The Products of Amino Acid Catabolism

Products of Glucogenic Amino Acids	Products of Ketogenic Amino Acids
Pyruvate	Acetyl CoA
Oxaloacetate	Acetoacetyl CoA
Fumarate	
Succinyl CoA	
α-Ketoglutarate	

Ketogenic Amino Acids

Ketogenic amino acids are degraded to acetyl CoA or acetoacetyl CoA, and their carbon skeletons can either be oxidized to carbon dioxide and water or used for the synthesis of

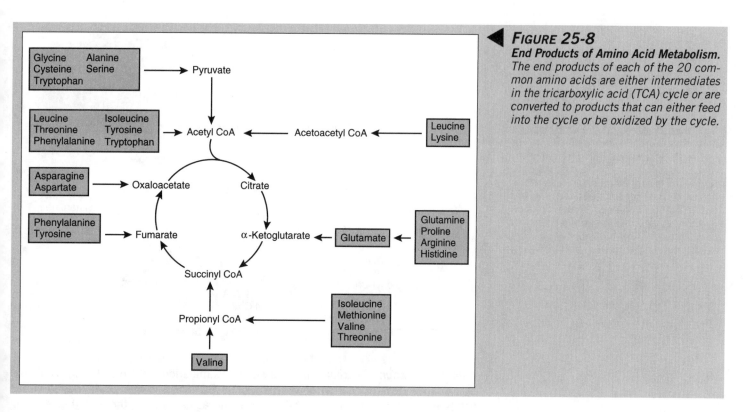

FIGURE 25-8
End Products of Amino Acid Metabolism.
The end products of each of the 20 common amino acids are either intermediates in the tricarboxylic acid (TCA) cycle or are converted to products that can either feed into the cycle or be oxidized by the cycle.

ketone bodies or fatty acids. In humans, only two of the amino acids are strictly ketogenic, lysine and leucine.

Ketogenic and Glucogenic Amino Acids

Four of the common amino acids are both ketogenic and glucogenic. Isoleucine and the three aromatic amino acids, phenylalanine, tyrosine, and tryptophan, give rise to products that can be used for both the synthesis of ketones and glucose. The glucogenic amino acids are degraded to intermediates in either glycolysis or the TCA cycle and can be used as a substrate for gluconeogenesis.

Glucogenic Amino Acids

The remaining 14 amino acids are strictly glucogenic and are degraded either to pyruvate, the end product of glycolysis, or to α-ketoglutarate, succinyl CoA, fumarate, or oxaloacetate, all intermediates in the TCA cycle.

BRANCHED-CHAIN AMINO ACID METABOLISM

Although the catabolism of most amino acids begins in the liver with either transamination or deamination, the catabolism of valine, isoleucine, and leucine begins in skeletal muscle where the concentration of BCAA transaminase is high. This enzyme is not expressed to a significant extent in the liver. Following a meal, these three amino acids make up more than half of the total amino acid pool in the blood that leaves the liver. Following transamination of the BCAAs in muscle tissue, alanine is the major carrier of amino groups from muscle to the liver, where they are incorporated into urea and excreted. The branched-chain keto acids (BCKAs) that result from transamination are oxidized as fuel by muscle, liver, kidney, and brain tissue.

Pathways for BCAA Degradation

The key features of the pathways by which valine, isoleucine, and leucine are degraded are shown in Figure 25-9.

FIGURE 25-9

Pathway for Branched-Chain Amino Acid (BCAA) Catabolism. *The first two reactions convert valine, isoleucine, and leucine to the corresponding branched-chain acyl CoA derivatives. A single transaminase and branched-chain keto acid (BCKA) dehydrogenase catalyze the first two reactions, respectively. The further degradation of the branched-chain acyl CoA derivatives involves separate enzymes for each product. Transamination occurs primarily in muscle, and the remaining reactions can occur in several tissues, including heart, muscle, liver, brain, and kidney.*

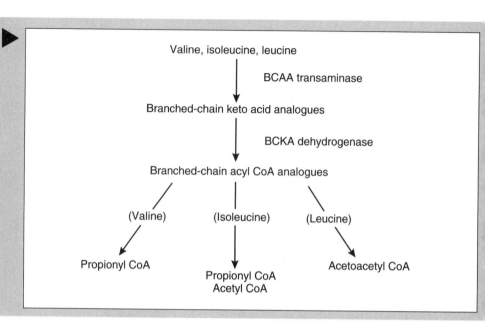

Common Reactions. Degradation starts with transamination of the BCAAs and is followed by oxidative decarboxylation of the respective BCKAs. A single *BCAA transaminase* catalyzes the transamination of all three amino acids, and all three of the resulting BCKAs are decarboxylated by the same *BCKA dehydrogenase*, resulting in the corresponding acyl CoA thioesters.

The BCKA dehydrogenase is similar in structure and mechanism to that of the pyruvate dehydrogenase complex and the α-ketoglutarate dehydrogenase complex. All are multienzyme complexes localized in the mitochondria, and all catalyze oxidative decarboxylation reactions, requiring five coenzymes (thiamine pyrophosphate, lipoic acid, CoA, NAD^+, and flavin adenine dinucleotide [FAD]).

End Products. The three acyl CoA thioesters resulting from the BCKA dehydrogenase reaction are further degraded in separate but parallel pathways (see Figure 25-9). The reactions involved are similar to those in the pathway of fatty acid oxidation. The end product of valine catabolism is propionyl CoA, while that of leucine is acetoacetyl CoA. Isoleucine is degraded to both propionyl CoA and acetyl CoA.

Regulation. The rate-limiting step in BCAA catabolism is catalyzed by the BCKA dehydrogenase complex. The enzyme is regulated allosterically by end-product inhibition. Both NADH and acyl CoA inhibit the enzyme. A specific protein kinase and a protein phosphatase are associated with the BCKA dehydrogenase complex and regulate its activity. Phosphorylation of BCKA dehydrogenase results in its inhibition. The BCKA dehydrogenase kinase is inhibited by the accumulation of BCKA.

Assimilation of Propionyl CoA into the TCA Cycle

The glucogenic nature of valine and isoleucine are attributed to the ability of propionyl CoA to be converted to succinyl CoA, an intermediate in the TCA cycle (Figure 25-10). Propionyl CoA is carboxylated to methylmalonyl CoA in a reaction that requires ATP as a substrate and biotin as a coenzyme. Methylmalonyl CoA subsequently undergoes a

Defects in Propionyl CoA and Methylmalonyl CoA Metabolism
The major source of propionyl CoA is from the degradation of valine, isoleucine, threonine, and methionine. Propionyl CoA is normally converted to succinyl CoA by reactions involving propionyl CoA carboxylase and methylmalonyl CoA mutase. Defects in either of these enzymes result in metabolic acidosis and the excretion of organic acids in the urine. Some cases of acidosis caused by high levels of methylmalonic acid respond to high doses of vitamin B_{12}.

itamin B$_{12}$–dependent rearrangement reaction, resulting in succinyl CoA. The latter reaction is catalyzed by methylmalonyl CoA mutase.

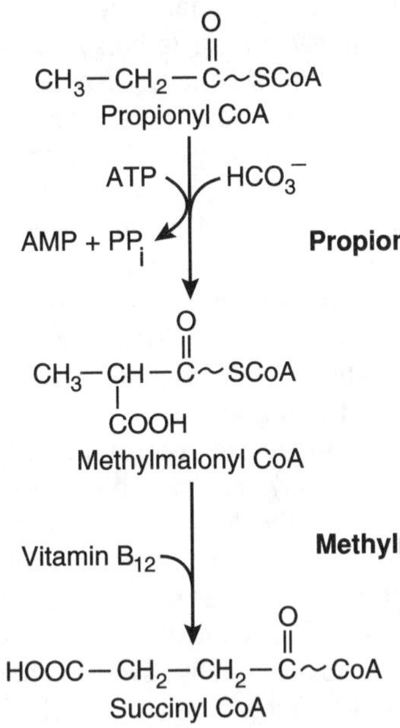

FIGURE 25-10
Conversion of Propionyl CoA to Succinyl CoA. The conversion of propionyl CoA to methylmalonyl CoA is catalyzed by propionyl CoA carboxylase, an enzyme requiring biotin. The structure of methylmalonyl CoA is rearranged by methylmalonyl CoA mutase in a reaction that is dependent on vitamin B$_{12}$. Both enzymes are mitochondrial enzymes.

Transfer of Amino Nitrogen from BCAAs to Urea

Most of the amino groups in the BCAAs are transported to the liver by alanine (Figure 25-11). The initial transamination reaction in muscle is catalyzed by BCAA transaminase and is followed by a second transamination catalyzed by alanine transaminase. Alanine is released by muscle and carried to the liver, where the amino group is transferred back to glutamate. Glutamate is used for the synthesis of aspartate and NH$_4^+$, both substrates for urea synthesis.

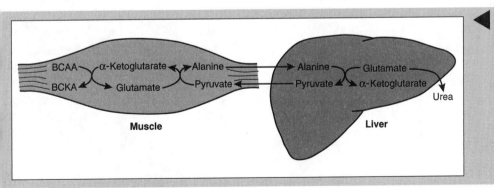

FIGURE 25-11
Flow of Nitrogen from Branched-Chain Amino Acids (BCAAs) to Urea. Alanine is the primary carrier of amino nitrogen from BCAAs in skeletal muscle to the liver, where it is incorporated into urea. Muscle contains both BCAA transaminase and alanine transaminase, whereas liver contains only alanine transaminase. BCKA = branched-chain keto acid.

Maple Syrup Urine Disease (MSUD)

A genetic defect in BCKA dehydrogenase is responsible for MSUD. The symptoms appear early in infancy, and death often occurs by 1 year of age. Symptoms include vomiting, lethargy, and severe brain damage. Autopsy shows brain edema, lack of myelin, and a reduction in the total lipids. Urine and plasma contain elevated levels of the BCAAs and the corresponding α-ketoacids and α-hydroxyacids. Diagnosis is confirmed by assaying for BCKA dehydrogenase in fibroblasts or leukocytes. As the name implies, the urine has a characteristic odor similar to that of burnt sugar.

Incidence of MSUD
MSUD, an autosomal recessive disorder, occurs in about 1 in 185,000 newborns throughout the world. The disease is particularly prevalent in the inbred Mennonite population of Lancaster county, Pennsylvania, where it occurs in about 1 in 175 newborns [2]. Screening of newborns is performed in about half of the states in the United States.

RESOLUTION OF CLINICAL CASE

The patient presented at the beginning of this chapter was suffering from an episode of hyperammonemia. In most cases of neonatal hyperammonemia, the infant appears normal for at least 2–5 days, when vomiting, lethargy, hypothermia, and hyperventilation begin to appear. Hyperammonemia is usually associated with elevated levels of glutamine and alanine. Both of these amino acids are nontoxic carriers of amino groups from extrahepatic tissues to the liver, where they can be incorporated into urea and excreted. The presence of orotic acid in the urine, together with undetectable levels of serum citrulline and decreased serum arginine, suggest a genetic deficiency in OTC. The presence of orotic acid in the urine is secondary to an accumulation of carbamoyl phosphate. Carbamoyl phosphate normally stays within the mitochondria, where it is made. However, when there is a deficiency in OTC, it accumulates and spills over into the cytosol, where it enters the pathway of pyrimidine biosynthesis, resulting in orotic acid. The patient was treated by restricting amino acids to those that are essential and by giving sodium benzoate to promote the excretion of hippuric acid, which is a conjugate of benzoic acid and glycine. Since glycine is in equilibrium with the NH_4^+ pool, the excretion of hippuric acid lowers the NH_4^+ concentration. Measurement of plasma glutamine levels is considered to be the best single indicator of effective therapy [1]. An increase in the NH_4^+ concentration increases the activity of glutamine synthetase. The gene for OTC is found on the X chromosome and is expressed only in the liver and small intestine. Women who are carriers are usually asymptomatic, although they often experience migraines, vomiting, and lethargy when they eat meat. In newborn males, OTC deficiency is manifested by hyperammonemic coma, which, if untreated, can lead to death or mental retardation. The child presented in this case suffered no mental retardation. Dietary amino acid restriction, together with sodium benzoate administration, have been effective in maintaining his NH_4^+ levels within the normal range.

REVIEW QUESTIONS

Directions: For each of the following questions, choose the **one best** answer.

1. Which of the following pairs of enzymes participate in the major route of nitrogen transfer from amino acids to urea?
    - **(A)** Glutaminase and asparaginase
    - **(B)** Transaminases and glutamate dehydrogenase
    - **(C)** Glutamate dehydrogenase and glutaminase
    - **(D)** Transaminases and glutaminase
    - **(E)** Amino acid oxidases and glutamate dehydrogenase

2. Which of the following amino acids is excreted when benzoic acid is used for the treatment of urea cycle disorders?
    - **(A)** Aspartate
    - **(B)** Arginine
    - **(C)** Ornithine
    - **(D)** Glycine
    - **(E)** Glutamine

3. Which of the following characteristics best describes the urea cycle?
    - **(A)** All of the enzymes are localized in the cytosol of hepatocytes
    - **(B)** The enzymes are present in high concentration in the perivenous hepatocytes
    - **(C)** Arginine is the end product of the urea cycle
    - **(D)** The cleavage of argininosuccinate releases fumarate
    - **(E)** Asparagine is a substrate in the urea cycle

4. Maple syrup urine disease (MSUD) is a genetic disorder in the catabolism of which of the following compounds?
    - **(A)** Aromatic amino acids
    - **(B)** Nonessential amino acids
    - **(C)** Branched-chain amino acids
    - **(D)** Urea
    - **(E)** Propionic acid

5. A deficiency in vitamin B_{12} will impair the catabolism of which of the following amino acids?
    - **(A)** Leucine
    - **(B)** Valine
    - **(C)** Phenylalanine
    - **(D)** Arginine
    - **(E)** Histidine

6. Which of the pairs of amino acids are the most ammoniagenic?

   (A) Histidine and glutamine

   (B) Aspartate and glycine

   (C) Glutamate and valine

   (D) Serine and alanine

   (E) Threonine and isoleucine

ANSWERS AND EXPLANATIONS

1. The answer is B. Many transaminases use α-ketoglutarate as an amino acceptor, resulting in glutamate. The NH_4^+ used in urea synthesis is released from glutamate by glutamate dehydrogenase.

2. The answer is D. Benzoic acid conjugates only with glycine, forming hippuric acid, which is excreted in the urine.

3. The answer is D. Argininosuccinate lyase catalyzes the cleavage of argininosuccinate to arginine and fumarate. The first two enzymes in the urea cycle are in the mitochondria, and all of the enzymes are enriched in the periportal hepatocytes. The end product of the cycle is urea. Aspartate, but not asparagine, is a direct substrate for urea synthesis.

4. The answer is C. A defect in branched-chain keto acid dehydrogenase results in MSUD. This enzyme is required for the catabolism of valine, isoleucine, and leucine, the three branched-chain amino acids.

5. The answer is B. Valine is degraded to propionyl CoA, which is assimilated into the TCA cycle by the sequential action of propionyl CoA carboxylase and methylmalonyl CoA mutase. The latter reaction requires vitamin B_{12} as a coenzyme.

6. The answer is A. Amino acids that are directly deaminated are more ammoniagenic than those that are transaminated. Both histidine and glutamine are deaminated. Each of the other possible answers contains one, but not two, amino acids that are directly deaminated. Glycine, serine, and threonine are all deaminated.

REFERENCES

1. Brusilow SW, Horwich AL: Urea cycle enzymes. In *Metabolic and Molecular Bases of Inherited Disease*, 7th ed. Edited by Scriver CR, Beaudet AL, Sly WS, et al. New York, NY: McGraw-Hill, 1995, pp 1187–1221.
2. Chuang DT, Shih VE: Disorders of branched chain amino acid and keto acid metabolism. In *Metabolic and Molecular Bases of Inherited Disease*, 7th ed. Edited by Scriver CR, Beaudet AL, Sly WS, et al. New York, NY: McGraw-Hill, 1995, pp 1239–1267.

26

ONE-CARBON METABOLISM AND THE SYNTHESIS OF NONESSENTIAL AMINO ACIDS

CHAPTER OUTLINE

INTRODUCTION OF CLINICAL CASE

A 14-month-old girl was brought to the hospital because her parents were concerned about her development. She had been well developed and healthy at birth, but she was still unable to walk and had only a few words in her vocabulary. By 1 year, she had become very hyperactive and often screamed, but no words were discernible. She had a musty body odor, and her skin was fair and soft except for isolated areas of dermatitis. An acidified urine sample turned a deep green color when ferric chloride was added. Her urinary levels of 5-hydroxyindoleacetic acid and vanillylmandelic acid were normal. Her fasting serum phenylalanine levels were markedly elevated (32 mg/dL). She was placed on a formula for 2 weeks that contained no phenylalanine, and during this time, both her urinary phenylketoacids and plasma phenylalanine levels decreased, but her weight also decreased. Low amounts of phenylalanine were added back to her formula, and over the next several weeks, she was maintained at a serum phenylalanine level of about 4 mg/dL [1]. Her hyperactivity decreased moderately, her attention span increased, and her dermatitis disappeared. She is currently 2 years old and has continued to grow on a diet that restricts phenylalanine intake.

CARRIERS OF SINGLE-CARBON FRAGMENTS IN METABOLISM

Many reactions in metabolism involve the transfer of a single-carbon atom from a donor to an acceptor. In these metabolic reactions, three compounds serve as carriers of the single-carbon (C_1) units: biotin, S-adenosylmethionine (SAM), and tetrahydrofolate (THF). The C_1 units can exist in four oxidation states (Table 26-1). Biotin transfers carboxyl groups; SAM transfers methyl groups; and THF transfers carbon atoms at all other oxidation states.

TABLE 26-1 ▶
Carriers of Single-Carbon Atoms in Metabolism

Carrier	Source of Carbon Atoms	Oxidation State of Carbon	Types of Reactions
Biotin	Carbon dioxide	—COOH (carboxyl group)	Carboxylation reactions
S-Adenosylmethionine (SAM)	Methionine	—CH$_3$ (methyl group)	Methylation reactions
Tetrahydrofolate (THF)	Tryptophan	—CHO (formyl)[a]	Purine ring synthesis
	Histidine	—CH= (methenyl)[a]	Purine ring synthesis
	Serine and glycine	—CH$_2$$^-$ (methylene)	Thymidine synthesis
	Reduction of —CH$_2$$^-$	—CH$_3$ (methyl)[b]	Homocysteine to methionine

[a] The carbon atoms in the formyl and methenyl groups are in the same oxidation state.
[b] THF participates in only one methylation reaction; all others involve SAM.

Biotin

Biotin, a vitamin widely distributed in nature, serves as a coenzyme for several carboxylases. Carbon dioxide is attached to biotin in a reaction that requires energy. The energy is supplied by the hydrolysis of adenosine triphosphate (ATP) to adenosine diphosphate (ADP) and inorganic phosphate (P_i). The bond between carbon dioxide and biotin is a high-energy bond that is used in subsequent reactions in which the carboxyl group is transferred from biotin to an acceptor.

$$CO_2 + \text{biotin} + ATP \xrightarrow{\text{biotin carboxylase}} \text{biotin}{\sim}CO_2 + ADP + P_i$$

$$\text{Biotin}{\sim}CO_2 + \text{acceptor} \xrightarrow{\text{carboxylases}} \text{acceptor-}CO_2 + \text{biotin}$$

In metabolism, there are three major carboxylases that use biotin: (1) pyruvate carboxylase, the first enzyme in gluconeogenesis, (2) acetyl coenzyme A (CoA) carboxylase, the first enzyme in fatty acid synthesis, and (3) propionyl CoA carboxylase, a key enzyme in the catabolism of branched-chain amino acids.

S-Adenosylmethionine (SAM)

The major carrier of methyl groups in metabolism is SAM, which is formed from methionine and ATP. The synthesis of SAM is shown in the following reaction, which is catalyzed by methionine adenosyltransferase. In this reaction, the sulfur atom of methionine becomes linked to the 5'-carbon of adenosine. Two of the phosphate groups of ATP are released as pyrophosphate (PP_i) and one as inorganic phosphate (P_i). The sulfonium bond between the sulfur atom and the methyl carbon of SAM is a high-energy bond that drives subsequent methylation reactions.

$$\text{Methionine + ATP} \xrightarrow{\text{methionine adenosyltransferase}}$$

$$\text{S-adenosylmethionine} + PP_i + P_i$$

Methylation Reactions. A typical methylation reaction that uses SAM as a methyl donor is shown in the following equation. The enzymes that catalyze these reactions are known as methyltransferases. The removal of the methyl group from SAM results in *S*-adenosylhomocysteine. Some common acceptors in methylation reactions involving SAM are shown in Table 26-2.

$$\text{Acceptor + S-adenosylmethionine} \xrightarrow{\text{methyltransferase}}$$

$$\text{acceptor-CH}_3 + \text{S-adenosylhomocysteine}$$

Structure of S-Adenosylmethionine

Acceptor	Product	Metabolic Pathway
Guanidoacetic acid	Creatine	Creatine synthesis
Phosphatidylethanolamine	Phosphatidylcholine	Phospholipid synthesis
Ribosomal and transfer RNA	Methylated RNA	RNA synthesis
Norepinephrine	Epinephrine	Catecholamine synthesis
Protein-bound lysine	Trimethyllysine	Carnitine synthesis

◄ **TABLE 26-2**
Selected Methylation Reactions Involving S-Adenosylmethionine

Fate of S-Adenosylhomocysteine. S-*adenosylhomocysteine*, a by-product of all SAM-dependent methylation reactions, is hydrolyzed to adenosine and homocysteine. Homocysteine is either converted to methionine or used in the synthesis of cysteine.

Tetrahydrofolate (THF)

The major carrier of single-carbon atoms in metabolism is THF. Folic acid, the vitamin precursor of THF, is reduced to the active cofactor form in a reaction requiring the reduced form of nicotinamide-adenine dinucleotide phosphate (NADPH).

Structure and Function of THF. THF consists of a pteridine ring structure, *p*-aminobenzoic acid (PABA) and one or more glutamate residues. The carbon atoms that are transferred by THF are bound to the N^5 and N^{10} atoms of the THF. Carbon atoms in different oxidation states are attached to THF differently. For example, formyl groups are attached to N^{10}, and methyl groups are attached to N^5, whereas methenyl and methylene groups form carbon bridges between the N^5 and N^{10} atoms of THF (Figure 26-1).

Donors, Acceptors, and Interconversion of THF Derivatives. The carbon atoms transferred by THF originate in four amino acids: tryptophan, histidine, glycine, and serine. Intermediates in the degradation of these amino acids donate carbon atoms to THF. Most of the carbon acceptors are intermediates in the synthesis of purines and pyrimidines (Figure 26-2). All of the THF derivatives except 5-methyl-THF are easily interconverted by reversible reactions.

Sulfa Drugs, Folic Acid, and Bacterial Growth
All organisms require folic acid for growth and reproduction. Bacteria are able to synthesize folic acid from a pterin precursor and PABA, whereas humans must obtain folic acid from dietary sources. The basis for using sulfonamides as antibiotics resides in their ability to inhibit bacterial growth without affecting the growth of mammalian cells. They are structural analogs of PABA and act as competitive inhibitors of enzymes involved in the synthesis of folic acid.

Formiminoglutamate (FIGLU) and Folate Deficiency
FIGLU is an intermediate in histidine degradation that donates a carbon atom to THF, resulting in 5-formimino-THF, which can be converted to methenyl-THF. A deficiency in folate prevents this reaction from occurring and results in the excretion of FIGLU in the urine.

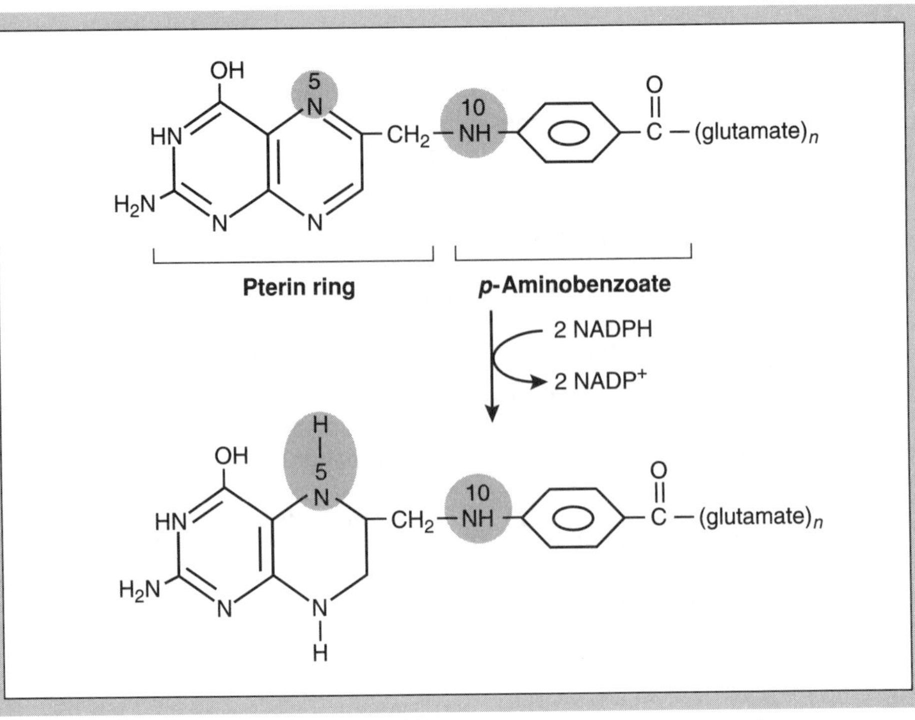

FIGURE 26-1 ▶

Structure and Formation of Tetrahydrofolate (THF). *Folic acid (upper structure) contains a pterin ring, p-aminobenzoic acid, and one or more molecules of glutamate. The coenzyme THF (lower structure) is generated by the reduction of folic acid.*

FIGURE 26-2 ▶

Role of Tetrahydrofolate (THF) as a Carrier of Carbon Atoms. *Carbon atoms are donated to THF in various states of oxidation, with the most oxidized form being a formyl group and the most reduced form a methyl group. The donors are intermediates in the degradation of the amino acids listed on the left, and the major acceptors of the carbon atoms are listed on the right.*

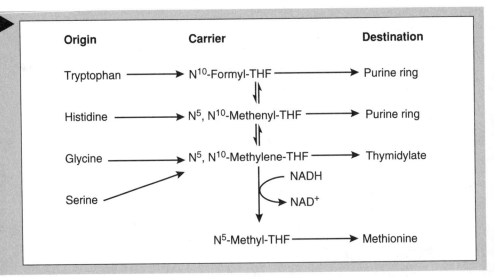

STRATEGIES USED TO SYNTHESIZE NONESSENTIAL AMINO ACIDS

The nonessential amino acids are considered nonessential only in the nutritional context. From a biologic perspective, these amino acids are necessary for protein synthesis and, therefore, are as important as the essential amino acids. Most of the nonessential amino acids are synthesized from intermediates in glycolysis or the tricarboxylic acid (TCA) cycle (Figure 26-3). Transamination and amidation reactions are important in these pathways. However, two of the nonessential amino acids, cysteine and tyrosine, are synthesized from the essential amino acids methionine and phenylalanine.

Transamination of α-Keto Acids

Pyruvate, the end product of glycolysis, together with oxaloacetate and α-ketoglutarate, intermediates in the TCA cycle, are the precursors for several of the nonessential amino acids.

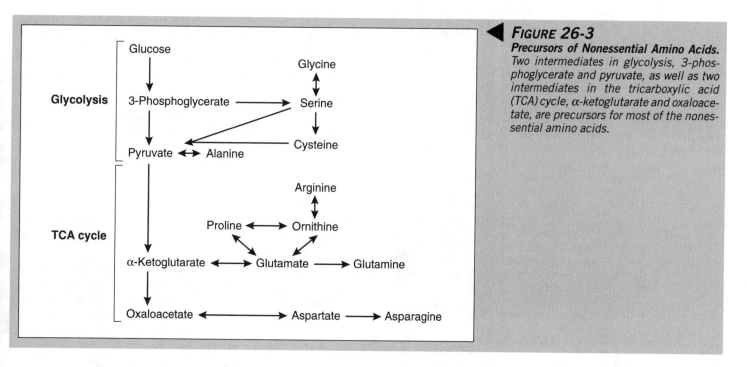

FIGURE 26-3
Precursors of Nonessential Amino Acids.
Two intermediates in glycolysis, 3-phosphoglycerate and pyruvate, as well as two intermediates in the tricarboxylic acid (TCA) cycle, α-ketoglutarate and oxaloacetate, are precursors for most of the nonessential amino acids.

Alanine, Aspartate, and Glutamate. Transamination of pyruvate, oxaloacetate, and α-ketoglutarate, results in the synthesis of alanine, aspartate, and glutamate, respectively. Transamination reactions are readily reversible, and they are used in both the synthesis and degradation of amino acids.

$$\text{Pyruvate + glutamate} \overset{\textbf{alanine transaminase}}{\rightleftharpoons} \text{alanine} + \alpha\text{-ketoglutarate}$$

$$\text{Oxaloacetate + glutamate} \overset{\textbf{aspartate transaminase}}{\rightleftharpoons} \text{aspartate} + \alpha\text{-ketoglutarate}$$

The synthesis of glutamate can occur either by reversing the reactions shown above or by reversing the reaction catalyzed by glutamate dehydrogenase shown below. When the glutamate dehydrogenase reaction is used for glutamate synthesis, it is a reductive amination reaction, and when it occurs in the opposite direction, it is an oxidative deamination reaction that generates ammonium ions (NH_4^+) for use in urea synthesis (see Chapter 25).

$$\alpha\text{-Ketoglutarate} + NH_4^+ + \text{NADH} \overset{\textbf{glutamate dehydrogenase}}{\rightleftharpoons}$$
$$\text{glutamate} + NAD^+ + H^+$$

Nonessential Amino Acids Derived from Glutamate. Glutamate is the precursor for several other nonessential amino acids, including proline, arginine, glutamine, and ornithine (see Figure 26-3). The reactions that interconvert these amino acids are reversible and participate both in synthesis and degradation.

Amidation of Glutamate and Aspartate

The addition of an amide group to the side chain of glutamate and aspartate results in the synthesis of glutamine and asparagine, respectively.

Glutamine Synthesis. The substrates for glutamine synthesis are ammonia and glutamate, and the reaction is catalyzed by glutamine synthetase. The energy required to form the amide bond is supplied by the hydrolysis of ATP.

$$\text{Glutamate} + NH_4^+ + \text{ATP} \overset{\textbf{glutamine synthetase}}{\longrightarrow} \text{glutamine} + \text{ADP} + P_i$$

Asparagine Synthesis. Asparagine is synthesized in humans by the transfer of an amide group from the side chain of glutamine to the side chain of aspartate. The energy for asparagine synthesis is provided by the hydrolysis of ATP to adenosine monophosphate (AMP) and PP$_i$. In bacteria, the synthesis of asparagine is analogous to that of glutamine, with the amide group originating in ammonia.

$$\text{Aspartate + glutamine + ATP} \xrightarrow{\text{asparagine synthetase}}$$

$$\text{asparagine + glutamate + AMP + PP}_i$$

Synthesis of Serine and Glycine

Both serine and glycine are synthesized from 3-phosphoglycerate (3-PG), an intermediate in glycolysis. Following the synthesis of serine, the transfer of a carbon atom from methylene-THF results in the production of glycine.

Serine Synthesis. The conversion of 3-PG to serine requires three reactions, which are shown below. The reactions involve the oxidation of 3-PG to 3-phosphopyruvate by nicotinamide adenine nucleotide (NAD$^+$), which is followed by transamination to give 3-phosphoserine. The hydrolysis of the phosphate ester results in serine.

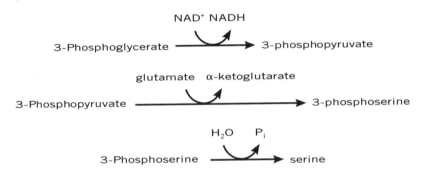

Glycine Synthesis. Glycine is formed from serine by the removal of the hydroxymethyl group from the side chain. The methylene carbon group is transferred to THF, and the hydroxyl group is released as water. This reaction is reversible, allowing glycine and serine to be interconverted.

$$\text{Serine + THF} \underset{}{\overset{\text{serine hydroxymethyltransferase}}{\rightleftarrows}}$$

$$\text{glycine + 5,10-methylene-THF + H}_2\text{O}$$

CYSTEINE SYNTHESIS

Relationships among Methionine, Homocysteine, and Cysteine

Methionine

$$\text{H}_3\text{C}-\text{S}-\text{CH}_2-\text{CH}_2-\overset{\overset{\text{NH}_2}{|}}{\text{CH}}-\text{COOH}$$

Homocysteine

$$\text{HS}-\text{CH}_2-\text{CH}_2-\overset{\overset{\text{NH}_2}{|}}{\text{CH}}-\text{COOH}$$

Cysteine

$$\text{HS}-\text{CH}_2-\overset{\overset{\text{NH}_2}{|}}{\text{CH}}-\text{COOH}$$

The two sulfur-containing amino acids are methionine and cysteine. Methionine, an essential amino acid, is the source of sulfur for cysteine synthesis, and the remainder of the cysteine molecule is derived from serine. Therefore, cysteine is a nonessential amino acid only if the diet contains an adequate supply of methionine.

Conversion of Methionine to Homocysteine

The synthesis of cysteine requires methionine and serine as substrates, and it involves homocysteine as a key intermediate. The metabolic relationship between methionine, homocysteine, and cysteine is shown in Figure 26-4.

Methionine is first converted to SAM, which is used only in methylation reactions. A by-product of these reactions is S-adenosylhomocysteine, which is hydrolyzed to adenosine and homocysteine. Homocysteine can either be used for the synthesis of cysteine, or it can be converted back to methionine.

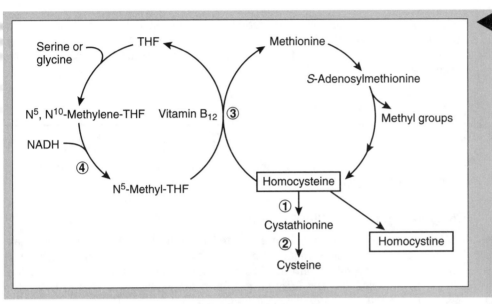

FIGURE 26-4
Formation and Fate of Homocysteine.
Homocysteine is formed from methionine in a two-step reaction that results in the removal of the methyl group from the side chain of methionine. Cystathionine is formed by the condensation of serine and homocysteine and is cleaved, releasing cysteine. Enzymes that catalyze the numbered reactions are: (1) cystathionine synthase; (2) cystathionase; (3) homocysteine-tetrahydrofolate methyltransferase (also known as methionine synthetase); and (4) 5,10-methylene-tetrahydrofolate reductase. A deficiency in enzymes 1, 3, or 4 results in the accumulation of homocysteine and homocystine. A deficiency in enzyme 2 results in cystathioninuria. THF = tetrahydrofolate.

Conversion of Homocysteine to Cysteine

The conversion of homocysteine to cysteine is accomplished by two consecutive reactions (see Figure 26-4). In the first reaction, homocysteine is condensed with serine, producing cystathionine. This reaction is catalyzed by *cystathionine synthase*. In the second reaction, cystathionine is cleaved by *cystathionase*, resulting in cysteine, α-ketobutyrate, and NH_4^+. The sulfhydryl group of cysteine is derived from homocysteine, and the remainder of the structure comes from serine. Both cystathionine synthase and cystathionase require pyridoxal phosphate as a coenzyme.

Recycling Homocysteine to Methionine

When adequate cysteine is available, excess homocysteine can be recycled to methionine in a reaction that is catalyzed by homocysteine-THF methyltransferase. This enzyme requires two cofactors, methylcobalamin, a derivative of vitamin B_{12}, and 5-methyl-THF (CH_3-THF). Methylcobalamin serves as the methylating agent for homocysteine, and CH_3-THF is used to convert cobalamin back to methylcobalamin, as shown in the following reactions.

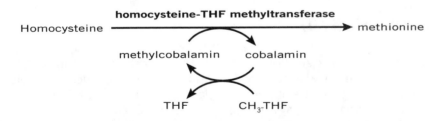

Abnormalities in Homocysteine Metabolism

Two conditions resulting from inherited defects in the pathway of homocysteine metabolism have been reported, homocystinuria and cystathioninuria.

Homocystinuria. Homocystine is the oxidized form of homocysteine, and it consists of two molecules of homocysteine linked together by a disulfide bond. A defect in *cystathionine synthase* leads to the accumulation of homocysteine and methionine in the blood and the excretion of homocystine in the urine. This disorder includes skeletal abnormalities, thrombosis, mental retardation, and dislocation of the lens. Homocystinuria is inherited as an autosomal recessive trait. Some forms of homocystinuria respond to vitamin B_6 administration.

Folate, Vitamin B_{12}, and Megaloblastic Anemia

Megaloblastic anemia results from abnormalities in DNA synthesis or in the synthesis of purine and pyrimidine metabolism, a branch of metabolism that is dependent on tetrahydrofolate as a carbon carrier. Some forms of megaloblastic anemia are responsive to vitamin B_{12}. In the absence of vitamin B_{12}, tetrahydrofolate gets trapped as methyl-THF and cannot be converted back to the other oxidation states of carbon atoms that are required for purine and pyrimidine nucleotide synthesis. A deficiency in vitamin B_{12} also results in the accumulation of methylmalonic acid in the blood and urine, a finding that is helpful in pinpointing the molecular basis of megaloblastic anemia.

Relationship Between Homocysteine and Homocystine

Homocysteine

$$HS-CH_2-CH_2-\underset{\underset{NH_2}{|}}{C}H-COOH$$

Homocystine

$$S-CH_2-CH_2-\underset{\underset{NH_2}{|}}{C}H-COOH$$
$$S-CH_2-CH_2-\underset{\underset{NH_2}{|}}{C}H-COOH$$

Cystathioninuria. A deficiency in *cystathionase* results in the accumulation of cystathionine and its excretion in the urine. Cystathioninuria is inherited as an autosomal recessive trait, although no specific clinical symptoms appear to be associated with this enzyme deficiency.

TYROSINE SYNTHESIS

Phenylalanine, an essential amino acid, is the precursor of tyrosine. Tyrosine synthesis occurs primarily in the liver and is catalyzed by phenylalanine hydroxylase.

Phenylalanine Hydroxylase Complex

Tetrahydrobiopterin (THB)
THB is a coenzyme that is used in the hydroxylation of the aromatic amino acids and the synthesis of nitric oxide. It is synthesized from guanosine triphosphate.

Tyrosine is formed by the addition of a hydroxyl group to the phenylalanine side chain (Figure 26-5). This reaction requires molecular oxygen; two enzymes, phenylalanine hydroxylase and dihydrobiopterin (DHB) reductase; and two cofactors, tetrahydrobiopterin (THB) and NADPH. The reaction results in the oxidation of THB to DHB. The regeneration of THB is catalyzed by DHB reductase and requires NADPH.

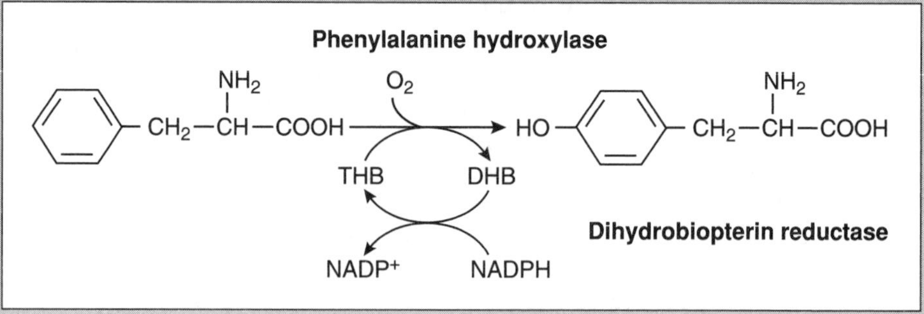

FIGURE 26-5
Conversion of Phenylalanine to Tyrosine. The hydroxylation of phenylalanine involves the reduction of molecular oxygen by tetrahydrobiopterin (THB) to hydroxyl groups. One hydroxyl group is incorporated into the ring of tyrosine, and the other appears in water. The catalytic cycle is completed by the reduction of dihydrobiopterin (DHB) back to tetrahydrofolate.

The formation of tyrosine is an irreversible reaction that is catalyzed by a multi-enzyme complex consisting of phenylalanine hydroxylase and DHB reductase. Although phenylalanine hydroxylase is found only in the liver, DHB reductase is also found in the brain and adrenal medulla, where it is involved in the synthesis of serotonin and the catecholamines (see Chapter 27).

Phenylketonuria (PKU)

A deficiency in phenylalanine hydroxylase, DHB reductase, or THB results in the accumulation of phenylalanine and leads to PKU. In PKU, phenylalanine is metabolized by pathways that are normally latent in the liver, resulting in the production of phenylpyruvate, phenyllactate, phenylacetate, and phenylacetylglutamine (Figure 26-6).

In PKU, the levels of phenylalanine in both blood and urine may be increased as much as 30-fold. Phenylpyruvate is normally not detected in either the plasma or the urine, but in PKU, the levels in blood are between 0.3 and 1.8 mg/dL, and the levels in urine are between 300 and 2000 mg/dL. Phenyllactate, phenylacetate, and phenylacetylglutamine are also excreted in the urine. Severe mental retardation occurs unless phenylalanine is restricted in the diet. It cannot be eliminated, however, because it is an essential amino acid. The dietary goal is to maintain blood phenylalanine levels between 2 and 6 mg/dL.

Nutrasweet
Nutrasweet, also known as aspartame, is a dipeptide that is widely used as a synthetic sweetener. It contains aspartic acid and phenylalanine methyl ester. The use of Nutrasweet by pregnant women who are either homozygous or heterozygous for PKU may cause brain damage to the fetus.

Classic PKU. An inherited deficiency in phenylalanine hydroxylase is known as classic PKU. The incidence of PKU is about 1 in 10,000 live births. Diagnosis can be made within a few days after birth by measuring the level of phenylalanine in the blood. Screening newborns for PKU is mandated by law. Treatment involves a diet that is low in phenylalanine.

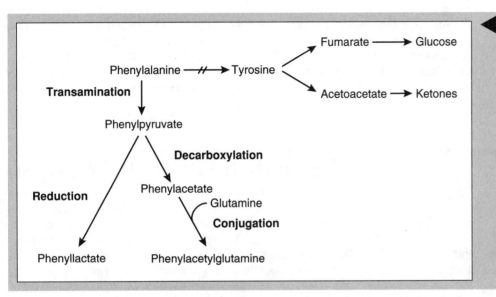

FIGURE 26-6
Pathways of Phenylalanine Excretion in Phenylketonuria (PKU). *The end products of phenylalanine and tyrosine normally are fumarate and acetoacetate. In PKU, a defect in the conversion of phenylalanine to tyrosine leads to the accumulation of phenylalanine, which is transaminated to phenylpyruvate. Phenylpyruvate can be reduced to phenyllactate, decarboxylated to phenylacetate, and conjugated with glutamine to give phenylacetylglutamine.*

Atypical PKU. An inherited defect in DHB reductase or a deficiency in THB results in a form of PKU known as atypical PKU. About 2% of the infants born with PKU have atypical PKU. Treatment of this form of PKU requires both the restriction of dietary phenylalanine and supplementation with dopamine and 5-hydroxytryptophan. These supplements provide the intermediates in catecholamine and serotonin synthesis, which is impaired in PKU patients with a defect in DHB reductase.

Maternal PKU. Maternal PKU occurs in unborn children of phenylketonuric mothers whose diets are not restricted in phenylalanine. During pregnancy, the dietary goal is to maintain the mother's blood phenylalanine level between 2 and 4 mg/dL. Phenylketones produced in the mother readily cross the placenta, resulting in brain damage in the unborn child.

INTERORGAN SYNTHESIS OF ARGININE

The synthesis of arginine requires two reactions that occur in the small intestine and two that occur in the kidney. The enzymes involved are normally considered participants in the urea cycle. Although the liver is the only organ that can synthesize urea (see Chapter 25), the enzymes that catalyze the first two reactions in urea synthesis are expressed in intestinal cells, resulting in the accumulation of citrulline.

$$NH_4^+ + HCO_3^- + 2\ ATP \xrightarrow{\textbf{carbamyol phosphate synthetase-1}}$$

$$\text{carbamyol phosphate} + 2\ ADP + P_i$$

$$\text{Carbamyol phosphate} + \text{ornithine} \xrightarrow{\textbf{ornithine transcarbamoylase}} \text{citrulline} + P_i$$

Citrulline is released by intestinal cells and taken up by the kidney, where it is converted to arginine by the two reactions shown below. Argininosuccinate synthetase and argininosuccinate lyase, enzymes that are a part of the urea cycle in the liver, are also expressed in the kidney, where arginine accumulates as the end product.

$$\text{Citrulline} + \text{aspartate} + ATP \xrightarrow{\textbf{argininosuccinate synthetase}}$$

$$\text{argininosuccinate} + AMP + PP_i$$

$$\text{Argininosuccinate} \xrightarrow{\textbf{argininosuccinate lyase}} \text{arginine} + \text{fumarate}$$

Arginase, the urea cycle enzyme that cleaves arginine to urea and ornithine, is found in very low concentrations in the kidney, whereas in the liver, it is present in extremely high concentrations. Thus, essentially all of the arginine produced in the urea cycle is immediately cleaved, releasing urea, whereas arginine that is formed in the kidney accumulates and can be released into the blood for use by various tissues for protein synthesis.

RESOLUTION OF CLINICAL CASE

The patient introduced at the beginning of this chapter has phenylketonuria. The green color observed when ferric chloride was added to the urine sample indicates the presence of urinary phenylpyruvate. The diagnosis of PKU was based on the quantitative measurement of plasma phenylalanine (32 mg/dL). A concentration of over 20 mg/dL is considered positive for PKU. The urinary levels of 5-hydroxyindoleacetic acid and vanillylmandelic acid were normal. These compounds are degradation products of catecholamine and serotonin. Since the synthesis of catecholamine and serotonin require tetrahydrobiopterin and dihydrobiopterin reductase, the results suggest that the cause of PKU in this child is a phenylalanine hydroxylase deficiency, rather than a tetrahydrobiopterin or dihydrobiopterin reductase deficiency.

PKU is the most common disease resulting from an enzyme deficiency in amino acid metabolism. If untreated, symptoms of mental retardation are seen usually within the first year. Tyrosine becomes an essential amino acid in PKU and must be provided in the diet. The low IQ and neurologic symptoms seen in this patient can be attributed to the toxic effects of phenylalanine [2]. It has been suggested that high concentrations of phenylalanine may inhibit the transport of other amino acids into the brain. Fair skin is often seen in PKU and results from a deficiency in tyrosine. The characteristic musty body odor is the result of the presence of phenylacetate. The conventional treatment of PKU is to restrict protein in the diet until the age of puberty, when most of the brain development is believed to be complete. The goal of treatment is usually to maintain plasma phenylalanine levels between 2 and 6 mg/dL. Women with PKU who live to childbearing age must resume a phenylalanine-restricted diet during pregnancy to avoid damage to the fetus in utero.

REVIEW QUESTIONS

Directions: For each of the following questions, choose the **one best** answer.

1. Which of the following combinations of substrates and cofactors is required for recycling methionine in humans?
    (A) Thiamine, vitamin B_{12}, and homocysteine
    (B) Vitamin B_{12}, biotin, and S-adenosylmethionine
    (C) Cysteine, pyridoxine, and 5,10-methylene-tetrahydrofolate (THF)
    (D) Homocysteine, vitamin B_{12}, and 5-methyl-THF
    (E) Homoserine, 5-methyl-THF, and vitamin B_{12}

2. Which of the following organs contribute arginine to the amino acid pool?
    (A) Skeletal muscle and intestine
    (B) Small intestine and kidney
    (C) Liver and kidney
    (D) Skeletal muscle and liver
    (E) Kidney and skeletal muscle

3. Which of the following pairs of compounds participates in the transfer of methyl groups?
    (A) Biotin and tetrahydrofolate (THF)
    (B) Methylcobalamin and formyl-THF
    (C) 5-Methyl-THF and S-adenosylmethionine (SAM)
    (D) SAM and folic acid
    (E) Tetrahydrobiopterin and methylcobalamin

4. Which of the following statements about phenylketonuria (PKU) is correct?
    (A) The diagnosis relies on the presence of tyrosine in the blood
    (B) Following puberty, a normal diet with no restrictions can be followed throughout life
    (C) Newborn screening must occur before the infant has ingested protein
    (D) Elevated levels of phenylalanine are found in the blood, and high levels of phenylpyruvate are found in the urine
    (E) Treatment involves a diet that is void of protein

5. Which of the following nonessential amino acids are synthesized from essential amino acids?
    (A) Glutamate and proline
    (B) Phenylalanine and cysteine
    (C) Glycine and asparagine
    (D) Tyrosine and cysteine
    (E) Methionine and alanine

ANSWERS AND EXPLANATIONS

1. The answer is D. Homocysteine is converted to methionine in a reaction that requires both methylcobalamin (a derivative of vitamin B_{12}) and 5-methyl-THF as cofactors. Methylcobalamin methylates homocysteine, and 5-methyl-THF is used to regenerate methylcobalamin. The conversion of homocysteine to cysteine requires pyridoxine. Thiamine and homoserine are not involved in methionine and homocysteine metabolism.

2. The answer is B. The first two reactions in urea synthesis occur in the small intestine and are catalyzed by carbamyol phosphate synthetase-1 and ornithine transcarbamoylase. The product of these two reactions is citrulline, which is released into the blood. Citrulline is extracted by the kidney and converted to arginine by the action of argininosuccinate synthetase and argininosuccinate lyase. Although all of these enzymes are found in the liver as part of the urea cycle, arginine does not accumulate in the liver because the high concentration of arginase converts it to urea and ornithine.

3. The answer is C. SAM is the primary donor of methyl groups in biochemical reactions. The only reaction in human biochemistry known to use methylcobalamin and 5-methyl-THF is the reaction that recycles homocysteine to methionine. Biotin transfers only carboxyl groups, and formyl-THF transfers only carbon atoms that are oxidized to aldehydes. Tetrahydrobiopterin is involved in the hydroxylation of aromatic amino acids, but it has no role in carbon transfer reactions.

4. The answer is D. Phenylalanine and phenylpyruvate are elevated in blood and urine, respectively, in patients with PKU. Treatment involves a diet that is low in protein but not void of protein. Some protein is required since phenylalanine is an essential amino acid. Although the dietary restriction may be lifted at puberty, it should be reinstated during pregnancy to avoid brain damage to the fetus that results from phenylketones produced by the mother. Newborn screening for PKU is mandated by law. Diagnosis is based on elevated levels of phenylalanine and decreased levels of tyrosine in the blood. However, within the first 24 hours, a false negative value of blood phenylalanine may be obtained because the mother clears increased phenylalanine prior to birth. Therefore, diagnosis is performed within 2–3 days after the infant has first received protein in either breast milk or formula.

5. The answer is D. Tyrosine and cysteine are synthesized from two essential amino acids, phenylalanine and methionine, respectively. Glutamate, proline, glycine, asparagine, and alanine are nonessential amino acids that are synthesized from intermediates in glycolysis or the tricarboxylic acid cycle.

REFERENCES

1. Armstrong MD, Tyler FH: Dietary treatment of phenylketonuria. *J Clin Invest* 34:565–580, 1955.
2. Scriver CR, Kaufman S, Eisensmith RC, et al: The hyperphenylalaninemias. In *The Metabolic and Molecular Bases of Inherited Disease*, 7th ed. Edited by Scriver CR, Beaudet AL, Sly WS, et al. New York, NY: McGraw-Hill, 1995, pp 1015–1075.

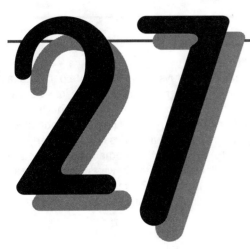

SPECIALIZED PRODUCTS DERIVED FROM AMINO ACIDS

INTRODUCTION OF CLINICAL CASE

A 3-year-old boy was admitted to the hospital because of weight loss, vomiting, constipation, irritability, and abdominal pain. A physical examination revealed no abnormalities. The patient had been showing signs of weakness and gradual weight loss for several months. The vomiting and abdominal pain, however, had started 3 weeks ago, just before the family moved from London to the United States. Examination of a blood smear showed numerous reticulocytes. His red blood cell (RBC) count was $3.6 \times 10^6/mm^3$ (normal: $4.5-6.2 \times 10^6/mm^3$), and his hemoglobin level was 8.5 g/dL (normal: 14–18 g/dL). An analysis of a 24-hour urine specimen showed elevated levels of coproporphyrin and Δ-aminolevulinic acid (Δ-ALA). The level of coproporphyrin was elevated 10-fold, and Δ-ALA was elevated 400-fold over normal levels. X-rays revealed opaque particles in the intestinal tract and bands of increased density in the growing areas of the long bones. When questioned, the patient's mother said that her son had a habit of chewing on furniture, toys, doors, and window sills. The family was currently living in a condemned house that had not been painted for many years. Analysis of a blood sample showed lead to be present in a concentration of 0.71 µmol/dL. Calcium ethylenediaminetetraacetate (CaEDTA) was administered intravenously, and a day after treatment was started, the lead in a 24-hour urine specimen increased from 0.5 µmol to 28 µmol [1]. The patient's condition began to improve, and he was dismissed from the hospital a week after being admitted.

AMINO ACIDS: PRECURSORS OF NEUROTRANSMITTERS AND HORMONES

Several neurotransmitters and hormones are biogenic amines, which are derived from amino acids by a few simple modifications. The aromatic amino acids, tyrosine and tryptophan, are important precursors. Catecholamines and the thyroid hormones are derived from tyrosine, whereas serotonin and melatonin are derived from tryptophan. The neurotransmitters and hormones derived from these amino acids are tissue specific, with the product of a particular type of cell being determined by the complement of enzymes found in that cell (Figure 27-1). Other amino acids that are precursors of biogenic amines include glutamate and histidine. In most cases, the conversion of amino acids to biogenic amines involves three types of reactions: decarboxylation, hydroxylation, and S-adenosylmethionine (SAM)–dependent methylation.

FIGURE 27-1

Products Derived from Tyrosine and Tryptophan. The products derived from tyrosine are shown in the upper portion of the figure, and those derived from tryptophan in the lower portion. Most of the excess tyrosine and tryptophan is catabolized by the liver, giving rise to products that can be used either for gluconeogenesis or ketogenesis. An intermediate in tryptophan can be converted to nicotinamide, a precursor of nicotinamide adenine dinucleotide (NAD+). The products of extrahepatic tyrosine and tryptophan metabolism are tissue or cell specific.

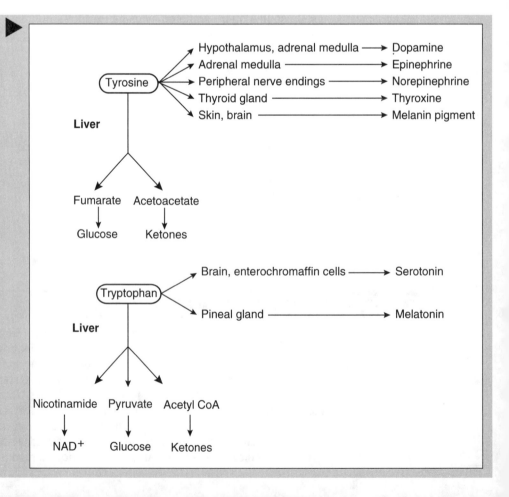

Catecholamines

The major catecholamines are dopamine, norepinephrine, and epinephrine. These compounds are derived from tyrosine and are synthesized by chromaffin cells in the central nervous system (CNS) and the adrenal medulla.

Synthesis of Catecholamines. The pathway for synthesis is identical in both the CNS and the adrenal medulla Figure 27-2. The initial reaction in the pathway is the hydroxylation of tyrosine, which is followed by sequential decarboxylation, hydroxylation, and methylation reactions. *Tyrosine hydroxylase* catalyzes the first reaction in the pathway, resulting in 3,4-dihydroxyphenylalanine (dopa). This reaction requires oxygen and tetrahydrobiopterin (THB) as substrates. Dihydrobiopterin reductase and reduced nicotinamide adenine dinucleotide phosphate (NADPH) are required to maintain THB in the reduced state. Decarboxylation of dopa results in dopamine. *Dopa decarboxylase* requires pyridoxal phosphate as a cofactor. This enzyme, also known as aromatic amino acid decarboxylase, has a broad specificity and catalyzes the decarboxylation of several aromatic amino acid derivatives.

In some cells of the CNS, synthesis stops with dopamine. In other cells, dopamine is further hydroxylated by *dopamine-β-hydroxylase*, resulting in norepinephrine. This enzyme is found in secretory granules that store norepinephrine and epinephrine. It requires oxygen, ascorbic acid, and copper for activity. Most of the norepinephrine present in organs is synthesized by sympathetic nerves that innervate the organs.

In the adrenal medulla, norepinephrine is converted to epinephrine in a methylation reaction that is catalyzed by *phenylethanolamine*-N-*methyltransferase* (PNMT). Epinephrine is the major catecholamine synthesized by the adrenal medulla. It is not synthesized by extramedullary tissues.

Regulation of Catecholamine Synthesis. The rate-limiting step in catecholamine synthesis is catalyzed by tyrosine hydroxylase. This enzyme is found only in tissues that synthesize catecholamines and is subject to feedback inhibition by both dopamine and

Chromaffin Cells
The cells that synthesize catecholamines are referred to as chromaffin cells because they contain granules that turn a red-brown color when exposed to potassium dichromate. Catecholamines that are stored in the granules have a high affinity for dichromate.

L-Dopa and Treatment of Parkinson's Disease
Parkinson's disease is caused by an inadequate supply of dopamine in the brain. Replacement therapy with dopamine is ineffective because dopamine does not cross the blood–brain barrier. Treatment with L-dopa, however, is effective because it enters the brain where it is decarboxylated to dopamine.

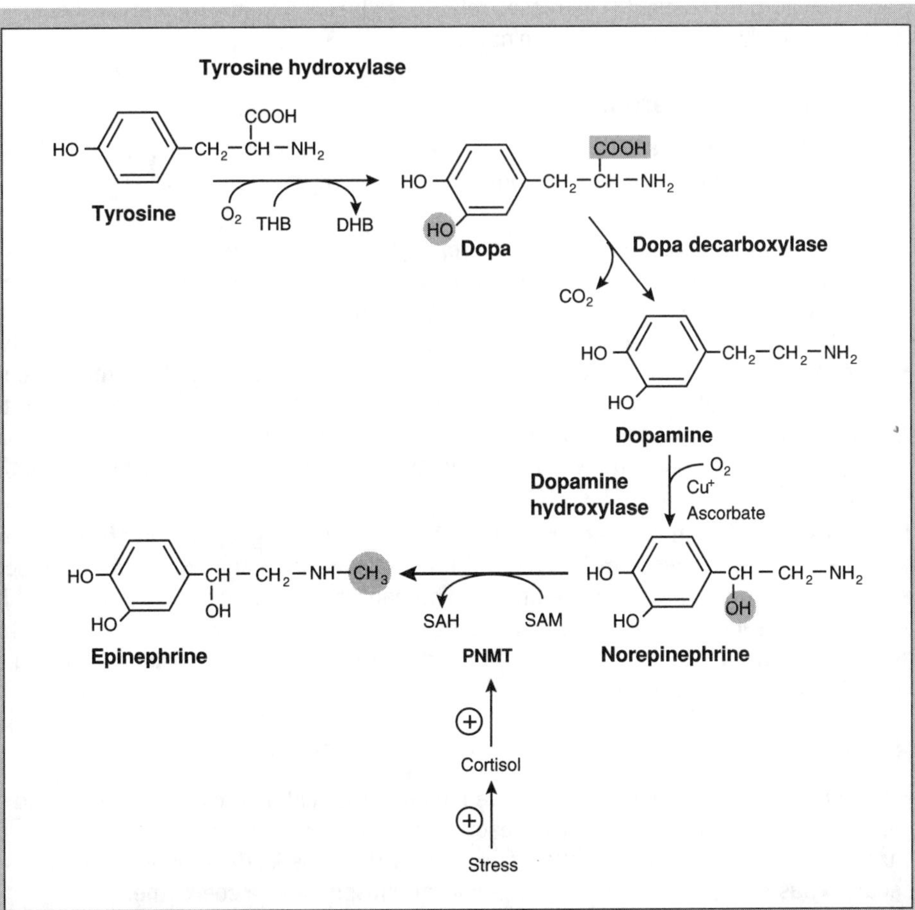

◀ **FIGURE 27-2**
Synthesis of Catecholamines. *Phenylethanolamine-N-methyltransferase (PNMT) is present only in the adrenal medulla. The synthesis of PNMT is induced by cortisol, which is made in the adjacent cortical tissue of the adrenal gland. Cortisol is released from the adrenal cortex in response to stress. Dopa = dihydroxyphenylalanine; THB = tetrahydrobiopterin; DHB = dihydrobiopterin; SAM = S-adenosylmethionine; SAH = S-adenosylhomocysteine; Cu⁺ = copper ion.*

norepinephrine. Tyrosine hydroxylase is activated by cyclic adenosine monophosphate (cAMP)–dependent phosphorylation. In the adrenal medulla, the synthesis of PNMT is induced by cortisol in response to stress.

Catecholamine Release. The release of catecholamine from the adrenal medulla is stimulated by the binding of acetylcholine (ACh) to nicotinic receptors on the surface of the cells. ACh stimulates calcium (Ca^{2+})-dependent exocytosis of secretory granules that contain catecholamines, adenosine triphosphate (ATP), and dopamine-β-hydroxylase.

Inactivation of Catecholamines. Catecholamines have half-lives between 15 and 30 seconds, and they are metabolized rapidly. Most tissues contain two enzymes that inactivate catecholamines. *Catechol*-O-*methyltransferase (COMT)*, a cytosolic enzyme, catalyzes the SAM-dependent methylation of all three catecholamines, and *monoamine oxidase (MAO)*, a mitochondrial enzyme, catalyzes the oxidative deamination of monoamines. These two enzymes act sequentially to inactivate catecholamines, although the reactions can occur in either order. The end product of dopamine degradation is homovanillic acid, while that of norepinephrine and epinephrine degradation is vanillylmandelic acid (VMA). About 70% of the catecholamines found in the urine are VMA.

Functions of Catecholamines. The catecholamines prepare the body for a "fight or flight" response. They exert their effect by binding to receptors on the surface of cells and altering the intracellular concentration of Ca^{2+} and cAMP. There are two broad classes of receptors, α-adrenergic and β-adrenergic receptors. The binding of catecholamines to α-adrenergic receptors activates phospholipase C, leading to the production of inositol triphosphate and subsequent release of Ca^{2+} from intracellular stores. In contrast, the binding of catecholamines to β-receptors activates adenylate cyclase, leading to increased cAMP production. Most of the actions of the catecholamines are mediated by these two second messengers. Some of the effects of the catecholamines are: (1) increased cardiac output and decreased peripheral resistance to blood flow, (2) increased glycogen degradation and release of glucose into the blood, (3) increased triglyceride hydrolysis and release of fatty acids from adipose tissue, (4) increased release of glucagon from pancreatic α-cells, and (5) increased glycogen degradation in muscle.

Serotonin and Melatonin

In addition to being an essential amino acid required for protein synthesis, tryptophan is the precursor of serotonin and melatonin. The synthesis of each of these compounds is tissue specific.

Synthesis. Serotonin, also known as 5-hydroxytryptamine, is found in brain cells, intestinal cells, and platelets. It is synthesized and stored in brain and intestinal cells, but platelets take up serotonin from the plasma. Serotonin synthesis involves the *hydroxylation* of tryptophan, followed by *decarboxylation* (Figure 27-3). In the pineal gland, two additional reactions convert serotonin to melatonin. Acetylation of the amino group, followed by methylation of the hydroxyl group of serotonin produces melatonin. The rate-limiting step in the synthesis of both serotonin and melatonin is catalyzed by *tryptophan hydroxylase*, which, like phenylalanine and tyrosine hydroxylase, requires molecular oxygen and THB.

Functions. Serotonin has several biologic functions, including regulation of sleep, temperature, and blood pressure. It is a powerful vasoconstrictor and stimulator of smooth muscle contraction. The role of melatonin in humans is not well understood, although its synthesis appears to be regulated by the light–dark cycle. It has been proposed that melatonin plays a role in establishing circadian rhythms. It may also be involved in normal reproductive functions.

Histamine

Histamine, a chemical messenger involved in numerous cellular responses, is formed by the decarboxylation of histidine. This reaction is catalyzed by histidine decarboxylase, an enzyme that is found in most cells, as well as by the nonspecific aromatic amino acid, decarboxylase. Both enzymes require pyridoxal phosphate as a coenzyme.

Pheochromocytomas
Pheochromocytomas are tumors of chromaffin tissue that produce large amounts of catecholamines. These tumors are usually not detected until they secrete enough epinephrine or norepinephrine to result in severe hypertension [4].

Carcinoid Tumors and Serotonin Secretion
Endocrine cells are distributed throughout the small intestine. Neoplastic transformation of enterochromaffin cells that synthesize serotonin results in excessive production of serotonin, which results in diarrhea, abdominal cramps, and flushing. Patients may also have symptoms of pellagra because of the decreased availability of tryptophan for NAD^+ synthesis.

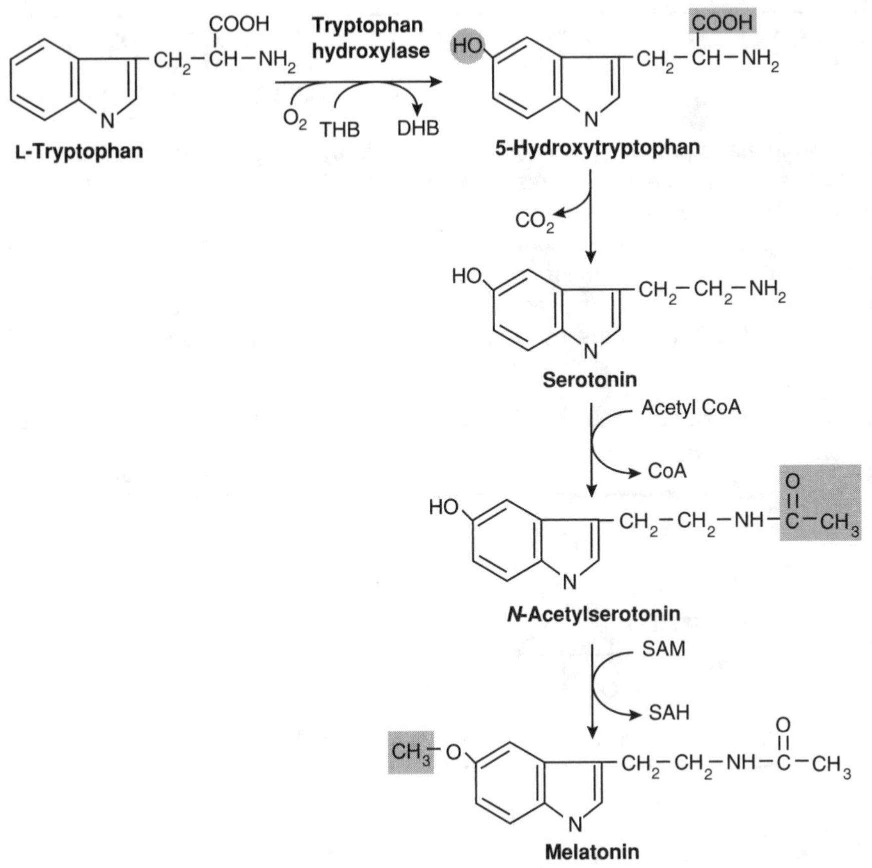

FIGURE 27-3
Synthesis of Serotonin and Melatonin. The last two enzymes in the pathway are found only in the pineal gland. In brain cells and the enterochromaffin cells, the end product is serotonin. THB = tetrahydrobiopterin; DHB = dihydrobiopterin; SAM = S-adenosylmethionine; SAH = S-adenosylhomocysteine.

$$\text{Histidine} \xrightarrow[\text{pyridoxal phosphate}]{\textbf{histidine decarboxylase}} \text{histamine} + CO_2$$

Histamine plays an important role in mediating allergic and inflammatory reactions. It is stored in mast cells and released during an inflammatory response. It is a powerful vasodilator, resulting in expansion of the capillaries, localized edema, and a drop in blood pressure. In the lungs, histamine causes constriction of the bronchioles, and in the stomach, it stimulates the secretion of hydrochloric acid.

γ-Aminobutyric Acid (GABA)

GABA is formed by the release of the α-carboxyl group of glutamate. The reaction is catalyzed by L-glutamate decarboxylase and requires pyridoxal phosphate.

$$\text{Glutamate} \xrightarrow[\text{pyridoxal phosphate}]{\textbf{L-glutamate decarboxylase}} \gamma\text{-aminobutyrate} + CO_2$$

GABA is found in high concentrations in the brain, where it functions as an inhibitory neurotransmitter. It is also found in lower concentrations in the kidney and pancreatic islet cells.

GABA and Huntington's Disease
Huntington's disease is a progressive and fatal disease characterized by brief involuntary movements (chorea). The degeneration of GABAergic neurons and the decreased levels of GABA in affected individuals suggest that the loss of inhibitory neurotransmitter pathways may be responsible for the uncontrolled movements [5].

PROTEIN-BOUND TYROSINE: THE PRECURSOR OF THYROID HORMONES

The thyroid gland produces two hormones, triiodothyronine (T_3) and tetraiodothyronine (T_4). The synthesis of each requires three substrates, thyroglobulin, iodine, and *hydrogen peroxide*. Thyroglobulin is a large glycoprotein, which is synthesized by the follicular cells of the thyroid and contains about 120 tyrosine residues, which can be used for the synthesis of T_3 and T_4. Iodine is supplied by the diet, primarily in the form of inorganic iodide (I^-). Before I^- can be used in thyroid hormone synthesis, it must be oxidized to the I^+ form. The major steps involved in T_3 and T_4 synthesis are shown in Figure 27-4.

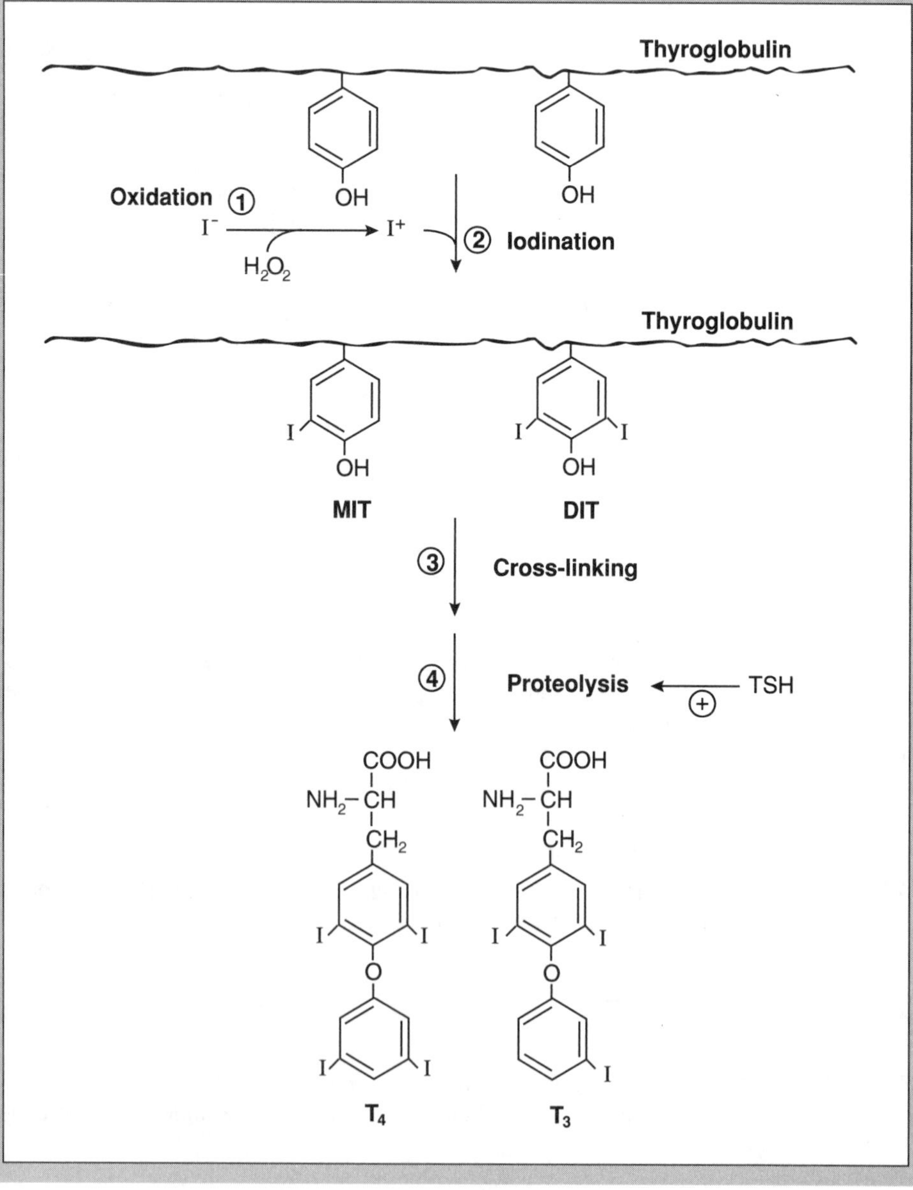

FIGURE 27-4 ▶
Major Steps in the Synthesis of Thyroid Hormones. Steps 1, 2, and 3 represent the oxidation of iodide, the iodination of tyrosine side chains in thyroglobulin, and the cross-linking of iodinated side chains. All of these steps are catalyzed by thyroid peroxidase. In step 4, tetraiodothyronine (T_4) and triiodothyronine (T_3) are released by proteolysis, which is activated by thyroid-stimulating hormone (TSH). MIT = monoiodotyrosine; DIT = diiodotyrosine.

Uptake and Oxidation of Iodide

The follicular cells take up I^- against a strong electrochemical gradient. The uptake requires energy, which is supplied by the hydrolysis of ATP and is linked to the sodium

(Na^+), potassium (K^+)-ATPase in the plasma membrane. The uptake of I^- is the rate-limiting step in the synthesis of T_3 and T_4, and it is regulated by thyroid-stimulating hormone (TSH), which is produced by the pituitary gland. The oxidation of I^- is catalyzed by *thyroid peroxidase*, which uses hydrogen peroxide as the oxidizing agent. The oxidation of I^- to I^+ is obligatory to the synthesis of the thyroid hormones.

Iodination of Tyrosine

The incorporation of oxidized iodide into the side chains of tyrosine residues of thyroglobulin is described as the organification of iodine, and it is catalyzed by thyroid peroxidase. Either one or two atoms of I^+ can be added to a tyrosine ring, resulting in monoiodotyrosine (MIT) or diiodotyrosine (DIT), respectively.

Cross-linking of Iodinated Tyrosine Residues

Following the addition of I^+ to the tyrosine side chains of thyroglobulin, *thyroid peroxidase* catalyzes a reaction that cross-links two iodinated tyrosine side chains. The cross-linkage must include one DIT residue. The second residue can be either MIT or DIT, resulting in protein-bound T_3 and T_4, respectively. Formation of T_4 is preferred over that of T_3. The protein-bound forms of T_3 and T_4 are inactive.

Release of T_3 and T_4 from Thyroglobulin

The last step in thyroid hormone synthesis is the release of T_3 and T_4 from thyroglobulin by proteolysis. This reaction is stimulated by the binding of TSH to follicular cells. Proteolysis releases T_4, MIT, DIT, and a small amount of T_3. Both T_3 and T_4 are released into the blood, whereas MIT and DIT are deiodinated within the cell, a reaction that allows I^- to be recycled. Normally, the amount of T_4 released is 20–30 times higher than T_3. The biologic activity of T_3, however, is much greater than that of T_4. In the target tissues for thyroid hormones, most of the T_4 is converted to T_3 by deiodination.

Mechanism of T_3 and T_4 Action

Target tissues that respond to T_3 and T_4 have intracellular receptors that bind the hormone. Thyroid hormone receptors are both structurally and functionally homologous to steroid hormone receptors. The hormone-receptor complex binds to specific regions in target genes, resulting in a change in the rate at which the genes are transcribed.

Physiologic Effects of T_3 and T_4

Thyroid hormones affect many pathways in carbohydrate, lipid, and protein metabolism, and they are required for normal development. Some of the metabolic responses to thyroid hormones are: increased oxygen consumption and thermogenesis; stimulation of protein synthesis, particularly enzymes involved in oxidative metabolism; promotion of positive nitrogen balance; increased release of fatty acids from adipose tissue; and increased glycogen degradation and fatty acid oxidation in the liver.

Antithyroid Drugs
The thioureas are a class of drugs used to inhibit the synthesis of thyroid hormones. The target for these drugs is thyroid peroxidase, and they inhibit the oxidation of I^- but have no effect on its uptake. Examples of these drugs are thiouracil, propylthiouracil, and methimazole.

Graves' Disease
One of most common causes of hyperthyroidism is the production of an antibody that mimics the action of TSH by binding to the TSH receptor, resulting in enlargement of the thyroid gland and uncontrolled production of T_3 and T_4.

Cretinism
This is a condition caused by low levels of thyroid hormones prior to birth or in the neonatal stages of development. The appearance of numerous congenital defects and severe mental retardation underscore the requirement for thyroid hormones for normal development.

PORPHYRIN AND HEME METABOLISM

Porphyrins are cyclic compounds that have a high affinity for binding metal ions, usually ferrous iron (Fe^{2+}) or ferric iron (Fe^{3+}). They contain four pyrrole rings, which are linked together by single-carbon bridges. All of the atoms in porphyrins are derived from glycine and succinyl coenzyme A (CoA). Heme, the prosthetic group for hemoglobin, myoglobin, and the cytochromes, is the most common metalloporphyrin in humans (Figure 27-5). The degradation of heme results in bilirubin, which is secreted in the bile and reduced to urobilinogen by intestinal bacteria. Abnormalities in the synthesis of heme result in a group of diseases known as porphyrias, whereas abnormalities in the degradation and secretion of heme result in jaundice.

FIGURE 27-5

Structure of Heme. The heme structure is shown in the upper portion of the figure. An abbreviated form of the heme structure is shown below, where each arm of the cross represents a pyrrole ring. Substituents on the pyrrole rings are methyl (M), vinyl (V), and propionyl (P) groups.

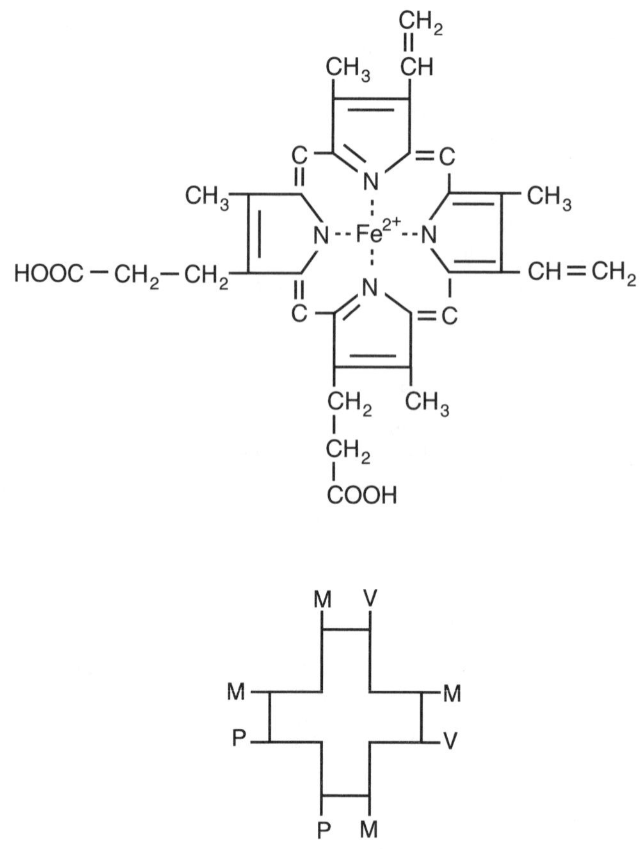

Key Steps in Heme Synthesis

Most heme synthesis in the body occurs in the bone marrow and liver, although all nucleated cells have the capacity to synthesize heme. The initial reaction and the last three reactions in the pathway occur in the mitochondria, and the intermediate steps are extramitochondrial. An overview of heme synthesis is provided in Figure 27-6.

Synthesis of Δ-Aminolevulinic Acid (Δ-ALA). The initial step in heme synthesis is the condensation of glycine and succinyl CoA, resulting in the formation of Δ-ALA. This reaction is catalyzed by Δ-ALA synthase, which requires pyridoxal phosphate as a coenzyme. Formation of Δ-ALA is the rate-limiting step in the synthesis of heme.

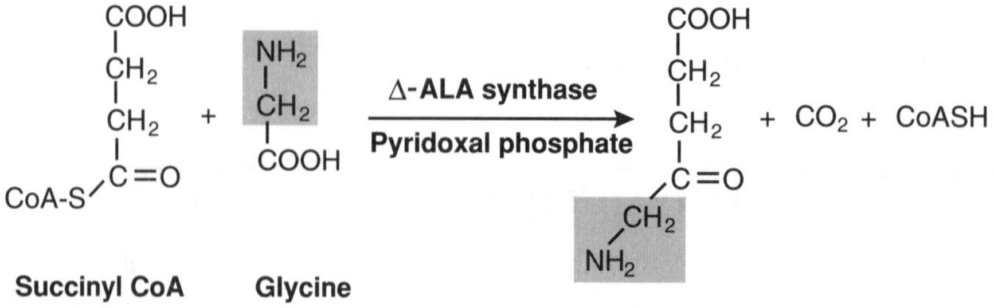

Synthesis of Porphobilinogen (PBG). The condensation of two molecules of Δ-ALA results in PBG. The formation of PBG is catalyzed by Δ-ALA dehydratase, an enzyme that is strongly inhibited by lead. This reaction provides the pyrrole ring system that is used to assemble porphyrins.

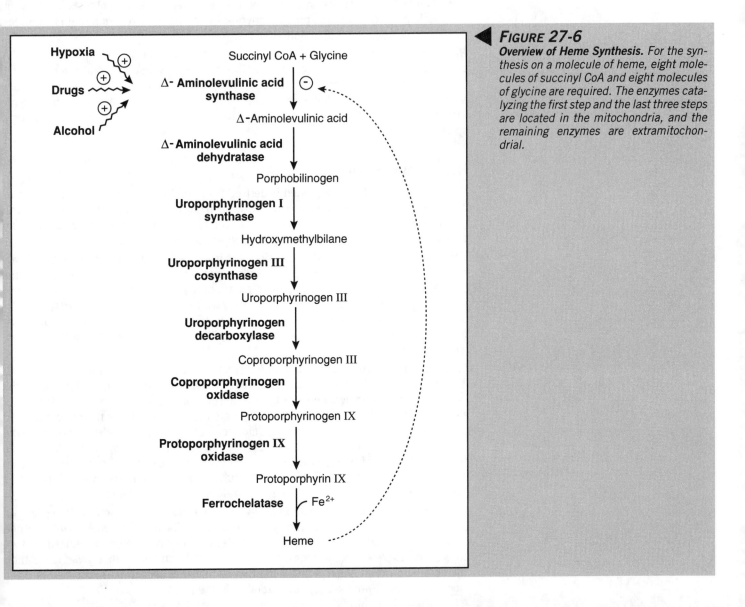

Formation of Uroporphyrinogen III. Four molecules of PBG are converted to uroporphy-rinogen III by the action of two enzymes, *uroporphyrinogen I synthase* and *uroporphyrinogen III cosynthase*. Uroporphyrinogen I synthase catalyzes the condensation of four molecules of PBG, resulting in a linear tetrapyrrole. Each pyrrole ring has an acetyl group (A) and a propionyl group (P) attached as side chains. In the absence of uroporphyrinogen III cosynthase, the linear tetrapyrrole spontaneously cyclizes, resulting in uroporphyrino-gen I. However, in the presence of uroporphyrinogen III cosynthase, the product is

FIGURE 27-6

Overview of Heme Synthesis. *For the synthesis on a molecule of heme, eight molecules of succinyl CoA and eight molecules of glycine are required. The enzymes catalyzing the first step and the last three steps are located in the mitochondria, and the remaining enzymes are extramitochondrial.*

uroporphyrinogen III. The only difference between these isomers is in the ordering of the A and P side chains. The sequence of A and P in uroporphyrinogen I is symmetric, whereas in uroporphyrinogen III it is asymmetric. Only uroporphyrinogen III is used in the pathway of heme synthesis.

PBG

Type III   **Type I**

Uroporphobilinogens

Conversion of Uroporphyrinogen III to Heme. Uroporphyrinogen III is converted to proto-porphyrin IX through a series of decarboxylation and oxidation reactions that alter the side chains attached to the pyrrole rings. The final step in heme synthesis involves the introduction of Fe^{2+} into the protoporphyrin-IX ring system, a reaction that is catalyzed by *ferrochelatase*, which is inhibited by lead.

Regulation of Heme Synthesis. The rate-limiting enzyme in heme synthesis is Δ-ALA synthase. This enzyme is inducible and turns over rapidly, having a half-life of about 1 hour. Synthesis of the enzyme is induced by hypoxia and repressed by free heme. Many drugs, including alcohol, that are metabolized by microsomal cytochrome P-450 enzyme systems induce the synthesis of Δ-ALA synthase in the liver, resulting in increased heme synthesis.

Heme Degradation

Most of the heme that is degraded is derived from the turnover of hemoglobin. Approximately 6 grams of hemoglobin are degraded each day in the normal adult. The porphyrin ring system of heme is degraded in the reticuloendothelial cells of the liver, spleen, and bone marrow. The steps in heme degradation are shown in Figure 27-7.

Conversion of Heme to Bilirubin. The first step in heme degradation is catalyzed by *heme oxygenase*, a microsomal enzyme that oxidizes one of the carbon bridges that connect the pyrrole rings. The products of this reaction are biliverdin, carbon monoxide, and Fe^{3+}. This is the only reaction in humans that is known to result in carbon monoxide production. Biliverdin, a green pigment, is reduced to bilirubin, a reddish-yellow pigment by *biliverdin reductase*. The colors of biliverdin and bilirubin are responsible for the characteristic tones of bruises.

Conjugation of Bilirubin with Glucuronic Acid. Bilirubin is a hydrophobic compound that is relatively insoluble in aqueous media and is transported from peripheral tissues to the liver by albumin. The liver conjugates free bilirubin with either one or two molecules of glucuronic acid to form glucuronides, which are much more soluble than unconjugated bilirubin. The transfer of glucuronic acid from uridine diphosphate–glucuronic acid (UDP–glucuronic acid) to bilirubin is catalyzed by *bilirubin glucuronyltransferase*. The conjugated forms of bilirubin are secreted into the bile by an active transport mechanism, which is the rate-limiting step in bilirubin metabolism in the liver. Bilirubin and other heme degradation products are often referred to as bile pigments.

Metabolism of Bilirubin Diglucuronide by Intestinal Bacteria. In the intestine, the glucuronic acid groups are removed from bilirubin by bacterial enzymes, and the bile pigment is reduced to *urobilinogen*, a colorless compound, which is oxidized to *stercobilin* and excreted in the feces. Stercobilin is the compound that gives feces their characteristic brown color. A small fraction of the urobilinogen is reabsorbed into the blood, extracted by the kidney, and excreted in the urine.

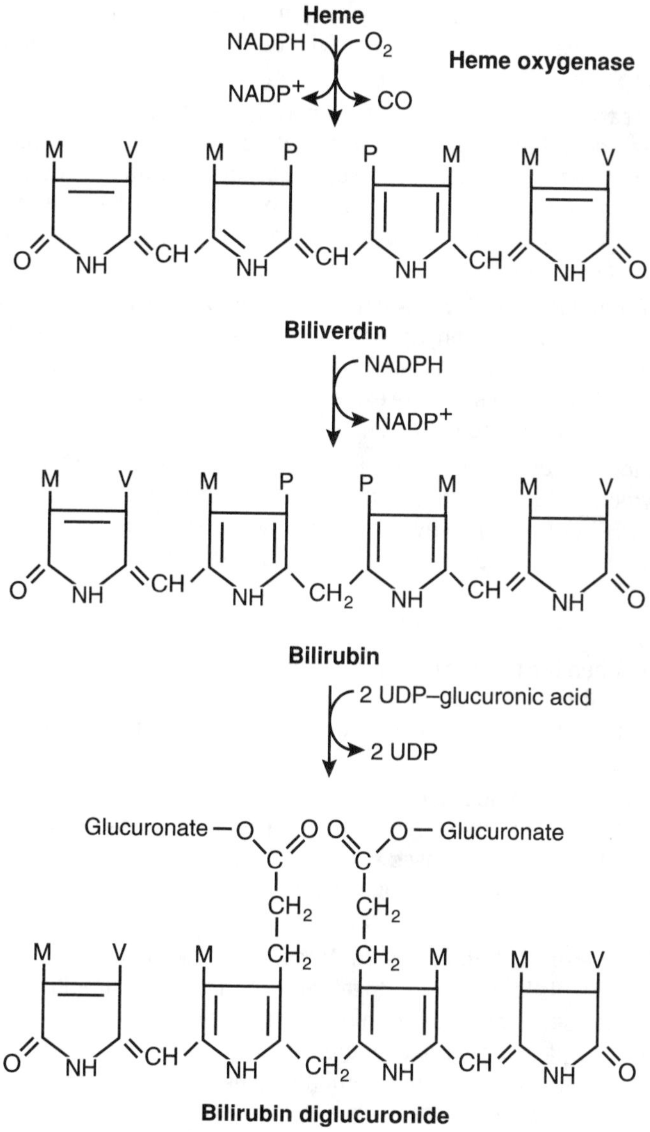

► FIGURE 27-7
Heme Degradation. *The conversion of heme to bilirubin occurs in the reticuloendothelial cells of the spleen and liver. Heme oxygenase catalyzes the first step, in which a carbon bridge connecting two pyrrole rings is cleaved, resulting in biliverdin and the release of Fe^{3+} and carbon monoxide (CO). Following reduction of biliverdin, bilirubin is transported to the liver by albumin where it is conjugated with glucuronic acid. $NADP^+$ and NADPH = the oxidized and reduced forms of nicotinamide-adenine dinucleotide phosphate, respectively; UDP = uridine diphosphate; M = methyl; V = vinyl; P = propionyl.*

Abnormalities in Heme Metabolism

The two major classes of abnormalities in heme metabolism are the porphyrias, which result from defects in heme synthesis, and jaundice, which results from increased bilirubin levels in the blood.

PORPHYRIAS

The porphyrias are a family of diseases resulting from a defect in heme synthesis. The defect may be either inherited or acquired. The most common form of acquired porphyria is lead poisoning. Porphyrias are characterized by the accumulation of intermediates behind the defective enzyme and a decrease in the intermediates beyond the block. In all of the porphyrias, the production of heme is decreased, resulting in increased Δ-ALA synthase activity, thereby exacerbating the accumulation of intermediates. Patients with defects leading to the accumulation of tetrapyrroles or porphyrins are usually sensitive to light, whereas patients with defects that lead to the accumulation of Δ-ALA and PBG experience intermittent bouts of abdominal pain and neuropsychiatric disturbances, but they are not photosensitive. Treatment of the porphyrias involves the administration of hematin (heme with iron in the Fe^{3+} state) to repress the synthesis of Δ-ALA synthase, and strict avoidance of alcohol, drugs, or anesthetics that induce the synthesis of

Relationship Between Glucose Intake and Heme Synthesis
Glucose inhibits heme synthesis by a mechanism that is not well understood. When placed on a low-calorie diet, some patients develop symptoms of porphyria for the first time.

cytochrome P-450. Descendents of King George III have been shown to have porphyria, resulting from a deficiency in protoporphyrinogen oxidase (see Figure 27-6), and it has been suggested that his periodic erratic behavior during the American revolution may be attributed to porphyria.

Porphyria Cutanea Tarda. The most common porphyria results from a genetic defect in *uroporphyrinogen decarboxylase*, an enzyme that converts four of the acetic acid side chains attached to methyl groups. This disease has an autosomal recessive inheritance pattern, and its clinical manifestations include photosensitivity, liver disease, and excretion of large quantities of uroporphyrinogens in the urine. Acute episodes can be precipitated by alcohol consumption.

Congenital Erythropoietic Porphyria. A defect in *uroporphyrinogen III cosynthase* results in congenital erythropoietic porphyria, which is transmitted as an autosomal recessive trait. Patients with this disease are sensitive to light, and large quantities of uroporphyrinogen I accumulate in tissues and are excreted in the urine. The teeth, bones, and urine of patients often have a pink to red color.

Acute Intermittent Porphyria. A defect in *uroporphyrinogen I synthase* results in the inability to polymerize PBG, resulting in the accumulation and excretion of large amounts of Δ-ALA and PBG. Affected individuals have acute symptoms that include neuropsychiatric disorders and abdominal pain. The disease is inherited as an autosomal dominant trait.

JAUNDICE

Jaundice occurs when the plasma levels of bilirubin exceed 2–2.5 mg/dL. When bilirubin reaches this level, it begins to accumulate in the skin, sclera (whites of the eyes), and other tissues. Although jaundice is not a disease, it is an important symptom of some underlying disease.

Causes of Jaundice. Jaundice can result either from overproduction of bilirubin or decreased excretion of bilirubin. Overproduction is usually associated with excessive breakdown of erythrocytes. Decreased excretion may result either from liver damage or obstruction of the bile duct. Liver damage can result in decreased uptake of bilirubin or in a decreased ability to conjugate bilirubin.

Measurement of Serum Bilirubin Levels. Measurement of conjugated, unconjugated, and total bilirubin levels in the serum, together with the level of urobilinogen excreted in the urine, provides useful information in determining the underlying cause of jaundice. For example, liver damage results in an increased proportion of unconjugated bilirubin in the serum and increased excretion of urobilinogen in the urine. On the other hand, obstruction of the bile duct results in an elevated level of conjugated bilirubin in the serum and decreased excretion of urobilinogen in the urine.

The various forms of bilirubin in the serum can be measured by van den Bergh's test, in which conjugated bilirubin reacts directly and rapidly with diazotized sulfanilic acid, producing a red color that can be quantitated spectrophotometrically. Therefore, the conjugated bilirubin is frequently referred to as *direct bilirubin*. Unconjugated bilirubin is bound to albumin and does not react with this reagent unless the serum is first treated with methanol to release the bound bilirubin. Therefore, when the reaction is carried out in the presence of methanol, the concentration of total bilirubin is measured. The concentration of unconjugated bilirubin, known as *indirect bilirubin*, is equal to the difference between the total and the direct bilirubin levels.

Neonatal Jaundice
The immature liver of premature infants is frequently unable to conjugate bilirubin with glucuronic acid, resulting in an increase in the circulating level of free bilirubin. When the bilirubin level reaches a concentration of 2–2.5 mg/dL, it begins to accumulate in the skin and the sclera, resulting in the yellow color seen in jaundice. Jaundice in newborns is treated by phototherapy, which facilitates the degradation of bilirubin to products that are more soluble and can be excreted in the urine.

Kernicterus
Kernicterus refers to neurologic dysfunction that results from the toxic effects of bilirubin on the brain. Bilirubin is hydrophobic and readily crosses the blood-brain barrier. It accumulates in the brain, leading to motor and cognitive defects or death. When the level of unconjugated bilirubin exceeds the binding capacity of albumin, which is approximately 20 mg/dL, a newborn child is at risk for kernicterus.

OTHER SPECIALIZED PRODUCTS DERIVED FROM AMINO ACIDS

Melanins

Melanins are insoluble polymers of varying lengths that are synthesized from tyrosine. They are synthesized in melanocytes, the pigment-producing cells of the skin. Color variation in the skin of different people reflects different levels of melanin synthesis. The conversion of tyrosine to melanin is initiated by tyrosinase, a copper-containing enzyme that converts tyrosine sequentially to dopa and dopaquinone. Subsequent reactions involve nonenzymatic oxidation reactions that lead to polymerization and the formation of brown and black pigments.

$$\text{Tyrosine} \xrightarrow[\text{copper, oxygen}]{\text{tyrosinase}} \text{dopa} \xrightarrow[\text{copper, oxygen}]{\text{tyrosinase}} \text{dopaquinone}$$

$$\xrightarrow{\text{spontaneous}} \text{melanins}$$

Albinism and Defective Melanin Production
The term albinism refers to several inherited defects in melanin production. Some forms of albinism result from a genetic defect in tyrosinase. Affected individuals have an increased susceptibility to sunlight and an increased incidence of several types of carcinoma [2].

Creatine

Creatine is found in muscle and brain tissue where it serves as a reservoir of high-energy phosphate groups. Creatine phosphate is used to maintain the intracellular concentration of ATP during short periods of intense muscle contraction. The synthesis and degradation of creatine and creatine phosphate are shown in Figure 27-8.

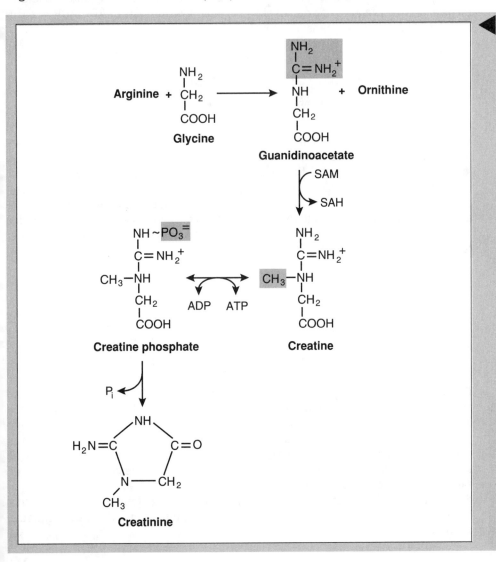

◀ **FIGURE 27-8**
Synthesis and Degradation of Creatine. The first step in creatine synthesis occurs in the kidney and the second step in the liver. Creatine is released into the blood and extracted by the muscle and brain, where it is converted to creatine phosphate. Creatine phosphate cyclizes, forming creatinine.

Creatine Synthesis. The synthesis of creatine requires three amino acids: glycine, arginine, and methionine. Methionine is required for the synthesis of SAM which is used as a methylating agent during creatine synthesis. In the first reaction, the guanidinoacetate group ($NH_2-C=NH_2^+$) is transferred from the arginine side chain to glycine, resulting in guanidinoacetate. Methylation of guanidinoacetate results in creatine. Creatine and creatine phosphate can be rapidly interconverted by the reaction shown below.

$$\text{Creatine} + \text{ATP} \xrightleftharpoons[\hspace{3cm}]{\text{creatine kinase}} \text{creatine phosphate} + \text{ADP}$$

Creatine Degradation. Creatine phosphate is unstable and is spontaneously converted to creatinine, which is excreted in the urine. The formation of creatinine is nonenzymatic and irreversible, and the amount of creatinine excreted in the urine during a 24-hour period is proportional to the muscle mass. The amount of creatinine produced is very constant from day to day.

Glutathione

Glutathione, a tripeptide containing glutamate (Glu), cysteine (Cys), and glycine (Gly), is the most abundant sulfur-containing compound in cells. The concentration of glutathione in animal cells is about 5 mM.

Synthesis of Glutathione. The synthesis of glutathione involves two consecutive steps in which peptide bonds are formed. These reactions are catalyzed by glutathione synthetase, and they require energy, which is supplied by hydrolysis of ATP (ADP = adenosine diphosphate; P_i = inorganic phosphate).

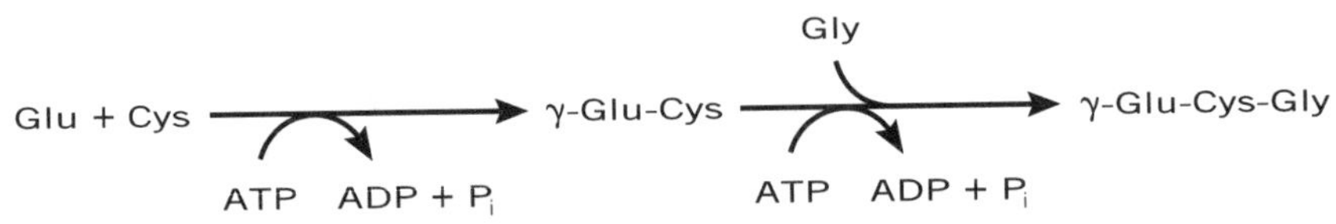

$$\text{Glu} + \text{Cys} \xrightarrow[\text{ATP} \quad \text{ADP} + P_i]{} \gamma\text{-Glu-Cys} \xrightarrow[\text{ATP} \quad \text{ADP} + P_i]{\text{Gly}} \gamma\text{-Glu-Cys-Gly}$$

Oxidized and Reduced Forms of Glutathione. Many of the functions of glutathione are dependent on its ability to cycle between oxidized and reduced forms, as shown in the following equation. Normally, the reduced form constitutes about 98% of the total glutathione pool. Its free sulfhydryl group provides protection against oxidative stress. This ratio is maintained by *glutathione reductase* and the reduced form of nicotinamide-adenine dinucleotide phosphate (NADPH), which is supplied by the pentose phosphate pathway. Reduced glutathione is commonly abbreviated as GSH, and oxidized glutathione as GSSG.

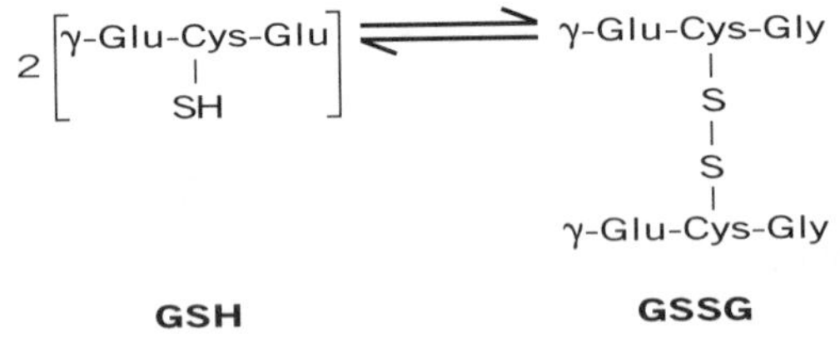

$$2\begin{bmatrix} \gamma\text{-Glu-Cys-Glu} \\ | \\ SH \end{bmatrix} \rightleftharpoons \begin{matrix} \gamma\text{-Glu-Cys-Gly} \\ | \\ S \\ | \\ S \\ | \\ \gamma\text{-Glu-Cys-Gly} \end{matrix}$$

$$\text{GSH} \qquad\qquad\qquad \text{GSSG}$$

Functions of Glutathione. One of the most important functions of glutathione is to maintain protein sulfhydryl groups in their reduced state. In the RBC, glutathione is essential in reducing hydrogen peroxide levels and preventing oxidative damage and hemolysis (see Chapter 14). It plays an important role in eicosanoid synthesis, serving as a reductant in the cyclooxygenase reaction and as a substrate in peptidyl-leukotriene synthesis (see Chapter 22). In the liver, glutathione is used in the detoxification of toxic electrophilic xenobiotics that gain access to the body as food additives, pollutants, or drugs. Many of these compounds form conjugates with glutathione and are further metabolized to a family of compounds known as mercapturic acids, which are excreted in the urine.

Nitric Oxide

Nitric oxide, a powerful vasodilator and a neurotransmitter, is generated from arginine by nitric acid synthase, an enzyme that catalyzes the reaction shown below. Nitric oxide synthase is activated by Ca^{2+} and requires molecular oxygen and THB for catalytic activity. Dihydrobiopterin (DHB) reductase and NADPH are also required to regenerate THB. Nitric oxide is a free radical gas that can readily diffuse in and out of cells.

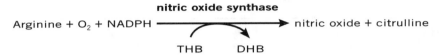

Arginine + O_2 + NADPH $\xrightarrow[\text{THB \quad DHB}]{\text{nitric oxide synthase}}$ nitric oxide + citrulline

Nitric oxide synthase is found primarily in brain cells, endothelial cells, and macrophages. Different isozymes are found in each of these locations, and the nitric oxide generated in each location has a different function.

Endothelial-Derived Nitric Oxide. Nitric oxide diffuses out of endothelial cells and into vascular smooth muscle cells where it activates cytosolic guanylate cyclase, resulting in increased synthesis of cyclic guanosine monophosphate (cGMP). Activation of cGMP-dependent protein kinase leads to the phosphorylation of smooth muscle contractile proteins and relaxation.

Brain-Derived Nitric Oxide. Nitric oxide that is synthesized in the brain affects several different types of neurons. The receptor for nitric oxide in neurons is cytosolic guanylate cyclase, resulting in cGMP synthesis. The proteins that are phosphorylated and the consequence of phosphorylation in neurons are not well understood.

Macrophage-Derived Nitric Oxide. The activity of nitric oxide synthase in macrophages is normally low but is stimulated in response to bacterial infection. The synthesis of nitric oxide in macrophages is part of the mechanism used by these cells for killing bacterial and tumor cells.

RESOLUTION OF CLINICAL CASE

The patient introduced at the beginning of the chapter was suffering from lead poisoning. This diagnosis was suspected on the basis of information provided by the patient's mother and was confirmed by the presence of lead in the plasma at a concentration of 0.71 µmol/dL. Clinical symptoms of lead poisoning become evident when the concentration exceeds 0.24 µmol/dL [1]. The source of lead was paint on doors and window sills that the patient ingested. X-ray analysis indicated that fragments of paint were still present in his intestinal tract. Lead salts have been widely used in paints, and although it is illegal in the United States to use more than 600 parts per million of lead in paint, in the United Kingdom, manufacturers are required only to label paint products that contain large quantities of lead [3]. Lead has a high affinity for sulfhydryl groups of proteins and inactivates a number of enzymes by reacting with cysteine side chains. The low RBC count and the low level of hemoglobin indicate that this patient is anemic. Lead leads to anemia by inhibiting Δ-ALA dehydratase and ferrochelatase, two enzymes in the pathway of heme synthesis. Inhibition of these enzymes results in the accumulation and excretion of Δ-ALA and coproporphyrin. The pattern of increased density seen in x-rays of the long bones is the result of the accumulation of lead, which has a high affinity for bone, particularly in the rapidly growing areas. Treatment of a patient with lead poisoning involves giving chelating compounds that have a high affinity for lead and will form complexes that can be excreted. The chelator used to treat this patient was CaEDTA, although other chelators such as penicillamine are also commonly used. The chelator was given intravenously to this patient to avoid dissolving the paint fragments in the intestine.

REVIEW QUESTIONS

Directions: For each of the following questions, choose the **one best** answer.

1. Which of the following compounds is the major end product of tyrosine metabolism in the adrenal medulla?
    (A) Dopamine
    (B) Epinephrine
    (C) Norepinephrine
    (D) Phenylalanine
    (E) Melanin

2. Which of the following statements describes Δ-aminolevulinic acid (Δ-ALA) synthase?
    (A) It is a cytosolic enzyme found in the liver and bone marrow
    (B) It is inhibited by drugs that induce the synthesis of cytochrome P-450
    (C) It is inhibited by lead
    (D) It catalyzes the rate-limiting step in heme synthesis
    (E) It requires tetrahydrobiopterin (TBH) as a cofactor

3. Which of the following neurotransmitters is a catecholamine?
    (A) Serotonin
    (B) γ-Aminobutyric acid (GABA)
    (C) Dopamine
    (D) Histamine
    (E) Acetylcholine (ACh)

4. Which of the following compounds is a degradation product of heme?
    (A) Δ-Aminolevulinic acid (Δ-ALA)
    (B) Bile salts
    (C) Porphobilinogen
    (D) Biliverdin
    (E) Coproporphyrinogen

5. Which of the following compounds is synthesized by macrophages for killing bacterial cells?
    (A) Nitric oxide
    (B) Glutathione
    (C) Melatonin
    (D) Melanin
    (E) Carbon monoxide

6. Which of the following statements about bilirubin is correct?
    (A) Direct bilirubin is the same as unconjugated bilirubin
    (B) Conjugated bilirubin is transported in the blood by albumin
    (C) Treatment of neonatal jaundice with phototherapy facilitates the excretion of bilirubin
    (D) Bilirubin is reduced to biliverdin by the reticuloendothelial cells of the liver and spleen
    (E) Damage to the liver results in increased levels of direct bilirubin

ANSWERS AND EXPLANATIONS

1. The answer is B. The major product derived from tyrosine in the adrenal medulla is epinephrine. Dopamine and norepinephrine are end products in the brain, and melanin is synthesized in melanocytes. Phenylalanine is not derived from tyrosine but is the precursor of tyrosine.

2. The answer is D. Δ-ALA synthase catalyzes the rate-limiting step in heme synthesis and is the site where heme synthesis is regulated. It is a mitochondrial enzyme found in liver and bone marrow, and it requires pyridoxal phosphate, not TBH, for activity. The synthesis of the enzyme is induced by drugs that stimulate the synthesis of cytochrome P-450. Lead inhibits Δ-ALA dehydratase but has no effect on Δ-ALA synthase.

3. The answer is C. Dopamine is the only neurotransmitter listed that is derived from tyrosine, the precursor for the catecholamines. Serotonin, GABA, histamine, and ACh are synthesized from tryptophan, glutamate, histidine, and serine, respectively.

4. The answer is D. Biliverdin is produced in the first step of heme degradation. This reaction, catalyzed by heme oxygenase, results in the opening of the cyclic porphyrin ring, giving biliverdin, a linear tetrapyrrole. Δ-ALA, porphobilinogen, and coproporphyrinogen are intermediates in the synthesis of heme. Bile acids result from the degradation of cholesterol, and the bile pigments are bilirubin and other intermediates in the degradation of heme.

5. The answer is A. Bacterial lipopolysaccharide stimulates the synthesis of nitric oxide in macrophages. Nitric oxide is a free radical that participates in the oxidative killing of bacteria and tumor cells. In other tissues, nitric oxide acts as a second messenger or as a neurotransmitter. The major function of glutathione is to serve as a reducing agent in many types of reactions that protect cells against oxidative damage. Melatonin is synthesized only in the pineal gland; melanin is synthesized only in melanocytes; and carbon monoxide is synthesized only in reticuloendothelial cells that degrade heme.

6. The answer is C. Phototherapy results in the degradation of bilirubin to products that are more water soluble and can be excreted. In van den Bergh's test, direct bilirubin corresponds to conjugated bilirubin, and indirect bilirubin is unconjugated bilirubin that is bound to albumin. In the catabolism of heme, biliverdin is reduced to bilirubin in the reticuloendothelial cells. Conjugation of bilirubin occurs only in the liver, and liver damage often results in decreased levels of direct (conjugated) bilirubin.

REFERENCES

1. Schwarz, V: *A Clinical Companion to Biochemical Studies*, San Francisco, CA: W. H. Freeman, 1978, pp 46–50.
2. Bhagavan, NV: *Medical Biochemistry*, Boston, MA: Jones and Bartlett, 1992, p 382.
3. Gillham B, Papachristodoulou DK, Thomas JH: *Wills' Biochemical Basis of Medicine*, Boston, MA: Butterworth-Heinemann, 1997, p 362.
4. Murray RH, Granner DK, Mayes PA, et al: *Harper's Biochemistry*, 24th ed. Stamford, CT: Appleton and Lange, 1996, p 564.
5. Gillham B, Papachristodoulou DK, Thomas JH: *Wills' Biochemical Basis of Medicine*, Boston, MA: Butterworth-Heinemann, 1997, pp 294–295.

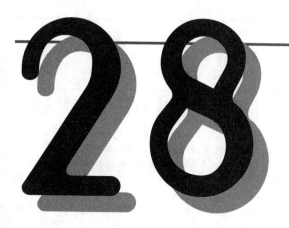

28 NUCLEOTIDE METABOLISM

INTRODUCTION OF CLINICAL CASE

A 52-year-old lawyer was admitted to the hospital after collapsing at a celebration following his successful campaign for state senator. Upon admission, he appeared inebriated. Analysis of a blood sample showed his blood alcohol level was 51 mmol/dL (about 0.24%). Other laboratory values obtained on the blood sample were: glucose, 56 mg/dL (normal: 70–110 mg/dL); lactate, 26 mg/dL (normal: 4–16 mg/dL); uric acid, 12.2 mg/dL (normal: 3–8 mg/dL). When the patient awoke the next morning, he complained of severe pain in his big toe. He said that he had experienced this same pain in both his toe and hand several times earlier. The joints of his big toe were inflamed and very tender. Nodules (tophi) were visible in his earlobes. When questioned about his drinking, he admitted that he had been a heavy drinker for several years, although he did not believe that he had a problem with alcohol. Blood samples taken 24 hours after admission showed that his plasma lactate level had returned to within the normal range, although his uric acid level remained high (10.8 mg/dL). Treatment with allopurinol was started, and within 3 days his plasma uric acid level was within the normal range. He was dismissed from the hospital with instructions to continue taking allopurinol.

INTRODUCTION TO NUCLEOTIDE METABOLISM

Nucleotides perform a variety of functions in cells. They are the building blocks for deoxyribonucleic acid (DNA) and ribonucleic acid (RNA), and they play numerous roles in energy transduction reactions. The hydrolysis of adenosine triphosphate (ATP) supplies the energy needed to drive many endergonic reactions in the body. Nucleotides also act as activated carriers of monosaccharides, lipids, amino acids, sulfate, and methyl groups in numerous metabolic pathways. They are structural components of several coenzymes, including coenzyme A (CoA), flavin adenine dinucleotide (FAD), and nicotinamide adenine dinucleotide (NAD). The adenine nucleotides are important allosteric regulators of key enzymes in metabolism, whereas cyclic adenosine monophosphate (cAMP) and cyclic guanosine monophosphate (cGMP) are second messengers that mediate the effect of many peptide hormones. The nucleotides can be synthesized from small molecules that are available in cells, or they can be synthesized by salvage pathways that recycle the purine and pyrimidine rings. In rapidly dividing cells that are synthesizing large quantities of DNA and RNA, the need for nucleotides is greater than in nondividing cells. In nondividing cells, most of the nucleotides can be supplied by the salvage pathways. Several drugs that are used as chemotherapeutic agents interfere with the synthesis of nucleotides.

Components of Nucleotides

Nucleotides consist of a nitrogen-containing ring (frequently referred to as a nitrogenous base), a pentose, and one or more phosphate groups.

Nitrogenous Bases: Purines and Pyrimidines. The common nucleotides contain two types of nitrogenous bases, purines and pyrimidines. Two purines, adenine and guanine, and three pyrimidines, uracil, cytosine, and thymine, are found in the nucleic acids. The structures of these purines and pyrimidines are shown in Figure 28-1. Thymine is found only in DNA, and uracil only in RNA. Adenine, guanine, and cytosine are present in both DNA and RNA. The atoms in a purine ring are identified by numbers 1 to 9, whereas the atoms in the pyrimidine ring are identified by numbers 1 to 6.

Pentoses: Ribose and Deoxyribose. The nucleotides found in DNA contain deoxyribose, whereas those in RNA contain ribose. The carbon atoms in the pentoses are numbered 1' to 5' to distinguish them from atoms in the purine and pyrimidine rings. Ribose and deoxyribose differ only at the 2'-carbon. Ribose has a hydroxyl group attached to the 2'-carbon which is replaced by a hydrogen (H) atom in deoxyribose.

Structure and Numbering System for Purine and Pyrimidine Rings

Purine ring

Pyrimidine ring

Components of a Nucleotide

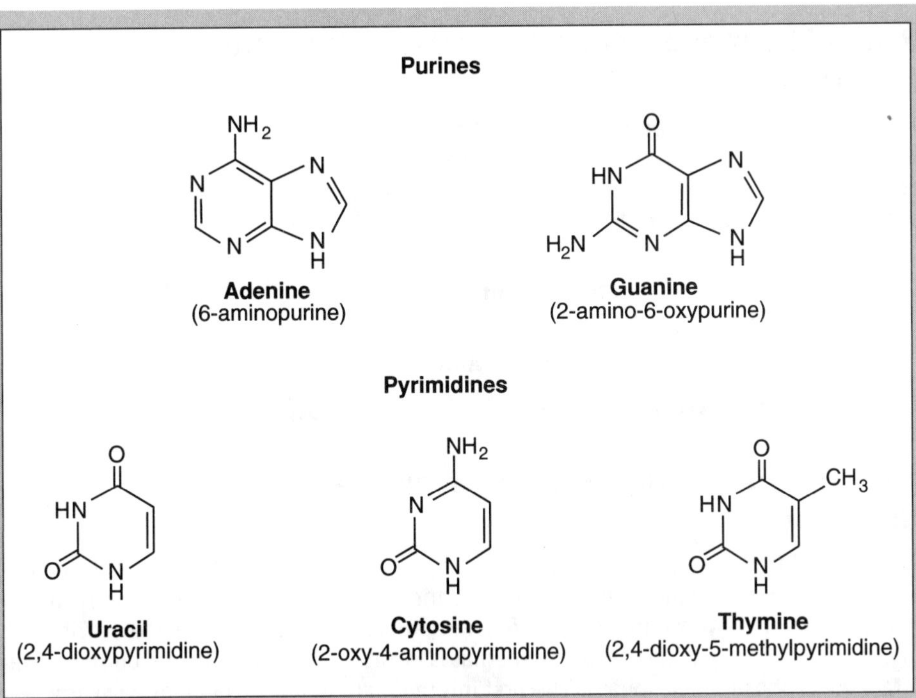

FIGURE 28-1
Structures of Purines and Pyrimidines.
The purines and pyrimidines are nitrogenous bases that are found in nucleic acids. Thymine is found only in DNA, and uracil is found only in RNA. Adenine, cytosine, and guanine are found in both DNA and RNA.

Phosphate Groups. The phosphate groups are linked to the 5'-carbon of the pentose. If more than one phosphate is present, the first is attached to the pentose by an ester linkage, while additional phosphate groups are attached to one another through an anhydride linkage.

Nomenclature

The attachment of a pentose to a nitrogen-containing base results in a nucleoside. The addition of a phosphate group to a nucleoside results in a nucleotide. If the nucleoside contains adenine and ribose, it is known as adenosine. If one phosphate group is attached to adenosine, the nucleotide is known as either adenosine monophosphate (AMP) or adenylate. If two or three phosphate groups are attached to the 5'-carbon of adenosine, the nucleotides are known as adenosine diphosphate (ADP) and adenosine triphosphate (ATP), respectively. The nomenclature for all the common nucleosides and nucleotides is summarized in Table 28-1.

Nomenclature	
Base:	purine or pyrimidine
Nucleoside:	base-pentose
Nucleotide:	base-pentose-phosphate

TABLE 28-1
Nomenclature of Nucleosides and Nucleotides

Base	Ribonucleoside	Ribonucleotide
Adenine (A)	Adenosine	Adenylate or adenosine monophosphate (AMP)
Guanine (G)	Guanosine	Guanylate or guanosine monophosphate (GMP)
Cytosine (C)	Cytidine	Cytidylate or cytidine monophosphate (CMP)
Uracil (U)	Uridine	Uridylate or uridine monophosphate (UMP)

Base	Deoxyribonucleoside	Deoxyribonucleotide
Adenine (A)	Deoxyadenosine	Deoxyadenylate or deoxyadenosine monophosphate (dAMP)
Guanine (G)	Deoxyguanosine	Deoxyguanylate or deoxyguanosine monophosphate (dGMP)
Cytosine (C)	Deoxycytidine	Deoxycytidylate or deoxycytidine monophosphate (dCMP)
Thymine (T)	Deoxythymidine	Deoxythymidylate or deoxythymidine monophosphate (dTMP)

Note. A nucleotide with two or three phosphates is named as the corresponding nucleoside diphosphate (NDP) or nucleoside triphosphate (NTP), where N is the name of the specific nucleoside.

Role of Phosphoribosylpyrophosphate (PRPP) in Nucleotide Metabolism

PRPP is the donor of ribose-5-phosphate in the synthesis of all nucleotides. The synthesis of PRPP is catalyzed by PRPP synthetase, which uses ribose-5-phosphate and ATP as substrates. PRPP synthetase is activated by inorganic phosphate (P_i) and inhibited by purine nucleotides.

$$^=O_3POH_2C \quad \xrightarrow[\text{ATP} \quad \text{AMP}]{\text{PRPP synthetase}} \quad ^=O_3POH_2C$$

Ribose-5-phosphate   Phosphoribosylpyrophosphate

Strategies Used in the Synthesis of Purine and Pyrimidine Nucleotides

A strategic difference in the synthesis of purine and pyrimidine nucleotides is the point at which ribose-5-phosphate is introduced into the pathway. In the synthesis of pyrimidine nucleotides, the pyrimidine ring is first assembled and then attached to ribose-5-phosphate. In contrast, all of the intermediates involved in assembling the purine ring are attached to ribose-5-phosphate. The first intermediate in purine nucleotide synthesis is 5′-phosphoribosylamine. This amino group ultimately becomes N-9 of the purine ring.

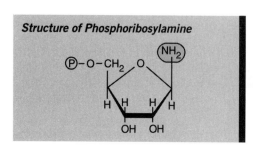

Structure of Phosphoribosylamine

PYRIMIDINE NUCLEOTIDE METABOLISM

Pyrimidines are specialized products that are derived from amino acids. The atoms in the pyrimidine ring come from aspartic acid, glutamine, and carbon dioxide (CO_2). An overview of the pathway is shown in Figure 28-2. The synthesis can be considered in three phases: the synthesis of the parent nucleotide, the conversion of the parent nucleotide to uridine triphosphate (UTP), and the conversion of UTP to cytidine triphosphate.

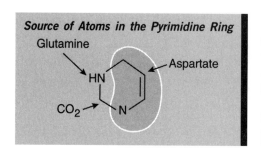

Source of Atoms in the Pyrimidine Ring

Synthesis of the Parent Nucleotide: Orotidine-5′-Monophosphate (OMP)

The synthesis of the parent nucleotide involves the assembly of the pyrimidine ring and the subsequent transfer of ribose-5-phosphate onto the ring.

Carbamoyl Phosphate Synthesis. The first step in the pathway results in the synthesis of carbamoyl phosphate from carbon dioxide, glutamine, and ATP. This reaction, catalyzed by carbamoyl phosphate synthetase-2 (CPS-2), is shown in the following equation. The mixed anhydride bond between the carbon and phosphate groups is a high-energy bond that is used to drive the next reaction in the pathway. CPS-2, a cytosolic enzyme, is distinct from CPS-1, the mitochondrial enzyme that is a part of the urea cycle.

Comparison of CPS-1 and CPS-2		
	CPS-1	*CPS-2*
Pathway	Urea cycle	Pyrimidine synthesis
Location	Mitochondria	Cytosol
Source of nitrogen	NH_4^+	Glutamine
Allosteric activators	N-Acetyl-glutamate	ATP and PRPP
Allosteric inhibitors	...	UTP

$$CO_2 + 2\ ATP + glutamine \xrightarrow{CPS-2} H_2N-\overset{\overset{\displaystyle O}{\|}}{C}\sim OPO_3^= + 2\ ADP + P_i + glutamate$$

Carbamoyl Aspartate Synthesis. Aspartate transcarbamoylase (ATCase) catalyzes the transfer of the carbamoyl group from phosphate to the amino group of aspartate, resulting in carbamoyl aspartate. The energy for forming the C–N bond comes from the hydrolysis of the high-energy bond in carbamoyl phosphate.

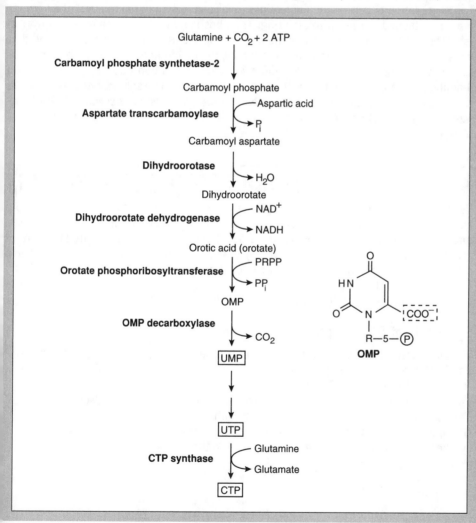

Conversion of Carbamoyl Aspartate to OMP. Three sequential reactions are required to convert carbamoyl aspartate to the parent nucleotide, OMP (see Figure 28-2). The first reaction, catalyzed by dihydroorotase, involves the elimination of water from the amino and carboxyl groups of carbamoyl phosphate, forming dihydroorotate, a cyclic pyrimidine. Oxidation of dihydroorotate to orotic acid is followed by the transfer of ribose-5-phosphate from PRPP to N-1 of orotic acid, resulting in the parent nucleotide, OMP.

FIGURE 28-2
Pathway of Pyrimidine Nucleotide Synthesis. The first step, catalyzed by carbamoyl phosphate synthetase-2, is the rate-limiting step in eukaryotes. This enzyme is inhibited by uridine triphosphate (UTP) and activated by adenosine triphosphate (ATP). CO_2 = carbon dioxide; P_i = inorganic phosphate; NAD^+ and NADH = oxidized and reduced forms of nicotinamide adenine dinucleotide, respectively; PRPP = phosphoribosylpyrophosphate; PP_i = pyrophosphate; OMP = orotidine monophosphate; UMP = uridine monophosphate; CTP = cytidine triphosphate.

Conversion of OMP to UTP and CTP

The reactions by which the parent nucleotide is converted to uridine and cytidine nucleotides are shown in Figure 28-2. The decarboxylation of OMP results in UMP, which is phosphorylated by two sequential reactions to give UTP. The synthesis of CTP is catalyzed by CTP synthase. This reaction involves the transfer of an amide group from the side chain of glutamine to C-4 of the ring, resulting in CTP.

Regulation of Pyrimidine Nucleotide Synthesis

The regulation of pyrimidine nucleotides is markedly different in eukaryotic and prokaryotic cells. In mammalian cells, *CPS-2* is allosterically inhibited by UTP and activated by ATP and PRPP. The activation by ATP allows cells to achieve a balance in the synthesis of purine and pyrimidine nucleotides, a factor that is important in DNA synthesis. In prokaryotes, ATCase is the primary site of regulation. It is allosterically inhibited by CTP and activated by ATP.

In mammalian cells, the first three enzymes of the pathway, CPS-2, ATCase, and dihydroorotase, are organized on the same *multifunctional protein*. This protein, known as *CAD* (from the first letter in the names of the enzymes), consists of three distinct catalytic domains, all encoded by the same gene. Similarly, the two enzymes that convert orotate to UMP, orotate phosphoribosyltransferase and OMP decarboxylase, are found as two separate domains on the same multifunctional protein.

Degradation of Pyrimidine Nucleotides

The degradation of pyrimidine nucleotides involves the sequential removal of all groups that are attached to the pyrimidine ring. The phosphate groups are removed by hydrolysis. The pentoses are removed by the addition of P_i across the *N*-glycosidic bond that links the pentose to the pyrimidine. And finally, the pyrimidine ring is degraded to small soluble molecules, including ammonium ion (NH_4^+), carbon dioxide, β-alanine, and β-aminoisobutyrate. Alternatively, the pyrimidine rings can be salvaged and used for the resynthesis of nucleotide monophosphates. *Pyrimidine phosphoribosyltransferase* catalyzes the transfer of ribose-5-phosphate from PRPP to N-1 of the pyrimidine ring.

PURINE NUCLEOTIDE METABOLISM

Purines, like pyrimidines, can be thought of as specialized products that are derived from amino acids. The atoms in the purine ring are contributed by glutamine, glycine, aspartate, carbon dioxide, and formyl-tetrahydrofolate (formyl-THF). The entire structure of glycine is incorporated into the ring, whereas aspartate and glutamine only donate nitrogen atoms to the ring. The formyl groups that are donated by THF during synthesis are derived from the degradation of amino acids (see Chapter 26). An overview of the pathway of purine nucleotide synthesis is shown in Figure 28-3.

Synthesis of 5'-Phosphoribosylamine

The first step that is committed to purine synthesis is catalyzed by glutamine:PRPP amidotransferase. In this reaction, the amide group from the side chain of glutamine is transferred to C-1 of PRPP, producing 5'-phosphoribosylamine and releasing pyrophosphate (PP_i). The amino group is attached to C-1 of ribose by an *N*-glycosidic linkage. Through several subsequent reactions, this nitrogen becomes N-9 of the purine ring. Glutamine:PRPP amidotransferase catalyzes the rate-limiting step in purine nucleotide synthesis and is the primary site of regulation in the pathway.

Synthesis of Parent Nucleotide: Inosine Monophosphate (IMP)

The next nine steps in the pathway convert 5'-phosphoribosylamine to IMP, the parent purine nucleotide. These steps involve two reactions in which amide groups are trans-

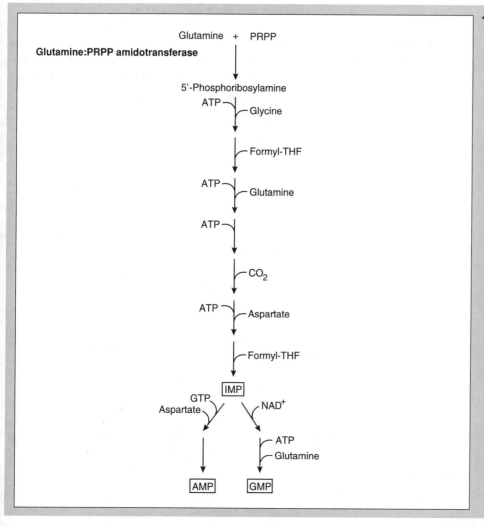

FIGURE 28-3
Pathway of Purine Nucleotide Synthesis.
The initial step in the pathway is the primary site of regulation. Nine steps are required to convert 5'-phosphoribosylamine to inosine monophosphate (IMP). The substrates that donate one or more atoms to the ring system and the order in which they are used are listed on the right. The synthesis of IMP requires two amide transfer reactions, in which glutamine is the nitrogen donor, and two one-carbon transfer reactions, in which formyl-THF is the donor; the energy required is supplied by the hydrolysis of four molecules of adenosine triphosphate (ATP). The pathway branches at IMP to give adenosine monophosphate (AMP) and guanosine monophosphate (GMP). The synthesis of both AMP and GMP from IMP requires a source of energy, either guanosine triphosphate (GTP) or ATP, and an amino donor, either aspartate or glutamine. PRPP = phosphoribosylpyrophosphate; THF = tetrahydrofolate; CO_2 = carbon dioxide.

ferred from glutamine to intermediates and two reactions in which one-carbon (C_1) fragments are transferred from formyl-THF into various intermediates in the pathway. Four molecules of ATP are required to convert 5'-phosphoribosylamine to IMP (see Figure 28-3).

Conversion of IMP to AMP and GMP

The pathway branches at IMP, with one pathway leading to the production of AMP and the other to GMP (Figure 28-4). Each pathway consists of two reactions that result in the attachment of amino groups to the purine ring, and each pathway requires a source of energy. The pathway leading to AMP uses aspartate as an amino donor and GTP as a source of energy. The pathway leading to GMP uses glutamine as an amino donor and ATP as a source of energy. The first step after the branch point in each pathway is inhibited by the end product of that pathway.

Conversion of Nucleoside Monophosphates to Diphosphates and Triphosphates

Nucleoside triphosphates are formed from monophosphates in two stages. All of these reactions are reversible, and the direction is dependent on the relative concentrations of the nucleotides.

Nucleoside Monophosphate Kinases. The nucleoside monophosphate kinases are a family of enzymes that are specific for different purines and pyrimidines but are not specific for the pentose. These enzymes are named for the nucleoside monophosphate. For example, the reaction shown below is catalyzed by guanylate kinase.

$$\text{GMP} + \text{ATP} \rightleftharpoons \text{GDP} + \text{ADP}$$

Nucleoside Diphosphate Kinase. The reaction catalyzed by nucleoside diphosphate kinase converts nucleoside diphosphates to the corresponding triphosphates. This enzyme has a broad specificity for both the phosphate donor and phosphate acceptor.

$$\text{CTP} + \text{ATP} \rightleftharpoons \text{CTP} + \text{ADP}$$

FIGURE 28-4
Conversion of Inosine Monophosphate (IMP) to Adenosine Monophosphate (AMP) and Guanosine Monophosphate (GMP). The conversion of IMP to AMP and GMP proceeds along separate and parallel pathways. Adenylosuccinate synthetase is inhibited by AMP and activated by GMP, whereas IMP dehydrogenase is inhibited by GMP and activated by AMP. P_i = inorganic phosphate; NAD+ and NADH = the oxidized and reduced forms of nicotinamide adenine dinucleotide; ADP and ATP = adenosine diphosphate and triphosphate, respectively; GDP and GTP = guanosine diphosphate and triphosphate, respectively.

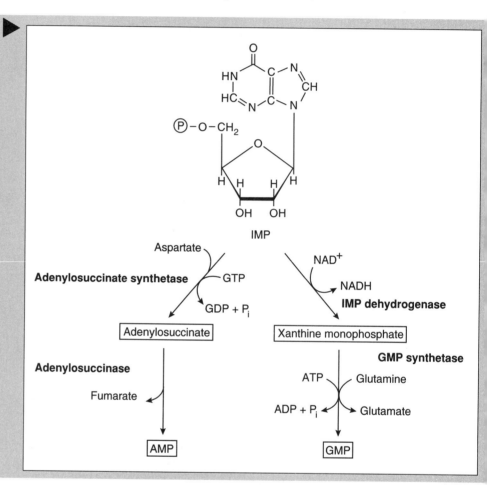

Regulation of Purine Nucleotide Synthesis

The rate-limiting step in purine nucleotide synthesis is catalyzed by glutamine:PRPP amidotransferase, the enzyme that synthesizes 5'-phosphoribosylamine. The most important factor in regulating the rate of this reaction is the concentration of PRPP. The concentration of PRPP in cells is 10–100 times lower than the Michaelis constant (K_m) of the enzyme for PRPP. Therefore, small changes in the concentration of PRPP result in a proportional increase in the rate of 5'-phosphoribosylamine synthesis. This enzyme is also inhibited by the accumulation of AMP, GMP, and IMP. Other sites at which feedback inhibition by the purine nucleoside monophosphates occurs are the synthesis of PRPP and the synthesis of adenylosuccinate and xanthine monophosphate, the immediate precursors of AMP and GMP, respectively (Figure 28-5).

Purine Nucleotide Degradation

The end product of purine nucleotide degradation is uric acid. The pathway of degradation is similar to the early stages in the pathway of pyrimidine nucleotide degradation. Substituents attached to the purine ring are sequentially removed from AMP and GMP by parallel pathways (Figure 28-6). Phosphate groups are removed by nucleotidase. Amino groups attached to the purine rings are released by the base-specific enzymes, *adenosine deaminase* and *guanine deaminase*, and the pentoses are removed by *purine nucleoside*

Gout
Gout is a heterogeneous group of genetic and acquired diseases characterized by high levels of uric acid in the blood and urine. Virtually everyone who has gout has a blood uric acid level greater than 7 mg/dL, which is the maximum solubility in plasma. All of the clinical symptoms arise from its low solubility in biologic fluids [1]. Uric acid is in equilibrium with its anionic form urate. The pK_a for the dissociation of uric acid is about 5.7.

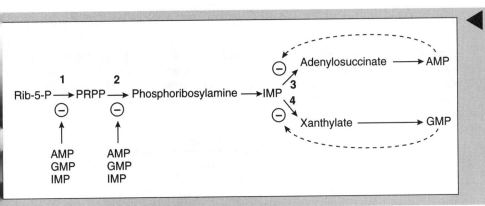

FIGURE 28-5
Regulation of Purine Nucleotide Synthesis. The enzymes that are subject to feedback inhibition are numbered as: (1) phosphoribosylpyrophosphate (PRPP) synthetase; (2) glutamine:PRPP phosphoribosyltransferase; (3) adenylosuccinate synthetase; and (4) inosine monophosphate (IMP) dehydrogenase. Rib-5-P = ribose-5-phosphate; GMP = guanosine monophosphate; AMP = adenosine monophosphate.

phosphorylase. The sum of these reactions converts AMP and GMP to hypoxanthine and xanthine, respectively. The terminal stage of purine nucleotide degradation is the oxidation of hypoxanthine and xanthine to uric acid, reactions that are both catalyzed by xanthine oxidase. The ring system of purines, unlike that of pyrimidines, cannot be opened up and degraded to smaller products, and it is excreted intact as uric acid. Xanthine oxidase is a flavoprotein that requires molybdenum as an essential cofactor.

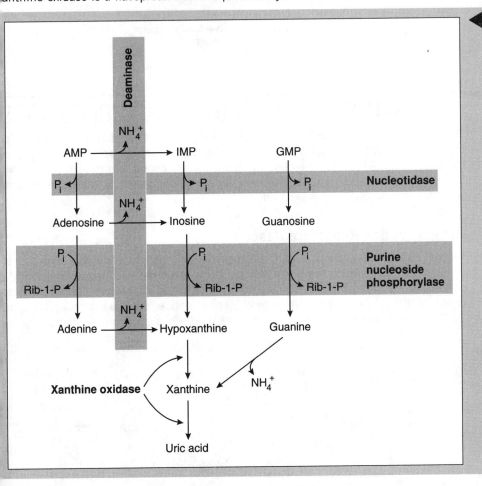

FIGURE 28-6
Degradation of Purine Nucleotides to Uric Acid. Four types of reactions are involved in the degradation of purine nucleotides, as indicated by the shaded areas. Nucleotidase releases inorganic phosphate (P_i) from all of the nucleoside monophosphates; purine nucleoside phosphorylase adds P_i across the bond, joining the base with ribose (or deoxyribose) and releasing ribose-1-phosphate (Rib-1-P); and a family of deaminases releases ammonium ion (NH_4^+) from the purine rings. The deaminases, in contrast to other enzymes in the pathway, are specific, with a different deaminase for each reaction that releases NH_4^+. The deaminases are named for the substrate (adenosine monophosphate [AMP] deaminase, adenosine deaminase, adenine deaminase, guanine deaminase). Xanthine oxidase catalyzes the two steps that convert hypoxanthine to uric acid. IMP = inosine monophosphate; GMP = guanosine monophosphate.

Salvage Pathways in Purine Metabolism

In most cells, pathways are available that allow hypoxanthine and guanine to be recycled. The function of these pathways is to avoid the high-energy demand placed on the cell by the de novo synthesis of nucleotides. Most of the energy expenditure in the de novo pathway is used to synthesize the ring system. The substrates for the salvage reactions may come either from dietary sources or from the intracellular nucleic acid turnover. The

critical step in the salvage pathway of purines is catalyzed by one of two enzyme
depending on the base being recycled.

Hypoxanthine-Guanine Phosphoribosyltransferase (HGPRT). Hypoxanthine and guanine
are both substrates for HGPRT, an enzyme that transfers ribose-5-phosphate from PRP
onto the purine ring, resulting in IMP and GMP, respectively. Any hypoxanthine that is n
salvaged is converted to uric acid.

$$\text{Hypoxanthine} \xrightarrow[\textbf{HGPRT}]{\text{PRPP} \quad \text{PP}_i} \text{IMP}$$

$$\text{Guanine} \xrightarrow[\textbf{HGPRT}]{\text{PRPP} \quad \text{PP}_i} \text{GMP}$$

Adenine Phosphoribosyltransferase (APRT). APRT is responsible for recycling adenine t
AMP in a reaction that is analogous to that catalyzed by HGPRT. The specific activity o
APRT in most cells, however, is only a fraction of that of HGPRT.

$$\text{Adenine} \xrightarrow[\textbf{APRT}]{\text{PRPP} \quad \text{PP}_i} \text{GMP}$$

SYNTHESIS OF DEOXYRIBONUCLEOTIDES

The synthesis of DNA requires deoxyribonucleotides. The conversion of ribonucleotide
to deoxyribonucleotides occurs only at the diphosphate level. This reaction is catalyze
by ribonucleotide reductase, an enzyme found in all species and tissues. The deoxy
ribonucleoside diphosphates are subsequently phosphorylated to the correspondin
triphosphates for use in DNA synthesis.

Ribonucleotide Reductase Reaction

Ribonucleotide reductase is a multienzyme complex that is active only prior to cel
division when cells are actively synthesizing DNA. The enzyme converts all four of the
ribonucleoside diphosphates (NDP) to the corresponding deoxyribonucleoside diphos
phates (dNDP). The reaction catalyzed by ribonucleotide reductase is shown in Figure
28-7. The reducing agent in the reaction is *thioredoxin*, a small protein containing two

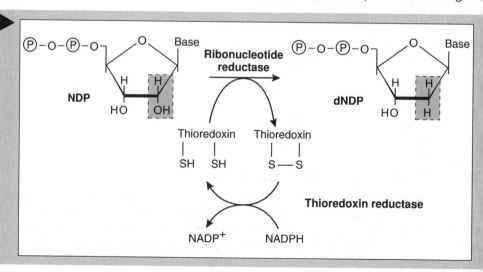

FIGURE 28-7 ▶
Reduction of Ribonucleotides to Deoxyribonucleotides. *The reduction of ribose to deoxyribose occurs at the nucleoside diphosphate level. A ribonucleoside diphosphate (NDP) is converted to the corresponding deoxyribonucleoside diphosphate (dNDP). Thioredoxin is oxidized in the reaction, and its regeneration requires the reduced form of nicotinamide-adenine dinucleotide phosphate (NADPH) and thioredoxin reductase. NADP⁺ = oxidized form of nicotinamide-adenine dinucleotide phosphate.*

ysteine residues that are located close to one another in the peptide chain. Reduction of
e 2'-hydroxyl group by thioredoxin results in the oxidation of the cysteine sulfhydryl
roups to a disulfide. The catalytic cycle is completed by *thioredoxin reductase*, which
ses the reduced form of nicotinamide-adenine dinucleotide phosphate (NADPH) to
egenerate the reduced form of thioredoxin.

Regulation of Ribonucleotide Reductase

ibonucleotide reductase is subject to a complex pattern of allosteric regulation, which
nsures that the pool of deoxyribonucleotides has the balanced composition that is
equired for DNA synthesis. There are two types of allosteric sites on ribonucleotide
eductase.

Type I Regulatory Site. The overall catalytic activity of the enzyme is regulated by binding
TP and dATP to this site. ATP is an allosteric activator, and dATP is an allosteric inhibitor
f the enzyme. The binding of ATP and dATP to this site affects the overall rate of
eoxyribonucleotide synthesis.

Type II Regulatory Site. This site confers substrate specificity on the enzyme and is
esponsible for maintaining balance in the cellular pool of dADP, dGDP, dCDP, and dUDP.
arious nucleotides, including ATP, dATP, dGTP, and dTTP, bind to the site and either
ncrease or decrease the affinity of other deoxyribonucleotides for the catalytic site.

SYNTHESIS OF THYMIDYLATE

DNA contains thymine rather than uracil. The pathway for de novo synthesis of thymine
nvolves only deoxyribonucleotides. The immediate precursor of deoxythymidine monophosphate (dTMP) is deoxyuridine monophosphate (dUMP).

Thymidylate Synthase and Dihydrofolate Reductase

The reaction catalyzed by thymidylate synthase involves the addition of a methyl group to
the ring of dUMP, resulting in dTMP (Figure 28-8). The methyl group is supplied by
methylene-THF. Following the transfer of the methylene group to the ring, it is reduced by
THF to a methyl group. The reduction results in the concomitant oxidation of THF to
dihydrofolate (DHF). The completion of the catalytic cycle requires that THF be regenerated, a reaction that is catalyzed by dihydrofolate reductase.

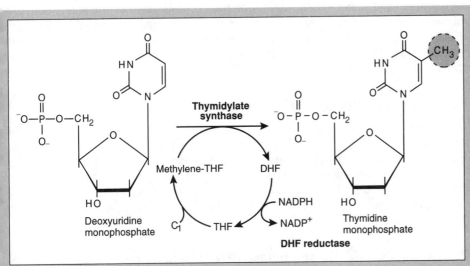

FIGURE 28-8
Conversion of Deoxyuridine Monophosphate (dUMP) to Thymidine Monophosphate (dTMP). Thymidylate synthetase catalyzes the addition of a methyl (CH_3) to carbon-5 of the ring. A methylene group is transferred from tetrahydrofolate (THF) and subsequently reduced, resulting in the release of dihydrofolate (DHF). Regeneration of THF requires NADPH and DHF reductase before another one-carbon fragment (C_1) can be added. $NADP^+$ and NADPH = oxidized and reduced forms of nicotinamide-adenine dinucleotide phosphate, respectively.

Antitumor Agents That Interfere with dTMP Synthesis

The thymidylate synthase and dihydrofolate reductase reactions provide the only pathway for synthesis of thymine nucleotides. Therefore, inhibitors of these enzymes de-

crease the rate of DNA synthesis and cell division, and they are commonly used in the treatment of tumors. Although the division of all cells is affected by these compounds, cancer cells grow and divide more rapidly than most normal cells and, therefore, are more sensitive to these drugs.

5-Fluorouracil (5-FU). The synthesis of dTMP is inhibited by 5-FU. Salvage pathways convert 5-FU to 5-fluorodeoxyuridine monophosphate (5-F-dUMP), which binds to the active site of thymidylate synthase and inactivates the enzyme. The structure of 5-F-dUMP is sufficiently similar to the natural substrate so that it begins to undergo catalysis but it is unable to complete the catalytic cycle. Therefore, this compound is sometimes referred to as a mechanism-based inhibitor or a suicide substrate.

Methotrexate. Methotrexate is a structural analog of folic acid and is a powerful competitive inhibitor of DHF reductase. The affinity of DHF reductase for methotrexate is about 100 times greater than for DHF.

ABNORMALITIES IN PURINE NUCLEOTIDE METABOLISM

Disorders in purine nucleotide metabolism leading to disease occur in the de novo synthetic pathway, the salvage pathway, and the pathway of purine degradation.

Superactive PRPP Synthetase

Several mutations have been identified in the gene encoding PRPP synthetase. Paradoxically all of these defects are characterized by overproduction of purines. Some of the mutants have an increased maximum velocity (V_{max}), while others do not respond to feedback inhibition by nucleotides. Therefore, purines are synthesized at a rate that exceeds the needs of the cell, resulting in increased degradation and uric acid production. The gene coding for PRPP synthetase is located on the X chromosome.

HGPRT Deficiency

An absence of HGPRT results in Lesch-Nyhan syndrome, a severe neurologic disease characterized by mental retardation, jerky involuntary movements, compulsive self-mutilation, and the overproduction of uric acid. Virtually all of the intermediates beyond hypoxanthine and guanine in the salvage pathway are converted to uric acid. About one-third of the cases of Lesch-Nyhan syndrome result from spontaneous mutations in the HGPRT gene, which is located on the X chromosome and is inherited as a X-linked recessive trait. Therefore, a new mutation may occur in an asymptomatic mother and remain silent until transmitted to a male child.

Adenosine Deaminase (ADA) Deficiency

ADA is involved in the conversion of adenosine and deoxyadenosine to hypoxanthine. Patients with a deficiency in ADA have impaired function of both T cells and B cells, resulting in severe combined immunodeficiency disease (SCID). The accumulation of dATP inhibits ribonucleotide reductase, thereby blocking the formation of deoxyribonucleotides and DNA synthesis. Numerous methylation reactions, which are important in protecting purine and pyrimidine bases in DNA and RNA, are also inhibited by deoxyadenosine [2].

Purine Nucleoside Phosphorylase (PNP) Deficiency

The removal of pentoses from ribo- and deoxyribonucleosides is catalyzed by PNP. In the absence of this enzyme, nucleosides accumulate. T cells are particularly vulnerable to a deficiency in PNP because the deoxyguanosine that accumulates is converted to dGTP, which inhibits ribonucleotide reductase and, therefore, DNA synthesis in these cells [2].

Allopurinol
Allopurinol, a drug used to treat gout, is a structural analog of hypoxanthine. It binds to the active site of xanthine oxidase and is converted to alloxanthine, an inhibitor of the enzyme. Therefore, in the presence of allopurinol, uric acid production is decreased and hypoxanthine and xanthine accumulate. Hypoxanthine and xanthine are more soluble than uric acid and can be more readily excreted.

Hypoxanthine

Allopurinol

ANTIMETABOLITES, NUCLEOTIDE SYNTHESIS, AND CHEMOTHERAPY

Antimetabolites are compounds that resemble a normal metabolite and interfere with its utilization in a cell. Several antimetabolites are useful as chemotherapeutic agents because of their ability to interfere with the synthesis or utilization of purine and pyrimidine nucleotides. The inhibition of thymine nucleotide synthesis by 5-FU and methotrexate has been described earlier in this chapter. The structures of some drugs commonly used in chemotherapy are shown in Figure 28-9.

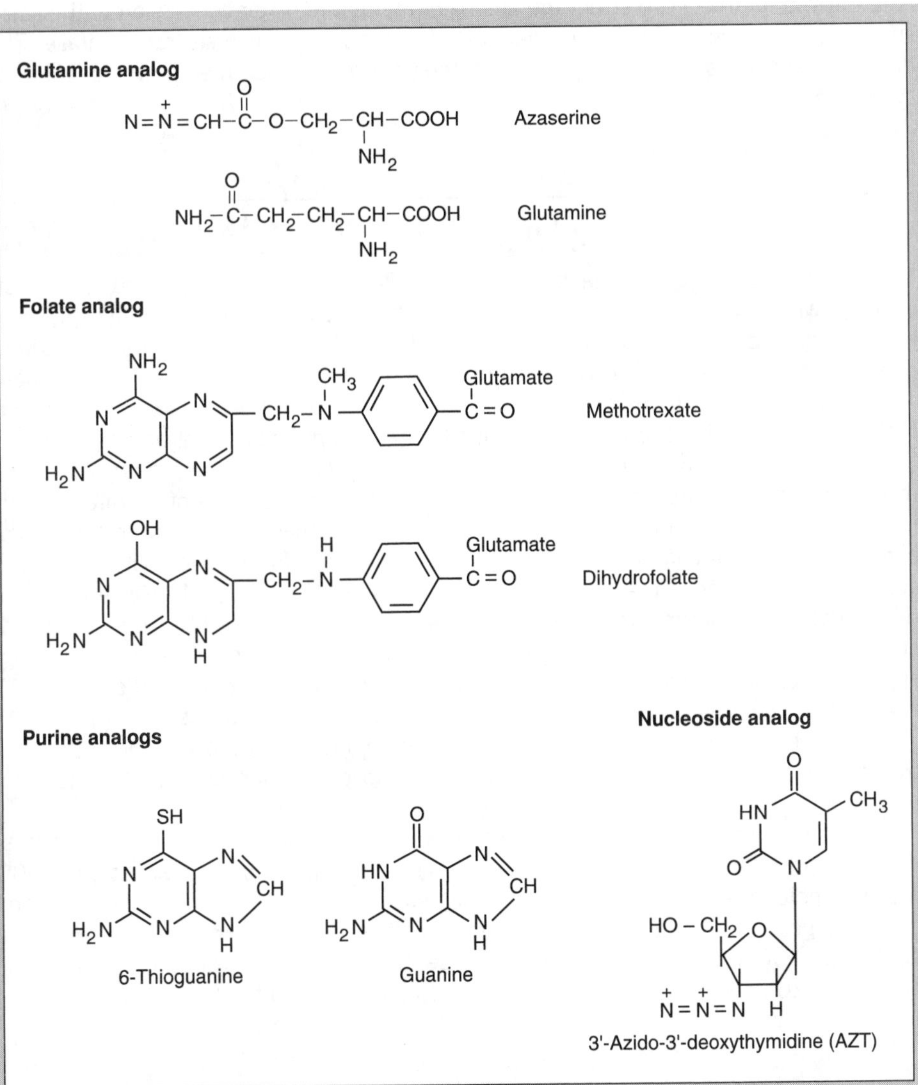

FIGURE 28-9
Antimetabolites That Interfere with Nucleotide Synthesis or Utilization. The major types of antimetabolites shown are structural analogs of glutamine, folic acid, purines, and nucleosides. Azaserine inhibits amide transferases; methotrexate inhibits dihydrofolate reductase; 6-thioguanine is converted by hypoxanthine-guanine phosphoribosyltransferase (HGPRT) to the corresponding nucleotide, which inhibits inosine dehydrogenase and the synthesis of guanosine monophosphate; 3'-azo-3'-deoxythymidine terminates DNA synthesis by reverse transcriptase.

Analogs of Glutamine

Azaserine and 6-diazo-5-oxy-L-norleucine (DON), structural analogs of glutamine, inhibit several steps in the pathway of purine nucleotide synthesis. These compounds inactivate amidotransferases by binding to the glutamine site and becoming covalently attached to sulfhydryl groups, which are essential for enzyme activity.

Analogs of Folic Acid

Methotrexate and aminopterin are structural analogs of folic acid. These drugs inhibit DHF reductase, which converts both DHF and dietary folate to THF.

Analogs of Purines and Pyrimidines

6-Mercaptopurine and 6-thioguanine are structural analogs of inosine and guanine, respectively. The first step in the conversion of IMP to AMP is inhibited by 6-mercaptopurine, while the first step in the conversion of IMP to GMP is inhibited by 6-thioguanine. These analogs are converted by HGPRT to the corresponding mononucleotides, which inhibit the formation of 5′-phosphoribosylamine. The effect of 5-FU, a pyrimidine analog, on thymine nucleotide synthesis was discussed earlier in this chapter.

Analog of Nucleosides

Azidothymidine (AZT) is a structural analog of thymidine. After conversion to the corresponding 5′-triphosphate, it terminates DNA synthesis by reverse transcriptase. This drug, also known as zidovudine, is used in the treatment of acquired immunodeficiency syndrome (AIDS).

RESOLUTION OF CLINICAL CASE

The patient introduced at the beginning of this chapter was diagnosed with gouty arthritis, which was exacerbated by chronic alcoholism. The symptoms of hypoglycemia and lactic acidemia are secondary to the effect of alcohol metabolism on gluconeogenesis (see Chapter 13). The accumulation of uric acid is enhanced by lactic acid. The metabolism of large quantities of alcohol places a heavy demand on the supply of NAD^+. Consequently, reactions that require NAD^+ are impaired. In particular, the oxidation of lactate to pyruvate, an important substrate for gluconeogenesis, occurs very slowly in the presence of large quantities of ethanol. The accumulation of lactate, in turn, inhibits the excretion of uric acid, resulting in an increase in the plasma uric acid concentration [3]. All of the clinical symptoms of gout arise from the low solubility of uric acid in biologic fluids. The maximum solubility at 37°C is 7 mg/dL. However, in the peripheral tissues, where the temperature is below 37°C, the solubility is decreased, and crystals form easily, particularly in joint cavities and in cartilaginous tissue. Deposits of aggregated crystals, known as tophi, initiate an inflammatory reaction that causes swelling, redness, heat, and severe pain in the affected areas [1]. Classic symptoms of acute gouty arthritis are inflammation in the big toe and tophi in the earlobes. The patient was treated with allopurinol, which decreased uric acid production by inhibiting xanthine oxidase.

Gout is a group of metabolic diseases associated with hyperuricemia and the deposition of monosodium urate crystals in tissues [4]. It has a prevalence of about 3 in 1000, with the incidence being about 10 times higher in men than in women. The symptoms usually appear in the fourth decade in men and after menopause in women. Plasma uric acid levels, however, are usually elevated for several years before symptoms appear. Only about 1 in 20 people with hyperuricemia develop clinical gout [4].

REVIEW QUESTIONS

Directions: For each of the following questions, choose the **one best** answer.

1. Which of the following events occurs in the reaction catalyzed by ribonucleotide reductase?
    - **(A)** Inhibition by ribonucleotides
    - **(B)** Reduction of ribonucleotides by thioredoxin and NAD
    - **(C)** Reduction of purine and pyrimidine ribonucleoside diphosphates
    - **(D)** Regeneration of tetrahydrofolate (THF) by NADPH
    - **(E)** Activation by dATP

2. Which of the following statements correctly describes the de novo synthesis of pyrimidines in humans?
    - **(A)** Phosphoribosylpyrophosphate (PRPP) is required in the first step
    - **(B)** Formyl-tetrahydrofolate (formyl-THF) donates two carbon atoms to the pyrimidine ring
    - **(C)** The conversion of UTP to CTP requires NH_4^+
    - **(D)** The rate-limiting step is activated by UTP and inhibited by ATP
    - **(E)** Aspartate donates both carbon and nitrogen atoms to the ring

3. Which of the following compounds has the greatest effect on the rate-limiting step in purine nucleotide synthesis?
    - **(A)** Ribose-1-phosphate
    - **(B)** Phosphoribosylpyrophosphate (PRPP)
    - **(C)** ADP
    - **(D)** Glutamine
    - **(E)** Aspartate

4. Which of the following enzymes is deficient in Lesch-Nyhan syndrome?
    - **(A)** Adenine phosphoribosyltransferase (APRT)
    - **(B)** Adenosine deaminase (ADA)
    - **(C)** Hypoxanthine-guanine phosphoribosyltransferase (HGPRT)
    - **(D)** Phosphoribosylpyrophosphate (PRPP) synthetase
    - **(E)** Purine nucleoside phosphorylase (PNP)

5. Which of the following statements about gout is true?
    - **(A)** It results from the overproduction of orotic acid
    - **(B)** It can result from a deficiency in phosphoribosylpyrophosphate (PRPP) synthetase
    - **(C)** It can be treated with inhibitors of xanthine oxidase
    - **(D)** It occurs more frequently in women than men
    - **(E)** The symptoms appear in early adolescence

ANSWERS AND EXPLANATIONS

1. The answer is C. Both purine and pyrimidine ribonucleoside diphosphates are reduced to the corresponding deoxyribonucleotides in the reaction catalyzed by ribonucleotide reductase. This reaction requires thioredoxin and NADPH as reducing agents but does not involve NAD. NADPH is required to regenerate the reduced form of thioredoxin. THF is not involved in the reaction. Ribonucleotide reductase is activated by ATP and inhibited by dATP.

2. The answer is E. The nitrogen atom and all three carbon atoms of aspartate are incorporated into the pyrimidine ring. The other nitrogen and carbon atoms in the ring come from glutamine and carbon dioxide. PRPP is not used in the synthesis of the pyrimidine ring, but when the ring is completed it becomes attached to ribose-5-phosphate, which is provided by PRPP. Formyl-THF is required in the synthesis of purine, but not pyrimidine, rings. The rate-limiting step in pyrimidine synthesis is catalyzed by carbamoyl phosphate synthetase-2 (CPS-2) in eukaryotes and by ATCase in prokaryotes. CPS-2 is inhibited by UTP and activated by ATP.

3. The answer is B. The rate-limiting step in purine nucleotide synthesis is catalyzed by glutamine:PRPP amidotransferase. The concentration of PRPP is the most important factor in determining the rate of this reaction. PRPP is present in cells at a concentration that is 10–100 times lower than the Michaelis constant (K_m) of the enzyme for PRPP. This enzyme is also subject to feedback inhibition by AMP, GMP, and IMP. Although glutamine is required as a substrate, it is present in cells at concentrations that have little effect on the rate of the reaction. Ribose-1-phosphate, ADP, and aspartate have no significant effect on the enzyme.

4. The answer is C. Lesch-Nyhan syndrome results from an absence of HGPRT. Abnormalities in all of the other enzymes listed have also been reported. A deficiency in ADA results in severe combined immunodeficiency disease (SCID), with impairment in both T and B cells. The aberrant forms of PRPP all result in increased, rather than decreased, activity and are characterized by excessive purine nucleotide synthesis, leading to increased uric acid production. A deficiency in PNP results in an immunodeficiency disease that only affects T cells but has no effect on B cells. A deficiency in APRT results in the inability to salvage adenine, although the neurologic disorders that are associated with HGPRT are not seen with APRT deficiency.

5. The answer is C. Allopurinol, one of the most effective drugs for treating gout, inhibits xanthine oxidase. Gout results from the accumulation of crystals of sodium urate (the ionized form of uric acid) in joints. Orotic acid accumulates from a deficiency in the synthesis of pyrimidines or from a deficiency in ornithine transcarbamoylase, an enzyme in the urea cycle. Gout can result from superactive forms of PRPP synthetase but not from a deficiency in this enzyme. Lesch-Nyhan syndrome is characterized by impaired T and B cell function and by gout, but the gout associated with overproduction of uric acid and dysfunction of B and T cells is associated with the inability to synthesize deoxyribonucleotides. Gout is much more prevalent in men than in women, and the symptoms do not appear until well into adulthood.

REFERENCES

1. Bhagavan NV: *Medical Biochemistry*. Boston, MA: Jones and Bartlett, 1992, p 654.
2. Cohn RM, Roth KS: *Biochemistry and Disease*. Baltimore, MD: Williams and Wilkins, 1966, p 290.

3. Schwarz V: *A Clinical Companion to Biochemical Studies*. San Francisco, CA: W. H. Freeman, 1978, pp 27–30.
4. Becker MA, Roessler BJ: Hyperuricemia and gout. In *The Metabolic and Molecular Bases of Inherited Disease*, 7th ed. Edited by Scriver CR, Beaudet AL, Sly WS, et al. New York, NY: McGraw-Hill, 1995, pp 1655–1677.

INDEX

NOTE: An f after a page number denotes a figure; a t after a page number denotes a table.